Clinical Reasoning in the Health Professions

Clinical Reasoning in the Health Professions

Edited by

Joy Higgs BSc, Grad Dip Phty, MHPEd, PhD
Professor and Head of School of Physiotherapy, The University of Sydney, New South Wales, Australia

and

Mark Jones BSc (Psych), PT, M App Sc
Coordinator, Senior Lecturer, Postgraduate Programs in Manipulative Physiotherapy, School of Physiotherapy, University of South Australia, South Australia, Australia

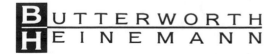

Butterworth-Heinemann Ltd
Linacre House, Jordan Hill, Oxford OX2 8DP

℞ A member of the Reed Elsevier plc group

OXFORD LONDON BOSTON
MUNICH NEW DELHI SINGAPORE SYDNEY
TOKYO TORONTO WELLINGTON

First published 1995
Reprinted 1995

British Library Cataloguing in Publication Data
A catalogue record for this book is available from the British Library

Library of Congress Cataloguing in Publication Data
A catalogue record for this book is available from the Library of Congress

ISBN 0 7506 0787 4

Typeset by TecSet Ltd, Wallington, Surrey
Printed and bound in Great Britain by The Bath Press, Avon

Contents

Section Four   Approaches to teaching clinical reasoning

Section Five   Directions for the future

Contributors

Roger D. Adams PhD
Senior Lecturer, School of Physiotherapy, University of Sydney, Lidcombe, New South Wales, Australia

José F. Arocha Lic, MA, PhD
Postdoctoral Fellow, Centre for Medical Education, McGill University, Montreal, Quebec, Canada

Henny P. A. Boshuizen PhD
Associate Professor, Program Coordinator (Health Professions Education), Department of Education, University of Limburg, Maastricht, The Netherlands

Doris L. Carnevali RN, BSN, MN
Associate Professor Emeritus, School of Nursing, University of Washington, Seattle, Washington, USA

Judi Carr Dip Physio, Grad Dip F Ed
Senior Lecturer, School of Physiotherapy, University of South Australia, Adelaide, South Australia, Australia

Christine Chapparo MA, Dip OT
Senior Lecturer, School of Occupational Therapy, University of Sidney, Lidcombe, New South Wales, Australia

Allan Christie M App Sc, Grad Dip Physio (Orthop)
Senior Lecturer, School of Physiotherapy (Orthopaedics), University of South Australia, Adelaide, South Australia, Australia

Sheila A. Corcoran-Perry PhD, RN, FAAN
Professor, School of Nursing, University of Minnesota, Minneapolis, USA

Jancis K. Dennis
Department of Physical Therapy, Medical College of Georgia, Augusta, Georgia, USA

Janet Doyle BA, Dip Aud, M App Sc, PhD, M Aud SA
Head, School of Communication Disorders, La Trobe University, Bundoora, Victoria, Australia

Helen Edwards MA
Senior Lecturer, Education Development, Lincoln School of Health Sciences, La Trobe University, Bundoora, Victoria, Australia

Arthur S. Elstein PhD
Professor, Department of Medical Education, University of Illinois at Chicago, Chicago, Illinois, USA

Marsha E. Fonteyn RN, PhD, CCRN
Assistant Professor and Adjunct Nurse Researcher, School of Nursing, University of San Franciso, San Francisco, California, USA

Miranda Franke B App Sc (Speech Pathology), Grad Dip (Communication Disorders)
Clinical Education Coordinator and Associate Lecturer, Department of Communication Disorders, La Trobe University, Bundoora, Victoria, Australia

Robert P. Graby Ed D
Associate Dean, School of Education, University of San Francisco, San Francisco, California, USA

Gail Hart RN, DCHN, BA, MHP, PhD
Associate Professor, School of Nursing, Queensland University of Technology, Red Hill, Queensland, Australia

Brett K. Hayes PhD, MPsych(Clin), MAPsS
Senior Lecturer in Psychology, Department of Psychology, The University of Newcastle, Callaghan, Australia

Joy Higgs BSC, Grad Dip Phty, MHPEd, PhD
Professor and Head of School of Physiotherapy, University of Sydney, Lidcombe, New South Wales, Australia

Gail Jensen PT, PhD
Associate Professor, Department of Physical Therapy, School of Pharmacy and Allied Health, Creighton University, Omaha, Nebraska, USA

Mark Jones BSc (Psych), PT, M App Sc
Coordinator and Senior Lecturer, Postgraduate Programs in Manipulative Physiotherapy, School of Physiotherapy, University of South Australia, Adelaide, South Australia, Australia

David R. Kaufman BA, MA, PhD
Postdoctoral Fellow in Cognitive Studies in Medicine, McGill University, Montreal, Quebec, Canada

Bella J. May Ed D, PT, FAPTA
Professor, Department of Physical Therapy, Medical College of Georgia, Augusta, Georgia, USA

Bill McGuiness Dip T, B Ed, RN
Lecturer, School of Nursing, La Trobe University, Bundoora, Victoria, Australia

Linda McKenzie Dip App Sc (Orth), DOBA
Lecturer, Division of Orthoptics, La Trobe University, Bundoora, Victoria, Australia

Suzanne M. Narayan BA, BS, MS, PhD, RN
Professor, Nursing Department, Metropolitan State University, St Paul, Minnesota, USA

David Newble BSc, MD, FRACP, Dip Ed
Associate Professor of Medicine, University of Adelaide, Queen Elizabeth Hospital, Woodville, South Australia, Australia

Geoffrey Norman BSc, MA, PhD
Professor, Department of Clinical Epidemiology and Biostatistics, McMaster University, Hamilton, Ontario, Canada

Vimla L. Patel BSc, MA, PhD
Professor, Department of Medicine, Director McGill Cognitive Science Centre, Associate Director Centre for Medical Education, McGill University, Montreal Quebec, Canada

Susan Prion RN, MS, MA
Instructor, College of Professional Studies, University of San Francisco, San Francisco, California, USA

Judy Ranka BSc (OT), MA (Educ and Work), OTR
Lecturer, School of Occupational Therapy, University of Sydney, New South Wales, Australia

Kathryn Refshauge Dip Physio, Grad Dip Manip Ther, M Biomed Engineer
Senior Lecturer, School of Physiotherapy, University of Sydney, Lidcombe, New South Wales, Australia

Jules Rothstein PT, PhD, FAPTA
Head of Department of Physical Therapy, University of Illinois at Chicago, Chicago, USA

Susan Ryan MSc, B App Sc, OTR, SROT, AAOT
Senior Lecturer, Department of Rehabilitation Sciences, University of East London, London, UK

Henk G. Schmidt PhD
Professor of Educational Psychology and Health Professions Education, Dean of the Faculty of Health Sciences, University of Limburg, Maastricht, The Netherlands

Angie Titchen MSc, MCSP
Research and Development Fellow, National Institute for Nursing, Oxford, UK

Cees van der Vleuten MA, PhD
Associate Professor, Department of Educational Development and Research, University of Limburg, Maastricht, The Netherlands

Nancy T. Watts PT, PhD
Professor Emerita, Graduate Program in Physical Therapy, MGH Institute of Health Professions, Massachusetts General Hospital, Winchester, Massachusetts, USA

Acknowledgements

We would like to acknowledge each of the authors who have contributed to this text. Their commitment to quality, their sharing of research experiences and their creative ideas have helped to produce a work which we believe can stimulate and inspire its readers.

Our thanks are also due to our families for their support and encouragement and to several friends and colleagues who have provided invaluable help. Our special thanks go to Helen, Judi, Annie, Phil and Dave.

Introduction

Joy Higgs and Mark Jones

Clinical reasoning is the foundation of professional clinical practice. In the absence of sound clinical reasoning, clinical practice becomes a technical operation requiring direction from a decision maker. It is the role of professional health care practitioners to practise in a manner which demonstrates professional autonomy, competence and accountability, to engage in lifelong learning and to contribute to the development of the knowledge base of their discipline (Higgs, 1993). In order to achieve these outcomes health professionals need to be able to reason effectively, to make sound and defensible clinical decisions and to learn through their clinical experience and other avenues in order to continually develop their knowledge as the basis for making effective clinical decisions and useful contributions to the knowledge of the field.

This is a multidisciplinary text written for the health professions. It has relevance across the health disciplines and we hope that the rich and varied contributions in the book by many of the world's leading and emerging scholars in this field will add to the development of clinical reasoning. Throughout the text, international scholars, researchers and teachers have contributed their ideas, research findings and experiences to promote discussion on the nature and teaching of clinical reasoning. Models, guidelines and strategies are presented. These aim to promote effective clinical reasoning in practice, creative and successful clinical reasoning learning programs and directions for future research.

One of the controversies which exists in relation to the field of clinical reasoning and problem solving is whether such skills can, and indeed should be 'taught', or whether they need to emerge in the process of developing clinical experience. Harris (1993, p. 19) addresses this question as follows:

> The possibility of guiding a practitioner, initiating a novice, or enhancing the competence of an expert . . . depends on the validity of two assumptions. The first assumption is that human experience is sufficiently regular and repeatable that one can learn from others' (and one's own) experiences. The second assumption is that in order to introduce a novice to the ethos of an activity or to improve the practice of a person already initiated, an order or method in the practice must be conveyed, as distinguished from random events.

He goes on to say (pp. 20–21):

> . . . the possibility of guiding a practitioner also depends on the validity of the corollary assumption that the repeatable elements in human experience, that is, the methods, are *expressible*, although not necessarily in direct written or oral precepts. . . . (and) on the validity of a final assumption that an increase in a practitioner's understanding of a practice leads to improvement in that practice, or better, more successful outcomes of the practice.

This book builds on the acceptance of the validity of these assumptions and clearly supports the argument that not only can clinical reasoning be learned, but that teachers, mentors and experienced clinicians can help others, both novices and peers to develop their clinical reasoning expertise. In reflecting on these assumptions, we present several arguments. Firstly, the regularities of human experience are more unpredictable and multi-faceted than those of the physical sciences. This makes reasoning in human contexts both complex and challenging. Experience is a profound source of learning. This has long been the foundation of educational systems. In relation to the second assumption, we argue that with clinical reasoning there is no one method to be learned. Rather, alternative methods or more general strategies can be learned, or indeed created, to suit the client, the context and the clinician.

We contend that, on the one hand, there may well be several viable paths to a successful outcome, while on the other, part of the skill of clinical reasoning lies in matching the reasoning strategy to the variables in the given situation. In relation to the ability to express (describe, explain, teach) methods of clinical reasoning, this provides a significant challenge to teachers. Clinical reasoning is not something which can be neatly described like a method for conducting a simple chemical experiment. Throughout this book Harris' (1993) argument that professional practice involves science/technology, art and craft and the use of the corresponding forms of knowledge (propositional, reflective and practical), is strongly supported. We argue that teaching clinical reasoning can involve many approaches (e.g. explanations, providing opportunities for experience and prompting reflection and self-directed learning). Each of these activities would be aimed at enhancing the learner's understanding, and ability to perform clinical reasoning. Finally, we contend that effective teaching of a cognitive skill such as clinical reasoning, involves enhancing the learner's *ability* to perform clinical reasoning as well as his/her *understanding* of this phenomenon (with the latter often being achieved through the former). Therefore, given that clinical reasoning is the keystone of effective, autonomous clinical practice, the final assumption that improved practice will result, and thus this teaching/learning endeavour is worthwhile, is strongly defensible.

Moving beyond the question 'Should we teach clinical reasoning?' we come to the questions 'What is to be taught, and how?'. To examine the concept and practice of clinical reasoning across the health professions is not a simple task, largely because such thinking is a rather inaccessible phenomenon which is not always conscious, let alone observable. Also, this is a phenomenon which results from a complex interaction of many factors including contextual and disciplinary parameters, emotions, knowledge, experience, cognitive skill and personal frames of reference. Four main disciplines: medicine, nursing, occupational therapy and physiotherapy, have been selected to guide the discussion. In addition, other disciplines, including speech pathology, orthoptics and psychology, have been involved in the examination of strategies for understanding and teaching clinical reasoning. The inclusion of the varied disciplines brings a range of perspectives to the discussion as well as evident similarities. Readers will find an extensive variety of ideas here to stimulate, expand and challenge their current notions of clinical reasoning and their approaches to applying or teaching it.

Understanding clinical reasoning

Clinical reasoning is a highly complex phenomenon. This is evident in examining the growing body of literature in this field of study. There is no one accepted theoretical or research-based model of clinical reasoning. Indeed this text encourages readers to construct their own personal interpretation of clinical reasoning from the spectrum of ideas and perspectives that are presented, and invites clinicians, scholars and researchers to take today's literature and ideas and turn them into tomorrow's visions and explorations.

At the same time, in the midst of this complexity, and mindful of the need for clinical reasoning to operate within a context and rules of the relevant disciplinary paradigm, we consider that clinical reasoning also has an essential simplicity. *We have defined clinical reasoning as the thinking and decision making processes which are integral to clinical practice.* This definition is compatible with the various key perspectives presented in this text. In Chapter 2, in discussing clinical reasoning expertise, Boshuizen and Schmidt have referred to clinical reasoning as 'the thinking process occurring while dealing with a clinical case'. Elstein refers to solving clinical diagnostic problems in Chapter 4 which deals with clinical reasoning in medicine. In Chapter 5 Fonteyn defines clinical reasoning in nursing as 'the cognitive processes and strategies that nurses use to understand the significance of patient data, to identify and diagnose actual or potential patient problems, and to make clinical decisions to assist in problem resolution and to enhance the achievement of positive patient outcomes'. Jones et al in Chapter 6 refer to clinical reasoning in physiotherapy as 'the thought processes associated with a clinician's examination and management of a patient or client'. In Chapter 7 Chapparo and Ranka describe clinical reasoning as the fundamental process involved in collecting, classifying and analysing information concerning the client's ability and life situation, and then using these data in order to define client problems, goals and occupational therapy treatment focus.

A similar interpretation of clinical reasoning to ours is presented in the recently released text on clinical reasoning for occupational therapists written by the internationally renowned scholars in this field, Cheryl Mattingly and Maureen Fleming (Mattingly and Fleming, 1994). These authors emphasize the interdependence of thought (clinical reasoning) and action (clinical practice). They describe reasoning as 'judgement in action' leading to 'action based upon judgement' and argue that 'the confluence of action and judgement may also be the basis for the therapists' conviction that evaluation and treatment are reciprocal and continuous, not distinct, processes' (Fleming and Mattingly, 1994, p. 342).

As the illustration on the front cover demonstrates, we have conceptualized clinical reasoning as a spiralling thinking process; a search for a growing understanding of the clinical situation as the basis for clinical intervention. Within this process we contend that three elements (cognition, knowledge and metacognition) operate in harmony. That is, to reason effectively clinicians need a sound discipline-specific knowledge base from which they can derive context-relevant knowledge, and they need to be able to effectively utilize cognitive or thinking skills (such as analysis, synthesis and evaluation of data collected) and metacognition (i.e. monitoring or awareness of thinking processes).

The nature and operation of clinical reasoning will be further explored in Sections One and Two in the book. Section One deals with what clinical reasoning is and how it develops. In Chapter 1 the editors present our interpretation of clinical reasoning relating this to three key models which appear in the literature: hypothetico-deductive reasoning, pattern recognition and a knowledge-driven interpretation of clinical reasoning. In Chapter 2 Boshuizen and Schmidt discuss their model of the development of clinical reasoning expertise.

Section Two provides an overview of the methods of investigating clinical reasoning and then examines clinical reasoning in the practice of medicine, nursing, physiotherapy and occupational therapy. These chapters combine to present the image of a rapidly developing field of literature with a growing emphasis on the interdependence between clinical knowledge and clinical reasoning and on the importance of higher level cognitive functions in the effective operation of clinical reasoning. The four disciplines examined here, along with others discussed in Section Four, approach clinical reasoning in unique as well as related ways. This illustrates the existence of common or core features of clinical reasoning (such as the role of clinical knowledge) and the context-dependent nature of clinical reasoning which is created by such factors as the conceptual framework of the discipline and the role these professions play in health care. For instance, the dominance of the 'illness model' or the 'wellness model', or the relative emphasis on diagnostic and management decisions in a given profession, can significantly influence the nature of clinical reasoning within that profession.

Teaching clinical reasoning

In Section Three the focus of the text moves away from the nature of clinical reasoning to the teaching of clinical reasoning on the health sciences. The seven chapters in Section Three deal with multidisciplinary issues and dimensions of teaching clinical reasoning. Chapter 8 provides a broad introduction to designing health science curricula or learning programs which will enable students to develop their clinical reasoning abilities. In Chapter 9 the role of biomedical knowledge in clinical reasoning expertise is examined along with a discussion on teaching implications. Chapter 10 focuses on the importance of knowledge in clinical reasoning, on its generation and the value of including a variety of ways of knowing in health science education programs. In Chapter 11 the nature of clinical reasoning as a process of cognition is examined through a correlation between clinical reasoning and categorization. This analysis provides valuable directions for teaching. Chapter 12 examines the role of educational technology, in particular computer-aided learning, in teaching clinical reasoning. Chapters 13 and 14 examine the difficult area of assessment of clinical reasoning behaviours. Chapter 13 looks broadly at the assessment of student performance while Chapter 14 provides guidance for teachers, clinicians and students in the self-assessment and development of clinical reasoning ability.

In Section Four twelve chapters portray a wealth of experience from educators who have already constructed and implemented learning programs to help students develop their clinical reasoning skills. These chapters are program and/or discipline-specific.

The chapters in both Sections Three and Four emphasize an adult learning approach to teaching clinical reasoning. In part this was an intention of the editors and in part it has emerged from the educational philosophy and practices of the teachers who have presented their programs in Section Four. As will be demonstrated in these chapters, the adult learning approach, through its emphasis on such elements as learning through experience, the search for personal meaning, learner responsibility, empowerment of the learner, an internal motivation to solve problems and the autonomy of self-reward through enquiry, is highly compatible with the nature of the phenomenon (clinical reasoning) which is to be learned. These cognitive and humanist perspectives and strategies which underpin adult learning are very evident in clinical reasoning education lit-

erature. They are highlighted in the essentially cognitive nature of clinical reasoning and the particularly human and humanistic context of health care. A further link between both clinical reasoning and adult learning is the notion of higher level cognitive processes. In both situations the quality of the cognition, decision making and resulting action will be enhanced through the application of such higher level cognitive processes as reflection (both after and during action), metacognition (or the processing of cognition) and evaluation. Each of these themes is developed in many chapters in this book.

The future

The final chapter draws our attention to the future of the practice, teaching and study of clinical reasoning. For readers and authors alike, this chapter asks us to build upon our current ideas, interpretations and strategies and continue to explore this fundamental element of clinical practice.

References

Fleming, M.H. and Mattingly, C. (1994) Action and inquiry: Reasoned action and active reasoning. In *Clinical Reasoning: Forms of Inquiry in a Therapeutic Practice* (eds C. Mattingly and M.H. Fleming). F.A. Davis, Philadelphia, pp. 316–342

Harris, I.B. (1993) New expectations for professional competence. In *Educating Professionals: Responding to New Expectations for Competence and Accountability* (eds L. Curry, J. Wergin et al). Jossey Bass, San Francisco, pp. 17–52

Higgs, J. (1993) Physiotherapy, professionalism and self-directed learning. *Journal of the Singapore Physiotherapy Association*, **14**, 8–11

Mattingly, C. and Fleming, M.H. (1994) *Clinical Reasoning: Forms of Inquiry in a Therapeutic Practice*. F.A. Davis, Philadelphia

Section One

Clinical reasoning

1

Clinical reasoning

Joy Higgs and Mark Jones

Members of the professions must build and maintain a formidable store of knowledge and skills; they must learn to absorb information through the various senses and to assess its validity, reliability and relevance; and they must acquire the art and culture of their calling. And, most importantly, they must learn to use these qualities to solve practical problems. (Heath, 1990, p. 198)

Each of the skills to which Heath refers above, is essential to the role of the health science professional. In particular solving clinical problems or making clinical decisions is a critical skill and it defines to a large extent the concept of professional autonomy. The broad term we predominantly use throughout this text is clinical reasoning. This term refers to the thinking and decision making processes associated with clinical practice. We contend that the three core elements of clinical reasoning are the use of knowledge, the act of cognition or thinking and the process of metacognition (which refers to the awareness and monitoring of cognition). Metacognitive skills can also be thought of as higher order cognitive skills that are necessary for the management of knowledge and the management of other cognitive skills.

The importance of utilizing a metacognitive approach is, we believe, an essential part of effective clinical reasoning, and of critical self-evaluation and responsible practice, which together provide the foundation for reflective practice (as per Schon, 1987) and professional autonomy. We argue that the ability to reason knowingly, and to justify articulately our decisions and intervention, is essential for effective clinical practice and for the development of the knowledge bases of our professions. We aim to promote the development and utilization of metacognition in learning, practice and research and to encourage those involved in such activities to make the process of clinical reasoning more transparent and accessible to understanding and communication. By bringing a 'higher level of attention' (as per Torbert, 1978) to our reasoning and decision making processes we are able to enhance our understanding of the clinical problem, to become more aware of, and more able to deal effectively with the many complex factors influencing reasoning and decision making, to enhance communication, and to decrease the level of potential bias and error in our reasoning.

In the introduction to this text we presented clinical reasoning as an obscure and complex phenomenon (i.e. the process of attempting to structure meaning from a mass of confusing data and experiences occurring within a specific clinical context and then make decisions based on this understanding) as well as a rather simple construct, i.e. *the thinking underlying clinical practice*. A similar simple interpretation of clinical reasoning is to consider it as a thinking process directed towards enabling the clinician to take 'wise' action, meaning taking the best judged action in a specific context (Cervero, 1988; Harris, 1993).

This chapter pursues our exploration of the paradox inherent in the complex simplicity of clinical reasoning. We will first examine the context within which clinical reasoning occurs and the important role it plays in clinical practice. From this background emerges our interpretation of clinical reasoning. This model (or analogy) will be initially presented as a simple vision of reasoning occurring in search of understanding as the basis for clinical intervention. Next we examine our interpretation of clinical reasoning from several perspectives: in relation to methods of investigating clinical reasoning; in comparison to three existing dominant interpretations of clinical reasoning (i.e. hypothetico-deductive reasoning, pattern recognition and contemporary models of knowledge–reasoning interdependence); and in consideration of the notion of clinical reasoning expertise. Finally, we will consider the implications of our model/analogy for the teaching of clinical reasoning.

The context of clinical reasoning

Clinical reasoning occurs within several contexts: the immediate personal context of the individual patient/client (1), the unique multi-faceted context of the client's clinical problem within the actual clinical setting in question, the personal and professional framework of the clinician, the broad context of health care delivery and the complex context of professional decision making. In order to understand and address the reasoning behind clinical decisions the various contextual factors that influence reasoning need to be appreciated.

The personal context of individual clients includes such factors as their unique cultural, family, work and socioeconomic frames of reference, each of which contributes to the client's beliefs, values and expectations, and their perceptions and needs in relation to their clinical problems. Within their particular contexts people who receive health care services are living in varying conditions of health and illness. The problems that these people present can be 'confusing and contradictory, characterized by imperfect, inconsistent, or even inaccurate information' (Kassirer and Kopelman, 1991, p. vii). In addition, the consumers of health care are becoming increasingly well informed about their health and about health care services. Terms such as self-help and holistic health care are becoming more central to health care and the goal of achieving effective participation by consumers in their health care is widespread, requiring that health care professionals actively involve their clients in clinical decision making wherever desirable.

Health professionals need to develop a broad understanding of the environment in which they work, including knowledge of the factors influencing health (e.g. the environment, socioeconomic conditions, cultural beliefs and human behaviour). The Pew Health Professions Commission (1992) identified a number of future trends influencing health care in the USA including: efficiency and effectiveness through co-ordinated care, diversity and aging in the population, tensions in the expansion of science and technology, consumer empowerment and values (e.g. access, individual rights) that shape health care. Familiarity with such trends (as applicable to the region concerned) will promote effective clinical reasoning and decision making.

As well as processing clinical data and information concerning the personal needs and preferences of their clients, health care professionals need to be able to deal effectively with an increasing body of scientific, technical and professional knowledge. This knowledge explosion poses a very real dilemma for clinicians. On the one hand it can be argued that 'rapid social change and technological changes have become so commonplace that their ability to shock has diminished' and that people's capacity to cope with constant high-level change is limited (Candy, 1991, p. xiii). On the other hand, we need to enable students and graduate health care professionals to learn to manage change and to process complex information within the context of changes in their own knowledge and knowledge of the field. Developing a sound individual understanding of clinical reasoning and a capacity to reason effectively will facilitate this ability to manage complex and

(1) These terms will be used interchangeably throughout this chapter.

changing information. This is one of the goals of this text.

Within the context of professional decision making, the term health professional implies a qualified health care provider who demonstrates professional autonomy, competence and accountability (Higgs, 1993). Professional status incorporates the responsibility to make independent and accountable clinical decisions. This is particularly important where health professionals act in a first-contact practitioner role. There is an increasing demand for such accountability from all sectors of society, including consumers, the health professions themselves, from health care authorities, and where relevant, from registration bodies (Higgs, 1990).

To meet the expectations of society and the demands of a changing health care service, autonomous health care professionals need to be skilled in making clinical decisions. Indeed, the ability to make sound clinical judgements could be described as the most important factor in effective clinical practice. The importance placed upon clinical reasoning by the health professions is evident in the increasing level of clinical reasoning teaching in health science curricula (Elstein, 1981; Margolis et al, 1982; Neame et al, 1985; Tanner, 1987; Burnett and Pierson, 1988; Jones, 1988; Higgs, 1990; Kassirer and Kopelman, 1991; Rogers et al, 1991; Schwartz, 1991).

The contexts of health care are many and varied, ranging from programs of mass media health promotion, to high technology intensive care hospital units. Despite this diversity, a number of commonalities do exist. Firstly, in each case the focus is on the health of people. Secondly, since the services provided occur in human contexts, the health care environment is typically characterized by complexity, uncertainty and subjectivity. These factors have a strong influence on the nature of reasoning and on the impact of decisions made.

Health care systems could be described as 'soft systems', a term introduced by Checkland (1981) to refer to systems in which goals may be unrecognizable and outcomes ambiguous. In clinical settings, clinicians frequently face ill-defined problems, goals that are complex and outcomes that are difficult to predict clearly. Professional people dealing with, and immersed in the 'messiness' of reality in the clinic, need to develop the ability to cope with the uniqueness, uncertainty and conflict inherent in real problems. They need to be able to perform competently in situations which are often unclear or indeterminate (Schon, 1983; Kennedy, 1987; Cervero, 1988).

To achieve this outcome, Schon (1987) contends that clinicians need to be *reflective practitioners* and thereby shape and reshape actions as required by the context. The dominant positivistic view of professional knowledge, *technical rationality*, argues that professional activity consists of 'instrumental problem solving made rigorous by the application of scientific theory and technique'. Health professionals need to proceed beyond the limitations of this view to develop 'an epistemology of practice which places technical problem solving within a broader context of reflective inquiry, shows how reflection-in-action may be rigorous in its own right, and links the art of practice in uncertainty and uniqueness to the scientist's art of research' (Schon, 1988, p. 60).

Kennedy (1987) argues that professional judgement within the ambiguous or uncertain situations of health care is an inexact science and that judging clinical decisions by a priori standards of rationality is inappropriate. Thus the importance of individual perspectives rather than a priori criteria (Jungermann, 1986) and the defensibility of these perspectives could be more valuable evaluation criteria in the case of professional clinical judgements/decisions. Skills of professional judgement and critical self-evaluation are also needed to cope with information processing constraints or 'bounded rationality' (as per Newell and Simon, 1972) which result in limitations on the individual's ability to access knowledge and solve problems (Feltovich, 1983; Bransford et al, 1986; Hassebrock and Johnson, 1986).

One way to interpret how professionals cope with the uncertainties and challenges of clinical reasoning is to look beyond science. Harris (1993) for instance, presents the concept of professional practice as comprising a blend of art, craft and technology. Similarly, Evans (1989, p. 9) argues:

> we have heard many times that the (older) practice of clinical medicine is an 'art' – not reducible to the axioms of science. Clearly, what makes an essentially empirical discipline an art rather than a science is nothing more than the need to overcome the limitations of

inadequate models – the need to negotiate the complex waters of uncertainty. The art emerges from the master of techniques that, at least superficially, defy explanation, appear not to be rule-governed, and yet, when practised well, resonate with intuition.

The nature of professional craft knowledge and personal knowledge as well as the propositional knowledge of science are discussed in depth in Chapter 10. In Section Four many strategies and guidelines are presented as examples of how students and clinicians can learn the craft and science, and develop the art of clinical reasoning.

An interpretation of clinical reasoning

Based upon the above discussion it could well be concluded that clinical reasoning can be characterized as a process of reflective inquiry, in collaboration with the client (if possible), which seeks to promote a deep and contextually relevant understanding of the clinical problem, in order to provide a sound basis for clinical intervention. The essential elements of effective clinical reasoning could be described as cognition (reflective inquiry), a strong underpinning of discipline-specific knowledge and metacognition (which provides the integrative element between cognition and knowledge). Figure 1.1 illustrates the essential interaction of these three core elements in the process of clinical reasoning.

This model or analogy of clinical reasoning has been developed by the authors as a result of examination of the research, theories and experiences of others working in this field, and from our own scholarship and experience. It seeks to cross disciplinary boundaries and contexts to present both the essence and core elements of clinical reasoning. A simple outline is presented here and further detail will be explored throughout the chapter.

In this analogy, clinical reasoning is represented by an upward and outward spiral. This image is intended to demonstrate clinical reasoning as both a cyclical and a developing process. Each loop of the spiral incorporates data input, data interpretation (re-interpretation) and problem formulation (re-formulation) to achieve a progressively broader and deeper understanding of the clinical problem (see Figure 1.2). Based on this deepening under-

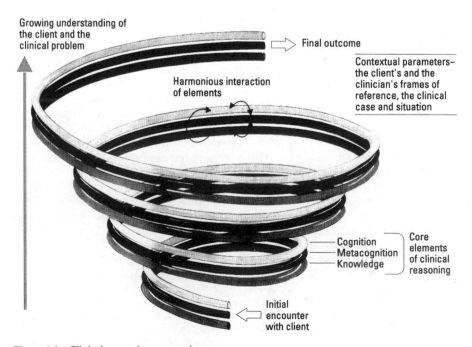

Figure 1.1   Clinical reasoning – overview

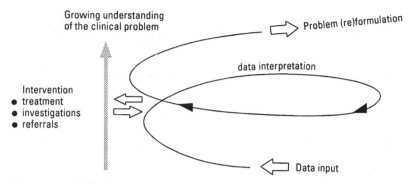

Figure 1.2   Clinical reasoning – within a loop

standing, decisions are made concerning intervention, and actions are taken. For instance, the clinician can decide to refrain from intervention, to collect further data, to conduct a treatment or to provide care, etc. The clinician's (or student's) proficiency in clinical reasoning can be represented by parameters such as the speed with which they ascend the spiral and the validity and depth of understanding of the clinical problem that is achieved. These outcomes are influenced by both internal factors (e.g. knowledge base, familiarity/experience with this type of case, reasoning skills) and external factors (e.g. institutional expectations, profession-specific frameworks of operation, complexity of the case).

Throughout the reasoning process the core elements of knowledge, cognition and metacognition interact. That is, cognitive or thinking skills (such as analysis, synthesis and evaluation of data collected) are utilized to process clinical data against the clinician's existing discipline-specific and personal knowledge base. At the same time metacognition is employed to monitor the clinician's thinking processes and conclusions, in order to detect links or inconsistencies between clinical data and existing clinical patterns or expectations based upon prior learning, to reflect on the soundness (accuracy, reliability, validity) of observations and conclusions and to critique the reasoning process itself (for logic, scope, efficiency, creativity, etc.). The process of clinical reasoning occurs throughout the clinician's interaction with the client, each decision or intervention producing a clearer picture of the

clinical problem which in turn generates further findings/data and/or questions in the continuing process of data interpretation and decision making.

Process versus content orientation in the investigation and interpretation of clinical reasoning (2)

To examine the above model we will firstly consider the field of clinical reasoning research. Clinical reasoning can be investigated via both a process and a content orientation. The former emphasizes behaviours and cognition, and the latter, clinical knowledge.

Process-oriented perspective

Process-oriented research into clinical reasoning can be closely linked to the field of psychology. Much of the early clinical reasoning research of the 1950s and 1960s focused on attempting to analyse the behaviours (and steps) involved in problem solving via the psychometric paradigm (e.g. Rimoldi, 1961). The focus of these studies was the assessment of physician/student performance. The research of this era supported the notion of the generic nature and transferability of effective problem solving skills (Grant, 1992).

Along with the rise of cognitive psychology, research into clinical reasoning also adopted a cognitive (rather than behavioural) focus with an emphasis on understanding the nature of clinical reasoning and on the development of clinical reasoning expertise. This cognitive

(2) Refer to Chapter 3 for a comprehensive discussion of methods used in the study of clinical reasoning.

psychology approach to clinical reasoning research included information processing, simulation, decision theory and categorization studies (3). In each of these approaches, use of knowledge derived from the clinical knowledge base of the individual was an important factor, as well as the active processing of received data, in enabling interpretation and solution of the clinical problem. Examples of research in this area include work by Barrows et al (1978), Elstein et al (1978), Gale (1982), Bordage and Zacks (1984), Feltovich and Barrows (1984), Feltovich et al (1984), Payton (1985), Corcoran (1986), Putzier et al (1985) and Fonteyn (1991). Recent developments in the cognitive tradition have included the use of propositional analysis (e.g. Patel and Groen, 1986; Schmidt et al, 1988).

For some time in nursing and occupational therapy, and more recently in physiotherapy, clinical reasoning research has challenged the domination of the empirico-analytical research paradigm (4) (to which much of the above research belongs). Newer research models are being adopted which operate within the interpretive research paradigm and the critical research paradigm (which emphasizes awareness of the reality and influence on behaviour of the social and historical construction of our thinking).

Research paradigms in the interpretive tradition include hermeneutics (based on the theory of interpretation) (Gadamer, 1975; Skinner, 1985), constructivism (where the emphasis is on people making sense of their worlds) (Candy, 1991), phenomenology (which seeks to understand lived experiences) (Swanson-Kauffman and Schonwald, 1988; Van Manen, 1990), grounded theory (which focuses on the world of the research subject) (Bowers, 1988) and ethnography (providing descriptions of phemonena from a given cultural perspective) (Omery, 1988). Knowledge gained through these approaches enhances the learner's depth of understanding of the perspectives of the key actor, the wholeness of human experiences and the interactions between these experiences and the context in which they occur.

The critical paradigm advocates becoming aware of how our knowledge is socially and historically constructed and how this limits our actions, with a goal of helping us to challenge the restrictions and habits of these limitations (Freire, 1970; Kemmis, 1985; Mezirow, 1981). In practical terms, such an approach in the health care context would encourage the clinician to look beyond accepted or seemingly unchangeable rules and situations, and in the spirit of lifelong learning, the clinician would engage in critical self-reflection and be open to transformation of his/her perspectives.

Work in the interpretive paradigm has been conducted by Benner (1984) in nursing (with an emphasis on seeking understanding of behaviours and context), by Crepeau (1991) and Fleming (1991a) in occupational therapy (with an emphasis on structuring meaning and interpreting the problem from the patient's perspective) and by Jensen et al (1992) in physiotherapy (with a focus on elucidating the complex and unknown processes that occur during therapeutic interventions). The clinical reasoning processes which such approaches describe, focus on strategies which seek a deep understanding of the client's perspective and the influence of contextual factors, in addition to the more traditional and 'clinical' understanding of the 'patient's' condition. Chapparo (1993) describes clinical reasoning in occupational therapy as a multi-strategy process incorporating procedural, interactive (with the client) and conditional reasoning (5).

As the volume and depth of research into clinical reasoning grows it is becoming more and more apparent that existing clinical reasoning models do not encompass the varying dimensions or reflect the diverse discipline-specific practice paradigms which exist across the health professions. Our model does not attempt to describe the precise processes of

---

(3) The categorization process of grouping objects or events can be related to the process of recognizing the similarity between a set of signs and symptoms and a previously experienced or learned clinical pattern or diagnosis. Similarly, when a clinician uses an expectation derived from past experience to make a treatment decision, that a particular plan of intervention is likely to be more appropriate or successful than others, given the patient's condition and prognosis, then this too is categorization. Refer to Chapter 11 for a detailed discussion of this literature.

(4) In Chapters 1 and 10 three major research paradigms (the empirico-analytical, interpretive and critical paradigms) which stem from the philosophical stances of positivism, idealism and realism, respectively, will be considered.

(5) Refer to Chapter 7 for a further discussion of clinical reasoning in occupational therapy.

clinical reasoning. Rather it has focused on the fundamental elements of reasoning which are common across the models favoured by and relevant to the different disciplines, i.e. information processing involving cognition and metacognition, use of clinical knowledge and a search for understanding (including the client's perspective) to enable decision making and intervention.

As portrayed in Figures 1.1 and 1.2, our model accommodates the cognitive, interpretive and critical traditions. We have emphasized the place of the clinician's knowledge base, and of their cognition and metacognition, in processing information in order to achieve understanding of the clinical problem as the basis for intervention. In relation to the use of mathematical models and probability in clinical decision making we do not describe the overall process of clinical reasoning as decision analysis. Neither would we see clinical decision making as resulting in prescriptive decisions, except in a limited number of more technical decision making contexts (e.g. radiology). Yet, the concept and practice of critically analysing both data and decisions, utilizing metacognition, is an important aspect of our model. We see this occurring within an interpretive and critical approach which we argue is more compatible with the majority of clinical situations (where the emphasis is on client context-specificity) the varied conceptual frameworks of diverse professions and the complexity and ambiguity inherent in human situations (6).

Our model supports the interpretive and critical paradigms, not only for the relevance of these approaches to the clinical context, but also because we emphasize that clinical reasoning, and the understanding or interpretation which results from this process in a given situation, is unique to the clinician (and client) involved. This argument rests on the following premises: that clinical reasoning occurs within the frame of reference of the individual; that the knowledge base of the clinician is unmatched, being derived from personal and professional experiences of the clinician as well as from the

learning of propositional knowledge; and that the engagement of an individual (within their particular frame of reference and knowledge base) with another individual (the client) within the client's specific context must result in a unique understanding of and proposed solution to the client's clinical problem. This is not to argue that we support whimsical, unsupported or potentially irresponsible problem understanding and solutions. Rather, we recognize that human problems can have multiple interpretations and solutions. The key to effective and accountable clinical practice, we contend, is that the clinician's understanding of the problem should be substantial in order to avoid potential harmful or ineffective intervention outcomes, and that their solutions should be justifiable in terms of sound arguments based upon propositional, professional and personal knowledge (7) of the clinician (and as appropriate, personal knowledge of the client).

Content (knowledge)-oriented perspective

A recent trend in the study of clinical reasoning and problem solving is the emerging conviction that clinical reasoning and clinical knowledge are interdependent, rather than being factors which can be learned separately. Norman (1990) for instance writes that in an endeavour to deal effectively with the knowledge explosion, many educational programs over the last few decades adopted the goal of developing problem-solving skills, and diminished their curricular emphasis on knowledge acquisition. In doing so they neglected to recognize that effective problem solving requires a large store of relevant knowledge. Norman et al (1990) contend that, on the whole, programs which have aimed to teach problem-solving skills have been unsuccessful (as demonstrated by Perkins and Salomon, 1989). They cite evidence (Schmidt et al, 1989) which supports the argument that problem-based learning for instance, rather than being a mechanism for teaching inquiry skills, is more successful in promoting the development of knowledge

---

(6) In Chapter 16 Nancy Watts presents a clinical decision analysis model. It can be seen that the fundamental goal of processing information (clinical data and knowledge) to understand the clinical problem as a basis for action is similar in both Watts' model and ours. An important aspect of teaching via this model is helping students learn to critically analyse information and to recognize and avoid judgemental errors. Clinical knowledge is used in the selection of the intervention strategy with the best probability of cost and outcome effectiveness.

(7) Chapter 10 discusses the nature and validity of these three forms of knowledge in depth.

which is related to clinical problems. This argument is supported in the model of clinical reasoning expertise developed by Boshuizen and Schmidt (8) in which expertise is linked to depth of clinical knowledge. Similarly, Grant (1991) argues that rather than over-emphasizing problem-solving skills, greater attention needs to be directed towards learner self-reliance in knowledge acquisition with problem solving being seen as part of the broader notion of reflective inquiry (as per Schon, 1988). In our model knowledge and thinking are clearly interdependent.

The interpretive and critical paradigms add an important dimension to the search for (and use of) knowledge in the human sciences. The empirico-analytical paradigm (9) relies on rules and causal laws more appropriate to the natural sciences, and the knowledge produced is insufficient for operation within human contexts (Kneller, 1958; Polanyi, 1958; Habermas, 1974; Schon, 1983; Skinner, 1985; Manley, 1991). This argument is well summarized by Barnett (1990) who contends that in a world where problems are not discrete nor solutions definite, we need knowledge beyond traditional science. Such a context occurs in the health sciences (as described at the beginning of this chapter). The human sciences need a view of knowledge that accords validity to both propositional (theoretical/scientific) knowledge and non-propositional knowledge (e.g. professional craft knowledge and personal knowledge/ knowledge of self), that seeks both personal and public validation, and that recognizes that knowledge is a dynamic phenomenon (10). Such a view is embodied in our model.

The notion of knowledge which we have incorporated into our model rests on three main arguments. Firstly, we have adopted a constructivist approach which regards knowledge as a construction of the human mind seeking to make sense of the world, rather than something that is 'discovered' (Novak and Gowin, 1984). Secondly, we argue that much of the knowledge which underpins health care is emerging, dynamic and imprecise, and is context-dependent. As such, it frequently provides the basis for justification rather than verification, for variability rather than one correct answer, for interpretation rather than conviction, and for a breadth of choice which challenges the decision maker. At the same time, knowledge in any discipline is grounded in the conceptual frameworks, philosophies, ideologies and practices of that group, which allows for a desirable range of approaches to health care delivery. In this text the professions examined provide evidence of such variation and it is within this range of contexts (e.g. illness versus wellness frameworks) and approaches (e.g. self-help versus compliance to prescribed treatment) that clinical reasoning needs to be explored to provide a multidisciplinary perspective.

Thirdly, we strongly support Schon's (1987) argument that, beyond research-based propositional knowledge, professionals today need practical knowledge, which we would term professional craft knowledge. The search for such knowledge and for personal knowledge or wisdom is the subject of considerable interest in current research and scholarship. Carper (1978) for instance, has produced a landmark paper on the structure of the domain of nursing knowledge, identifying four fundamental patterns of knowing: empirics (science), aesthetics (art), personal knowledge and ethics (moral knowledge). Likewise, Sarter (1988) has produced a most informative text which illustrates a multitude of paths to knowledge. Many of these paths have followed the interpretive and critical paradigms, recognizing the value of these approaches in producing knowledge of real value to the human context of clinical practice.

Interpretations of clinical reasoning in the literature

In this section our model of clinical reasoning will be compared to three existing dominant models of clinical reasoning, i.e. hypothetico-deductive reasoning, pattern recognition and contemporary models of knowledge–reasoning interdependence.

(8) Refer to Chapter 2 for a discussion of this model.

(9) The scientific paradigm or empiricist model of knowledge relies on observation and experiment in the empirical world, resulting in generalizations about the content and events of the world, which can be used to predict future experience (Moore, 1982). Only statements publicly verifiable by sense data are valid.

(10) Chapter 10 presents such a view of knowledge.

Hypothetico-deductive reasoning

Hypothetico-deductive reasoning as a model of clinical reasoning originated in medical research (Elstein et al, 1978; Kassirer and Gorry, 1978; Barrows et al, 1978; Gale, 1982; Feltovich et al, 1984). This reasoning approach involves the generation of hypotheses based on clinical data and knowledge, and testing of these hypotheses through further inquiry. The hypothetico-deductive reasoning model is illustrated in Figure 1.3a.

This interpretation of and approach to clinical reasoning is supported across the health professions. It has been seen as the dominant model of clinical reasoning in medicine for some time (Elstein et al, 1978; Gale, 1982; Feltovich and Barrows, 1984), as a commonly used approach in physiotherapy (Jones, 1992), as one of the modes of reasoning in occupational therapy (where it is linked to the concept of 'procedural reasoning') (Fleming, 1991b), and as an approach used by nurses as part of diagnostic reasoning (Padrick et al, 1987). However, in a number of the health professions other models and modes of reasoning are gaining prominence. In occupational therapy clinical reasoning is currently viewed as involving multiple strategies such as procedural, interactive, conditional and ethical reasoning (Fleming, 1991b; Chapparo, 1993). In nursing there is growing evidence that much of nurses' reasoning does not focus on either diagnosis or hypothesis generation (Fonteyn, 1991a and b; Fonteyn et al, 1991). In physiotherapy clinical reasoning models are emphasizing decision making in relation to many aspects of clinical practice beyond diagnosis (e.g. Jones, 1992) and the role of metacognition in clinical reasoning (e.g. Higgs, 1992).

Hypothesis generation and testing involves both inductive reasoning (moving from a set of specific observations to a generalization) and deductive reasoning (moving from a generalization to a conclusion in relation to a specific case) (Dewey, 1938; Ridderikhoff, 1989). Induction is used to generate hypotheses, and deduction to test hypotheses (Hopkins, 1980). Albert et al (1988) describe inductive reasoning as probabilistic reasoning, since a conclusion is reached (e.g. concerning a diagnostic hypothesis) on the basis of the probability of that conclusion in relation to the evidence available. This evidence is evaluated in relation to existing knowledge. Deductive reasoning is widely used in the health sciences in the presentation of arguments to defend our decisions and actions. Such reasoning follows the 'if . . . then' mode, with the 'if' referring to an implicit or explicit premise (or supporting statement) and the 'then' to the conclusion that is derived from that premise in relation to the situation and evidence in question.

Figure 1.3b demonstrates the similarities between the hypothetico-deductive reasoning model (Figure 1.3a) and our model (Figures 1.1 and 1.2). In each case a growing understanding of the case is occurring as a result of ongoing interpretation of data in comparison with existing knowledge. The inclusion of monitoring and the critical appraisal of thinking (metacognition) in clinical reasoning models is a relatively recent aspect of hypothetico-deductive reasoning models (as illustrated in Figure 1.3a, derived from Jones (1992)).

Pattern recognition

Pattern recognition or inductive reasoning, as an interpretation of the clinical reasoning process (in particular, diagnostic reasoning), has been supported by a number of researchers (e.g. Hamilton, 1966; Gorry, 1970; Scadding, 1967). Elstein et al (1990, p. 10) report on the work of Groen and Patel (1985) and Johnson (1983) which concluded that 'expert reasoning in non-problematic situations looks . . . like pattern recognition or direct automatic retrieval from a well-structured network of stored knowledge'. Elstein et al (1990, p. 10) argue, however, that experts 'clearly do consider and evaluate alternatives when confronted with problematic situations'.

Cox (1988, p. 103) describes pattern recognition or intuitive reasoning as follows: 'When a picture is strongly pathognomic, the limp of a stroke, the stare of exophthalmos, the colour and shape of a melanoma, the slump of depression, the facies (presentation) of Parkinsonism, the recognition from a pattern stored in "clinical memory" is so immediate as to be called "intuitive"'. To recognize patterns, he argues, it is first necessary to have experienced the pattern.

Inductive reasoning has both strengths and weaknesses. While it lacks certainty, inductive reasoning enables conclusions to be reached in the face of imprecise data and limited premises.

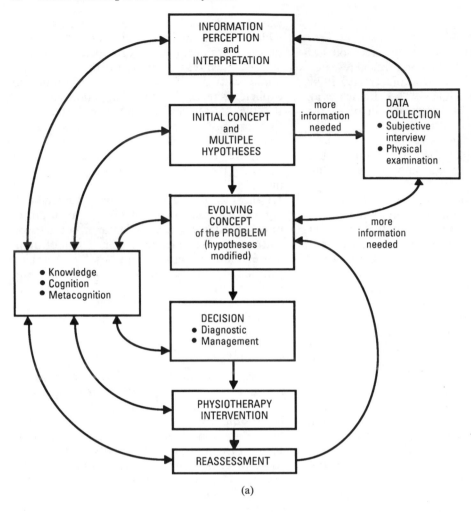

(a)

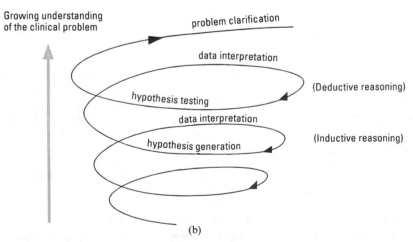

(b)

Figure 1.3   (a) The clinical reasoning process (adapted from Barrows and Tamblyn, 1980). (b) Analysis of the hypothetico-deductive reasoning model

Albert et al (1988, p. 100) describes this as follows: 'Of course we would all prefer to deal with certainties rather than probabilities. Unfortunately, in most instances in medicine and science, sufficient information for correct deductive arguments from acceptable premises is lacking. We must then rely on inductive inferences from premises accepted as true.'

Recently Patel and Groen (1986) and Arocha et al (1993) have used the terms 'backward reasoning' where hypotheses elicit the re-interpretation of data or the acquisition of new clarifying data in order to test a hypothesis, and 'forward reasoning' to equate to inductive reasoning in which data analysis results in hypothesis generation or diagnosis, utilizing a sound knowledge base. Forward reasoning is more likely to occur in familiar cases with experienced clinicians, and backward reasoning with inexperienced clinicians or in atypical or difficult cases (Patel and Groen, 1986).

Pattern recognition could be thought of as pattern interpretation. Through the use of inductive reasoning pattern recognition/interpretation is a process characterized by speed and efficiency (Ridderikhoff, 1989; Arocha et al, 1993). This is illustrated in Figure 1.4. By comparison, hypothetico-deductive reasoning, particularly the phase of backward/deductive reasoning, is generally regarded as being a slower, more demanding and more detailed process than inductive reasoning (Patel and Groen, 1986; Ridderikhoff, 1989; Patel and Groen, 1991; Arocha et al, 1993). This is pictorially represented in Figure 1.3b by the extra loops in the process, prior to the clinician gaining sufficient understanding of the case to take appropriate action.

Explanations of how pattern recognition occurs include categorization and the use of prototypes. Categorization involves grouping of objects or events. It can be related to the process of recognizing the similarity between a set of signs and symptoms and a previously experienced clinical pattern or case. The new case is placed in the same category as the past case(s) and is given the same label (diagnosis) (Schmidt et al, 1990; Brooks et al, 1991; Norman et al, 1992). Both diagnostic and non-diagnostic patterns (e.g. recognition of psychological, social, cultural client cues) exist. Similarly, when a clinician makes a treatment decision based on past experience that a particular plan of intervention was successful, given the patient's situation, condition and prognosis, then this too is categorization. An important aspect of the use of categorization in clinical reasoning is the link made by the clinician between the context of the condition, events or situation with previous cases. In the prototype model experience results in the construction of abstract associations which convey the meanings assigned to symptoms and signs (Bordage and Zacks, 1984) or semantic relationships consisting of links between clinical features (e.g. local versus general location of pain) (Elstein et al, 1990). The use of prototypes enhances the ability of clinicians to interpret clinical data since the recognition of the clinical pattern is matched against learned abstractions rather than specific instances which may be difficult to match clearly.

In our model, reasoning occurs throughout clinical practice, not merely to the point of diagnosis. Thus, Figure 1.4 represents an act of pattern recognition or interpretation, rather than the whole process of reasoning which occurs throughout the encounter with the client. Decision making (regarding diagnoses, prognoses, contra-indications, interventions,

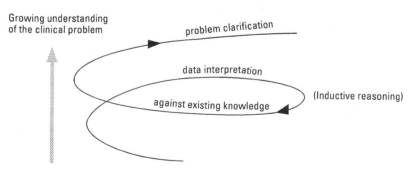

Figure 1.4 Analysis of the pattern recognition model

etc. (11)) occurs throughout the clinician's involvement with a case. Such decisions may be made using inductive or deductive reasoning. Repeated instances of pattern recognition, for instance, may occur in familiar cases as the clinician makes various decisions based largely on perceived connections between the current case and previous experiences stored in memory.

Knowledge–reasoning integration

Recent research in the health sciences has demonstrated that clinical reasoning is not a separate skill that can be developed independently of relevant professional knowledge and other clinical skills, such as investigative skills (e.g. Schmidt et al, 1990). Similar findings have occurred in other fields (e.g. chess: De Groot, 1965; Chase and Simon, 1973; physics: Larkin et al, 1980; Chi et al, 1981). There is increasing evidence to support the importance of domain-specific knowledge and an organized knowledge base (12) in clinical problem-solving expertise (Greeno, 1980; Hayes, 1981; Bordage and Zacks, 1984; Bordage and Lemieux, 1986; Patel and Groen, 1986; Grant and Marsden, 1987; Norman, 1988; Norman et al, 1989; Elstein et al, 1990; Schmidt et al 1990; Patel et al, 1990; Hassebrock and Prietula, 1992; Hassebrock et al, 1993a). However, it is the interaction between such knowledge and skills in reasoning which lies at the heart of clinical reasoning expertise. Both domain-specific knowledge and skills in cognition (critical, creative, reflective and logical/analytical thinking) and metacognition are essential for effective thinking and problem solving (Nickerson et al, 1985; Baron and Sternberg, 1987; Alexander and Judy, 1988; Barrows and Pickell, 1991).

Boshuizen, Schmidt and colleagues (Boshuizen and Schmidt, 1992; Schmidt et al, 1992; Schmidt and Boshuizen, 1992) have developed a stage theory on the development of expertise which emphasizes the parallel development of knowledge acquisition and clinical reasoning expertise. This model is based upon the notion and observation that developing knowledge and resultant reasoning expertise is largely the result of changes in knowledge structure. The first stage relates to (medical) students' acquisition of a great deal of biomedical knowledge within the framework of the basic and medical sciences. At this stage clinical reasoning relies heavily on biomedical knowledge and the generation and testing of multiple hypotheses. With experience of using knowledge in clinical reasoning the student's (or clinician's) knowledge is restructured, with knowledge elements becoming encapsulated into concept clusters with clinically-relevant foci. Knowledge is structured around illness scripts or abstract categories of illness features which include enabling conditions, faults and consequences (Feltovich and Barrows, 1984). This encapsulated knowledge now provides the basis for clinical reasoning in which whole illness scripts along with considerable associated information and expectations are used in a streamlined operation, with some unfolding of encapsulated biomedical knowledge occurring as needed, for instance, in difficult clinical cases. Ongoing clinical experience results in the accumulation of 'instantiated scripts' (i.e. actual detailed cases/specific instances) in the clinician's knowledge base. These are used during clinical reasoning with similar cases in the future. Where the current clinical case matches a learned/experienced illness script, clinical reasoning is prompt and automatic. Conscious reasoning and recourse to less clinically-structured and more basic knowledge occurs in complex situations.

Patel and Kaufman (see Chapter 9) regard the above interpretation as 'idealized' and cite biomedical misconceptions held by physicians and the different structure of the biomedical and clinical sciences as evidence that the biomedical sciences and clinical medicine constitute two distinct and not fully compatible worlds,

---

(11) For further discussion on types of hypotheses see Jones (1992) and Chapter 6.

(12) Understanding of knowledge base structure can be enhanced through the study of research into schemata and memory. 'A schema is conceived of as a modifiable information structure that represents generic concepts stored in memory. Schema represent knowledge that we experience – interrelationships between objects, situations, events and sequences of events that normally occur.' (Glaser, 1984, p. 100). Rumelhart and Ortony (1977) describe schemata as prototypes stored in memory, of situations which have been experienced frequently and which the individual uses to interpret instances characterized by related knowledge. For a detailed discussion of memory see Chapter 14.

with distinct modes of reasoning and knowledge. They suggest that the key role played by basic sciences may be in facilitating explanation and coherent communication rather than in facilitating clinical reasoning itself. Clearly, further research is needed to clarify the role of both biomedical knowledge and all knowledge types in professional practice. In our interpretation the roles of knowledge in clinical reasoning are numerous and the roles of various forms of knowledge are closely linked to the context (of the client, profession, situation) in which the knowledge is being utilized.

In our model the major function of clinical reasoning is to enhance the clinician's understanding of the clinical problem (and to some extent the client's understanding) to provide the basis for clinical intervention. A number of the more recent approaches to understanding clinical reasoning have been based upon interpretative investigation approaches. In nursing, a number of studies (Pyles and Stern, 1983; Agan, 1987; Rew and Barrow, 1987; and Rew, 1990) have emphasized the role of intuitive skills in clinical reasoning, linking intuitive knowledge to past experience with specific patient cases. In this sense 'intuitive knowledge' could be another way of describing 'instance scripts' which can be used unconsciously in inductive reasoning. Fonteyn and Fisher (1992) have linked nurses' experience and associated intuition to the use of advanced reasoning strategies or heuristics. Such heuristics include 'pattern matching' and 'listing' (or listing items relevant to the working plan) (Fonteyn and Grobe, 1993). In occupational therapy, Fleming (1991b) proposes a reasoning theory of an occupational therapist with a 'three track mind' in which clinical reasoning involves an integration of three reasoning strategies, i.e. procedural, conditional (projected) and interactive reasoning. In representing clinical reasoning as a process involving a growth in understanding (of the client's needs and condition, and of the situation), our model recognizes and addresses these newer interpretative approaches to understanding clinical reasoning.

Clinical reasoning expertise

Expertise in clinical practice and clinical reasoning

Simon (1980) has suggested that it takes at least ten years' experience to obtain proficiency in any profession. While experience is obviously necessary to obtain expert status, it is equally recognized that clinicians with comparable years of experience can have markedly different levels of expertise. What characteristics, then, are associated with clinical expertise in general, and clinical reasoning in particular? It is reasonable to assume the most important characteristic associated with clinical expertise is effectiveness and appropriateness in clinical outcome. Experts are expected to achieve better clinical results. And when outcome is considered with respect to diagnostic accuracy and clinical results, few would question this assertion. However, other dimensions of outcome, particularly as viewed from the patient's perspective may find some peer-judged experts wanting.

The clinical reasoning behind clinical performance encompasses not only diagnostic and management-oriented problem solving but also deals with clients' unique personal experience of their problems (i.e. the specific meaning and influences of their clinical problems). As such, clinical performance and the associated clinical reasoning cannot be judged solely on the basis of clinical results, such as whether the surgery or therapeutic intervention worked. Recipients of health care may have regained their health or function yet still feel the care giver's performance was inadequate. A premise of this chapter, and indeed of many chapters throughout this book, is that clinical reasoning cannot be fully understood when only the clinician's perspective is considered. Shared decision making between client and clinician is important if 'success' is to be realized from the client's perspective.

In our model, clinical expertise, of which clinical reasoning is a critical component, is viewed as a continuum along multiple dimensions. These dimensions include clinical outcomes, and also personal attributes such as intuition, clinical skills (e.g. manual and technical ability, communication and interpersonal skills), personality characteristics (e.g. empathy), and knowledge, cognitive and metacognitive proficiency (e.g. logical, creative and reflective reasoning).

To examine the nature of clinical reasoning expertise in further detail we will consider the seven knowledge and cognitive dimensions of expertise identified by Glaser and Chi (1988, pp. xvii–xx) and add an eighth dimension dealing with the client's perspective. These characteristics of expertise are consistent with the three components portrayed in our spiral model of clinical reasoning (i.e. knowledge, cognition, metacognition) and with the way we have interpreted these elements to include such factors as knowledge of the client's needs and perspectives and shared decision making.

1. *'Experts excel mainly in their own domains.'*
2. *'Experts perceive large meaningful patterns in their domain.'*

In terms of clinical reasoning these first two characteristics can largely be related to experts' superior levels and organization of knowledge in their own domain. The importance of domain-specific knowledge was discussed earlier in this chapter.

3. *'Experts are fast: they are faster than novices at performing the skills of their domain, and they quickly solve problems with little error.'*

This factor has been explained, in part, by the ability of experts to perform some tasks automatically thereby freeing up their memory and cognitive capacity for simultaneous processing of additional information or other tasks. It has also been related to experts' ability to reach a solution without having to conduct an extensive search of their knowledge base. This is possible because of the experts' superior organization of knowledge. Years of reflective practice has enabled the expert to acquire a large store of 'if . . . then . . .' production rules (Newel and Simon, 1972; Greeno and Simon, 1986) which specify that if certain features or conditions are present then certain decisions or actions are most probable or desirable (e.g. diagnoses, management plans, explanations, etc.). In this sense schemata (information structures stored in memory) include composite pictures comprising the clinical features of cases and information pertaining to the situations and the associated clinical interventions, which have been linked through experience.

4. *'Experts have superior short-term and long-term memory.'*

The examples offered by Glaser and Chi (1988) as evidence for this characteristic relate to well-structured situations such as chess playing and recall of digits by experts. This notion that experts have superior memory may be too simplified when considered in the context of the health professions where problems are ill-structured and complex and are capable of being represented, and hence recalled, along multiple dimensions. In fact findings associated with the superior memory skills of chess experts (de Groot, 1965; Chase and Simon, 1973) have not been replicated when applied to medical problems (Muzzin et al, 1982; 1983). This inability to replicate the superior memory findings of chess in the medical domain was in part related to the methodology utilized by Muzzin et al (1982; 1983) which relied on verbatim recall.

Later research by Patel et al (1986) re-analysed data from the Muzzin et al (1982) study and by using different techniques of linguistic analysis, these authors were able to demonstrate superior recall of material relevant to the diagnosis of a case by experts when the recall occurred in the form of inferences ('minor changes that preserved the semantics of the proposition'). However, even when inferences rather than verbatim recall were used, the picture is further complicated by additional research reported by Patel and Groen (1991) which demonstrated that recall is not proportionally related to the length of training period or the degree of expertise. For example, Patel and Groen (1991, p. 111) described the results of one experiment where 'fourth-year medical students recalled and inferred significantly more information than did either second-year students or internists on the comprehension of two clinical-problems texts: infectious endocarditis and gastrointestinal cancer'. This finding may be related to the more experienced internists' different organization of knowledge which allowed for unnecessary information to be filtered out. While these results suggest knowledge cannot be accurately reflected by outcome measures which emphasize recall, of greater significance to this chapter is the implication that expertise cannot be simply characterized through the use of pattern recognition.

As Patel and Groen (1991) pointed out, if expertise were simply a process of pattern recognition, one would expect a direct relationship between recall and diagnostic accuracy. This is not the case as diagnostic accuracy increases directly with expertise where recall does not.

5. *'Experts see and represent a problem in their domain at a deeper (more principled) level than novices; novices to tend to represent a problem at a superficial level.'*

As with other characteristics of expertise this factor is largely related to experts' organization of knowledge. It is also related to the depth of understanding gained by the clinician as a result of personal experience in managing the clinical problem (as per Boshuizen and Schmidt, 1992). This characteristic also suggests that the concept of pattern recognition as a process whereby a clinician simply matches the present case with a similar case from previous experience, is an incomplete account of what actually occurs (13). Bordage and colleagues (Bordage and Zacks, 1984; Bordage et al, 1990; Bordage and Lemieux, 1991) have demonstrated that better diagnosticians possess a broad range of problem representations which include categorizations of similar and opposing information within multiple dimensions of a problem (e.g. location of pain: such as local versus general; duration of pain: such as intermittent versus constant; cause of pain: such as trauma versus inflammation). Bordage and Lemieux (1991) argued that these 'semantic axes' are a fundamental and clinically significant component of a clinician's organization of knowledge. They suggest that for education to facilitate students' acquisition of deeper levels of knowledge representation, greater attention is needed regarding the semantic qualitative relationships which characterize the presenting symptoms and signs (e.g. 'Did the symptoms appear slowly or rapidly, recently, or some time ago? Are they constant or intermittent, unilateral or bilateral, focal or diffuse, superficial or deep, peripheral or central?') (Lemieux and Bordage, 1992, p. 203).

6. *'Experts spend a great deal of time analysing a problem qualitatively.'*

Glaser and Chi (1988) discuss how experts at the start of a problem-solving situation will generally attempt to 'understand' a problem in contrast to novices who are much quicker to jump in and apply strategies in search for a solution. This characteristic of the expert is particularly important in the more ill-defined problems where considerable inquiry and clarification is often necessary before the problem(s) themselves can be identified.

7. *'Experts have strong self-monitoring skills.'*

Glaser and Chi (1988) discussed studies which demonstrate that experts are more aware than novices of when they have made errors, why they lack understanding, and when they need to review their problem solutions. This advanced level of awareness is included in the skill of metacognition.

The use of higher level cognitive skills, including metacognition, as part of clinical reasoning is an important strategy for dealing with the variabilities, uncertainties, cognitive limitations and ambiguities in clinical decision making. Hassebrock et al (1993b) argue that metacognition (self-monitoring) is needed within these limitations to plan, control and evaluate the knowledge and strategies involved in clinical reasoning. According to Swanson (1990) metacognition provides an interface between general problem-solving skills and domain-specific knowledge.

Research on the role of metacognition in problem solving has focused on two areas, i.e. awareness of cognitive processes and the nature of metacognitive processes involved in reasoning (Bransford et al, 1986; Sternberg, 1988; Glaser, 1990; Swanson, 1990). Flavell (1979) has focused on the processes involved in metacognition and has identified such elements as: realizing that important problem solving (task) information is missing or ambiguous, recognizing that solving the problem will be difficult, planning strategies to manage the clinical problem, being aware that reasoning errors have been committed, evaluating the effectiveness

(13) For further discussion of pattern recognition in the context of prototype theory, see Chapter 11.

of reasoning strategies, modifying reasoning strategies and allocating cognitive resources.

In addition, Flavell (1979) developed a model of metacognition which included three categories of metacognitive knowledge: person knowledge (awareness of the capacity and limitation of the individual as a cognitive processor), task knowledge (awareness of available task data quality, relevance, etc.), and strategy knowledge (awareness of plans and strategies for goal achievement). In investigating these categories Hassebrock et al (1993b) found that physicians' metacognitive ability commonly involved combinations of all three metacognitive knowledge types. They advocate the teaching and assessment of metacognition in programs aiming to foster medical problem solving.

8. 'Experts have a depth of understanding of the clinical problem which includes the client's perspective'

The authors of this chapter add this challenging criterion to the description of clinical reasoning expertise. In a sense this is an attitudinal feature of expertise since it involves recognizing and valuing the place of the client in the decision making process (if possible) or at least giving consideration to the client's needs as a person. We would argue that this determinant of clinical expertise is applicable throughout clinical practice. It is particularly important in situations or professional contexts where the professional framework/paradigm expects clinical care to involve a partnership approach between clinician and client. In occupational therapy, for instance, considerable emphasis is placed on the utilization of a client-centred approach in which the focus is on people's rights to develop skills and habits required for a balanced, wholesome life (Shannon, 1977).

The eight characteristics presented above have emphasized the different levels and focus of knowledge and cognitive/metacognitive skills which exist behind the clinical reasoning inherent in clinical expertise. Less expert clinicians may only possess general knowledge of their profession while experts possess specialized knowledge. While this may account for superior expert outcomes with regard to diagnostic accuracy, other non-domain-specific knowledge and personal attributes will play a large role in determining how clinicians are perceived and

judged by health care recipients. Similarly, while domain-specific knowledge and associated cognitive skills such as pattern recognition are characteristic of experts, cognitive strategies such as hypothetico-deductive reasoning, which are less dependent upon domain-specific knowledge and skills, are crucial when clinical patterns are not easily recognized. Acquisition of expertise must be approached with consideration of all aspects influencing clinical outcomes as viewed from both the clinician's and the client's perspectives.

Implications of our model for the development and teaching of clinical reasoning expertise

An important question facing health science educators is whether clinical reasoning skills can and should be taught. Gale (1982) argues that the range of diagnostic thinking processes as presented in hypothetico-deductive reasoning, is characteristic of mature adult cognition in general (as per Inhelder and Piaget, 1958; Peel, 1971; Bruner, 1973). Albert et al (1988), similarly, describe the tacit employment of thinking skills, particularly, deductive reasoning, in clinical situations. That is, clinicians frequently employ reasoning skills, learned through life experience, without conscious thought. If clinical reasoning is indeed similar to adult thinking in general, then health science students do not need to learn this process, rather they simply need time to experience and develop their ability to apply their knowledge in clinical practice. Gale (1982, p. 64), however, contends that while medical education does not need to teach normal adult thinking processes, it 'must facilitate in the student self-awareness and self-monitoring skills for the entire range of potential thinking processes, some subset of which might be employed at any one time'.

We would argue that health science educators should facilitate the development of students' awareness of their clinical reasoning and of their learning (knowledge generation) processes. We strongly recommend the practice of helping students (and clinicians) to learn about thinking and learning, to learn to value cognition and knowledge as valuable tools to facilitate effective clinical practice and to develop expertise in the use of higher level cognitive skills (including metacognition and critical reflection-in-action). Through these means the students/clinicians can learn how to manage their reasoning rather than acquiring expertise (or perhaps erroneous thinking practices and knowledge) via trial and error or chance. Experience alone is rarely a sufficient teacher. It needs to be processed through reflection and critical appraisal, to make sense of this experience and to learn effectively from it (Schon, 1987; Boud, 1988; Boud and Walker, 1991).

Another important argument in favour of teaching clinical reasoning is that effective clinical reasoning is dependent upon the depth and organization of clinicians' knowledge bases, and upon their ability to use this knowledge effectively. The latter is dependent upon the clinician's ability to use knowledge in a way which is relevant to his or her disciplinary and client contexts. We support the teaching of clinical reasoning, preferably in conjunction with the acquisition of domain-specific knowledge (as well as personal knowledge). This stance is also supported by Barrows and Pickel (1991) in their recent text *Developing Clinical Problem-Solving Skills: A Guide to More Effective Diagnosis and Treatment*. We advocate the practice of clinical reasoning in application to clinical problems in both simulated and real clinical contexts, with active reflection-in-action and retrospective reflection on the reasoning process in order to enhance both reasoning ability and knowledge. It is the role of teachers to facilitate this learning. Strategies for achieving this goal will be explored at length in Sections 3 and 4 of this text.

Conclusion

This chapter has argued that clinical reasoning is central to clinical practice and has explored the nature of clinical reasoning and the criteria for demonstrating expertise in clinical reasoning. Throughout these discussions there has been an emphasis on three key elements: knowledge, cognition and metacognition operating within the frame of reference of the clinician, the context of the client and the complex, variable world of health care, to achieve a growing understanding of the clinical problem which provides the basis for clinical intervention. These interacting factors comprise the interpretation of clinical reasoning presented by the authors. This interpretation provides a means of integrating key messages and frameworks pertaining to major professional frameworks across the health professions with current theories/interpretations of clinical reasoning.

References

Agan, R. (1987) Intuitive knowing as a dimension of nursing. *Advances in Nursing Science*, **10**, 63–70

Albert, A.D., Munson, R. and Resnik, M.D. (eds) (1988) *Reasoning in Medicine: An Introduction to Clinical Inference*. The Johns Hopkins University Press, Baltimore

Alexander, P.A. and Judy, J.E. (1988) The interaction of domain-specific and strategic knowledge in academic performance. *Review of Educational Research*, **58**, 375–404

Arocha, J.F., Patel, V.L. and Patel, Y.C. (1993) Hypothesis generation and the coordination of theory and evidence in novice diagnostic reasoning. *Medical Decision Making*, **13**, 198–211

Barnett, R. (1990) *The Idea of Higher Education*. The Society for Research into Higher Education and Open University Press, Buckingham

Baron, J.B. and Sternberg, R.J. (1987) *Teaching Thinking Skills: Theory and Practice*. W.H. Freeman and Co, New York

Barrows, H.S., Feightner, J.W., Neufield V.R. and Norman G.R. (1978) *An Analysis of the Clinical Methods of Medical Students and Physicians*. Report to the Province of Ontario Department of Health, McMaster University, Hamilton, Ontario

Barrows, H.S. and Pickell, G.C. (1991) *Developing Clinical Problem-Solving Skills: A Guide to More Effective Diagnosis and Treatment*. Norton and Comp, New York

Barrows, H.S. and Tamblyn, R.M. (1980) *Problem-Based Learning: An Approach to Medical Education*. Springer, New York

Benner, P. (1984) *From Novice to Expert: Excellence and Power in Clinical Nursing Practice*. Addison-Wesley, London

Bordage, G. and Lemieux, M. (1986) Some cognitive characteristics of medical students with and without diagnostic reasoning difficulties. In *Proceedings of the 25th Annual Conference of Research in Medical Education of the American Association of Medical Colleges*. American Association of Medical Colleges, New Orleans, Louisiana, pp. 185–190

Bordage, G. and Lemieux, R. (1991) Semantic structures and diagnostic thinking of experts and novices. *Academic Medicine*, **66**, S70–S72

Bordage, G. and Zacks, R. (1984) The structure of medical knowledge in the memories of medical students and general practitioners: Categories and prototypes. *Medical Education*, **18**, 406–416

Bordage, G., Grant, J. and Marsden, P. (1990) Quantitative assessment of diagnostic ability. *Medical Education*, **24**, 413–425

Boshuizen, H.P.A. and Schmidt, H.G. (1992) On the role of biomedical knowledge in clinical reasoning by experts, intermediates and novices. *Cognitive Science*, **16**, 153–184

Boud, D. (1988) How to help students learn from experience. In *The Medical Teacher*, 2nd edn (eds K. Cox and C.E. Ewan). Churchill Livingstone, Edinburgh, pp. 68–73

Boud, D. and Walker, D. (1991) *Experience and Learning: Reflection at Work*. Deakin University Press, Geelong, Victoria

Bowers, B.J. (1988) Grounded theory. In *Paths to Knowledge: Innovative Research Methods For Nursing*, (ed. B. Sarter). National League for Nursing, New York, pp. 33–60

Bransford, J., Sherwood, R., Vye, N. and Rieser, J. (1986) Teaching thinking and problem solving: Research foundations. *American Psychologist*, **41**, 1078–1089

Brooks, L.R., Norman, G.R. and Allen, S.W. (1991) Role of specific similarity in a medical diagnostic task. *Journal Experimental Psychology, General*, **120**, 278–287

Bruner, J.S. (1973) *Beyond the Information Given*. Allen and Unwin, London

Burnett, C.N. and Pierson, F.M. (1988) Developing problem-solving skills in the classroom. *Physical Therapy*, **68**, 1381–1385

Candy, P.C. (1991) *Self-Direction for Lifelong Learning*. Jossey-Bass, San Francisco

Carper, B.A. (1978) Fundamental patterns of knowing. *Advances in Nursing Science*, **1**, 13–23

Cervero, R.M. (1988) *Effective Continuing Education for Professionals*. Jossey-Bass, San Francisco

Chapparo, C. (1993) Clinical reasoning: A model for occupational therapy in the practice area of neurology. Unpublished PhD Thesis, Macquarie University, Sydney

Chase, W. and Simon, H. (1973) Perception in chess. *Cognitive Psychology*, **4**, 55–81

Checkland, P.B. (1981) *Systems Thinking: Systems Practice*. John Wiley and Sons, New York

Chi, M.T.H., Feltovich, P.J. and Glaser, R. (1981) Categorization and representation of physics problems by experts and novices. *Cognitive Science*, **5**, 121–152

Corcoran, S. (1986) Planning by expert and novice nurses in cases of varying complexity. *Research in Nursing and Health*, **9**, 155–162

Cox, K. (1988) How to teach clinical reasoning. In *The Medical Teacher*, 2nd edn (eds K. Cox and C.E. Ewan). Churchill Livingstone, Edinburgh, pp. 102–107

Crepeau, E.B. (1991) Achieving intersubjective understanding: Examples from an occupational therapy treatment session. *American Journal of Occupational Therapy*, **45**, 1016–1025

De Groot, A.D. (1965) *Thought and Choice in Chess*. Mouton, The Hague

Dewey, J. (1938) *Logic: The Theory of Inquiry*. Holt, Rinehart and Winston, New York

Elstein, A.S. (1981) Educational programs in medical decision making. *Medical Decision Making*, **1**, 70–73

Elstein, A.S., Shulman, L.S. and Sprafka, S.A. (1978) *Medical Problem Solving. An Analysis of Clinical Reasoning*. Harvard University Press, Cambridge, MA

Elstein, A.S., Shulman, L.S. and Sprafka, S.A. (1990) Medical problem solving: a ten year retrospective. *Evaluation and the Health Professions*, **13**, 5–36

Evans, D.A. (1989) Issues of cognitive science in medicine. In *Cognitive Science in Medicine* (eds D.A. Evans and V.L. Patel). The Massachusetts Institute of Technology Press, Cambridge, Massachusetts, pp. 1–19

Feltovich, P.J. (1983) Expertise: Reorganizing and refining knowledge for use. *Professions Education Researcher Notes*, **4**, 5–9

Feltovich, P.J. and Barrows, H.S. (1984) Issues of generality in medical problem solving. In *Tutorials in Problem-Based Learning; A New Direction in Teaching the Health Professions* (eds H.G. Schmidt and M.L. De Volder). Van Gorcum, Assen

Feltovich, P.J., Johnson, P.E., Moller, J.H. and Swanson, D.B. (1984) LCS: The role and development of medical knowledge in diagnostic expertise. In *Readings in Medical Artificial Intelligence: The First Decade* (eds W.J. Clancey and E.H. Shortliffe). Addison-Wesley, Reading, pp. 275–319

Flavell, J. (1979) Metacognition and cognitive monitoring: A new area of cognitive–developmental inquiry. *American Psychologist*, **34**, 906–911

Fleming, M.H. (1991a) Clinical reasoning in medicine compared with clinical reasoning in occupational therapy. *American Journal of Occupational Therapy*, **45**, 988–996

Fleming, M.H. (1991b) The therapist with the three track mind. *American Journal of Occupational Therapy*, **45**, 1007–1014

Fonteyn, M. (1991a) A descriptive analysis of expert critical care nurses' clinical reasoning. Doctoral Dissertation, The University of Texas, Austin, Texas, USA

Fonteyn, M. (1991b) Implications of clinical reasoning studies for critical care nursing. *Focus on Critical Care. AACN*, **18**, 322–327

Fonteyn, M. and Fisher, S. (1992) The study of expert nurses in practice. Unpublished paper presented at *Transformation Through Unity: Decision-Making and Informatics in Nursing* in Portland, Oregon on October 17, 1992 at the University of Oregon Health Science Centre, Portland, Oregon

Fonteyn, M. and Grobe, S. (1993) Expert critical care nurses' clinical reasoning under uncertainty: Representation, structure and process. In *Sixteenth Annual Symposium on Computer Applications in Medical Care* (ed. M. Frisse). McGraw-Hill, New York, pp. 405–409

Fonteyn, M., Grobe, S. and Kuipers, B. (1991) A descriptive

analysis of expert critical care nurses' clinical reasoning. In *Nursing Informatics '91* (eds E. Hovenga, K. Hannah, K. McCormick and J. Roland). Springer-Verlag, New York, pp. 765–768

Freire, P. (1970) *Cultural Action for Freedom*. Harvard Educational Review, Massachusetts.

Gadamer, H.G. (1975) Hermeneutics and social science. *Cultural Hermeneutics*, **2**, 312

Gale, J. (1982) Some cognitive components of the diagnostic thinking process. *British Journal of Educational Psychology*, **52**, 64–76

Glaser, R. (1984) Education and thinking: the role of knowledge. *American Psychologist*, **39**, 93–104

Glaser, R. (1990) The re-emergence of learning theory within instructional research. *American Psychologist*, **45**, 29–39

Glaser, R. and Chi, M.T.H. (1988) Overview. In *The Nature of Expertise* (eds M.T.H. Chi, R. Glaser and M.J. Farr). Lawrence Erlbaum Associates, Hillsdale, New Jersey, pp. xvi–xxviii

Gorry, G.A. (1970) Modelling the diagnostic process. *Journal of Medical Education*, **45**, 293–302

Grant, J. and Marsden, P. (1987) The structure of memorized knowledge in students and clinicians: an explanation for diagnostic expertise. *Medical Education*, **21**, 92–98

Grant, R. (1992) Obsolescence or lifelong education: choices and challenges. *Physiotherapy*, **78**, 167–171

Grant, R. (1991) Professional obsolescence. *Physiotherapy Theory and Practice*, **7**, 81–82

Greeno, J.G. (1980) Trends in the theory of knowledge for problem solving. In *Problem Solving and Education: Issues in Teaching and Research* (eds D.T. Tuma and R. Reif). Lawrence Erlbaum Associates, Hillsdale, New Jersey, pp. 9–23

Greeno, J.G. and Simon, H.A. (1986) Problem solving and reasoning. In *Steven's Handbook of Experimental Psychology* 2nd edn, Vol 2: *Learning and Cognition* (eds R.C. Atkinson, R.Hernstein, G. Lindsey and R.D. Luce). John Wiley and Sons, New York, pp. 572–589

Habermas, J. (1974) *Theory and Practice* (translated by J. Viertel). Heinemann, London

Hamilton, M. (1966) *Clinicians and Decisions*. Leeds University Press, Leeds

Harris, I.B. (1993) New expectations for professional competence. In *Educating Professionals: Responding to New Expectations for Competence and Accountability* (eds L. Curry, J. Wergin et al). Jossey-Bass, San Francisco, pp. 17–52

Hassebrock, F. and Johnson, P.E. (1986) Medical knowledge and cognitive effort in diagnostic reasoning. Paper presented at the *Annual Meeting of the American Educational Research Association*. American Educational Research Association, San Francisco

Hassebrock, F. and Prietula, M. (1992) Protocol-based coding scheme for the analysis of medical reasoning. *International Journal of Man/Machine Studies*, **37**, 613–652

Hassebrock, F., Johnson, P.E., Bullemer, P., Fox, P.W. and Moller, J.H. (1993a) When less is more: Representation and selective memory in expert problem solving. *American Journal of Psychology*, **106**, 155-189

Hassebrock, F., Jonas, A.P. and Bauer, L. (1993b) Metacognitive aspects of medical problem solving. Paper presented to the *Annual Meeting of the American Educational Research Association*. American Educational Research Association, Atlanta

Hayes, J.R. (1981) *The Complete Problem Solver*. Franklin Institute Press, Philadelphia

Heath, T. (1990) Education for the professions: Contemplations and reflections. In *Higher Education in the Late Twentieth Century: Reflections on a Changing System – A Festschrift for Ernest Roe* (ed. I. Moses). Higher Education Research and Development Society of Australia, Sydney

Higgs, J. (1990) Fostering the acquisition of clinical reasoning skills. *New Zealand Journal of Physiotherapy*, **18**, 13–17

Higgs, J. (1992) Developing knowledge: a process of construction, mapping and review. *New Zealand Journal of Physiotherapy*, **20**, 23–30

Higgs, J. (1993) Physiotherapy, professionalism and self-directed learning. *Journal of the Singapore Physiotherapy Association*, **14**, 8–11

Hopkins, C.D. (1980) *Understanding Educational Research: An Inquiry Approach*. Charles E. Merrill, Columbus, Ohio

Inhelder, B. and Piaget, J. (1958) *The Growth of Logical Thinking from Childhood to Adolescence*. Routledge and Kegan Paul, London

Jensen, G.M., Shepard, K.F. and Hack, L.M. (1992) Attribute dimensions that distinguish master and novice physical therapy clinicians in orthopedic settings. *Physical Therapy*, **72**, 711-722.

Jones, M.A. (1988) Clinical reasoning in manipulative therapy education. Unpublished masters thesis, South Australian Institute of Technology, Adelaide

Jones, M.A. (1992) Clinical reasoning in manual therapy. *Physical Therapy*, **72**, 875–884

Jungermann, H. (1986) The two camps on rationality. In *Judgment and Decision Making: An Interdisciplinary Reader* (eds H.R. Arkes and K.R. Hammond). Cambridge University Press, New York, pp. 627–641

Kassirer, J.P. and Gorry, G.A. (1978) Clinical problem solving: a behavioral analysis. *Annals of Internal Medicine*, **89**, 245–255

Kassirer, J.P. and Kopelman, R.I. (1991) *Learning Clinical Reasoning*. Williams and Wilkins, Baltimore

Kemmis, S. (1985) Action research and the politics of reflection. In *Reflection: Turning Experience Into Learning* (eds D. Boud, R. Keogh and D. Walker). Kogan Page, London, pp. 139–163

Kennedy, M. (1987) Inexact sciences: Professional education and the development of expertise. In *Review of Research in Education*, **14**, 133–168. American Education Research Association, Washington, DC

Kneller, G.F. (1958) *Existentialism and Education*. Science Editions, John Wiley and Sons, New York

Larkin, J., McDermott, J., Simon, D.P. and Simon, H.A. (1980) Expert and novice performance in solving physics problems. *Science*, **208**, 1335–1342

Lemieux, M. and Bordage, G. (1992) Propositional versus structural semantic analysis of medical diagnostic thinking. *Cognitive Science*, **16**, 185–204

Manley, K. (1991) Knowledge for nursing practice. In *Nursing: A Knowledge Base for Practice* (eds A. Perry and M. Jolley). Edward Arnold, London, pp. 1–27

Margolis, C.Z., Barnoon, S. and Barak, N. (1982) A required course in decision-making for pre-clinical medical students. *Journal of Medical Education*, **57**, 184–190

Mezirow, J. (1981) A critical theory of adult learning and education. *Adult Education*, **32**, 3–24

Moore, T.W. (1982) *Philosophy of Education: An Introduction*. Routledge and Kegan Paul, London

Muzzin, L.J., Norman, G.R., Feightner, J.W. and Tugwell, P. (1983) Expertise in recall of clinical protocols in two specialty areas. In *Proceedings of the 22nd Annual Conference on Research in Medical Education of the American Association of Medical Colleges*. American Association of Medical Colleges, New Orleans, Louisiana, pp. 122–127

Muzzin, L.J., Norman, G.R., Jacoby, L.L., Feightner, J. W., Tugwell, P. and Guyatt, G.H. (1982) Manifestations of expertise in recall of clinical protocols. In *Proceedings of the 21st Conference on Research in Medical Education of the American Association of Medical Colleges*, pp. 163–168

Neame, R.L.B., Mitchell, K.R., Feletti, G.I. and McIntosh, J. (1985) Problem-solving in undergraduate medical students. *Medical Decison Making*, **5**, 312–324

Newell, A. and Simon, H.A. (1972) *Human Problem Solving*. Prentice-Hall, Englewood Cliffs, NJ

Nickerson, R.S., Perkins, D.N. and Smith, E.E. (1985) *the Teaching of Thinking*. Lawrence Erlbaum Associates, Hillsdale, New Jersey

Norman, G., Brooks, L.R. and Allen, S.W. (1989) Recall by expert medical practitioners and novices as a record of processing attention. *Journal of Experimental Psychology: Learning, Memory and Cognition*, **15**, 1116–1174

Norman, G.R. (1988) Problem-solving skills, solving problems and problem-based learning. *Medical Education*, **22**, 279–286

Norman, G.R. (1990) Editorial: problem-solving skills and problem-based learning. *Physiotherapy Theory and Practice*, **6**, 53–54

Norman, G.R., Coblentz, C.L., Brooks, L.R. and Babcock, C.J. (1992) Expertise in visual diagnosis: a review of the literature. *Academic Medicine*, **66**, S78–S83

Norman, G.R., Patel, V.L. and Schmidt, H.G. (1990) Clinical inquiry and scientific inquiry. *Medical Education*, **24**, 396–399

Novak, J.D. and Gowin, D.B. (1984) *Learning How to Learn*. Cambridge University Press, Cambridge

Omery, A. (1988) Ethnography. In *Paths to Knowledge: Innovative Research Methods for Nursing* (ed. B. Sarter). National League for Nursing, New York, pp. 17–32

Padrick, K., Tanner, C., Putzier, D. and Westfall, U. (1987) Hypothesis evaluation: a component of diagnostic reasoning. In *Classification of Nursing Diagnosis: Proceedings of the Seventh Conference* (ed. A. McClane). C.V. Mosby, Toronto, Canada, pp. 299–305

Patel, V.L. and Groen, G.J. (1986) Knowledge-based solution strategies in medical reasoning. *Cognitive Science*, **10**, 91–116

Patel, V.L. and Groen, G.J. (1991) The general and specific nature of medical expertise: A critical look. In *Toward a General Theory of Expertise: Prospects and Limits* (eds A. Ericsson and J. Smith). Cambridge University Press, New York, NY, pp. 93–125

Patel, V.L., Groen, G.J. and Arocha, J.F. (1990) Medical expertise as a function of task difficulty. *Memory and Cognition*, **18**, 394–406

Patel, V.L., Groen G.J. and Frederiksen, C.H. (1986) Differences between medical students and doctors in memory for clinical cases. *Medical Education*, **20**, 3–9

Payton, O.D. (1985) Clinical reasoning process in physical therapy. *Physical Therapy*, **65**, 924–928

Peel, E.A. (1971) *The Nature of Adolescent Judgment*. Staples Press, London

Perkins, D.N. and Salomon, G. (1989) Are cognitive skills context-bound? *Educational Researcher*, **18**, 16–25

Pew Health Commission (1992) Executive summary from the Pew Health Commission. 'Healthy America: Practitioners for 2005'. *Journal of Allied Health*, **Fall**, 3–22

Polanyi, M. (1958) *Personal Knowledge: Towards a Post-Critical Philosophy*. Routledge Kegan Paul, London

Putzier, D., Padrick, K., Westfall, U. and Tanner, C. (1985) Diagnostic reasoning in critical care nursing. *Heart and Lung*, **14**, 430–436

Pyles, S. and Stern, P. (1983) Discovery of nursing gestalt in critical care nursing: the importance of the grey gorilla syndrome. *Image: The Journal of Nursing Scholarship*, **15**, 51–57

Rew, L. (1990) Intuition in critical care nursing practice. *Dimensions of Critical Care Nursing*, **9**, 30–37

Rew, L. and Barrow, E. (1987) Intuition: A neglected hallmark of nursing knowledge. *Advances in Nursing Science*, **10**, 49–62

Ridderikhoff, J. (1989) *Methods in Medicine: A Descriptive Study of Physicians' Behaviour*. Kluwer Academic Publishers, Dordrecht

Rimoldi, H.J.A. (1961) The test of diagnostic skills. *Journal of Medical Education*, **36**, 73–79

Rogers, J.C., Swec, D.E. and Ullian, J.A. (1991) Teaching medical decision making and students' clinical problem solving skills. *Medical Teacher*, **13**, 157–164

Rumelhart, D.E. and Ortony, A. (1977) The representation of knowledge in memory. In *Schooling and the Acquisition of Knowledge* (eds R.C. Anderson, R.J. Spiro, W.E. Montague). Lawrence Erlbaum Associates, Hillsdale, New Jersey

Sarter, B. (ed.) (1988) *Paths to Knowledge: Innovative Research Methods for Nursing*. National League for Nursing, New York

Scadding, J.G. (1967) Diagnosis: The clinician and the computer. *Lancet*, **1**, 877–882

Schmidt, H., Boshuizen, H.P.A. and Hobus, P.P.M. (1988) Transitory stages in the development of medical expertise: The 'intermediate effect' in clinical case representation studies. In *Proceedings of the Tenth Annual Conference of the Cognitive Science Society* (eds V.L. Patel and G.J. Groen). Lawrence Erlbaum Associates, Hillsdale, NJ, pp. 139–145

Schmidt, H.G. and Boshuizen, H.P.A. (1992) Encapsulation of biomedical knowledge. In *Advanced Models of Cognition for Medical Training and Practice* (eds A.E. Evans and V.L. Patel). Springer Verlag, New York

Schmidt, H.G., Boshuizen, H.P.A. and Norman, G.R. (1992) Reflections on the nature of expertise in medicine. In *Deep Models for Medical Knowledge Engineering* (ed. E. Keravnou). Elsevier, Amsterdam, pp. 231–248

Schmidt, H.G., De Grave W.S., De Volder, M.L., Moust, J.H.C. and Patel, V.L. (1989) Explanatory models in the processing of science text: the role of prior knowledge activation through small-group discussion. *Journal of Educational Psychology*, **81**, 481–491

Schmidt, H.G., Norman, G.R. and Boshuizen, H.P.A. (1990) A cognitive perspective on medical expertise: theory and implications. *Academic Medicine*, **65**, 611–621

Schon, D.A. (1983) *The Reflective Practitioner: How Professionals Think in Action*. Temple Smith, London

Schon, D.A. (1987) *Educating the Reflective Practitioner*. Jossey-Bass, San Franciso

Schon, D.A. (1988) From technical rationality to reflection-in-action. In *Professional Judgement* (eds J. Dowie and A. Elstein). Cambridge University Press, Cambridge, pp. 60–77

Schwartz, K.B. (1991) Clinical reasoning and new ideas on intelligence: implications for teaching and learning. *The American Journal of Occupational Therapy*, **45**, 1033–1037

Shannon, P. (1977) The derailment of occupational therapy. *American Journal of Occupational Therapy*, **31**, 229–234

Simon, H.A. (1980) Problem solving and education. In *Problem Solving and Education: Issues in Teaching and Research* (eds D.T. Tuma and F. Reif). Lawrence Erlbaum Associates, Hillsdale, New Jersey, pp. 81–96

Skinner, Q. (1985) Introduction: The return of grand theory. In *The Return of Grand Theory in the Human Sciences* (ed. Q. Skinner). Cambridge University Press, Cambridge, pp. 1–20

Sternberg, R.J. (1988) *The Triarchic Mind: A New Theory of Human Intelligence*. Viking, New York

Swanson, H.L. (1990) Influence of metacognitive knowledge and aptitude on problem solving. *Journal of Educational Psychology*, **82**, 306–314

Swanson-Kauffman, K. and Schonwald, E. (1988) Phenomenology. In *Paths to Knowledge: Innovative Research Methods for Nursing* (ed. B. Sarter). National League for Nursing, New York, pp. 97–110.

Tanner, C.A. (1987) Teaching clinical judgement. *Annual Review of Nursing Research*, **5**, 153–173

Torbert, W.R. (1978) Educating toward shared purpose, self-direction and quality work – the theory and practice of liberating structure. *Journal of Higher Education*, **49**, 109–135

Van Manen, M. (1990) *Researching Lived Experience: Human Science for an Action Sensitive Pedagogy*. State University of New York Press, New York

2

The development of clinical reasoning expertise

Henny P. A. Boshuizen (1) and Henk G. Schmidt

The main objective of medical schools is to turn relative novices into knowledgeable and skilled professionals. Therefore students gather in classes to acquire knowledge, have practicals for demonstration purposes, follow skills training programs and have their clerkships. Yet, clinical teachers are not always content with the outcomes or their teaching. One complaint is that students might have knowledge about subjects X or Y, but that they do not demonstrate that knowledge in contexts where it has to be applied. Another complaint is that students are not able to solve clinical problems, especially in practical settings. Maybe they can in classroom settings, but in the face of real patients, they seem to lose their competence. Over the years, these observations have been made by many teachers inspiring a great deal of research (e.g., Barrows et al, 1978; Elstein et al, 1978) and the introduction of new approaches to teaching medicine, such as problem-based learning (Norman and Schmidt, 1992) aiming at the improvement of clinical reasoning in medicine.

This chapter seeks to answer the question whether clinical reasoning can be taught to medical students. It starts by describing the development from novice in medicine to expert, providing a theoretical framework for this development. Furthermore, it discusses several approaches to clinical reasoning skills

training and it delineates the implications of this theory for the way medical education can improve students' clinical reasoning.

A theory on the development of medical expertise

For a long time, it has been thought that the human mind can be trained in logical thinking, problem-solving or creativity. For that purpose children are encouraged to play chess, or to learn Latin in school. Polya's (1957) problem-solving training program also cherishes this general idea about the human mind. In the same vein, it was thought that experts in an arbitrary domain had trained their minds and had developed general problem-solving and thinking skills. This opinion has, however, been superseded, since research outcomes have shown that experts in a specific domain have not developed separate problem-solving skills that can be applied across domains. This is even the case with experts in chess, a mental activity that has always been thought to sharpen the mind. Instead, domain knowledge and associated skills to use this knowledge in problem solving develop simultaneously. This phenomenon has been observed in very different domains (chess: De Groot, 1965; engineering: Ackerman and Barbichon, 1963; statistics:

(1) Preparation of this chapter has been enabled by a grant to the first author from the Spencer Foundation, National Academy of Education, USA.

Allwood and Montgomery, 1981, 1982; mathematics: Bloom and Broder, 1950; physics: Chi et al, 1981).

In medicine, research groups in Canada, the USA, the UK and the Netherlands have shown that clinical reasoning is no separate skill that is acquired independent of medical knowledge and other diagnostic skills. Instead, their joint research efforts suggest a stage theory on the development of medical expertise, in which knowledge acquisition and clinical reasoning go hand in hand (see Boshuizen and Schmidt, 1992; Schmidt et al, 1992; Schmidt et al, 1990; Schmidt and Boshuizen, 1992).

This theory on medical diagnosis is essentially a theory on the acquisition and development of knowledge structures a student or a physician operates upon while diagnosing a case. Structural changes in knowledge result in dramatic changes in problem solving or clinical reasoning. During the first stage, medical students acquire large amounts of knowledge about the biomedical, basic sciences. They acquire concepts linked together in a knowledge network. By and by, more concepts are added and refined, and more and better connections are made. Knowledge accretion and validation are the students' main concerns in this period of their study. During this stage their clinical reasoning process is characterized by lines of reasoning consisting of chains of small steps commonly based on detailed, biomedical concepts. Another consequence of this knowledge reorganization is that students tend to generate a large number of hypotheses. Every new finding seems to trigger the activation of a new hypothesis, while they have difficulties to integrate this information in the representation already developed (Joseph and Patel, 1990).

An example of detailed reasoning is given in Table 2.1. It has been taken from a longer protocol in which a fourth year medical student is dealing with a case of pancreatitis. His initial hypothesis set contained gall bladder and pancreas disease. Apparently, this student is entertaining the hypothesis of biliary tract obstruction. First, he reasons whether the new finding about the patient's stools affects this hypothesis and decides that this is not the case. Next, three items later, he combines the information acquired and concludes that there is no inflammation (causing this obstruction) ⟨step 1⟩, hence, no cholecystitis ⟨step 2⟩, hence the biliary tract must be obstructed by something else, a stone for instance ⟨step 3⟩, or a carcinoma ⟨step 4⟩, which might be the case because the patient has lost weight ⟨step 5⟩. Later, it turns out that the hypothesis pancreas is still contemplated, which is then combined with biliary tract obstruction in a very detailed way.

By the end of the first stage of knowledge acquisition, students have a knowledge net-

Table 2.1 Lines of reasoning by a 4th year medical student

Case item (number and text)	Think-aloud protocol

31. (History)
    Defecation: paler and more malodorous stools
    according to the patient
	. . not so much undermines that idea . . er . . their frequency . . and their pattern compared with colour and . the like . . their smell er . . . yes . . no problems with defecation, that means in any case no constipation, which you wouldn't expect with an obstruction of the biliary tract . . . well yes

32. (History) Last bowel movement was yesterday	. . .
32. (History) Temperature: 37°C at 6 p.m.	. . . so no temperature
33. (Physical examination) Pulse rate: regular, 72/min	. . . er . . yes . . the past two . . together . . means that there's er no inflammation . . and that would eliminate an er . . an er . . cholecystitis . . and would rather mean an . . er . . obstruction of the biliary tract . . caused by a stone, for instance . . or, what may be the case too, by a carcinoma, but I wouldn't . . although, it might be possible, lost 5 kilograms in weight . .

Protocol fragment obtained from a 4th year medical student working on a pancreatitis case showing detailed reasoning steps. See Boshuizen and Schmidt (1992) for a detailed description of the experiment.

work that allows them to make direct lines of reasoning between different concepts within that network. The more often these direct lines are activated the more these concepts cluster together and students become able to make direct links between the first and last concept in such a line of reasoning, skipping intermediate concepts. In our first publication about this knowledge restructuring process we termed it 'knowledge compilation' (Schmidt et al, 1990), a term emphasizing the short-cuts in the lines of reasoning (Anderson, 1987). In later articles we introduced the term 'knowledge encapsulation', a term that better denotes the clustering aspect of the process (e.g. Boshuizen and Schmidt, 1992; Schmidt and Boshuizen, 1993). Many of these concept clusters have (semi-) clinical names, such as micro-embolism, aorta-insufficiency, forward failure, or extra-hepatic icterus, providing a powerful reasoning tool.

Encapsulation of biomedical knowledge results in the next stage of development of clinical reasoning skills, in which biomedical knowledge has been integrated into clinical knowledge. At this stage, students' clinical reasoning processes involve hardly any biomedical concepts. Students tend to make direct links between patient findings and clinical concepts that have the status of hypotheses or diagnoses in their reasoning process. However, if needed, this encapsulated biomedical knowledge can be unfolded again, for instance when dealing with a very complicated problem.

At the same time, a transition takes place from a network-type of knowledge organization to another type of structure we referred to as 'illness scripts'. Illness scripts have three components. The first component refers to Enabling Conditions of disease: i.e., the conditions or constraints under which a disease occurs. These are the personal, social, medical, hereditary and environmental factors that affect health in a positive or a negative way, or which affect the course of a specific disease. The second component is the Fault: i.e., the pathophysiological process that is taking place in a specific disease, represented in encapsulated form. The third component consists of the Consequences of the Fault: i.e., the signs and symptoms of a specific disease (also see Feltovich and Barrows (1984) who introduced this theoretical notion).

Contrary to knowledge networks, illness scripts are activated as a whole. After an illness script has been activated, no active, small-step search within that script is required; the other elements of the script are activated immediately and automatically. Therefore, people whose knowledge is organized in illness scripts have an advantage over those who have only semantic works at their disposal. While solving a problem, a physician activates one or a few illness scripts. Subsequently the illness script elements (Enabling Conditions and Consequences) are matched to the information provided by the patient. Illness scripts do not only incorporate matching information volunteered by the patient, they also generate expectations about other signs and symptoms the patient might have. Activated illness scripts provide a list of phenomena to look for in history taking and in physical examination. In the course of this verification process the script becomes instantiated, i.e. expected values are substituted by real findings, while scripts that fail in this respect will de-activate. The instantiated script yields a diagnosis or a differential diagnosis when a few competing scripts remain active.

An example of script activation by an experienced physician, dealing with the same clinical case as the student in Table 2.1, is given in Table 2.2. The information he heard about the patient's medical past and psycho-social circumstances (summarized in the protocol) are combined with the presenting complaint, and activate a few competing illness scripts: pancreatic disease, liver disease and abdominal malignancy (which he considers implausible due to the patient's age) and stomach perforation. In addition, he thinks of cardiomyopathy as an effect of excessive drinking. In the course of the think-aloud protocol he seemed to monitor the level of instantiation of every illness script de-acted. Except for gall bladder disease, no new scripts were activated.

Instantiated scripts remain available in memory as episodic traces of previously analysed patients and will be used in the diagnosis of future similar problems. Finally, the knowledge structures acquired during the different stages of development, biomedical networks, encapsulated structures, illness scripts and instantiated scripts, do not decay, nor do they become inert or inaccessible. They sediment into multiple layers which are accessed when ontologically more recently acquired structures fail in producing an adequate representation of a clinical problem (Schmidt et al, 1990).

Table 2.2   Illness script activation by a family physician

Case item (number and text)	Think-aloud protocol
8. Complaint: Continuous pain in the upper part of the abdomen, radiating to the back	. . . well, when I am visiting someone who is suffering an acute . . continuous – since when? – pain in his upper abdomen, radiating to the back, who had pancreatitis a year before . . of whom I don't know for sure if he still drinks or not after that course of Refusal, but of whom I do know that he still has mental problems, so still receives a disability benefit, then I think that the first thing to cross my mind will be: well, what about that pancreas, . . how's his liver . . and also that – considering his age – eh it is not very likely that there will be other things wrong in his abdomen . . eh. . of a malign thing er nature . . of course eh if he's taking huge amounts of alcohol there's always the additional possibility of a stomach eh problem, a stomach perforation . . . . . excessive drinking can also cause eh serious cardiomyopathy, which eh may cause heart defects . . . mm I can't er judge the word continuous very well yet in this context

Protocol fragment obtained from an experienced family physician working on a pancreatitis case. Earlier, he had received information about enabling conditions such as mental problems and alcohol abuse. See Boshuizen and Schmidt (1992) for a detailed description of the experiment.

So far we have seen that expert and novice knowledge structures differ in many respects. As a consequence, their clinical reasoning differs as well. Medical experts, who have large numbers of ready-made illness scripts organizing many enabling conditions and consequences associated with a specific disease, will activate one or more of these illness scripts when dealing with a case. Activation will be triggered by information concerning enabling conditions and/or consequences. Expert hypothesis activation and testing can be seen as an epiphenomenon of illness script activation and instantiation. These are on average automatic and 'unconscious' processes. As long as new information matches an active illness script no active reasoning is required. Only in case of severe mismatches or conflict, the expert engages in active clinical reasoning. During this process either illness-script-based expectations are adjusted, based on specific features of the patient, or the expert reverts to pure biomedical reasoning, drawing on de-encapsulated biomedical knowledge. An example of the first process is given by Lesgold et al (1988) who describe expert radiologist interpretations of an enlarged heart shadow on an X-ray screen. These experts took into consideration the marked scoliosis of the patient's thoracic spine, affecting the position of his heart relative to the slide. Hence, they concluded that the heart was not actually enlarged. Students on the other hand can only rely on more or less extensive and elaborate knowledge networks, less rich and less easily activated than experts' illness scripts. For that reason they will require more information before a specific hypothesis will be generated, only because the disease labels in the network are linked to a very limited number of Enabling Conditions or Consequences. Semantic networks must be reasoned through, step by step. This is a time consuming process, often requiring active monitoring. Contrary to illness scripts, the knowledge structures students activate do not automatically generate a list of signs and symptoms that are expected. Active search through their networks is needed in order to generate such a list of symptoms that might verify or falsify the hypotheses entertained. In general, students' clinical reasoning is less orderly, less goal oriented, more time-consuming, but most importantly, it is based on less plausible hypotheses resulting in less accurate diagnoses than experts. Table 2.3 summarizes these differences between novices, intermediates and experts.

Table 2.3   Knowledge restructuring and clinical reasoning at subsequent levels of expertise level

Expertise level	Knowledge representation	Knowledge acquisition and (re)structuring	Clinical reasoning	Control required in clinical reasoning
Novice	Networks	Knowledge accretion and validation	Long chains of detailed reasoning steps through pre-encapsulated networks	Active monitoring of each reasoning step
Intermediate	Networks	Encapsulation	Reasoning through encapsulated network	Active monitoring of each reasoning step
Expert	Illness scripts	Illness script formation	Illness script activation and instantiation	Monitoring of the level of script instantiation
		(Instantiated scripts)		

Teaching clinical reasoning

Traditional approaches to enhancing clinical reasoning in students are based on the assumption that clinical reasoning or problem solving is a skill, separate from content knowledge. A typical example is described by Elstein et al (1978). In this training program students were taught a couple of heuristics that had been derived from analysis of the reported and observed errors of diagnostic reasoning committed by medical students. For instance, students were taught that each piece of information they requested should be related to a plan for solving the problem: the planning heuristic. They were also taught that they should have at least two or three competing hypotheses under consideration and that each piece of information should be evaluated with respect to all hypotheses presently considered. It was found, however, that this training program had no significant effects on the students' diagnostic accuracy and cost. Furthermore, they found that students varied widely in their ability to apply the heuristics recommended in different cases. This finding and outcomes of comparisons of experts and weaker problem solvers suggested to the investigators that differences are more to be found in the repertory of their experiences, organized in long-term memory than in differences in the planning and problem-solving heuristics employed.

Until this moment we have avoided defining the concepts of clinical reasoning and clinical reasoning skills, first giving attention to the knowledge structures these reasoning processes operate upon. Nor have we given attention to the question whether clinical reasoning can be taught. Generally, clinical reasoning equals the thinking process occurring while dealing with a clinical case. Most researchers differentiate between different stages in the clinical reasoning process: beginning with hypothesis generation, inquiry strategy, data analysis, problem synthesis or diagnosis, and finally ending with diagnostic and treatment decision-making. Most often these different stages are thought to require different skills: hypothesis generation skills, inquiry skills, data-analysis skills, etc. Experts, performing better, are supposed to have better skills than novices and intermediates. This position is taken by Barrows and Pickell (1991). From the description of our theory, it will be evident that our position deviates from Barrows' and Pickell's. Despite these differences, there are many correspondences as well. Therefore, in order to picture our position most clearly, we will compare our approach with and differentiate it from Barrows' and Pickell's.

In their book entitled *Developing clinical problem solving skills; A guide to more effective diagnosis and treatment* Barrows and Pickell (1991) emphasize:

> There are two components of expert clinical problem-solving that need to be considered separately, even though they can not be separated in practice. One is *content*, the rich, extensive knowledge base about medicine that resides in the long term memory of the expert. The other is *process*, the method of knowledge manipulation the expert uses to apply that knowledge to the patient's problem. In expert performance these components are inexorably

intertwined. Both are required; a well developed reasoning process appropriately bringing accurate knowledge to bear on a problem in a most effective manner . . . This book should help you *perfect the process of clinical reasoning* (italics added by Boshuizen and Schmidt) to best deliver the knowledge that you now have (and will acquire in the future) to the care of your patients . . . To develop these skills you must practice, analyse, and repractice them until they are automatic. More important, if you associate your medical-school learning with this regime, your knowledge will be organized for effective recollection in your clinical work. (Barrows and Pickell, 1991, pp. xii–xiii.)

So Barrows and Pickell propose that clinical reasoning skills and medical knowledge can be acquired separately, although it is better to do both simultaneously in order to improve the organization of medical knowledge. For instance, they suggest that students should practise their scientific clinical reasoning skills at every opportunity. They provide the following advice (Barrows and Pickell, 1991, pp. 215–216):

- 'To develop an accurate initial concept (2), look carefully for important initial information as the patient encounter begins.'
- 'Generate a complete set of hypotheses in every patient encounter, carefully watching their degree of specificity and their complementarity. Be sure to watch out for hidden biases.'
- 'Use your creativity, and your inductive skills, to develop these hypotheses.'
- 'Use your critical deductive skills to inquire in a manner that will establish the more likely hypothesis.'
- 'Generate new hypotheses whenever your inquiries become unproductive or new data make your present hypotheses less likely.'
- 'In both your hypothesis generation and in inquiry strategy, be guided by an awareness of the basic pathophysiologic mechanism that may be operative in your patient's problem.'

This advice suggests many correspondences with our theory. For instance, the authors' suggestion to look for important initial information as the patient encounter begins, agrees with our emphasis on the role of enabling conditions in script activation. But what if a student does not have any scripts? Furthermore, their proposition to be aware of the basic pathophysiologic mechanism that might play a role, goes with our conceptions of Fault. In our theory, applying biomedical knowledge would be helpful if a diagnostician cannot activate a matching illness script. In addition, students' active application of pathophysiological knowledge during clinical reasoning would result in knowledge encapsulation which in turn is instrumental in illness script development. However, the difference between our approach and Barrows' and Pickell's is that these authors suggest that every student and physician, independent of level of expertise, should always apply these skills, while our theory suggests that applying information about enabling conditions or activating basic science knowledge are not skills, but are phenomena associated with a person's knowledge structure. More importantly, as long as the student does not have the relevant knowledge, many of the suggestions given can be only counterproductive.

For instance, a student who is confronted with a 48 year old patient complaining of shortness of breath might be overwhelmed by the information available at the beginning of the doctor–patient contact: the patient's appearance, verbal and non-verbal behaviour, and medical and social background. The suggestion to look for important information will not be very helpful, unless the student knows which factors might cause shortness of breath. The experienced physician, on the other hand, will immediately select the information that this patient is a worker in the local pottery industry and might therefore be suffering from silicosis. Only those students who have this knowledge in a network kind of way, even if they do not have the complete illness script, might have benefit from such a suggestion.

This analysis generates the question of whether clinical reasoning skills can be taught and trained as such or whether other educational measures will be needed in order to improve a student's clinical reasoning. It might be evident that our theory and previous

---

(2) The term 'initial concept' refers to the first interpretation and representation of a patient's problem constructed by the doctor or student.

experiences with direct training programs suggest that other measures are needed, as far as the cognitive, the reasoning component of the diagnostic process is concerned. What is more important, our theory suggests that in order to improve clinical reasoning, education must focus on the development of adequate knowledge structures. Hence, teaching, training, coaching, modelling or supervising should adapt to the actual knowledge organization of the student.

During the first stage in which knowledge accretion and validation takes place, students should be given ample opportunity to test the knowledge they have acquired on its consistency and connectedness, and to correct concepts and their connections and to fill the gaps they have detected. Students will do many of these things by themselves if they are provided with stimuli for thinking and with appropriate feedback. This stuff for thinking does not necessarily have to consist of patient problems. One could also think of short descriptions of physiological phemomena that have to be explained. An example taken from the first year curriculum of the university of Limburg is the following. A 60 year old lady flies from Amsterdam to New York. The first few days after arrival she feels tired, while she is unable to fall asleep at night. Her appetitie is minimal and her stomach is upset. The impression made by the city is overwhelming. The noise, heat and commotion are too much for her. The student's task is to explain these phenomena. By doing so they will touch on subjects such as physiological regulation of sleep, hunger, etc. in relation to biorhythm. Similar problems could help students to integrate knowledge from different disciplines. An example of a problem stimulating students to integrate their knowledge about anatomy and pathophysiology, is the following (taken from Norman and Schmidt, 1992). A 55-year-old woman lies crawling on the floor in obvious pain. The pain emerges in waves and extends from the right lumbar region to the front side of the groin and to the front of the leg.

During the following stage of knowledge encapsulation, students should deal with (more elaborate) patient problems. By going through the process of diagnosing a patient and afterward explaining the diagnosis to a peer or a supervisor, biomedical knowledge will become encapsulated into higher level concepts. For instance, diagnosing a patient having an acute bacterial endocarditis will first require detailed reasoning about infection, fever reaction, temperature regulation, circulation, hemodynamics, etc. Later on, a similar case will be explained in terms of bacterial infection, sepsis, microembolisms and aortic insufficiency (Boshuizen, 1989). These problems do not necessarily have to be presented by real patients in real settings. Paper cases and simulated patients will serve the same goal, maybe even better. Especially earlier on during the stage of knowledge encapsulation, when students have to do a great deal of reasoning, it might be very helpful to work with paper cases that present all relevant information. Reasoning through their knowledge networks in order to build a coherent explanation of the information available, students do not have to bother whether the information they work on is complete and valid. Later in this stage, when knowledge has been restructured into a more tightly connected format, greater uncertainty can be allowed.

Finally, the stage of illness script acquisition requires experience with real patients in real settings. Research by Custers et al (1993) suggests that at this stage, practical experience with typical patients (i.e. patients whose disease manifestations resemble the textbooks) should be preferred over experiences with atypical patients. There are no empirical data that can help to answer the question of whether illness script formation requires active dealing with the patient or whether observing a doctor–patient contact could serve the same goal. On the other hand, since encapsulation and script formation go hand in hand, especially earlier on in this stage, it is probable that 'hands on' experience is to be preferred. Having to reason about the patient would result in further knowledge encapsulation, while direct interaction with the patient provides the opportunity for perceptual learning, adding 'reality' to the symbolic concepts learned from textbooks. During this phase students might initially be overwhelmed by the information available in reality. They can easily overlook information for as long as they do not know its relevance. This will especially affect their perception of Enabling Conditions. Therefore, it might be helpful to draw the student's attention to the Enabling Conditions operating in the specific patients to make sure that their illness scripts are completed with this kind of information. Boshuizen et al (1992) emphasize that in this stage of training a mix of practical experience and theoretical education is needed. They have found that during the clinical rotations students tend to shift toward the application of biomedical knowledge although it is not yet fully integrated in their knowledge base. A combination of the two ways of learning can help students to build a robust and flexible knowledge base.

So we see that working on problems and diagnosing and explaining patient cases, applying biomedical knowledge and feedback on the student's thinking might help them to form a knowledge system that enables efficient and accurate clinical reasoning that does not require all control capacity available, i.e. monitoring of reasoning on encapsulated concepts in a network requires less control than monitoring of reasoning on pre-encapsulated, detailed concepts (see Table 2.3). However, in practice, clinical reasoning has to be performed in a context of real patients. In the end, students should be able to collect information through history-taking, physical examination and laboratory, guided by their clinical reasoning process and find a (preliminary) diagnosis in the time available. A well organized knowledge base is a first requirement, along with well-trained social, perceptual and psychomotor skills (3). Hence, students must learn to do their clinical reasoning and to perform these skills in a co-ordinated way. This again necessitates training and practice (Patrick, 1992).

The reader might have observed a similarity between what has been proposed in this chapter and problem-based curricula. This similarity is not incidental. However, our suggestions for learning with cases and from practical experience do not necessarily require a problem-based curriculum. They can be applied in traditional course-based curricula as well. On the other hand, not every problem-based curriculum is structured in the way we have proposed. For example, a program that uses problems as a starting point for learning may neglect the encapsulation function of working with cases. In our opinion it is essential that students do not only have to work with problems and cases. They also need an educational program, based on an insight into the different problems students experience at successive stages of development toward expertise.

The question remains, whether the phases in knowledge structure development have to be translated into a curriculum in which a complete, coherent, and well-integrated knowledge base has to be required first, followed by a term in which knowledge is encapsulated, completed by a period in which illness scripts are formed. As far as our theory and the available empirical evidence are concerned, there is no need for such a strict separation. If students have developed a complete knowledge base of a specific subject, e.g. the effects of vitamin B12 deficiency on the cellular and organic level, there is no need to prevent encapsulation as long as students remain willing and able to adjust their knowledge base and re-encapsulate when new knowledge is acquired. For motivational reasons it would be preferable to construct a curriculum in which different phases overlap.

References

Ackermann, W. and Barbichon, G. (1963) Conduites intellectuelles et activité technique. *Bulletin CERP*, **12**, 1–16

Allwood, C.M. and Montgomery, H. (1981) Knowledge and technique in statistical problem solving. *European Journal of Science Education*, **3**, 431–450

Allwood, C.M. and Montgomery, H. (1982) Detection of errors in statistical problem solving. *Scandinavian Journal of Psychology*, **23**, 131–140

Anderson, J.R. (1987) Skill acquisition: compilation of weak-method problem solutions. *Psychological Review*, **94**, 192–210

Barrows, H.S. and Pickell, G.C. (1991) *Developing Clinical Problem-Solving Skills; A Guide to More Effective Diagnosis and Treatment*. Norton and Comp, New York

Barrows, H.S., Feightner, J.W., Neufeld, V.R. and Norman, G.R. (1978) *An Analysis of the Clinical Method of Medical Students and Physicians*. McMaster University, Hamilton, Ontario

Bloom, B.S. and Broder, L.J. (1950) *Problem Solving Processes of College Students*. University of Chicago Press, Chicago

Boshuizen, H.P.A. (1989) De ontwikkeling van medische expertise; een cognitief-psychologische benadering (The development of medical expertise; a cognitive-psychological approach). PhD thesis, University of Limburg, Maastricht

Boshuizen, H.P.A. and Schmidt, H.G. (1992) On the role

---

(3) These skills have a knowledge component that makes it difficult to train them in isolation, separate from knowledge acquisition.

of biomedical knowledge in clinical reasoning by experts, intermediates and novices. *Cognitive Science*, **16**, 153–184

Boshuizen, H.P.A., Hobus, P.P.M., Custers, E.J.F.M. and Schmidt, H.G. (1992) Cognitive effects of practical experience. In *Advanced Models of Cognition for Medical Training and Practice* (eds A.E. Evans and V.L. Patel). Springer Verlag, New York

Chi, M.T.H., Feltovich, P.J. and Glaser, R. (1981) Categorization and representation of physics problems by experts and novices. *Cognitive Science*, **5**, 121–152

Custers, E.J.F.M., Boshuizen, H.P.A. and Schmidt, H.G. (1993) The influence of typicality of case descriptions on subjective disease probability estimations. Paper presented at the Annual Meeting of the American Educational Research Association, Atlanta, GA

De Groot, A.D. (1965) *Thought and Choice in Chess*. Mouton, The Hague

Elstein, A.S., Shulman, L.S. and Sprafka, S.A. (1978) *Medical Problem Solving: An Analysis of Clinical Reasoning*. Harvard University Press, Cambridge, MA

Feltovich, P.J. and Barrows, H.S. (1984) Issues of generality in medical problem solving. In *Tutorials in Problem-Based Learning; A New Direction in Teaching the Health Professions* (eds H.G. Schmidt and M.L. De Volder). Van Gorcum, Assen

Joseph, G.M. and Patel, V.L. (1990) Domain knowledge and hypothesis generation diagnostic reasoning. *Journal of Medical Decision Making*, **10**, 31–46

Lesgold, A, Rubinson, H., Feltovich, P.J., Glaser, R. and Klopfer, D. (1988) Expertise in a complex skill: diagnosing X-ray pictures. In *The Nature of Expertise* (eds M.T. H. Chi, R. Glaser and M. Farr). Erlbaum, Hillsdale, NJ

Norman, G.R. and Schmidt, H.G. (1992) The psychological basis of problem-based learning: A review of the evidence. *Academic Medicine*, **67**, 557–565

Patrick, J. (1992) *Training: Theory and Practice*. Academic Press, London

Polya, G. (1957) *How to Solve it*. Doubleday, Garden City, NY

Schmidt, H.G. and Boshuizen, H.P.A. (1992) Encapsulation of biomedical knowledge. In *Advanced Models of Cognition for Medical Training and Practice* (eds A.E. Evans and V.L. Patel). Springer Verlag, New York

Schmidt, H.G. and Boshuizen, H.P.A. (1993) On acquiring expertise in medicine. *Educational Psychology Review*, **5**, 205–221

Schmidt, H.G., Boshuizen, H.P.A. and Norman, G.R. (1992) Reflections on the nature of expertise in medicine. In *Deep Models for Medical Knowledge Engineering* (ed. E. Keravnou). Elsevier, Amsterdam, pp. 231–248

Schmidt, H.G., Norman, G.R. and Boshuizen, H.P.A. (1990) A cognitive perspective on medical expertise: Theory and implications. *Academic Medicine*, **65**, 611–621

Section Two

Clinical reasoning in the health professions

3

Methods in the study of clinical reasoning

Vimla L. Patel and José F. Arocha

This chapter presents an overview of some of the methods used in the study of clinical reasoning. It does not constitute an exhaustive overview. Instead, it presents only the most common approaches used in the study of clinical reasoning. When planning this chapter, we had to face the choice between presenting detailed descriptions of the methods or, rather, presenting the foundations of the methods, while describing only the major features of the methods. We opted for the second approach in view of the length of the paper, and because we thought the chapter would be more interesting this way. We also faced the decision of whether to present the methods used only in clinical reasoning research or widen somewhat the range of approaches to include new, but promising, research methodologies. Again, we decided by the latter option.

The first section presents a historical sketch of the evolution of the methods used in the field. It begins with a brief characterization of the more important methods used during the 1950s up to the 1970s. During the first two decades, the main methods were derived from the psychometric tradition. The emphasis in this tradition was on assessment of performance, rather than on basic research. The latter decade saw a paradigm shift in the behavioural sciences: a shift marked by the change from the behaviourist to the cognitive paradigm. This shift had a profound impact on the methods used, leading to a broadening of the methodologies to include a multiplicity of new data gathering and analysis techniques and a change

of focus, from an emphasis on describing overt behaviour to an emphasis on describing and modelling cognitive processes.

The second section is an overview of quantitative methodologies. The main approach here is the decision–theoretic approach for investigating decisions under risk of uncertainty. The descriptive study of decision making has been carried out mostly by using a few models, all based on probability theory, namely the regression and the Bayesian approaches as well as the expected utility approach.

The third section discusses the use of qualitative methodologies, known under the label of information processing. Unlike the quantitative methods, the qualitative tradition has focused on the study of the processes that lead to successful problem solving. The first approach to be considered is derived from the study of verbal protocols. Two important orientations are discussed: 1) the computer simulations of thought processes and the methods derived from them, most notably protocol analysis; and 2) studies of language and knowledge structures and the methodologies developed therein, especially discourse analysis. Following the description of verbal protocol research, in the fourth section, we present a type of qualitative research that has evolved out of anthropology and discourse analysis. It is treated separately from the preceding section because it derives from a different philosophical tradition than the information processing approach. We also present some newer developments that attempt to harmonize some of the ideas in the information processing and interpretative research paradigms. The outcome of this, the so called situated cognition approach, promises to provide interesting answers to the question of cognitive interaction.

The fifth section presents a discussion of some problems and unsolved issues in the methodologies of clinical reasoning. The section also attempts to provide some clarification of these issues. Finally, the sixth section presents a look at the future of the methodologies and the possibilities for unification of the methods presented in the chapter.

Historical sketch

The development of the methodologies used in the study of clinical reasoning in the health sciences has followed from developments in other areas of thinking and reasoning. What started mostly as a study within the psychometric tradition, has evolved to include a variety of methods. The study of clinical reasoning is pluralistic. The evolution of this pluralism is reflected in this section.

We have found it useful to divide the historical development into two main periods. The first period covers the early investigations of clinical reasoning in the 1950s up to the 1970s. It was dominated by the psychometric approach and it was devoted mainly to assessment rather than to basic research. The second period covers from the 1970s to the present. The period has been dominated by the cognitive paradigm known as information processing. This period is also beginning to change, thanks to new theoretical and methodological developments.

The precognitive era

The topic of clinical reasoning has always drawn the attention of medical education researchers. The way the research has been carried out has been determined by the particular theoretical and methodological frameworks dominant at the time.

The first studies of medical reasoning had as their goal the assessment of the clinical skills of physicians and medical students, as these skills were viewed as extremely important for achieving mastery. To this end, the research paradigm dominant during the 1950s and 1960s was the psychometric paradigm in which emphasis was placed on the identification of general skills, defined in terms of observable behaviours, through the use of psychometric tests.

The purpose of most early studies of clinical reasoning was to develop instruments for assessing clinical performance, rather than characterizing clinical reasoning. An overview of methods for studying clinical reasoning is presented by Vu (1979), where she distinguished between observational, record-based, and simulation methods. For the purposes of the present chapter, simulation methods are the most interesting because they deal with the actual reasoning processes used by subjects, whereas the others attempt to re-construct these processes from either observations or past records.

Simulation methods, which consist of simulating the physician/patient encounter, are of various kinds, e.g. written patient descriptions, real patient simulations, and computer simulations (Vu, 1979). What is common to all of them is that the information about a problem to be solved is presented to the subjects. The problem posed to the subjects can take several forms, from written patient presentations to computerized presentation systems to the use of live patient simulations. Based on the information presented, an inquiry process begins, in which the subjects request new information and make a diagnosis.

Rimoldi's (1961) test of diagnostic skills, was among the first to study the diagnostic process from a psychometric perspective. The test consists of a clinical case which describes a preliminary report on a patient. The subject is then asked to inquire about the patient by requesting additional information. The information is given to the subject on cue-cards with a question presented on one side and the answer on the other side. By studying the nature and the chronological sequence of questions asked, it is possible to evaluate the subject's level of clinical reasoning skills. The results of Rimoldi's study (1961) served to characterize the behaviour of physicians as more focused (i.e. they asked fewer and more appropriate questions) than that of medical students.

A second form of simulation methods are those that are used in the assessment of reasoning skills (Barro, 1973; Elstein et al, 1978;

McGuire, 1985). These methods are variations of the Patient Management Problem (PMP). PMPs are tests to assess the clinical process. The procedure basically consists of presenting an unfolding patient problem that the subject studies and then attempts to solve it by making decisions about the course of action to be taken. In some forms of the PMPs, the subjects receive feedback about the results of their decisions. Different reasoning paths, then, could be followed depending on the previous choices made.

It is important to note that these simulation methods were developed for the purposes of assessment. Because of this, one of the criteria in their creation has been ease of administration. This may have limited their utility as research tools since they had to reconcile the practical goals of assessment with the conceptual goals of research. Furthermore, most of the literature on these methods concern psychometric issues such as reliability and various forms of validity.

The cognitive era

The study of clinical reasoning and problem solving in its current form had, as a background, a series of theoretical and methodological developments that took place in other areas of research, notably the development of computer science, and with it, the first simulations of thought processes (Newell et al, 1958; Hovland, 1960). This background suggested that a different approach to research in clinical reasoning was needed. The emphasis was not on testing isolated quantitative hypotheses, but on testing models of reasoning (Newell and Simon, 1972). This requires a more qualitative approach to research than is traditionally accepted. A second line of research was inaugurated with the publication, in 1956, of the book *A Study of Thinking* by Bruner, Goodnow, and Austin. The emphasis of this research was on concept formation. As it was the case with Newell and Simon's research, this work marked a departure from the behaviouristic framework that had dominated behavioural science at the time. In medicine, these new lines of research were exemplified by the work of Elstein et al (1978). What united all the investigations of clinical reasoning carried out since the work of Elstein and colleagues is the use of the contrastive method, in which performances

of experts are compared to that of novices. This method is a legacy of De Groot's (1965) work on chess masters which subsequently influenced the research done by Chase and Simon (1973) and Larkin et al (1980), on physics problem solving.

It is recognized that the beginning of the study of medical cognition in its current form, started with the publication by Elstein, Shulman, and Sprafka (1978) of their pioneering work, covering more than a decade. This work was largely influenced by the study of problem solving that Newell and Simon had carried out during the late 1950s and that was changing the way research was done in psychology.

Some characteristics serve to differentiate the new, cognitive, from the old, behaviouristic, approaches. One characteristic that differentiated this work from earlier work is that it was aimed at developing a characterization of clinical reasoning, in line with the work that was being conducted in other areas of research, such as chess and physics. As it was done in these other areas, one of the aims of the new cognitive research in the health sciences was to specify the knowledge structures and processes used during clinical reasoning. This research posed the questions about the cognitive strategies and the type of knowledge used in diagnosing patient problems. Contrarily, the aim of earlier research was mainly to develop assessment instruments for health care professionals. Another characteristic of the new cognitive approach was that this research was developed under the guidance of theoretical models of the development of expertise and clinical reasoning. Whereas the previous work started by defining the aspects of clinical reasoning in purely behavioural terms, the new approach was based on a theory of the cognitive process used in clinical reasoning.

The methodology that was used by Elstein et al (1978) consisted of several methods which varied in terms of their fidelity to the real-life clinical situations. They developed these various methods in order to maximize the information available as no one method could provide all the information needed to investigate clinical reasoning and problem solving. Whereas some high-fidelity methods (e.g. use of simulated patients) capture some real-life aspects of the process, they may fail to capture some hidden cognitive processes. The low-fidelity methods (e.g. recall tasks) have the advantage of allowing to isolate specific aspects of the clinical reasoning process and study them in more depth. This work exemplifies the methodological pluralism that is encountered today in the study of clinical reasoning.

Following the theoretical and experimental approach of Newell and Simon (1972), Feltovich's (1984) research investigated the clinical reasoning process. In his research, he uncovered some of the characteristics that differentiate novices from experts. The main difference identified was in terms of the quality of knowledge structures of experts.

The study of some conceptual aspects of clinical reasoning was investigated by Bordage and Zacks (1984). Borrowing from the traditional methods of cognitive psychology started by Bruner et al's (1956) work, these researchers investigated the nature of diagnostic categories used by physicians and medical students. Their research was influenced by the work of Rosch (1978), which she had used to investigate the psychological nature of categories. Although this work is influenced by a different tradition, its basic concepts and methods are compatible with the information processing approach to cognition. While more recent psychological research (MacNamara, 1982) has questioned the validity of Rosch's work, the study of categories has extended to include more than the effect of specific instances. This kind of research has also been carried out in the health sciences (Brooks et al, 1991), and it is still a very active area of inquiry.

A line of research which has also been influenced by the work of Chase and Simon has been conducted by Patel and Groen (Patel and Groen, 1986; Patel et al, 1990) at McGill University in Montreal and by Schmidt and his collaborators at the University of Limburg in Maastricht, Holland (Schmidt et al, 1988). These two research teams have investigated several aspects of expertise using somewhat similar methodologies derived from propositional analysis (Kintsch, 1974). Their research has focused on the knowledge differences between novices and experts and on the kinds of inductive inferences they use. Of particular importance has been the investigation of the intermediate effect (i.e. the finding that intermediate subjects, those between novice and experts, often perform more poorly than either experts or novices) and the identification of different kinds of expertise (e.g. general and specific expertise).

In conclusion, the study of clinical reasoning has diversified to include very different methodological commitments and techniques. From purely behaviouristic and psychometric roots, it has developed into a multiplicity of methods and continues to do so. This has had a profound impact on the quantity and quality of the research. Various topics such as conceptual understanding (Feltovich et al, 1992), which until not long ago were non-existent, are now active and promising areas of study.

Methods of studying clinical reasoning in the health sciences

In summary, there have been basically two main traditions in the study of clinical reasoning in the health sciences. One tradition has emphasized the study of clinical decision making. This tradition uses quantitative methodologies and models to describe or prescribe clinical decision making. Descriptive decision making has been based in very simple input/output models, such as linear regression. The assumption is that simple linear models account very well for the decision making of clinicians. Prescriptive decision making has been based on decision theory, with the assumption that this theory is a normative guide for successful action (as a prescriptive guide to how decision making ought to be done).

The second major tradition has aimed at an understanding of the cognitive processes used during problem solving. It differs from the first approach in that it describes the knowledge structures that are used during problem solving. Instead of looking at clinical reasoning only at the points of decisions between alternatives, it examines the whole process from the formulation of hypotheses to the reaching of a solution to the problem. It also examines the nature of the knowledge used and the cognitive operations used to reach the solution. This second tradition has been highly influenced by the field of Artificial Intelligence (AI). Artificial Intelligence aims at developing machines capable of reproducing some human cognitive functions, such as perception, reasoning, and problem solving (Barr and Feigenbaum, 1981).

A third research tradition emphasizes the study of interactions as a form of reasoning and understanding. This is the interpretive tradition, which has been applied mostly in nursing research (Benner, 1984). The interpretive tradition has also influenced a newer research approach, given such diverse labels as situated cognition, situated action, and interactionism (Greeno, 1989). This approach also borrows from the Artificial Intelligence approach some of its concepts and its problematics but interprets cognitive functions as part of an interaction between the human and its environment, rather than something happening inside someone's head.

Quantitative methods

Experimental methods

Traditional experimental methods from cognitive psychology have been used in the study of clinical reasoning by several investigators (Norman et al, 1989a; Norman et al, 1989b) in various clinical tasks. One of the most widely used tasks used by these researchers involves the study of perceptual aspects of expertise. In these studies, the subjects are presented a series of slides (e.g. X-rays, photographs of dermatological affections) and then, after some period, are asked to interpret or recall the information in the slides. These data are then quantified and subjected to statistical analysis.

Decision making methods

The study of decision making has been carried out in a variety of domains and it is a very active area of research. Typically, decision making researchers start with a formal model of decision making and then collect data which are compared to the model. The models can be of various types. The more common are simple regression models, Bayesian estimation models, and decision theoretic models. The latter are the most mathematically sophisticated (Christensen et al, 1991).

Decision theory has its roots in the work of von Neumann and Morgenstern (1944) on game theory. The theory deals with making decisions in situations of uncertainty. The basic principle of the theory is that a rational person should maximize his or her expected utility, which is defined as the product of probability by utility. Hammond (1967) gives the following example: a businessman faces the decision of either winning $500,000 or losing $100,000, both of which have the same probability, 0.5. The expected utility in this case would be of 200,000 dollars [0.5 (500,000) − 0.5 (100,000)]. Decision theory has been used mostly as a model for rational decision making. Previously, the theory was thought to describe actual human decision making, but empirical research on psychological bases of decision making has falsified its claims as a descriptive theory (Tversky and Kahneman, 1974). The theory also has been used as a normative theory under the assumption that the maximization of the expected utilities is rational. Under this assumption, to be rational, people's decisions must mirror those derived from the model. If people's decisions depart from those specified by the model, then this is taken as evidence that they are not behaving rationally. This assumption, and therefore, the normative character of the theory, has also been severely questioned (Allais and Hagen, 1979; Hammond, 1967; Bunge, 1985). In short, critics argue that it is not always rational to maximize one's expected utility and therefore the theory cannot be taken as a prescription for action.

Whatever its merits either as a descriptive or a prescriptive theory, decision theory has stimulated a great deal of research in medicine (Weinstein et al, 1980) and various other domains (Dawes, 1988; Carroll and Johnson, 1990). The research on decision theory uses a model that serves as comparison for the empirical studies. The model is assumed to be a model of rationality such that lack of agreement between the subjects' responses and the model is taken as evidence that the subjects do not make decisions rationally. As it was said, the model assumes the maximization of expected utilities as the criterion for rationality.

Decision theory, as well as other statistical approaches to investigating decision making, make use of explicit numerical models for the evaluation of human decisions. The most used models, beside the expected utility model, are the regression and the Bayesian models. These are called weighted additive models because of the assumption that the decision process has the form of an additive function, $Y_i = f(X_{ij})$, in which i represents the alternative, j represents the number of attributes, and f is the function that relates the decision to the set of weighted attributes.

Typically, in a decision-making study, the subject is asked to generate a series of attributes that are of most importance for a given situation (e.g. a clinical case), and rank them in order of importance or preference. Once this is done, a set of weights is gathered for each of the attributes. The data are then combined into a decision formula (i.e. the decision model) and a decision is generated from the model. This is then used either to help the human decision maker arrive at a good decision or is used as a description of the decision maker's behaviour.

These models, also called input/output models, do not consider any mediating process between the attributes and the decision. Most of these models also assume that the decision function is linear. The methods used within these approaches consist of collecting a series of responses to a limited set of choices. The method assumes that all the relevant information is available to the subject and that all the alternatives and their consequences are known. The subject's task is to choose among these alternatives.

It is important to note that for this model to apply, all the information has to be available to the subject (and to the model). Also note that only the selection of alternatives (e.g. diagnoses) is illustrated by this model. This has provoked some researchers (Fox, 1988) to argue for an expansion in the study of decision making to include also the intermediate processes between the selection of attributes and the reaching of the decision. The argument supports the developing of knowledge-based decision methods based on the techniques of artificial intelligence, which calls for the inclusion of heuristics (e.g. means-ends analysis) and knowledge structures in the decision model.

Although decision models have been used to describe human behaviour, psychological research (Tversky and Kahneman, 1974) has shown that subjects do not behave according to the models. People show various kinds of biases that depart systematically from the models' predictions.

Summary of quantitative methods

Quantitative methods, as they are used in the study of clinical reasoning, cover a large variety of different techniques. There are some similarities among them, however. Their use involves the collection of responses that can be easily scorable and are used mostly to investigate input/output connections with no direct examination of the processes mediating these connections. This does not mean that they do not allow claims about what goes on between stimulus and responses, but that there is no direct consideration of mediating reasoning processes. To investigate these processes more directly different methodologies are needed. These methods have been developed under the information processing framework and have been termed 'process-tracing', which will be discussed next.

Qualitative methods

This section deals with what are considered to be, overall, qualitative methods. The methods described in this section vary widely in terms of their origins and applications and cover methods such as the generation of think-aloud protocols, discourse analysis methods, and ethnographic methods. The first originates in the study of clinical reasoning and the computer simulation of thought processes; the second in the analysis of text comprehension and conversation and the third in the analysis of complex, mostly social, situations. A common theme to all these methods is that they deal with real-life, or as close to real-life as possible, situations. Another common aspect is that they have only recently become accepted as methods of scientific study by scientists. A third common feature is that they are applied to unique situations. By this we mean that each case, consisting of a physician solving a case or a pair of nurses discussing a patient problem, is taken as a unit. In contrast to the quantitative methods discussed in the previous section, qualitative researchers attempt to describe single episodes in detail rather than obtaining gross average measures of many situations (Newell and Simon, 1972). A precursor of such a method is the clinical interview method exemplified in the research carried out by Piaget (1950). This method has been one of the more fruitful in psychology and has had a tremendous influence on current research in thinking.

Verbal reports

A common method of data gathering used by psychologists at the turn of the century was the introspective method. This consisted of asking a previously trained subject to report on his or her thoughts while engaged in carrying out a cognitive task. With the advent of behavioural psychology, however, the method lost its appeal. The problem was that the method required the subject to theorize about his or her own thought processes. This theorizing introduces new information and cognitive processes that the subject may have not used at the time of performance, resulting in a distortion of the thinking process underlying performance.

Although during the behaviourist era, introspection was much attacked for its unscientific character and verbal report methods were not much used, some of the most influential behaviourists recognized the value of verbal data in the study of thinking (e.g. Watson, 1920), and some form of verbal data were used during that era, even by behaviourists. There are several kinds of verbal reports. One of the earliest in psychological research was the use of recall to investigate memory phenomena. A second kind are retrospective protocols, such as stimulated recall (Elstein et al, 1978). A third kind is the 'think-aloud' method used in clinical reasoning and expertise research (Kassirer et al, 1982). Still another kind is the use of a form of retrospective protocols, called explanation protocols, used to study knowledge structures (Patel and Groen, 1986).

In its accepted modern form, research that uses verbal reports as data, deals with the study of pieces of discourse about a problem or a situation, without introspection. That is, the subject is asked to verbalize his or her thoughts without 'theorizing' about his or her cognitive processes. Any theorizing is the responsibility of the experimenter and not of the subject. Verbalizations are taken as any other behavioural data. A further difference with introspection is that the method is supported by a theory of the human information processing system (Newell and Simon, 1972; Ericsson and Simon, 1984).

In summary, we can distinguish between simultaneous, or think-aloud protocols and retrospective protocols. In both cases the subject reports only whatever comes to his or her mind. The difference is that in simultaneous protocols, the subject is reporting his or her thoughts while solving a task, whereas in retrospective protocols, the subject is asked to report a previous situation. Analysis methods can be found in Ericsson and Simon (1984).

In typical think-aloud research, the subjects are presented with a clinical case, most frequently in written form, which may contain anything from a single sentence to a whole patient record including the clinical interview, the physical examination results and the laboratory results. The subject is asked to read the information and verbalize whatever thoughts come to his or her mind. If the subject pauses for a few seconds, the experimenter intervenes with questions such as 'What are you thinking about?' or demands such as 'Please, continue', which encourage the subject to carry on talking.

Once the protocol has been collected, it is subjected to an analysis which has as its aim uncovering the cognitive processes and the information that the subject used during the patient encounter. The analysis of the protocol is then compared to a reference or domain model of the task to be solved. This model is frequently taken either from an expert collaborator in the study or from printed information about the topic, such as textbooks or scholarly expositions. For instance, Kuipers and Kassirer (1984), in their study of causal reasoning, used a model of the Starling equilibrium mechanism which was compared to the protocols from subjects at different levels of expertise: medical students, residents, and expert physicians. In the same vein, work by Patel and her colleagues (Patel and Groen, 1986; Joseph and Patel, 1990) use a reference model of the clinical cases which serves as a standard for comparison with the subjects' protocols.

For verbal reports to be valid, it is necessary that some conditions be met. If these are met, then, as research has shown (White, 1988), the use of verbal data is empirically justified. The conditions pertain to the type of tasks that should be used, the kinds of instructions given to the subject, and the familiarity of the subject with the task. Ericsson and Simon (1984) have developed an extensive description of these conditions and there is also independent research that has shown the validity of the methods (White, 1988). The theory of protocol analysis is based on the idea that, in problem solving, the verbalizations are interpreted as a search through a problem space of hypotheses and data.

Retrospective protocols

Retrospective protocols are collected after the situation described has already happened. In most situations, they are collected and analysed in the same manner as think-aloud protocols but with different goals in mind. They differ in that in think-aloud protocols the subject is asked to report whatever comes to his or her mind without making any evaluation of his or her thinking. In this sense the verbalizations at time t are hypothesized to be the contents of short-term memory at time t_1. In retrospective protocols, the verbalizations do not refer to the contents in short-term memory alone but are probably a mixing of short-term and long-term memory information (Newell and Simon, 1972). Therefore, whereas think-aloud protocols can be reliably used to characterize clinical reasoning, retrospective protocols can be used to characterize processes that are not dependent on the concurrent presentation of the stimulus materials. They may be used as a complement to think-aloud protocols or may be used to investigate other cognitive aspects associated with reasoning such as comprehension, metacognitive activities, and the use of knowledge.

Explanation protocols

One of the more interesting types of verbal data collection and analysis is the use of explanation tasks. This has been used by Patel and Groen (1986), Schmidt et al (1988) and Norman et al (1989a and b). The research by Patel and her colleagues began by collecting recall protocols with the aim of obtaining expert/novice differences akin to those obtained in previous research in other domains, such as physics (Larkin et al, 1980). Research which had been studying expert/novice differences in medicine, had failed to detect differences between subjects at different levels of expertise. Patel, influenced by the research on text comprehension (Kintsch, 1974; Frederiksen, 1975), attempted to use the concept of a proposition (i.e. an idea unit) as a cognitive unit rather than the 'chunk'. It is important to note that the proposition had been used in comprehension research and was found to be the most useful unit for the analysis of linguistic discourse. By applying these methods, using the standard free-recall method of cognitive psychology, they were able to obtain similar results to those that Chase and Simon had obtained in the study of chess expertise (e.g. use of chunking and forward reasoning).

Following, Patel and colleagues developed the explanation protocol method. This method consists of asking the subject to explain the pathophysiology of a case. This explanation is then represented in the form of a propositional structure (see Table 3.1). The analysis consists of several steps: 1) segment the subject protocol (the explanation of the case) into clauses according to the clause analysis method of Winograd (1972); 2) determine the propositions in each clause. This is done by taking each idea unit separately as a proposition; 3) once the propositional analysis is completed, the propositions are related in a semantic network, in which the relations between propositions are labelled following the propositional grammar developed by Frederiksen (1975). A semantic network is a structure of concepts and relations among concepts. Concepts are represented as nodes and relations are represented as links between nodes, according to graph theoretic notions (Sowa, 1984). The relations in the semantic networks contain mostly conditional and causal links. Thus a semantic network is a connected graph in which the connections among concepts as well as the direction of reasoning are represented. A graph is connected if there exists a path, directed or undirected, between any two nodes. The types of nodes correspond either to data given in the problem or to hypothesized information. Reasoning is characterized in the following form. When the direction of the relations are from the given data in the problem to the hypothesized node, it is encoded as forward, or data-driven reasoning. When the link is from the hypothesized node to explain the data in the problem, then it is coded as backward reasoning, or hypothesis-driven reasoning. A series of inferences between the two is

Table 3.1 Example of propositional analysis

Sentence: Painless recurrent haematuria suggests a possible tumour of the urinary tract		

Propositional analysis		
Proposition number	*Predicate*	*Arguments*
1.0	COND	[1.1], [1.2]
1.1	HAEMATURIA	**ATT:**Painless, **ASPECT:ITER** (Recurrent)
1.2	SUGGEST	**THM:**1.3
1.3	TUMOUR	**LOC:**Tract, **MOD:QUAL** (Possible)
1.4	TRACT	**ATT:**Urinary

Propositions are numbered within segments and consist of a predicate and a series of labelled arguments. A predicate may be an action (e.g. examine), an object (e.g. system) or a relation which connects propositions (e.g. COND, a conditional relation). Arguments may be case relations, such as PAT, the patient of a processive action; AGT, the agent of the resultive action; THM, the theme of a cognitive process, and RSLT, the result of an action. Arguments can also be relations such as LOC, the location of an object or action, and TNS, the tense, ASPECT, the aspect, or MOD, the modality. ATT expresses an attribute of an object or an act; ITER expresses an iterative, repeatable event or act; QUAL, qualified relationship indicating a probabilistic truth value (between 0 and 1).

coded as an elaboration. With this methodology, it has been possible to investigate some aspects of expert and novice reasoning in diagnostic tasks. More specifically, the method has been used to uncover the kinds of reasoning patterns that are used by expert physicians, which has served to identify several kinds of expertise, such as general and specific expertise (Groen and Patel, 1988).

Discourse analysis

As it is the case with protocol analysis, discourse analysis techniques have been used to analyse verbal data. The theoretical tradition of discourse analysis originates in linguistics and psycholinguistics, more specifically in the study of texts. Discourse analysis developed against the traditional emphasis of linguistic and psycholinguistics research on simple forms of linguistic performance, such as morphemes and lexical units. The idea was to begin to investigate larger bodies of language in order to tackle issues hardly dealt with by traditional theories, such as text semantics. What started as ' a research program in linguistics was extended to other forms of human performance, such as memory and reasoning in medicine (Patel and Frederiksen, 1984).

A methodology that is also influenced by the theories of discourse is the phenomenological or phenomenographic approach (Marton and Saljö, 1976). The emphasis in the application of this method is to investigate general approaches and knowledge that individuals use to learn and understand a situation or problem. Thus, the emphasis is on finding individual differences in the way people approach the phenomena around them. Methodologically, the work has been influenced by Piaget's clinical method in which subjects (thus far mostly students) are asked a series of questions and are also asked to externalize their cognitive process by solving a problem task. This approach has been applied to medicine by Ramsden et al (1989). The data are collected by asking the subjects to study patient records, taking as much time as they need. They are, then, asked questions in a non-directed way with the aim of eliciting information about the subjects' understanding of the problem and their ways of solving it. The analysis consists of generating categories that can meaningfully characterize what the subjects are doing from their own perspective.

Interpretative methods

With the increasing acceptance of qualitative methodologies, scholars in the behavioural sciences have begun to be receptive to new forms of conducting research which stress the interpretive aspect of inquiry. Instead of taking quantitative measures and subjecting them to statistical analyses, ethnographic researchers attempt to describe whole real-life situations in order to grasp their meaning (Benner, 1984). These researchers argue that in quantitative research there are a great deal of meaningless numbers while the more important aspects are neglected or misunderstood. They also argue that the behavioural sciences need rich descriptive data that takes into account the context of behaviour. Without this context, human action is meaningless. This context-dependence of action requires then a methodology that takes a descriptive approach to research.

Some philosophers (Taylor, 1971) and researchers in the social sciences (Suchman, 1987) have argued that the traditional scientific approach to research based on natural sciences such as physics is inadequate for investigating human issues. These require a new conceptualization of science which takes into account the 'social construction of shared meaning'. An analogy is the reading of texts. That is, the same way that words in a text obtain their meaning from the context provided by other words in the text, situations involving human action are not comprehensible without the context in which they occur. In both cases, the reader/observer's task is to 'interpret' the meaning of the text/actions. Because of this contextual character, human action cannot be studied wholly objectively.

Rather than investigating from the outside, the researcher is also a participant of the 'community' he or she is studying. Rather than attempting to minimize any interaction between the researcher and subject, the interpretive researcher attempts to maximize it, since it is this very interaction which comprehensively informs the researcher about the phenomenon under investigation.

In a study by Benner (1984) on nursing expertise, paired interviews were conducted with novice and expert nurses about a situation that was common to both. Benner's research is based on the models of skill acquisition and expertise developed by Dreyfus and Dreyfus (1986), whose work is, in turn, inspired by the phenomenological philosophy of Martin Heidegger (Heidegger, 1962). The method used by Benner consists of interpreting each situation by independent observer/interpreters and then comparing their interpretations and reaching a consensus about the meaning of the situations. The idea behind this method is to capture the subjects'. experiences in terms of their interpretations of the problem.

In summary, interpretive research has had a somewhat long history in educational research (Glaser and Strauss, 1967). During the last ten or so years, this kind of research endeavour has been growing in popularity among people dissatisfied with the traditional research approaches. It has been mostly applied to investigate processes that involve social inter-action, such as classroom instruction. Its acceptance in medical education has been somewhat late, but it may also grow as medical educators become familiar with it.

Situated cognition methods

In recent years, an approach to thinking and reasoning has developed that emphasizes the contextual aspect of cognition. Although indirectly related to the interpretive approach, it has been developed by independent researchers. Greeno (1989) in an exposition of the new approach complains that contrary to the standard, domain-based view of thinking in specific tasks, such as diagnostic and arithmetic tasks, the study of critical, productive thinking has not produced major advances. He cites several of the framing assumptions of the standard view of thinking as the causes of this slow progress:

> First, the locus of thinking is assumed to be in an individual's mind, rather than in interaction between an agent and a physical and social situation. Second, processes of thinking and learning are assumed to be uniform across persons and situations. Different individuals are more or less capable of critical or creative thinking, and different situations are assumed to have approximately the same character wherever and in whomever they occur. Third, resources for thinking are assumed to be knowledge and skills that are built up from simple components, socially through instruction in school, rather than general conceptual capabilities that children may have as a result of their everyday experience or native endowment (Greeno, 1989, p. 134).

In the situated approach the methods involve rich ethnographic description of persons acting in their environment, as reasoning is conceived of taking place in interaction with situations, rather than conceiving of it as a set of processes occurring inside someone's mind (e.g. as a set of knowledge structures and operations on them). The shift proposed by the situated cognition approach involves a new consideration of the environmental aspect in theories of cognition.

The methodology used in situated cognition research has some similarities with the ones used in information psychology research, in the sense of consisting of 'thick' descriptions. However, since they consider any thinking to occur in a situation, they record not only verbal data, but also actions and the tasks the subjects perform. Methods are being developed to record and analyse videotapes that capture the situated character of reasoning and thinking.

Summary of qualitative methods

The last 20 years of research in clinical reasoning has seen an explosion of approaches for the study of cognition in most of their manifestations. Methodologically, it has meant a multiplication of methods and techniques, which has had a somewhat beneficial effect on research. More topics in and related to clinical reasoning have been investigated in this period than in any other before. A very large arsenal of methodologies have accumulated that are suitable to study clinical reasoning from very constrained experimental studies of perceptual aspects of reasoning, to the study of cognitive operations, to the investigations of shared understanding in social situations. On the other hand, this multiplicity should also be a stimulus for reflecting on what has been accomplished, where the field is moving, as well as to gathering a taxonomy of findings and a summary evaluation of the various theories and hypotheses developed to account for those findings.

Unsolved issues

In their 1990 article reviewing the progress of the field Elstein, Shulman, and Sprafka foresee several future orientations that can be taken by the study of clinical reasoning in the health sciences. Despite their earlier optimism regarding the unification of the decision making and the information processing approach (see also Elstein et al, 1978; Berner, 1984), the field has gone in different directions and has branched into several approaches. This has, in turn, generated a multiplicity of methods ranging from the more traditional psychometric-based methods still in much use, to the newer developments such as the phenomenological approach (Ramsden et al, 1989), the interpretive approach (Benner, 1984), and research based on traditional experimental psychology (Norman et al, 1989a and b).

The methodological pluralism is healthy as long as it is accompanied by the development of a theory of expertise, of which a theory of reasoning would be a major component. The pluralism brings also a needed awareness of what the methods are designed for, what questions should they answer, and what their limitations are.

Among the issues that remain to be solved are a clarification of the goal that a particular methodological approach is supposed to accomplish. It is common to criticize an investigation for failing to give answers that are relevant to that study. An objection frequently made about qualitative research concerns the generalizability of its research results. However this criticism misses the point of qualitative research, which uses either a single or a few subjects. Such research has as its goal to give a detailed description of a series of phenomena. Most research using qualitative methods attempts to do this in one way or other. Whereas some attempt only a description of a phenomenon, others go further by trying to develop more or less formal representations of the structures and processes involved. The basic idea behind these research studies, however, is to provide evidence for the existence of the phenomenon in question, not to determine its generality. This should, in turn, help develop theories which include what Simon (1979) has called 'laws of qualitative structure'.

Asking questions of generalizability of the results can be meaningfully made of studies which are based on statistical comparisons, because they invariably are designed to answer such questions. The interest in carrying out such studies is not in determining whether or not a phenomenon exists but how general it is. They are unsuitable for answering questions such as what are the mechanisms underlying performance, but answer only how general that performance is.

A second issue concerns the external validity of the research. Some critics argue that the artificiality of research conditions places serious doubts on the quality of research studies. This artificiality would severely distort what actually happens in the real-life situations, enough to make this kind of research meaningless. However, maybe because of the extreme empiricist biases of many behavioural scientists, these critics fail to see the whole point of artificiality. The claim is that it is the results of an experiment that should be judged as valid or invalid. But conducting research in artificial environments implies a very different view of what is valid or not. It is not the results of the study per se, but the theoretical conclusions that are logically tied to such results. Let us present an example. In a study carried out by Coughlin (1985) in which a clinical text describing a patient was presented with the sentences scrambled, it was found that expert physicians were able to reorganize the text in a way that novices were unable to do. Of course, this study could be criticized for failing to approximate the conditions where expert physicians work; after all, they are very unlikely to read patient reports in which the information has been scrambled. But criticizing the study for this reason would totally miss the point of the study. The conclusion of this study was not that expert physicians were better at unscrambling clinical cases, but rather that their memory for clinical information was organized differently from that of novices. Only this theoretical conclusion can be meaningfully made.

One of the main goals of any science is to generate laws that can account for the relevant phenomena. Some researchers believe that laws of behaviour and cognition are impossible to achieve; others, that these laws are not universal as is the case in the mature sciences. Others hold the belief that it is by inductive generalizations that laws are obtained. Empirical generalizations, if strongly confirmed, then become laws of the discipline. Although there is some truth to the last position, most laws in the hard sciences are much more than empirical generalizations. They are theoretical propositions which possess referential universality and that have no counterpart in empirical terms. That is, they explain, but are not, empirical regularities themselves. Rather, they refer to the unobservable underlying processes that produce the empirical regularities. The solution is to acknowledge that science admits several kinds of laws. We mentioned the laws of qualitative structure, which can be uncovered by proposing models and then testing these models by comparing them with human performance. The advantage of laws of this kind is that they not only describe a phemonenon, but also account for it.

Different methodologies serve different purposes. Early research on reasoning was too monolithic, giving primacy to the standard methods typically studied in research design courses. As research becomes more sophisticated, new methods and techniques become increasingly used and new approaches to research tried out. The methodological pluralism to be effective needs to be accompanied by a real effort in developing rigorous theories of reasoning. Theorizing about such a complex field of clinical reasoning is a challenging task, but one that cannot be postponed.

Conclusion: a look at the future

Despite promises of unification, then, the study of clinical reasoning has branched into diverse methodological and substantial areas. This diversity has been welcomed to the extent that it has encouraged investigators to study reasoning more freely, without much restriction. It has also obviously resulted in some lack of communication among researchers involved in different research programs.

The time may be ripe for attempting to provide some coherence to the field and evaluate what aspects can now be brought together and what aspects still need more clarification or development before a fruitful unification is possible. There are some signs that the field may be starting this process already. In a recent NATO Advanced Scientific Research Workshop where investigators interested in clinical reasoning and models of cognition got together to share their research and development efforts, it was concluded that areas related to artificial intelligence, cognitive psychology, and medical decision making are considerably closer in terms of their methods, their research priorities and their theoretical foundations (Evans and Patel, 1992).

It is up to us, researchers of clinical reasoning with diverse backgrounds from Artificial Intelligence to psychology to education, to promote the development of a unified theory of clinical reasoning and decision making. We believe that the tools are available to make faster progress.

Acknowledgements

The work for the preparation and writing of this chapter was supported by FCAR (93ER1177). We thank André Krushniurk for providing helpful comments and Susan St-Pierre for formatting the final copy of the manuscript.

References

Allais, M. and Hagen, O. (1979) *Expected Utility Hypothesis and the Allais Paradox*. D. Reidel, Dordrecht, Holland

Barr, A. and Feigenbaum, E.A. (1981) *The Handbook of Artificial Intelligence*. William Kaufmann, Los Altos, CA

Barro, A.R. (1973) Survey and evaluation of approaches to physician performance measurement. *Journal of Medical Education*, **48**, 1048–1093

Benner, P. (1984) *From Novice to Expert: Excellence and Power in Clinical Nursing Practice*. Addison-Wesley, Menlo Park, CA

Berner, E. (1984) Paradigms and problem solving: A literature review. *Journal of Medical Education*, **59**, 625–633

Bordage, G. and Zacks, R. (1984) The structure of medical knowledge in memories of medical students and practitioners: Categories and prototypes. *Medical Education*, **18**, 406–416

Brooks, L.R., Norman, G.R. and Allen, S.W. (1991) The role of similarity in a medical diagnostic task. *Journal of Experimental Psychology: General*, **120**, 278–287

Bruner, J.S., Goodnow, J.J. and Austin, G.A. (1956) *A Study of Thinking*. Wiley, New York

Bunge, M. (1985) *Treatise on Basic Philosophy. Philosophy of Science: Philosophy of Social Sciences and Technology*. D. Reidel, Dordrecht, Holland

Carroll, J.S. and Johnson, E.S. (1990) *Decision Research*. Sage, Newbury Park, CA

Chase, W.G. and Simon, H.A. (1973) Perception in chess. *Cognitive Psychology*, **4**, 55–81

Christensen, C., Elstein, A.S., Bernstein, L.M. and Balla, J.I. (1991) Formal decision support in medical practice and education. *Teaching and Learning in Medicine*, **3**, 62–70

Coughlin, L.D.J. (1985) *The Effects of Randomization on the Free Recall of Medical Information by Experts and Novices*. Department of Educational Psychology, McGill University, Montreal, Quebec

Dawes, R.M. (1988) *Rational Choice in an Uncertain World*. Harcourt Brace Jovanovich, New York

De Groot, A.D. (1965) *Thought and Choice in Chess*. Mouton, The Hague

Dreyfus, H.L. and Dreyfus, S.E. (1986) *Mind Over Machine: The Power of Human Intuition and Expertise in the Era of the Computer*. Free Press, New York

Elstein, A.S., Shulman, L.S. and Sprafka, S.A. (1978) *Medical Problem Solving. An Analysis of Clinical Reasoning*. Harvard University Press, Cambridge, MA

Elstein, A.S., Shulman, L.S. and Sprafka, S.A. (1990) Medical problem solving: A ten year retrospective. *Evaluation and the Health Professions*, **13**, 5–36

Ericsson, A. and Simon, H.A. (1984) *Protocol Analysis: Verbal Reports as Data*. MIT Press, Cambridge, MA

Evans, D.A. and Patel, V.L. (eds) (1992) *Advanced Models of Cognition for Medical Training and Practice*. NATO ASI. Series F: Computer and Systems Sciences, Vol 97. Springer-Verlag, Heidelberg, Germany

Feltourch, P.J., Johnson, P.E., Moller, J.H. and Swanson, D.B. (1984) LCS: The role and development of medical knowledge in diagnostic expertise. In *Readings in Medical Artificial Intelligence: The First Decade* (eds W.J. Clancey and E.H. Shortliffe) Addison-Wesley, Reading, MA, pp. 275-319

Feltovich, P.J., Coulson, R.L., Spiro, R.J. and Dawson-Saunders, B.K. (1992) Knowledge application and transfer for complex tasks in ill-structured domains: Implications for instruction and testing in biomedicine. In *Advanced Models of Cognition for Medical Training and Practice* (eds D.A. Evans and V.L. Patel), NATO ASI. Series F: Computer and Systems Sciences, Vol 97. Springer-Verlag, Heidelberg, Germany, pp. 213–244

Fox, J. (1988) Formal and knowledge-based methods in decision technology. In *Professional Judgment. A Reader in Clinical Decision Making* (eds J. Dowie and A. Elstein). Cambridge University Press, Cambridge, pp. 226–252

Frederiksen, C.H. (1975) Representing logical and semantic structure of knowledge acquired from discourse. *Cognitive Psychology*, **7**, 371–458

Glaser, B. and Strauss, A. (1967) *The Discovery of Grounded Theory*. Aldine, Chicago

Greeno, J. (1989) A perspective on thinking. *American Psychologist*, **44**, 134–141

Groen, G.J. and Patel, V.L. (1988) The relationship between comprehension and reasoning in medical expertise. In *The Nature of Expertise* (eds M. Chi, R. Glaser and M. Farr) Lawrence Erlbaum Associates, Hillsdale, NJ, pp. 287–310

Hammond, J.S. (1967) Better decision with preference theory. *Harvard Business Review*, **45**, 123–141

Heidegger, M. (1962) *Being and Time* (trans. J. Macquarrie and E. Robinson). Harper and Row, New York

Hovland, C.I. (1960) Computer simulation of thinking. *American Psychologist*, **15**, 687–693

Joseph, G.M. and Patel, V.L. (1990) Domain knowledge and hypothesis generation in diagnostic reasoning. *Medical Decision Making*, **10**, 31–46

Kassirer, J.P., Kuipers, B.J. and Gorry, G.A. (1982) Toward a theory of clinical expertise. *American Journal of Medicine*, **73**, 251–259

Kintsch, W. (1974) *The Representation of Meaning in Memory*. Erlbaum, Hillsdale, NJ

Kuipers, B.J. and Kassirer, J.P. (1984) Causal reasoning in

medicine: analysis of a protocol. *Cognitive Science*, **8**, 363–385

Larkin, J.H., McDermott, J., Simon, H.A. and Simon, D.S. (1980) Expert and novice performance in solving physics problems. *Science*, **208**, 1335–1342

MacNamara, J. (1982) *Names for Things. A Study of Human Learning.* MIT Press, Cambridge, MA

Marton, F. and Saljö, R. (1976) Qualitative differences in learning: I. Outcome and process. *British Journal of Educational Psychology*, **46**, 4–11

McGuire, C.H. (1985) Medical problem solving: A critique of the literature. *Journal of Medical Education*, **60**, 587–595

Newell, A. and Simon, H.A. (1972) *Human Problem Solving.* Prentice-Hall, Englewood Cliffs, NJ

Newell, A., Shaw, J.C. and Simon, H.A. (1958) Elements of a theory of human problem solving. *Psychological Review*, **65**, 151–166

Norman, G., Brooks, L.R. and Allen, S.W. (1989a) Recall by expert medical practitioners and novices as a record of processing attention. *Journal of Experimental Psychology: Learning, Memory, and Cognition*, **15**, 1116–1174

Norman, G., Brooks, L.R., Rosenthal, D., Allen, S.W. and Muzzin, L.J. (1989b) The development of expertise in dermatology. *Archives of Dermatology*, **125**, 1063–1068

Patel, V.L. and Frederiksen, C.H. (1984) Cognitive processes in comprehension and knowledge acquisition by medical students and physicians. In *Tutorials In Problem-Based Learning* (eds H.G. Schmidt and M.L. De Volder). van Gorcum, Assen, Holland, pp. 143–157

Patel, V.L. and Groen, G.J. (1986) Knowledge-based solution strategies in medical reasoning. *Cognitive Science*, **10**, 91–116

Patel, V.L., Groen, G.J. and Arocha, J.F. (1990) Medical expertise as a function of task difficulty. *Memory and Cognition*, **18**, 394–406

Piaget, J. (1950) *The Psychology of Intelligence* (trans. M. Piercy and E. Berlyne). Routledge and Kegan Paul, London

Ramsden, P., Whelan, G. and Cooper, D. (1989) Some phenomena of medical students' diagnostic problem solving. *Medical Education*, **23**, 108–117

Rimoldi, H.J.A. (1961) The test of diagnostic skills. *Journal of Medical Education*, **36**, 73–79

Rosch, E. (1978) Principles of categorization. In *Cognition and Categorization* (eds E. Rosch and B.B. Lloyd). Lawrence Erlbaum Associates, Hillsdale, NJ, pp. 27–48

Schmidt, H., Boshuizen, H.P.A. and Hobus, P.P.M. (1988) Transitory stages in the development of medical expertise: The 'intermediate effect' in clinical case representation studies. In *Proceedings of the Tenth Annual Conference of the Cognitive Science Society* (eds V.L. Patel and G.J. Groen). Lawrence Erlbaum Associates, Hillsdale, NJ, pp. 139–145

Simon, H.A. (1979) Information processing models of cognition. *Annual Review of Psychology*, **30**, 363–396

Sowa, J.F. (1984) *Conceptual Structures: Information Processes in Mind and Machine.* Addison-Wesley, Reading, MA

Suchman, L. (1987) *Plans and Situated Action: The Problem of Human/Machine Communication.* Cambridge University Press, Cambridge, MA

Taylor, C. (1971) Interpretation and the sciences of man. *Review of Metaphysics*, **25**, 3–51

Tversky, A. and Kahneman, D. (1974) Judgment under uncertainty: Heuristics and biases. *Science*, **185**, 1124–1131

von Neumann, J. and Morgenstern, O. (1944) *Theory of Games and Economic Behavior.* Princeton University Press, Princeton

Vu, N.V. (1979) Medical problem solving assessment. A review of methods and instruments. *Evaluation and the Health Professions*, **2**, 281–307

Watson, J.B. (1920) Is thinking merely the action of language mechanisms? *British Journal of Psychology*, **11**, 87–104

Weinstein, M.C., Fineberg, H.V., Elstein, A.S., Frazier, H.S., Neuhauser, D., Neutra, R.R. and McNeil, B.J. (1980) *Clinical Decision Analysis.* W.B. Saunders, Philadelphia, PA

White, P. (1988) Knowing more about what we can tell: 'Introspective access' and causal report accuracy 10 years later. *British Journal of Psychology*, **79**, 13–45

Winograd, T. (1972) Understanding natural language. *Cognitive Psychology*, **3**, 1–191

4

Clinical reasoning in medicine (1)

Arthur S. Elstein

How do physicians solve diagnostic problems? What is known about the process of diagnostic clinical reasoning? Diagnostic reasoning has been an active area of interdisciplinary research in medicine for about 15 years. The investigators have included cognitive psychologists, physicians, philosophers and computer scientists. This chapter sketches our current understanding of answers to these questions by outlining the cogntive processes involved in diagnostic reasoning in clinical medicine. It will describe and analyse the psychological processes and mental structures employed in identifying and solving diagnostic problems of varying degrees of complexity and will review common errors and pitfalls in diagnostic reasoning.

To solve a clinical diagnostic problem means, first, to recognize that some part of a person is not functioning properly and then to set about tracing or identifying the cause or causes of the malfunctioning. The diagnosis is thus an explanation of disordered function, where possible a causal explanation.

Some signs of malfunction are obvious, for example, high fever, severe pain, unusual fatigue, or shortness of breath; others are more subtle, for example, borderline laboratory tests or a slight abdominal discomfort. Very little of the data collected is self-explanatory. For example, most first-year medical students probably recognize that a body temperature of 40 °C is abnormally high and that a chronic cough is also not a normal physical finding, but they are unlikely to be able to enumerate many plausible causes of these phenomena or to identify the additional information needed to pin down a probable cause. An understanding of clinical manifestations must be constructed, stored in long-term memory, and linked to other understanding and explanation in an expanding body of personal knowledge. This understanding is a result of learning and involves judgement and reasoning.

In most cases, not all of the information needed to identify and explain the situation is available in the early stages of the encounter with the patient. Physicians must decide what information to collect, what needs attention, and what can be safely set aside. Thus, data collection is both sequential and selective. Experienced physicians often go about this task almost automatically, sometimes very rapidly; novices struggle to develop a plan. But both approach a problem by collecting detailed information and drawing inferences from these observations about the underlying causes. What plans are used to guide data collection?

(1) Preparation of this review was supported in part by grant RO1 LM4583 from the National Library of Medicine

The hypothetico-deductive method

Early hypothesis generation and selective data collection

Elstein et al (1978) found that diagnostic problems are solved by a process of generating a limited number of hypotheses or problem formulations early in the workup and using them to guide subsequent data collection. Each hypothesis can be used to predict what additional findings ought to be present, if it were true, and then the workup is a guided search for these findings; hence, the method is hypothetico-deductive. The process of problem structuring via hypothesis generation begins with a very limited data set and occurs rapidly and automatically, even if clinicians are explicitly instructed not to generate hypotheses. Given the complexity of the clinical situation, the enormous amount of data that could potentially be obtained, and the limited capacity of working memory, hypothesis generation is a psychological necessity. It transforms an unstructured problem into a structured problem by generating a small set of possible solutions; this is a very efficient way to solve diagnostic problems. Elstein et al (1978) found that novices and experienced physicians alike attempt to generate hypotheses to explain clusters of findings, although the content of the experienced group's productions are of higher quality.

Other researchers have concurred with this view (Kassirer and Gorry, 1978; Pople, 1982; Kuipers and Kassirer, 1984). In general, it has been favourably received by medical educators (e.g. Barrows and Pickell, 1991; Kassirer and Kopelman, 1991), while researchers in cognitive psychology have been more sceptical. We will return to these conflicting interpretations later.

Data collection and interpretation

Next, the data obtained must be interpreted in the light of the hypotheses being considered. How much should previous diagnostic opinions or hunches be revised? To what extent do the data strengthen or weaken belief in the correctness of a particular diagnostic hypothesis?

Accuracy of data interpretation and thoroughness of data collection are separate issues.

A clinician could collect data quite thoroughly but could nevertheless ignore, misunderstand or misinterpret a significant fraction. In contrast, a clinician may be very economical and efficient in data collection but could interpret whatever is available quite accurately. Elstein et al (1978) found no statistically significant correlations between thoroughness of data collection and accuracy of data interpretation. This was an important finding for two reasons:

a) Increased emphasis upon interpretation of data

It is possible to study clinical reasoning either by allowing physicians to collect their own data base or by controlling the content of the case and examining differences in interpretation. Most early research allowed subjects to select items from a large array or menu of items. This approach, exemplified in Patient Management Problems (Feightner, 1985), permits investigation of the amount and sequence of data collection but offers less insight into data interpretation and problem formulation. To deepen understanding of these processes, investigators then asked subjects to think aloud while problem solving and then analysed their verbalizations as well as their data collection (Elstein et al, 1978; Neufeld et al, 1981; Barrows et al, 1982). Considerable variability in acquiring and interpreting data was found, increasing the complexity of the research task. One way to minimize this variability is to control the data base. Consequently, investigators switched to controlling the sequential presentation of data to subjects in order to concentrate on data interpretation and problem formulation (e.g. Feltovich et al, 1984; Kuipers et al, 1988). This shift led naturally to the second major change in research tactics:

b) Study of clinical judgement separated from data collection

Controlling the data base facilitates analysis although a price is paid in terms of fidelity to clinical realities. This strategy is the most widely used in current research on clinical reasoning. Sometimes clinical information is presented sequentially to a subject, so that the case unfolds in a simulation of real time, but the subject is given few options or none in data collection. The analysis can focus on memory organization, knowledge utilization, data inter-pretation, or problem representation (e.g. Moskowitz et al, 1988; Joseph and Patel, 1990; Bordage and Lemieux, 1991). In other studies, clinicians are given all the data at once and asked to make a diagnostic or treat-ment decision (Patel and Groen, 1986; Elstein et al, 1992).

An emphasis on problem representation and diagnosis reflects the assumption that once a diagnosis is correctly made, treatment planning follows almost automatically. Matters are actu-ally more complex. It is now clear that physi-cians might know what to do without understanding why it should be done (Spiro et al, 1987), or they might understand the rational basis for a management plan and still not choose to implement it (Elstein et al, 1992). For example, a clinician may feel that the pos-sible risks of a therapy outweigh the potential benefits even though other clinicians might dis-agree with that assessment.

Case specificity

Problem solving expertise varies greatly across cases and is highly dependent on the clinician's mastery of the particular domain. This proposi-tion was first put forth by Elstein et al (1978). Initially, it was quite surprising but now it has become an accepted part of the understanding of clinical reasoning. To see how our perspec-tive has changed, we have to go back to the early 1970s.

At that time, cognitive psychology had not yet moved to explicitly recognizing the role of knowledge in expertise, a view now widely accepted (Waldrop, 1984). Most work in pro-blem solving focused on general strategies or abilities (Luchins and Luchins, 1950; Johnson, 1955; Polya, 1957; Newell and Simon, 1972) and down-played the role of experience. Experiments deliberately used novel problems to control for differences in prior experience by eliminating them. Transfer from one domain to another was not widely thought to be a problem, provided adequate practice was provided. Thus, cognitive psychology in the late 60s and early 70s had not yet come to grips with the role of practice and experience in the devel-opment of expertise, with some notable excep-tions (e.g. De Groot, 1965; Kleinmuntz, 1968; Chase and Simon, 1973). Research in computer-assisted diagnosis, consultation, expert systems

and artificial intelligence was just beginning. Within a decade, this line of work would make clear that an extensive knowledge base is needed to solve clinical problems (e.g. Pople, 1982; Clancey and Shortliffe, 1984; Larkin et al, 1980).

Medical educators had long recognized that the rapid growth of scientific knowledge made it impossible for the medical degree to signify comprehensive mastery of the domain and that life-long learning was necessary. What was needed, therefore, was instruction in clini-cal logic or technique which could be applied to a broad range of problems, irrespective of con-tent. The early work at Michigan State on 'focal problems', instructional materials for first- and second-year medical students built on paradig-matic clinical situations (Ways et al, 1973) and the development of a problem-based curriculum at McMaster (Neufeld and Barrows, 1974) were both motivated by the desire to highlight for novices the formal, systematic continuities believed to lie behind diverse medical special-ties.

The research program of Elstein et al (1978) sought to identify the strategies and intellectual operations (not content) that distinguished expert from less expert physicians. The metho-dological assumptions were that peer nomina-tions could identify these two groups cleanly and that relatively few clinical situations would be needed to reliably discriminate the strategic differences between them. The finding of case specificity clearly challenged both assumptions. Clinicians who employed a per-fectly successful strategy in one case often had difficulty in the next. They were not particularly consistent across cases and the differences between clinicians were to be found more in their understanding of the problem and their problem representations than in the strategies employed. Thus it made more sense to talk about reasons for success and failure in a parti-cular case than about generic traits or strategies that made for expert diagnosticians.

For the community of evaluators in medical education and the other health professions, the finding of case specificity raised the practical problem of how many case simulations (like Patient Management Problems or related for-mats) would be needed for a reliable and valid assessment of a student's problem-solving skill. Test developers are now much more concerned about the number and content of clinical simulations in an examination than they were prior to the discovery of this knowledge (e.g. Page et al, 1990). (For discussion of psychometric properties of clinical simulations, see van der Vleuten and Swanson, 1990.)

The role of experience in clinical reasoning

The finding of case specificity posed a severe challenge to the hypothetico-deductive model of clinical reasoning as an adequate account of the reasoning process. Both successful and unsuccessful diagnosticians appeared to employ a hypothesis-testing strategy. Success in problem solving (i.e. diagnostic accuracy) depended more on mastery of the content in a domain rather than on the strategy employed.

By the mid-1980s, the view of diagnostic reasoning as complex and systematic generation and testing of hypotheses was being criticized. Patel and her co-workers (e.g. Groen and Patel, 1985) and Norman and his colleagues (e.g. Schmidt et al, 1990; Brooks et al, 1991) pointed out that the clinical reasoning of experts in familiar situations frequently does not display explicit hypothesis testing. It is rapid, automatic, and often non-verbal. The speed, efficiency and accuracy of experienced physicians suggested that they might not even use the same reasoning processes as novices and that experience itself might make hypothesis-testing unnecessary. Not all cases seen by an experienced physician appear to require hypothetico-deductive reasoning. Once a physician has seen a case of chicken-pox, it is a relatively simple matter to diagnose the next case by recalling the characteristic appearance of the rash.

For experienced physicians, much of daily practice consists of seeing new cases that strongly resemble patients previously seen. For this reason, expert reasoning in non-problematic situations looks more like pattern recognition or direct automatic retrieval from a well-structured network of stored knowledge (Groen and Patel, 1985). Even the use of the hypothetico-deductive method could plausibly be affected by previous experience. Since experienced clinicians have a better sense of clinical realities and, therefore, what the likely diagnostic possibilities are, they can more efficiently generate an early set of plausible hypoth-

eses so as to avoid fruitless and expensive pursuit of unlikely diagnoses. These arguments, and the evidence supporting them, suggested that experts use pattern recognition or direct retrieval of needed strategies from a well-organized network of stored information and knowledge as much or more than hypothesis testing. The research emphasis shifted from the problem-solving process to the organization of knowledge in the long-term memory of experienced clinicians (Norman, 1988).

Pattern recognition, prototypes and semantic relations

In broad outline, two accounts of how organized knowledge is used in medical problem solving have been developed. Categorization of a new case can be based either on retrieval of and matching to specific instances or a more abstract prototype.

Instance-based recognition

According to this model, a new case is classified by resemblance to a particular patient seen previously and is therefore given the same diagnosis (Schmidt et al, 1990; Brooks et al, 1991; Norman et al, 1992). This model is supported by the fact that clinical diagnosis is strongly affected by the context of events (for example, the location of a skin rash on the body), even when this context is normatively irrelevant. These context effects suggest that clinicians are matching a new case to a previous case, not to an abstraction from several cases, since the abstraction would not include these irrelevant features. Expert–novice differences are mainly to be explained in terms of the size of the knowledge store of prior instances available for pattern recognition. This theory of clinical reasoning has been developed with particular reference to pathology, dermatology and radiology, all medical specialties where the clinical data are predominantly visual and where verbal or quantitative representation of knowledge is less than in say, internal medicine, nephrology, or endocrinology. It is unclear whether the theory is limited to the visual domain.

Semantic structures

The prototype model (and its variants) holds that abstractions are constructed, based on previous experience (Bordage and Zacks, 1984). Differences between stronger and weaker diagnosticians are to be explained mainly in terms of variation in the content and complexity of their prototypes. Better diagnosticians have constructed more diversified and abstract sets of semantic relations, ways of representing the links between clinical features or aspects of the problem (Bordage and Lemieux, 1991; Lemieux and Bordage, 1992). Examples of these semantic relations are: duration of pain: intermittent vs. constant; location of pain: local vs. general; cause of pain: trauma vs. inflammation; condition of patient: stable vs. worse. Support for this view of knowledge organization is found in the fact that experts in a domain are more able to relate findings to each other and to potential diagnoses, and to identify what additional findings are needed to complete a picture (Elstein et al, 1993). These capabilities suggest that experts are working with more abstract representations and are not simply trying to match a new case to a previous instance, although that matching process may occur with simple cases.

Both theories agree in placing emphasis upon the physician's knowledge representation and less emphasis upon the strategy employed in problem solving than does the hypothetico-deductive account. A plausible synthesis of all three views is that: (a) experts explicitly use the hypothesis-testing method whenever routine problem recognition methods fail; (b) semantic processes are used in hypothesis generation and testing, in conjunction with other processes; (c) if rapid problem classification is unpacked and dissected, it can be seen to be a mixture of pattern recognition, intuition, and hypothesis testing that is not explicitly verbalized. 'Intuition' includes the capacity to identify a puzzling case as an unusual presentation of a more familiar class and to select a few cues as keys or pivots to unlocking the diagnostic puzzle (Eddy and Clanton, 1982).

Some recent research supports this formulation. Norman et al (1994) have shown that experienced physicians use a hypothetico-deductive strategy only with difficult cases. When a case is perceived to be simple or not very challenging, more routine methods, such as pattern recognition or feature matching, are used because they are quicker and easier. Thus, the controversy about the methods used in diagnostic reasoning can be resolved by realizing that the method selected depends upon the perceived characteristics of the problem. There is an interaction between the clinician's level of skill and the perceived difficulty of the task (Elstein, 1994). Easy cases are solved by pattern recognition and going directly from data to diagnostic classification (what Groen and Patel, 1985 call forward reasoning). Difficult cases need systematic hypothesis generation and testing. Whether a problem is easy or difficult depends in part on the knowledge and experience of the clinician who is trying to solve it.

Educational implications

What can be done to help learners acquire expertise in clinical reasoning? Each of these theories offers some assistance.

Consider first the hypothetico-deductive model: Even if it were true that experts in non-problematic situations do not routinely generate and test hypotheses and do retrieve a solution (diagnosis) directly from their structured knowledge, they clearly do generate and evaluate alternatives when confronted with problematic situations. For novices, most situations will initially be problems, not solvable by routine methods, and generating a small set of hypotheses is a useful procedural guideline. Second, since much expert hypothesis-generation and testing is implicit, a model that explicitly calls it to the novice's attention will aid learning. Thirdly, the hypothetico-deductive model directs the learner's attention toward forming a conception of the problem and using this plan to guide the workup. This plan will include a set of competing diagnoses (see the idea of Logical Competitor Sets in Feltovich et al, 1984) and the semantic relationships that make it possible to order the diagnostic candidates as similar and different. This plan will make it possible to reduce unnecessary and expensive laboratory testing, a welcome emphasis in an era that stresses cost containment. Finally, educators generally look for broad transfer of principles or concepts to new situations (Perkins and Salomon, 1989). An approach that is applicable to many cases is bound to be welcomed by educators. One must guard against overemphasizing its virtues.

Because it minimizes expected transfer, the instance-based approach stresses the importance of clinical experiences in contexts closely related to future practice. Clinical training should be examined with an eye to improved design of opportunities for supervised practice and rehearsal. The implicit message is that expertise is very complex and acquired with time and practice, and that when the novice has been practising medicine as long as the expert, she will be expert too. This implication reinforces, in a way, a very traditional doctrine in medical education: practical arts are learned by supervised practice and rehearsal combined with progressively increasing professional responsibility, supplemented by instruction in case conferences, clinical rounds, reading and the like. There is not much that formal theories of problem solving, judgement and decision making can do to facilitate this slow process.

The prototype position offers a more optimistic view of the instructional potential of cognitive science approaches, since it holds that clinical experience is necessary but needs to be reviewed and analysed so that the correct general models and principles are abstracted from the experience. Although the desired level of elaboration and structure generally develops, one ought not to count upon its spontaneous occurrence. Well designed educational experiences can facilitate the development of the desired cognitive structures. Given the emerging consensus about characteristics distinguishing experts from novices, an effective route to the goal would be extensive focused practice and feedback with a variety of problems (Bordage, 1987; Lemieux and Bordage, 1992). Similarly, Rabinowitz and Glaser (1985) proposed that an adequate understanding of the expert's knowledge structure will lead to more effective instruction to assist novices in acquiring that structure.

Is there a role for general strategies? The fact that clinical expertise is so heavily case-specific raises a deep question as far as teaching clinical logic is concerned: if expert clinicians are not consistent in their approach across cases, what formal generalizable logic or operations can or should be taught to learners? For some educators, generalizable strategies are provided by decision analysis and prediction rules developed by multivariate analysis, but these techniques work only with well-structured problems. For others, clinical heuristics have been the preferred route. Some educational reformers (e.g. Barrows, 1983; Norman, 1988)

shifted from 'teaching problem-solving' to 'problem-based learning'. This change emphasizes the importance of clinically relevant contexts in facilitating learning and also implies that a general strategy might be beyond reach. For those with a more analytic disposition, the problem of teaching the logic of clinical decision making (Christensen et al, 1991) remains: how can medical students be effectively introduced to formal schemes for drawing inferences that are meaningfully linked to clinical materials and yet are analytically separable from them and generalize across cases? In the past ten years, much effort has gone into developing expositions of clinical logic based on information processing psychology and decision analysis (e.g. Weinstein et al, 1980; Balla, 1985; Griner et al, 1986; Goldman, 1987; Albert et al, 1988; Pauker, 1988; Sox et al, 1988; Kassirer and Kopelman, 1991).

Errors in everyday clinical inference

To summarize, clinical reasoning can proceed either by pattern recognition or by hypothesis-testing. Neither is an error-proof strategy, nor are they always consistent with statistical rules of inference with imperfect information. The errors that can occur in difficult cases in internal medicine are illustrated and discussed by Kassirer and Kopelman (1991). The frequency of errors in actual practice is unknown, but considering a number of studies as a whole, an error rate of 15% might be a good first approximation.

Looking at an instance of diagnostic reasoning retrospectively, it is easy to see that a clinician could err either by oversimplifying the reasoning about a complex problem or by taking a problem that could appropriately have been dealt with routinely and using the much more effortful strategy of multiple competing hypotheses. It has been far more difficult for researchers and teachers of diagnostic reasoning to prescribe the appropriate strategy in advance. Because so much depends on the interaction between case and clinician, prescriptive guidelines for the proper amount of hypothesis generation and testing are still unavailable for the student clinician. Perhaps the most useful advice is to emulate the hypothesis-testing strategy used by experienced clinicians when they are having difficulty, since novices will experience as problematic many situations that the latter solve by routine pattern-recognition methods. Gathering more data without having hypotheses in mind is less likely to pay off. Occasionally these searches are successful but more often than not, they waste money and time with little return. In an era that emphasizes cost-effective clinical practice, gathering data unrelated to diagnostic hypotheses cannot be readily recommended.

Problems in hypothesis generation and restructuring

Many diagnostic problems are so complex that the correct solution is not contained within the initial set of hypotheses. Restructuring and reformulating must occur through time as data are obtained and the clinical picture evolves. However, as any problem solver works with a particular set of hypotheses, psychological commitment takes place and it becomes more difficult to restructure the problem (Janis and Mann, 1977). Ideally, one might want to work purely inductively, reasoning only from the facts, but this strategy is never employed because it is very inefficient and produces high levels of cognitive strain. A purely inductive approach to clinical reasoning would be inefficient in two ways: (1) Early findings could lead to a very long list of preliminary hypotheses. The problem space would become steadily larger as new clusters of data are obtained, rather than becoming better structured. (2) Exhaustive data collection would be required until enough evidence had been obtained to point conclusively to one candidate. It is much easier to solve a problem with some boundaries and hypotheses to provide the needed framework. On the other hand, early problem formulation may also bias the clinician's thinking (Barrows et al, 1982).

The emphasis in internal medicine training on formally constructing and analysing a set of diagnostic alternatives, called the differential diagnosis, is designed to help correct these problems. This is a useful heuristic strategy, rather than one that guarantees success, because instructions to develop a differential diagnosis generally omit clearly defined rules stating the best alternatives for a given situation or even how many alternatives should be in the differential list. Everyday clinical reasoning would insist that such rules are too rigid and

that some artistry is needed. Room should be left for common sense, intuition, and flexibility. Thus, the strategy of working through a differential diagnosis can prevent premature closure on a single salient alternative, but it cannot guarantee that the correct diagnostic alternative is included on the list. The longer and more exhaustive the list, the more likely it is to include the correct diagnosis, but the workup will become correspondingly more inefficient, expensive and time-consuming.

Overemphasizing rare conditions

Several features of human thinking together imply that it will be tempting to search for exotic diseases ('long shots') at the expense of more probable ones. This phenomenon is often observed and clinicians are regularly urged to alter their behaviour, but change has been difficult. Basic psychological research suggests several mechanisms underlying its persistence:

Sampling biases

Rare conditions are over-represented in both the clinical literature and in academic training centres, and so novices, in particular, may be led to overestimate their likelihood in the environment of everyday practice. Unusual cases are also more memorable than routine problems (Nisbett et al, 1982). These context problems are aggravated by training in tertiary care settings in preparation for practice in primary-care or community-hospital settings, and so efforts are now being made to increase the time spent in these settings in clinical training.

Probability distortions

Small probabilities tend to be overestimated (Tversky and Kahneman, 1981); this tendency is exacerbated when the small probabilities are vague and not precisely known or stated (Einhorn and Hogarth, 1986).

Regret minimization

Clinicians may respond to the regret they would feel about missing the diagnosis and thus potentially causing some harm instead of to a weighted combination of probability and value (Feinstein, 1985).

Confounding probability and value of an outcome

It is difficult for everyday judgement to keep separate accounts of the probability of a particular disease and the benefits that accrue from detecting it. Probability revision errors that are systematically linked to the perceived cost of mistakes demonstrate the difficulties experienced in separating assessments of probability from values (Wallsten, 1981; Poses et al, 1985).

Acquiring redundant evidence

In collecting data, there is a tendency to seek information that confirms a hypothesis rather than the data that facilitates efficient testing of competing hypotheses. This tendency has been called 'pseudodiagnosticity' (Kern and Doherty, 1982) or 'confirmation bias' (Wolf et al, 1985). It is less a cause of concern with information obtained in the clinical interview than with costly laboratory work or special tests.

Incorrect interpretation

The most common error in interpreting findings is over-interpretation: data which should not support a particular hypothesis, and which might even suggest that a new alternative be considered, are interpreted as consistent with hypotheses already under consideration (Elstein et al, 1978). The data best remembered tend to be those that support the hypotheses generated. Where findings are distorted in recall, it is generally in the direction of making the facts more consistent with typical clinical pictures. Positive findings are overemphasized and negative findings tend to be discounted (Wason and Johnson-Laird, 1972; Elstein et al, 1978). The principle of bounded rationality helps us understand the adaptive function of these errors: (a) a problem must be structured, so hypotheses are required; (b) the representation must be simpler than the problem; generating more hypotheses would make matters more complex and require more information processing. In general, efforts are continually made to keep matters simple and within the capacity of working memory. Even when clinicians agree on the presence of certain clinical findings, wide variations have been found in the weights assigned to these findings in the course of developing an interpretation of their meaning (Bryant and Norman, 1980; Wigton et al, 1986).

Base rate neglect

Good clinical reasoning should avoid overlooking unusual conditions that are masked as common problems and not neglect rare conditions that are treatable and potentially harmful if untreated. For example, most headaches are not caused by benign operable tumours, but a good clinician would not want to miss the few that are. On the other hand, one must avoid false alarms, overcalling relatively rare diagnoses, causing the patient unnecessary anxiety and wasting money on futile diagnostic work-ups. The literature suggests that, unless trained to use Bayes' theorem and to recognize when it is appropriate, physicians are just as prone to misusing or neglecting base rates in diagnostic inference as anyone else (Elstein, 1988).

Decision supports

Until recently, medical educators paid little attention to formal quantitative methods for dealing with these problems. It was implicitly assumed that they would become insignificant as clinical experience was acquired. However, in the United States, recent criticism of the overall cost and inefficiency of medical care has emphasized the over-utilization of laboratory tests and of expensive technologies that provide little benefit to patients. In other cases, physicians have been criticized for adhering to older methods and not adopting new therapies that have been shown to be effective. These criticisms have led to increased interest in practice guidelines. Efforts are also under way to improve both diagnostic inference and therapeutic decision making by adding statistical methods to the clinical armamentarium. Formal statistical reasoning using Bayes' theorem and clinical prediction rules is now propounded in several current textbooks (Weinstein et al, 1980; Balla, 1985; Cebul et al, 1985; Griner et al, 1986; Goldman, 1987; Albert et al, 1988; Pauker, 1988; Sox et al, 1988; Kassirer and Kopelman, 1991; Sackett et al, 1991). The approach appears to be gaining support, particularly among general internists, but is not yet widely utilized (Detsky, 1987; Balla et al, 1989). Computer programs that run on microcomputers and can provide decision support have been developed (De Bliek et al, 1988; Applied Informatics, 1990). The role of these programs in medical education and in future clinical practice is still to be determined. Broader use of these programs, at least as instructional tools if not in routine clinical practice, may be anticipated as the cost of microcomputers declines while the machines and programs become steadily more powerful. A program that calculates posterior probabilities can be implemented on any microcomputer using a simple spreadsheet.

Conclusion

Research on the clinical reasoning of physicians has a broad range, including but not limited to differences between expert and novice clinicians, psychological processes in judgement and decision making, non-normative biases in judgement and decision making and factors associated with their production and maintenance, improving instruction and training to enhance acquisition of good reasoning, and the development, evaluation and implementation of decision support systems and guidelines. Many recent studies of physicians' decision making have used statistical decision theory as a standard by which to assess unaided, intuitive clinical decisions. The aims of these studies have included understanding the process of clinical reasoning, improving instructional programs designed for medical students and clinical training, assessing competence at the level of medical licensure and certification, analysing the cognitive processes employed in specific clinical situations, and developing practice guidelines and standards.

Clinicians have been understandably reluctant to share their decision making authority with impersonal guidelines. Yet the expansion of biomedical knowledge and the growth of technological capability have vastly increased both the range of possible actions for diagnosis and treatment and their associated costs. These forces have led to pressure to control the costs of medical care and to involve patients and families more meaningfully in decision making. Thus, these forces imply some limitation of professional authority, while simultaneously increasing the scope of professional capability. Research on reasoning in medicine thus stands at the intersection of the interests of psychologists, medical sociologists, health policy planners, economists, patients and clinicians. Given this conjunction, there should be continued pursuit of both normative and descriptive studies of clinical reasoning in medicine and how it might be improved.

Acknowledgements

I wish to thank my colleague, Georges Bordage, for several valuable suggestions and comments. Responsibility for differences or errors in interpretation of the literature reviewed is mine alone.

References

Albert, D.A., Munson, R. and Resnik, M.D. (1988) *Reasoning in Medicine: An Introduction to Clinical Inference.* Johns Hopkins University Press, Baltimore

Applied Informatics (1990) *ILIAD User Manual.* Salt Lake City, Utah

Balla, J.I. (1985) *The Diagnostic Process: A Model for Clinical Teachers.* Cambridge University Press, New York

Balla, J.I., Elstein, A.S. and Christensen, C. (1989) Obstacles to acceptance of decision analysis in clinical settings. *British Medical Journal*, **298**, 579–582

Barrows, H.S. (1983) Problem-based, self-directed learning. *Journal of the American Medical Association*, **250**, 3077–3080

Barrows, H.S. and Pickell, G.C. (1991) *Developing Clinical Problem-Solving Skills: A Guide to More Effective Diagnosis and Treatment.* Norton, New York

Barrows, H.S., Norman, G.R., Neufeld, V.R. and Feightner, J. W. (1982) The clinical reasoning process of randomly selected physicians in general practice. *Clinical and Investigative Medicine*, **5**, 49–56

Bordage, G. (1987) The curriculum: overloaded and too general? *Medical Education*, **21**, 183–188

Bordage, G. and Lemieux, M. (1991) Semantic structures and diagnostic thinking of experts and novices. *Academic Medicine*, **66**, S70–S72

Bordage, G. and Zacks, R. (1984) The structure of medical knowledge in the memories of medical students and general practitioners: categories and prototypes. *Medical Education*, **18**, 406–416

Brooks, L.R., Norman, G.R. and Allen, S.W. (1991) Role of specific similarity in a medical diagnostic task. *Journal Experimental Psychology, General*, **120**, 278–287

Bryant, G.D. and Norman, G.R. (1980) Expressions of probability: Words and numbers. *New England Journal of Medicine*, **302**, 411

Cebul, R.D., Beck, L.M. and Carroll, J.G. (1985) *Teaching Clinical Decision Making*. Praeger, New York

Chase, W. and Simon, H.A. (1973) The mind's eye in chess. In *Visual Information Processing* (ed. W.G. Simon). Academic Press, New York, pp. 215–281

Christensen, C., Elstein, A.S., Bernstein, L.M. and Balla, J.I. (1991) Formal decision supports in medical practice and education. *Teaching and Learning in Medicine*, **3**, 62–70

Clancey, W.J. and Shortliffe, E.H. (eds) (1984) *Readings in Medical Artificial Intelligence: The First Decade*. Addison-Wesley, Reading, MA

De Bliek, R., Miller, R.A. and Masarie, F.E. (1988) *QMR User Manual*. University of Pittsburgh, Pittsburgh

De Groot, A.D. (1965) *Thought and Choice in Chess*. Mouton, The Hague

Detsky, A.S. (1987) Decision analysis: what the prognosis is. *Annals of Internal Medicine*, **106**, 321–322

Eddy, D.M. and Clanton, C.H. (1982) The art of diagnosis: Solving the clinico-pathological exercise. *New England Journal of Medicine*, **306**, 1263–1268

Einhorn, H.J. and Hogarth, R.M. (1986) Decision making under ambiguity. *Journal of Business*, **59**, S225–S250

Elstein, S.A. (1994) What goes around comes around: the return of the hypothetico-deductive strategy. *Teaching and Learning in Medicine*, **6**, 121–123

Elstein, A.S. (1988) Cognitive processes in clinical inference and decision making. In *Reasoning, Inference and Judgment in Clinical Psychology* (eds D.C. Turk and P. Salovey). Free Press/Macmillan, New York, pp. 17–50

Elstein, A.S., Holzman, G.B., Belzer, L.J. and Ellis, R.D. (1992) Hormonal replacement therapy: Analysis of clinical strategies used by residents. *Medical Decision Making*, **12**, 265–273

Elstein, A.S., Kleinmuntz, B., Rabinowitz, M., McAuley, R., Murakami, J., Heckerling, P.S. and Dod, J.M. (1993) Diagnostic reasoning of high- and low-domain knowledge clinicians: a re-analysis. *Medical Decision Making*, **13**, 21–29

Elstein, A.S., Shulman, L.S. and Sprafka, S.A. (1978) *Medical Problem Solving: An Analysis of Clinical Reasoning*. Harvard University Press, Cambridge, MA

Feightner, J.W. (1985) Patient management problems. In *Assessing Clinical Competence* (eds V.R. Neufeld and G.R. Norman). Springer, New York, pp. 183–200

Feinstein, A.R. (1985) The 'chagrin factor' and qualitative decision analysis. *Archives of Internal Medicine*, **145**, 1257–1259

Feltovich, P.J., Johnson, P.E., Moller, J.H. and Swanson, D.B. (1984) LCS: The role and development of medical knowledge in diagnostic expertise. In *Readings in Medical Artificial Intelligence: The First Decade* (eds W. J. Clancey and E. H. Shortliffe). Addison-Wesley, Reading, MA, pp. 275–319

Goldman, L. (1987) Quantitative aspects of clinical reasoning. In *Harrison's Principles of Internal Medicine*, 11th edn. (eds E. Braunwald, K.J. Isselbacher, R.G. Petersdorf, J.D. Wilson, J.B. Martin and A.S. Fauci). McGraw-Hill, New York, pp. 5–11

Griner, P.F., Panzer, R.J. and Greenland, P. (eds) (1986) *Clinical Diagnosis and the Laboratory: Logical Strategies for Common Medical Problems*. Year Book Medical Publishers, Chicago

Groen, G.J. and Patel, V.L. (1985) Medical problem-solving: Some questionable assumptions. *Medical Education*, **19**, 95–100

Janis, I.L. and Mann, L. (1977) *Decision-Making*. Free Press, New York

Johnson, D.M. (1955) *The Psychology of Thought and Judgment*. Harper and Row, New York

Joseph, G.M. and Patel, V.L. (1990) Domain knowledge and hypothesis generation in diagnostic reasoning. *Medical Decision Making*, **10**, 31–46

Kassirer, J.P. and Gorry, G.A. (1978) Clinical problem solving: A behavioral analysis. Annals of Internal medicine, **89**, 245–255

Kassirer, J.P. and Kopelman, R.I. (1991) *Learning Clinical Reasoning*. Williams and Wilkins, Baltimore

Kern, L. and Doherty, M.E. (1982) 'Pseudodiagnosticity' in an idealized medical problem-solving environment. *Journal of Medical Education*, **57**, 100–104

Kleinmuntz, B. (1968) The processing of clinical information by man and machine. In *Formal Representation of Human Judgment* (ed. B. Kleinmuntz). Wiley, New York, 149–186

Kuipers, B., Moskowitz, A.J. and Kassirer, J.P. (1988) Critical decisions under uncertainty: representation and structure. *Cognitive Science*, **12**, 177–210

Kuipers, B.J. and Kassirer, J.P. (1984) Causal reasoning in medicine: analysis of a protocol. *Cognitive Science*, **8**, 363–385

Larkin, J., McDermott, J., Simon, D.P. and Simon, H.A. (1980) Expert and novice performance in solving physics problems. *Science*, **208**, 1335–1342

Lemieux, M. and Bordage, G. (1992) Propositional versus structural semantic analyses of medical diagnostic thinking. *Cognitive Science*, **16**, 185–204

Luchins, A.S. and Luchins, E.H. (1950) New experimental attempts at preventing mechanization in problem solving. *Journal of General Psychology*, **42**, 279–297

Moskowitz, A.J., Kuipers, B.J. and Kassirer, J.P. (1988) Dealing with uncertainty, risks, and tradeoffs in clinical decisions: a cognitive science approach. *Annals of Internal Medicine*, **108**, 435–449

Neufeld, V.R. and Barrows, H.S. (1974) The 'McMaster Philosophy': An approach to medical education. *Journal of Medical Education*, **49**, 1040–1050

Neufeld, V.R., Norman, G.R., Feightner, J.W. and Barrows, H.S. (1981) Clinical problem-solving by medical students: A cross-sectional and longitudinal analysis. *Medical Education*, **15**, 315–322

Newell, A. and Simon, H.A. (1972) *Human Problem Solving*. Prentice-Hall, Englewood Cliffs, NJ

Nisbett, R.E., Borgida, E., Crandall, R. and Reed, H. (1982) Popular induction: Information is not always informative. In *Judgment Under Uncertainty: Heuristics and Biases* (eds D. Kahneman, P. Slovic and A. Tversky). Cambridge University Press, New York, pp. 101–116

Norman, G.R., Trott, A.L., Brooks, L.R. and Smith, E.K. M. (1994) Cognitive differences in clinical reasoning related to postgraduate training. *Training and Learning in Medicine*, **6**, 114–120

Norman, G.R. (1988) Problem-solving skills, solving problems and problem-based learning. *Medical Education*, **22**, 279–286

Norman, G.R., Coblentz, C.L., Brooks, L.R. and Babcock, C.J. (1992) Expertise in visual diagnosis: a review of the literature. *Academic Medicine*, **66**, S78–S83

Page, G., Bordage, G., Harasym, P., Bowmer, I. and Swanson, D. (1990) A revision of the Medical Council of Canada's Qualifying Examination: Pilot test results. In *Teaching and Assessing Clinical Competence* (eds W. Bender, R. Hiemstra, A. Scherpbier and R. Zwierstra). BoekWerk Publications, Groningen, pp. 403–407

Patel, V.L. and Groen, G. (1986) Knowledge-based solution strategies in medical reasoning. *Cognitive Science*, **10**, 91–116

Pauker, S.G. (1988) Clinical decision making. In *Cecil Textbook of Medicine*. 18th edn. (eds J.B. Wyngaarden and L.H. Smith, Jr.). Saunders, Philadelphia, pp. 74–79

Perkins, D.N. and Salomon, G. (1989) Are cognitive skills context bound? *Educational Researcher*, **18**, 16–25

Polya, G. (1957) *How to Solve It*. 2nd edn. Doubleday, Garden City, NY

Pople, H.E. (1982) Heuristic methods for imposing structure on ill-structured problems: The structuring of medical diagnostics. In *Artificial Intelligence in Medicine* (ed. P. Szolovits). Westview Press, Boulder, Colorado, pp. 119–190

Poses, R. M., Cebul, R. D., Collins, M. and Fager, S. S. (1985) The accuracy of experienced physicians' probability estimates for patients with sore throats. *Journal of the American Medical Association*, **254**, 925–929

Rabinowitz, M. and Glaser, R. (1985) Cognitive structure and process in highly competent performance. In *The Gifted and Talented: Developmental Perspectives* (eds F. D. Horowitz and M. O'Brien). American Psychological Association, Washington, pp. 75–98

Sackett, D.L., Haynes, R.B. and Tugwell, P. (1991) *Clinical Epidemiology: A Basic Science for Clinical Medicine*. 2nd edn. Little Brown, Boston

Schmidt, H.G., Norman, G.R. and Boshuizen, H.P.A. (1990) A cognitive perspective on medical expertise: theory and implications. *Academic Medicine*, **65**, 611–621

Sox, H.C. Jr, Blatt, M.A., Higgins, M.C. and Marton, K.I. (1988) *Medical Decision Making*. Butterworths, Stoneham, MA

Spiro, R.J., Feltovich, P.J., Coulson, R.L. and Anderson, D.K. (1987) *Multiple Analogies for Complex Concepts: Antidotes for Analogy-Induced Misconception in Advanced Knowledge Acquisition*. Conceptual Knowledge Research Project, Technical Report No. 2. SIU School of Medicine, Springfield, IL

Tversky, A. and Kahneman, D. (1981) The framing of decisions and the psychology of choice. *Science*, **211**, 453–458

van der Vleuten, C.P.M. and Swanson, D.B. (1990) Assessment of clinical skills with standardized patients: State of the art. *Teaching and Learning in Medicine*, **2**, 58–76

Waldrop, M.M. (1984) The necessity of knowledge. *Science*, **223**, 1279–1282

Wallsten, T.S. (1981) Physician and medical student bias in evaluating information. *Medical Decision Making*, **1**, 145–164

Wason, P.C. and Johnson-Laird, P.N. (1972) *Psychology of Reasoning: Structure and Content*. Harvard University Press, Cambridge, MA

Ways, P., Loftus, G. and Jones, J. (1973) Focal problem teaching in medical education. *Journal of Medical Education*, **48**, 565–571

Weinstein, M.C., Fineberg, H. V., Elstein, A.S., Frazier, H. S., Neuhauser, D., Neutra, R.R. and McNeil, B.J. (1980) *Clinical Decision Analysis*. Saunders, Philadelphia

Wigton, R.S., Hoellerich, V.L. and Patil, K.D. (1986) How physicians use clinical information in diagnosing pulmonary embolism: an application of conjoint analysis. *Medical Decision Making*, **6**, 2–11. Reprinted in *Professional Judgment: A Reader in Clinical Decision Making* (1988) (eds J. Dowie and A. Elstein). Cambridge University Press, New York, pp. 130–149

Wolf, F.M., Gruppen, L.D., Billi, J.E. (1985) Differential diagnosis and the competing hypotheses heuristic: A practical approach to judgment under uncertainty and Bayesian probability. *Journal of American Medical Association*, **253**, 2858–2862. Reprinted in *Professional Judgment: A Reader in Clinical Decision Making* (1988) (eds J. Dowie and A. Elstein). Cambridge University Press, New York, pp. 349–359

5

Clinical reasoning in nursing

Marsha E. Fonteyn

Why seek to understand nurses' clinical reasoning? The answer to this question may seem obvious to many, but is none the less worthy of consideration at the beginning of a chapter devoted to this topic. Clinical reasoning represents the essence of nursing practice. It is intrinsic to all aspects of care provision, and its importance pervades nursing education, research and practice. An understanding of nurses' clinical reasoning is important to nursing research because of the need for a scientific basis to evaluate nursing practice and education and a need to develop and test theories of nurses' cognitive processes and reasoning skills. Research is also needed to describe and explain the relationship between nurses' reasoning and patient outcomes, in order to demonstrate to society the essential role that nursing plays in the health care delivery system.

Knowledge about clinical reasoning is important to nursing education because education is expensive, and teaching that is based on inappropriate or irrelevant models of reasoning can lead to waste, and can also result in graduates who are ill-prepared to reason well in practice. Clinical reasoning is also important to nursing practice because patient care provision is becoming increasingly more complex and difficult, requiring sound reasoning skills to maintain patient stability, provide high quality care with positive outcomes, and avoid the costly, even deadly, mistakes that can occur from faulty reasoning and errors in decision making.

Definition of clinical reasoning

The literature provides several definitions of nurses' clinical reasoning. Radwin (1990) sees nurses' reasoning as a form of clinical judgement that occurs in a series of stages: encountering the patient, gathering clinical information, formulating possible diagnostic hypotheses, searching for more information to confirm or reject these hypotheses, and ultimately reaching a diagnostic decision. Jones (1988) also describes clinical reasoning as a diagnostic process. Fonteyn (1991a) defines nurses' clinical reasoning as the cognitive processes that nurses use when reviewing and analysing patient data. Fonteyn's research examining expert nurses' clinical reasoning (1991b) demonstrated that nurses use their knowledge and experience from previous patient cases to form relationships between the elements of patient data, to determine patient status, to identify actual and potential patient problems, and, consequently, to plan care, and make decisions to achieve optimal patient outcomes. In summary then, nurses' clinical reasoning can be defined as the cognitive processes and strategies that nurses use to understand the significance of patient data, to identify and diagnose actual or potential patient problems, and to make clinical decisions to assist in problem resolution and to enhance the achievement of positive patient outcomes.

Distinguishing between nurses' reasoning process and the nursing process

The clinical reasoning process that nurses use during care provision should not be confused with the *nursing process* that has become an intrinsic part of nursing education over the last 30 years, and that is often used to describe what is believed by a significant proportion of the nursing profession to encompass the essential nature of nursing practice (Henderson, 1982). Johnson (1959) was among the first to use the term *nursing process* to describe the series of steps that comprise the process of nursing. Over time, this five-step process, consisting of *assessment*, *diagnosis*, *planning*, *implementation*, and *evaluation*, has become entrenched in both nursing practice and education. It often provides the framework both for how students are taught to reason about nursing care and for how nursing is evaluated in practice (Wilkinson, 1992).

All of the steps of the nursing process require reasoning skills. Although fundamental to providing care, nurses' reasoning and decision making has yet to be fully described in nursing research literature, but the descriptive work that has been done reveals a distinction between how nurses reason in practice and how they were taught to reason in school (by following the steps of the nursing process). In their classic study of nurses' clinical judgement, Benner and Tanner (1987) found that experienced nurses are less likely to use an analytical process during reasoning. Rather, experienced nurses have developed a method of reasoning that often provides them with an 'intuitive grasp' of the whole clinical situation, without having to follow the step-by-step approach of the nursing process. According to Benner and Tanner, the analytical focus of the nursing process in education has resulted in the exclusion of techniques that would foster students' skills in intuitive judgement.

In their study of experienced nurses' clinical reasoning, Grobe et al (1991) also found that the reasoning used by experienced nurses during a planning task differs from the analytical step-by-step process taught to nursing students. Experienced nurses link one patient problem to another of their problems and to interventions that would resolve both problems. This method of reasoning is different from that taught using the nursing process. The nursing process method teaches students to focus on each patient problem and its associated interventions separately, which is less efficient and does not seem to reflect the realities encountered in actual practice, where one patient problem is often associated with another.

In a study designed to identify nursing diagnoses and interventions associated with care of abused elderly, Phillips and Rempusheski (1985) also found that the processes that subjects used to reason were distinctly different from the nursing process, in that they were non-linear and reflected continuous movement from one thought to another. Holzemer and Henry (1991) found that nursing diagnoses (an important component of the nursing process) were not even used by their nurse–subjects when they reasoned about the care of HIV positive patients with pneumocystic pneumonia.

Hurst et al (1991) used interviews of both experienced and novice nurses, supported by written vignettes, to explore nurses' reasoning processes. They found that nurses use different styles of reasoning, and proposed that adherence to the rigidly linear nursing process may be alien to some nurses' thinking. The steps of the nursing process are so similar to the research process that they should not be seen as a unique or innovative approach to problem solving, nor do they represent the only explanatory models of nurses' reasoning. Thus, when discussing the cognitive processes and strategies that nurses use to reason about patient care, it is important to clearly distinguish these from the *nursing process*, which represents one of the many approaches that nurses use in problem solving.

Theoretical perspectives

Several different theoretical perspectives have been suggested to assist in understanding nurses' clinical reasoning: information processing, decision analysis, and hermeneutics.

Information Processing Theory

Information Processing Theory (IPT) has been used as a framework for guiding a variety of studies of clinical reasoning (Putzier et al, 1985; Corcoran, 1986; Johnson, 1988;

Norman, 1988; Glaser and Chi, 1988; Fonteyn, 1991b). IPT was first described by Newell and Simon (1972) in their work examining how individuals with a great deal of experience with a specific problem-solving task reasoned during the task. A fundamental premise of IPT is that human reasoning consists of a relationship between an information processing system (the human problem solver) and a task environment (the context in which problem solving occurs). A postulate of this theory is that there are limits to the amount of information that one can process at any given time, and that effective problem solving is the result of being able to adapt to these limitations. Miller's (1956) earlier classic work had demonstrated that an individual's working, short-term memory (STM) can only hold 7 ± 2 symbols at a time. Newell and Simon's (1972) research showed that the capacity of STM could be greatly increased, however, by 'chunking' simple units into familiar patterns. Individuals with a great deal of knowledge and experience in a particular domain can more easily chunk information pertaining to that domain, and thus can make more efficient use of their STM during reasoning. An example of 'chunking' in nursing would be when a nurse experienced with caring for patients with acute respiratory failure observes several of the symptoms that a patient in failure exhibits, and then 'chunks' them all together in his or her STM as 'respiratory failure'. In contrast, nurses with little experience with this patient case would try to hold each individual symptom of failure ('elevated pCO_2', 'decreased pO_2', 'cyanosis', 'tachypnea', 'tachycardia', etc.) in their STM, and would soon run out of room to concentrate on anything else.

Another memory bank identified by Newell and Simon (1972) was long term memory (LTM), which has infinite storage space for information. The theory proposes that information gained from knowledge and experience is stored throughout life in LTM, and that it takes longer to access LTM information than the small amount of information temporarily stored in STM. This theory also proposes that the information stored in LTM may need to be accessed by associating it with related information, which helps explain why experts reason so well within their domain. Indeed, previous research has demonstrated that experts possess an organized body of domain-specific conceptual and procedural knowledge that can be easily accessed using reasoning strategies (heuristics) and specific reasoning processes that are gradually learned through academic learning and through clinical experience (Putzier et al, 1985; Johnson, 1988; Norman, 1988; Glaser and Chi, 1988; Fisher and Fonteyn, 1994; Fonteyn and Grobe, 1993).

Grier (1984) reported findings from an extensive review of nursing studies guided by IPT, and concluded that there is beginning support for explaining nurses' reasoning using information processing theory. She emphasized the need for further research to identify and describe the clinical reasoning used by more experienced nurses, including how they process information while reasoning.

Jones (1988) described recent advances in understanding clinical reasoning that have resulted from research in artificial intelligence, using IPT. She suggests that IPT might be useful for studies designed to assist in the development of expert systems in nursing by revealing how expert nurses structure and process information while reasoning about patient care.

Decision Analysis Theory

Decision Analysis Theory (DAT) was introduced into medicine about 20 years ago as a method of solving difficult clinical problems (Kassirer et al, 1987). DAT methods include: use of Bayes' theorem, use of decision trees, sensitivity analysis, and utility analysis. Bayes' theorem application involves using mathematical formulas, tabular techniques, nomograms, and computer programs to determine the likelihood of meaning of clinical data (Gray et al, 1984; Sackett et al, 1985).

Several nursing studies have demonstrated the applicability of decision theory to nurses' decision making. In her classic study examining the relationship between the expected value (anticipated outcome) nurses assign to each of their outcomes and their ranking of nursing actions, Grier (1976) demonstrated that nurses select actions that are consistent with their expected values, which seems to support the use of decision trees in some instances of nurses' reasoning and decision making. For example, in a cardiac arrest situation, nurses follow decision trees to choose the appropriate actions for treating specific life-threatening dysrhythmias.

In a study using a hypothetical patient to examine nurses' diagnostic reasoning, Aspinall (1979) found that subjects who used a decision tree to assist with their reasoning were more often correct in their diagnoses than those not using one. Hughes and Young (1990) used a decision model to examine the relationship between task complexity and consistency of nurses' decision making. They used the Decision Analytic Questionnaire, an instrument designed to measure nurses' decision making under uncertain conditions. They administered the instrument to a stratified random sample of 101 paid volunteer medical–surgical nurses drawn from three public hospitals. The results demonstrated that nurses made decisions that corresponded to those recommended by a decision model, but that agreement with the model decreased as task complexity increased. The investigators recommended that their findings be verified by future studies examining nurses' use of a decision model in actual clinical situations. They stress the need to consider task complexity during model design when developing decision models for use in nursing.

Hermeneutics

In a review summarizing and evaluating nursing research related to teaching clinical judgement, Tanner (1983) noted that most of the research to date had been guided by either decision theory (to predict and explain optimal judgement) or information processing theory (to describe the judgement process). She proposed that a portion of the future studies of nurses' judgement be guided by a hermeneutic approach (to reveal the judgement knowledge embedded in nursing practice).

Hermeneutics is based on the phenomenological tradition that maintains that meaning is subjective and contextually constructed. The intent of studies of nurses' reasoning guided by this method is to understand nurses' clinical world, including their reasoning as they make decisions about patient care. Benner et al (1992) used a hermeneutic approach to study the development of expertise in critical care nursing practice. Using group interviews, the investigators obtained narrative accounts of exemplars from their subjects, who were practising in adult, paediatric, or newborn intensive care units. They also observed a subsample of nurses while they provided care. Later, the investigators conducted personal history interviews with this subsample. Their findings indicated that nurses at different levels of expertise 'live in different clinical worlds, noticing and responding to different directives for action' (Benner et al, 1992, p. 13). According to these investigators, this clinical world is shaped by experience that teaches nurses to make qualitative distinctions in practice. They also found that beginner nurses were more task-oriented, while those with more experience focused on understanding their patients and their illness states.

Research findings of studies related to clinical reasoning

Studies of nurses' clinical judgement, problem solving, decision making, and intuition have contributed to the understanding gained from studies of nurses' clinical reasoning.

Clinical judgement studies

Nurses' clinical judgement represents a composite of traits that assists them in reasoning (Tanner, 1987). Benner et al's (1992) previously cited hermeneutic study described characteristics of clinical judgement exhibited by critical care nurses with varying levels of practice experience when they reasoned about patient care. Characteristics of clinical judgement identified in the most experienced subjects included: (1) the ability to recognize patterns in clinical situations that fit with patterns they had seen in other similar clinical cases; (2) a sense of urgency related to predicting what lies ahead; (3) the ability to concentrate simultaneously on multiple, complex patient cues and patient management therapies; and (4) an aptitude for realistically assessing patient priorities and nursing responsibilities.

In an earlier study designed to identify the role of intuition in experienced nurses' clinical judgement, Benner and Tanner (1987) identified six characteristics of intuitive judgement: pattern recognition, similarity recognition, commonsense understanding, skilled know-how, sense of salience, and deliberative rationality. They proposed that: 'In real life, these aspects cannot be separated. They work together in synergy in what seems to be a necessary combination of conditions for expert intuitive judgement (Benner and Tanner, 1987, pp. 23–31). They describe *pattern recognition* as the ability to perceive relationships between concepts in order to identify a pattern that has relevance in care provision. *Similarity recognition* is defined as the ability to recognize resemblances of a patient case or a clinical problem to previously encountered cases and problems. *Commonsense understanding* is defined as the ability to grasp the cultural, and emotional meaning of a patient's illness in addition to the physiological. *Skilled know-how* represents cognitive abilities that were acquired through clinical experience. *Sense of salience* is described as the ability to distinguish between important and unimportant observations and events. Finally, *deliberative rationality* is described as a strategy for maximizing judgement by not limiting oneself to a single interpretation of a given situation, but instead considering several possible explanations.

The characteristics of clinical judgement that have been identified by Benner and Tanner (1987) and Benner et al (1992) assist in our understanding of nurses' clinical reasoning by identifying and describing some of the cognitive traits, or skills, that nurses use during reasoning. This will help further theoretical development related to nurses' clinical reasoning that is needed to improve nursing education and practice. Thus, if we can describe and explain the cognitive skills that experienced nurses use when reasoning, we can begin to devise ways to teach these skills to nursing students and to further develop these skills in nurses in practice.

Problem-solving and decision-making studies

One of the primary objectives of clinical reasoning is to make decisions to maintain patient stability and resolve clinical problems. Thus, research on nurses' problem solving and decision making provides understanding about the processes involved in nurses' clinical reasoning.

Baumann and Bourbonnais (1982) used semi-structured interviews to examine the decision making abilities of 50 critical care nurses at varying levels of expertise. They found that knowledge and experience were the most important factors influencing nurses' decision making. In a replication of that study, using 24 coronary care nurses, Bourbonnais and

Baumann (1985) found that experience was vital to effective decision making. Relying on their experience, the nurses in this study described how they 'anticipated' emergencies that might occur. This strategy is very similar to *predictive reasoning* (i.e. anticipating patient responses and outcomes based on current and past information and previous experience). Predictive reasoning is a process identified by Fonteyn and Fisher (1992) in their study of expert critical care nurses' decision making during the care of critically-ill patients immediately after major surgery. These investigators also described subjects' use of two other reasoning processes: *backward reasoning* (i.e. searching the available data for support or substantiation of a clinical hunch when the working plan of care fails to provide an explanation for new data), and *forward reasoning* (i.e. incorporating new facts into the working plan of care to further refine the plan in order to meet the goals of care). Studies such as these assist in identifying the specific processes that nurses commonly use to make clinical decisions and therefore further overall theoretical understanding of nurses' clinical reasoning.

Intuition studies

Several investigators have proposed that intuition is an important part of nurses' reasoning processes (Pyles and Stern, 1983; Rew, 1990). Pyles and Stern (1983) conducted a qualitative, exploratory study to examine the decision making in a group of critical care nurses with varying levels of expertise. The investigators described the 'gut feelings' their subjects experienced as 'the sensory impression of the patient' (Pyles and Stern, 1983, p. 54), which they felt was as important to nurses' reasoning as their formal knowledge about patient cases. Many of the subjects in this study said they used these gut feelings to temper information from specific clinical cues. The subjects also emphasized the importance of previous clinical experience in developing intuitive skills.

In a qualitative study of 25 expert critical care nurses, Rew (1990) demonstrated the important role that intuition played in their reasoning and decision making. Subjects described their intuitive experiences as strong feelings of perceptions about their patients, about themselves and responding to their patients, or about anticipated outcomes, that they sensed without going through an analytical reasoning process.

The applicability of findings from studies such as these (about nurses' use of intuition in reasoning) to theoretical understanding of nurses' clinical reasoning is limited because of an incomplete description of nurses' intuition. The findings of these and similar studies of nurses' intuition (Agam, 1987; Rew and Barrow, 1987) suggest that intuition is closely associated with nurses' experience with specific patient cases. Thus, it would follow that the more experience nurses have with particular cases, the more they will use their intuition to guide their reasoning and decision making, and vice versa.

A longitudinal study currently in progress will test this assumption (Fonteyn and Fisher, 1992). The investigators are examining clinical reasoning in a group of highly experienced critical care nurses during episodes when they care for patients representing clinical cases with which they have had a great deal of experience, and during episodes when they care for patients representing clinical cases with which they have had almost no experience. The subjects think aloud while reasoning during actual episodes of patient care provision, and these verbal data are captured on a small tape recorder that the nurses carry in their pocket. Preliminary findings from this study show that subjects use a repertoire of sophisticated reasoning strategies (heuristics) when caring for and reasoning about patients representing clinical cases with which they have had a great deal of experience, and use considerably fewer and less sophisticated strategies when caring for patients representing cases with which they have had almost no experience. The investigators believe that further analysis of their data may reveal the association between nurses' intuition and reasoning skills, as well as the extent to which experience with specific clinical cases enhances these skills.

Clinical reasoning studies

Findings from Padrick et al's (1987) study examining nurses' reasoning revealed that, similar to physicians, much of nurses' reasoning efforts focus on generating diagnostic hypotheses. The investigators found that nurses' diagnostic reasoning consists of: (1) narrowing the search field, or problem sensing; (2) activation of diagnostic hypotheses that explain some or all of the cues presented; (3) systematic data gathering related to each hypothesis; and (4) evaluation of the hypothesis. These results provide support for the usefulness of the nursing process in guiding nurses' reasoning, which is currently the subject of much debate (as was discussed earlier in this chapter).

In contrast, findings from a study of expert critical care nurses' clinical reasoning (Fonteyn, 1991b; Fonteyn et al, 1991; Fonteyn and Grobe, 1993) showed that most of nurses' reasoning tasks are not aimed at diagnosis and hypotheses generation. Rather, nurses reason to distinguish between relevant and irrelevant patient data, to determine the significance of patient data, and to make decisions that assist in accomplishing the overall treatment plan for each patient. This study also provides a description of nurses' reasoning strategies (heuristics).

Heuristics are mental rules of thumb that assist in reasoning and are acquired over time through multiple experiences with similar patient cases (Bourbonnaise and Baumann, 1985; Koloder and Koloder, 1987; Grant and Marsden, 1987; Patel et al, 1989; Joseph and Patel, 1990; Fonteyn and Grobe, 1993; Fisher and Fonteyn, 1993). The heuristics that were identified by Fonteyn and Grobe (1993) included: *pattern matching* (i.e. the recognition of similarities of patient conditions, problems, and responses to those encountered in caring for previous similar cases); *attending* (i.e. distinguishing, from all available data, those indicators that are most relevant to maintaining patient stability); and *listing* (i.e. enumerating a list of items considered relevant to the working plan of care).

Again, preliminary findings from Fonteyn and Fisher's (1992) longitudinal study examining the reasoning used by a group of expert critical care nurses while they care for critically ill patients immediately after surgery identified the above described heuristics, as well as several others: *focused questioning* (i.e. puzzling over information, searching for more information, or checking hunches to assist in meeting the goals of care), *weighing* (i.e. evaluating the importance or value of patient data in order to determine its meaning and to decide what actions to take), and *anchoring* (i.e. using knowledge from previous cases to determine which pattern best fits the current situation, in order to formulate initial clinical hunches).

Classic studies of heuristic use by cognitive psychologists Tversky and Kahneman (1974; 1977; 1981) have shown that although the use of heuristics may facilitate efficiency in reasoning, and usually results in more effective decision making, heuristic use can also lead to biases, and result in reasoning errors. These biases have yet to be demonstrated in nursing research.

Future directions of research examining nurses' clinical reasoning

Despite the research that has already been done, the nature of nurses' clinical reasoning remains unclear. One explanation for the lack of clarity may be the continued propensity for investigators to study nurses' clinical reasoning outside the clinical arena, using either simulation, questionnaires, or interviews. The fullest and most accurate description of nurses' clinical reasoning will be obtained when reasoning is studied in the clinical area at the time it is occurring during care provision. Until recently, however, investigators have avoided this approach because it was thought to be either logistically impossible or a risk to patient care.

Fisher and Fonteyn (1993) demonstrated that it is both logistically possible and safe to study nurses' clinical reasoning in the clinical setting during the time that care is being given. Using a triangulated method, consisting of guided interviews, participant observation, and think aloud technique, the investigators collected data from a group of expert critical care nurses while they were providing postoperative care to critically ill patients. Findings from this pilot study suggest that a tremendous amount of rich, relevant data about nurses' reasoning can be obtained using this method. Moreover, studying nurses' reasoning in the clinical setting does not appear to compromise patient care nor disrupt either subjects' or unit functioning.

Future studies of nurses' clinical reasoning that use methods that examine reasoning in the clinical setting while care is being given to real (not simulated) patients will assist in completing the description of this phenomenon. Subsequent to this, studies should be initiated that examine the relationship between nurses' clinical reasoning and other variables, such as level of expertise, domain knowledge, the climate in which the reasoning and decision making take place, patient stability, and patient outcomes. Some of the important questions that future studies should address are: How is nurses' reasoning related to their sense of autonomy and job satisfaction? How is clinical reasoning related to expertise and level of knowledge within a domain? What factors are associated with optimal reasoning? What is the relationship between nurses' clinical reasoning and patient outcomes? Later, as the state of the science evolves from research that provides answers to these questions, experimental studies can be undertaken to provide answers to additional questions, such as: Is nurses' reasoning improved with increased autonomy or job satisfaction? Can nurses be taught strategies that will improve their reasoning? Can methods be devised to improve nurses' reasoning outside their domain knowledge? Do strategies to improve nurses' reasoning result in improved patient outcomes?

Educational focus on clinical reasoning

Critical thinking

Nurses increasingly need well-developed reasoning skills to assist them in understanding and resolving the complex patient problems encountered in practice. In their test entitled *Developing Clinical Problem-Solving Skills*, Barrows and Pickell (1991, p. 3) remind us that: 'ambiguities and conflicting or inadequate information are the rule in medicine'. This is equally true in nursing, where dealing with complex patient problems with uncertain and unpredictable outcomes requires continuous astute reasoning and accurate and efficient decision making. The cognitive skills that today's nursing students need to learn in order to reason accurately and make decisions effectively in practice are causing nurse educators to adjust their teaching methods. They are beginning to shift from reliance on the more traditional didactic methods of teaching to more creative teaching methods designed to improve students' reasoning skills and to furnish them with a repertoire of creative approaches to care (Fitzpatrick, 1991; Parfitt, 1989; Shamian, 1991).

Much of nursing education literature has begun to focus on ways to teach critical thinking. In a review examining 'articles written and research conducted pertinent to critical thinking in nursing', Beck et al (1992, p. 3) formed the following conclusions:

(1) The variables that correlate most strongly with critical thinking abilities of nursing students are: maths and science ability and score on an instrument, the Watson Glaser Critical Thinking Appraisal (WGCTA), designed to measure critical thinking skills.
(2) Some studies have demonstrated that nursing education improves critical thinking ability, while others have not.
(3) There have been numerous studies that indicate that baccalaureate degree nursing students demonstrate higher critical thinking abilities than associate degree or diploma nursing students, as measured by the WGCTA.
(4) There have been studies that show a positive correlation between nurses' skills in critical thinking and in making moral judgement.

For greater detail regarding these studies, readers should read the original report by Beck et al (1992), but despite their finding similar results across most of the studies examined in this review, Beck et al (1992) warn educators against over reliance on any single study. Most of the studies reviewed had convenience samples composed of volunteers, and none of the studies replicated previous research. Additional concerns expressed by Beck et al (1992) were that a tool to measure critical thinking that is content-specific to nursing has yet to be developed, and that the outcome variable most commonly used to measure success in nursing education has been a passing score on the state board exams, which does not directly measure nurses' critical thinking skills. Additionally, the authors of this review perceived a need for clearer definitions of such terms as problem solving, thinking, reasoning, clinical judgement, and critical thinking, so that research examining nurses' reasoning can be organized to form a meaningful body of knowledge for the profession.

Current nursing education literature often focuses on efforts to improve students' critical thinking skills. Holbert and Abrahm (1988) recommended that nursing educators should strive to teach and reinforce the use of higher order thinking abilities. Casebeer (1991) and Fonteyn and Flaig (1994) proposed using case studies to improve nursing students' reasoning skills. From case studies, students can learn to identify potential patient problems, suggest nursing actions, and describe outcome variables that would allow them to evaluate the effectiveness of their actions. Case studies provide the advantage of allowing nurse educators to give continuous feedback in the safe environment of simulation, and many others have supported their use (Greener, 1988; Barrows and Pickell, 1991; Kassirer and Kopelman, 1991; Shamian, 1991; Tanner, 1991). To increase their realism, case studies can be designed to provide information in chronological segments that more closely reflect real-life cases, where clinical events and outcomes evolve over time (Fonteyn, 1991b).

Other methods that have been suggested by nurse educators to improve students' critical thinking skills include: clinical experience, conferences, computer simulations, clinical logs, decision analysis, discussion, reflection, role modelling, role playing, and writing position papers (Tanner, 1987; Thiele and Sloan, 1987; Shamian, 1991; Miller and Malcolm, 1992).

Future directions of educational efforts related to nurses' clinical reasoning

In the future, educators must strive to devise additional methods to develop and improve nurses' clinical reasoning. This will, no doubt, require further changes in the structure and function of nursing curriculum. Students need to learn to improve how they identify significant clinical data and how they determine the meaning of data in regard to patient problems. They also need to learn how to reason about patient problems in ways that facilitate decisions about problem resolution.

Educators are realizing that the body of clinical knowledge and information is increasing too rapidly to expect that students can possibly remember all of the information that they will need for practice. Moreover, possessing an encyclopedic memory of facts and concepts will not ensure effective clinical reasoning.

Problem-based learning develops students' ability to continuously reflect on their reasoning and decision-making during patient care, and leads to self-improvement through practice.

Once students have developed their reasoning skills in this manner, they can then apply them while caring for real patients in the clinical setting. Fonteyn and Flaig (1994) advocate that educators temper the practice of requiring nursing students to write lengthy care plans focusing on the nursing process. Rather, they suggest teaching students to reason and plan care in the same manner as practising nurses. In practice, nurses first identify (from data initially obtained in report form and confirmed by patient assessment) the most important patient problems to focus on during their nursing shift. They include information from the patient, their families, and other members of the health care team in a plan of care that will assist in resolving the problems identified. As their shift progresses, they continuously evaluate and refine their plan of care based on additional data obtained either from further patient assessment, additional clinical data, and information from all individuals involved in carrying out the plan of care.

The use of computer assisted instruction (CAI) is another way that students can improve their reasoning skills. CAI programs can save educators time and effort while, at the same time, providing high-quality instruction that is intellectually challenging (Junge and Assal, 1993). CAI offers another means of providing problem-based learning for students, by using an electronic computer to combine self-paced individual and small-group learning.

In addition to traditional CAI programs, an increasing number of interactive videodisk (IVD) programs are being developed that augment learning by demonstrating, explaining, and providing reviews of nursing skills and procedures (Caldwell, 1992). It is predicted that faculty will begin to place greater reliance on the use of IVD programs for teaching repetitive tasks so that they can concentrate on developing students' reasoning and problem-solving skills.

Practice

The ultimate goal of both research and educational endeavours related to clinical reasoning in nursing is to improve nurses' reasoning in practice and, ultimately, to achieve more positive patient outcomes. Nursing literature suggests that nurses' reasoning and interventions have a significant effect on patient outcome (Marek, 1989; Bond and Thomas, 1991;

Jennings, 1991; Naylor et al, 1991; Nielsen, 1992). The relationship between nurses' reasoning and patient outcome will remain unclear, however, until the specific patient outcome indicators associated with nurses' reasoning have been identified, until the measurements of these indicators have been explicated, and until their impact on patient mortality and morbidity has been demonstrated through research. If nursing is to continue to play a proactive role in health care provision, it is essential to identify the role that nurses' reasoning and decision making has regarding overall patient outcome.

In this chapter, outcome is seen as the expected changes in predetermined patient-related factors, such as health status, behaviour, or level of knowledge, following the completion of nursing care (Redfern and Norman, 1990). A major difficulty in demonstrating the influence of nurses' reasoning on patient outcomes is the complex nature of the outcomes, which span a broad range of effects or presumed effects that are influenced not only by nursing and other health care providers, but by many other variables, including time, environmental conditions, support systems and patient history.

Computer support of nurses' reasoning in practice

Decision support systems and expert systems are currently being developed to assist nurses in practice to reason more efficiently and to make better clinical decisions. Such systems help nurses to manage large amounts of patient data, to distinguish between relevant and irrelevant data, and to use data to reason and make decisions about patient care. Decision support systems assist nurses to aggregate data, identify options for clinical decisions, and select appropriate courses of action. Expert systems provide symbolic representation of expert specialist knowledge that users can consult for advice about how to reason through a patient care dilemma, and for suggested courses of action and their rationale. Such systems also provide a mechanism for the user to enter information about the effects of actions, which are then incorporated into the system's knowledge base for future use.

Expert system development began in research laboratories in the mid-1970s and was first implemented in commercial and practical endeavours in the early 1980s (Frenzel, 1987). A few systems are beginning to be used in nursing practice. Creighton Online Multiple Modular Expert System (COMMES) assists nurses in identifying nursing diagnoses and developing care plans (Evans, 1988; Petrucci and Petrucci, 1991; Ryan, 1985). Another system, Computer-Aided Nursing Diagnosis and Intervention (CANDI) also assists nurses to formulate nursing diagnoses (Chang, 1988). The HELP Patient Care Information System, developed at the University of Utah, facilitates the scheduling of nursing staff, and can also help with care planning (Bradshaw et al, 1988). A Research Knowledge System (ARKS) is a system being developed to store, manage, and restructure the knowledge from nursing's scientific literature into a more useful form for easy access and application. This system is already used by doctoral students and faculty (Graves, 1990), and is currently being tested in practice (Bostrom, 1993, personal communication).

Until recently, expert systems required special programming languages and were designed to cover broad, rather than specific, domains in nursing. Both of these factors made development complicated, expensive, and time consuming. Expert system shells, coupled with a trend to focus on the more concise nursing problems encountered within a specific area of nursing practice will provide a means to expedite and facilitate the growth and development of expert systems for use in nursing practice (Petrucci and Petrucci, 1991). Two systems that have already been developed using expert shells are: the Urological Nursing Information System (UNIS), a system designed to assist nurses in planning care for incontinent patients, and CAREPLAN, a system designed to assist nurses caring for postpartum patients (Petrucci and Petrucci, 1991).

Future directions in practice related to nurses' clinical reasoning

The relationship between nurses' reasoning and patient outcomes should receive greater attention in the future in order to demonstrate the important role that nurses play in health care delivery. There will be increasing need to develop meaningful data sets related to patient outcomes. These data sets should contain the nursing actions that nurses commonly choose after reasoning about specific patient pro-

blems, and their associated patient outcomes. Prior to the development of these data sets, the indicators of patient outcome that are related to nurses' reasoning and decision making need to be identified and described in a manner that facilitates their measurement.

Computerized support systems will play an increased role in assisting nurses to reason, make decisions about appropriate nursing actions, and evaluate their impact on patient outcome. Although only a select portion of the nursing profession will be directly involved in system development, all nurses need to be knowledgeable enough about these systems to be able to be actively involved in their design and implementation in practice. Additionally, all nurses should understand enough about these systems to be able to effectively use them in their practice.

Conclusion

Both nursing and society would benefit from an improvement in nurses' clinical reasoning that would result in improved patient care and more positive patient outcomes. There are currently no uniform models of nurses' reasoning, nor do we adequately understand the variation in performance across levels of expertise or areas of practice. The information presented in this chapter offers a comprehensive perspective on what is currently known about nurses' clinical reasoning, and provides suggestions about future directions in research, education, and practice that will increase our understanding of this important phenomenon.

References

Agam, R. (1987) Intuitive knowing as a dimension of nursing. *Advances in Nursing Science*, **10**, 63–70

Aspinall, M. (1979) Use of a decision tree to improve accuracy of diagnosis. *Nursing Research*, **28**, 182–185

Barrows, H. and Pickell, G. (1991) *Developing Clinical Problem-Solving Skills*. W. W. Norton, New York

Baumann, A. and Bourbonnais, F. (1982) Nursing decision making in critical care. *National Health Development Program*. File No. 66606-1938-55, Canada

Beck, S., Bennett, A., McLeod, R. and Molyneaux, D. (1992) Review of research on critical thinking in nursing education. In *Review of Research in Nursing Education*,

Vol V (ed. L. Allan). National League for Nursing, New York, Pub. No. 15-2448

Benner, P., Tanner, C. and Chesla, C. (1992) From beginner to expert: Gaining a differentiated clinical world in critical care nursing. *Advances in Nursing Science*, **14**, 13–28

Benner, P. and Tanner, C. (1987) Clinical judgement: How expert nurses use intuition. *American Journal of Nursing*, **87**, 23–31

Bond, S. and Thomas, L. (1991) Issues in measuring outcomes of nursing. *Journal of Advanced Nursing*, **16**, 1492–1502

Bourbonnais, F. and Baumann, A. (1985) Crisis decision making in coronary care: A replication study. *Nursing Papers Perspectives in Nursing*, **17**, 4–19

Bradshaw, K., Sitting, D., Gardner, R., Pryor, T. and Bredd, M. (1988) Improving efficiency and quality in a computerized ICU. In *Proceedings of Twelfth Annual Symposium on Computer Applications in Medical Care* (ed. R.A. Greenes). IEE Computer Society Press, Los Angeles, pp 763–768

Caldwell, J. (1992) Preparing for the next 5 years of instructional technology. *Microworld*, **6**, 9–11

Casebeer, L. (1991) Fostering decision making in nursing. *Journal of Nursing Staff Development*, **7**, 271–274

Chang, E. (1988) CANDI: A knowledge-based system for nursing diagnosis. *Computers in Nursing*, **7**, 222–227

Corcoran, S. (1986) Planning by expert and novice nurses in cases of varying complexity. *Research in Nursing and Health*, **9**, 155–162

Evans, S. (1988) Nursing applications of an expert system for nursing diagnosis. In *Integrating Computers into Nursing Care* (eds M. Ball, K. Hannah, H. Peterson and U. Gerdin-Jelger). Springer, New York, pp. 309–313

Fisher, S. and Fonteyn, M. (1993) Use of triangulated method to describe and compare two diverse clinical settings: Critical care and psychiatric emergency. In *1993 Nursing Research Congress Abstracts. Advances in International Nursing Scholarship*. Omnipress, Madison, Wisconsin, p. 92

Fisher, S. and Fonteyn, M. (1994) Heuristic use associated with nurses' clinical reasoning. (In review.)

Fitzpatrick, J. (1991) How can we enhance nursing knowledge and practice? *Nursing and Health Care*, **10**, 517–521

Fonteyn, M. (1991a) Implications of clinical reasoning studies for critical care nursing. *Focus on Critical Care*, **18**, 322–327

Fonteyn, M. (1991b) A descriptive analysis of expert critical care nurses' clinical reasoning. Doctoral dissertation, The University of Texas, Austin, Texas, USA

Fonteyn, M. and Cooper, L. (1994) The written nursing process: Is it still useful to nursing education? *Journal of Advanced Nursing*, **19**, 315–319

Fonteyn, M. and Fisher, S. (1992) The study of expert nurses in practice. Unpublished paper presented at Transformation Through Unity: Decision-making and Informatics in Nursing in Portland, Oregon on October 17, 1992 at the University of Oregon Health Science Centre, Portland, Oregon

Fonteyn, M. and Grobe, S. (1993) Expert critical care nurses' clinical reasoning under uncertainty: Representation, structure and process. In *Sixteenth Annual Symposium on Computer Applications in Medical Care* (ed. M. Frisse). McGraw-Hill, New York, pp. 405–409

Fonteyn, M., Grobe, S. and Kuipers, B. (1991) A descriptive analysis of expert critical care nurses' clinical reasoning. In *Nursing Informatics '91* (eds E. Hovenga, K. Hannah, K. McCormick and J. Roland). Springer-Verlag, New York, pp. 765–768

Frenzel, L. (1987) *Understanding Expert Systems*. Howard W. Sama & Company, Indianapolis, Indiana:

Glaser, R. and Chi, M. (1988) Overview. In *The Nature of Expertise* (eds M. Chi, R. Glaser and M. Farr). Lawrence Erlbaum, New Jersey, pp. XV–XXXVI

Grant, J. and Marsden, P. (1987) The structure of memorized knowledge in students and clinicians: An explanation for diagnostic expertise. *Medical Education*, **21**, 92–99

Graves, J. (1990) A research-knowledge system (ARKS) for storing, managing, and modeling knowledge from the scientific literature. *Advances in Nursing Science*, **13**, 34–45

Gray, R., Begg, C. and Greenes, R. (1984) Construction of receiver operating characteristic curves when disease verification is subject to selection bias. *Medical Decision Making*, **4**, 151–164

Greener, D. (1988) Clinical judgement in nurse midwifery. A review of the research with implications for education. *Journal of Nurse-Midwifery*, **33**, 261–268

Grier, M. (1976) Decision making about patient care. *Nursing Research*, **25**, 105–110

Grobe, S., Drew, J. and Fonteyn, M. (1991) A descriptive analysis of experienced nurses' reasoning during a planning task. *Research in Nursing and Health*, **14**, 305–314

Henderson, V. (1982) The nursing process – is the title right? *Journal of Advanced Nursing*, **7**, 103–109

Holbert, C. and Abrahm, C. (1988) Reflections on teaching generic thinking and problem solving. *Nurse Educator*, **13**, 23–27

Holzemer, W. and Henry, S. (1991) Care plans for people with HIV/AIDS: Confusion or consensus? *Journal of Advances in Nursing*, **16**, 1444–1455

Hughes, K. and Young, W. (1990) The relationship between task complexity and decision making consistency. *Research in Nursing and Health*, **13**, 189–197

Hurst, K., Dean, A. and Trickey, S. (1991) The recognition and non-recognition of problem-solving stages in nursing practice. *Journal of Advanced Nursing*, **16**, 1444–1455

Jennings, B. (1991) Patient outcome research: Seizing the opportunity. *Advances in Nursing Science*, **14**, 59–72

Johnson, D. (1959) A philosophy for nursing diagnosis. *Nursing Outlook*, **7**, 198–200

Johnson, E. (1988) Expertise and decision making under uncertainty: performance and process. In *The Nature of Expertise* (eds M. Chi, R. Glaser and M. Farr). Lawrence Erlbaum, New Jersey, pp. 209–228

Jones, J. (1988) Clinical reasoning in nursing. *Journal of Advanced Nursing*, 13, 185–192

Joseph, G. and Patel, V. (1990) Domain knowledge and hypothesis generation in diagnostic reasoning. *Medical Decision Making*, 10, 31–46

Junge, C. and Assal, J. (1993) Designing computer assisted instruction programs for diabetic patients: How can we make them really useful? In *Sixteenth Annual Symposium on Computer Applications in Medical Care* (ed. M. Frisse). McGraw-Hill, New York, pp. 215–219

Kassirer, J. and Kopelman, R. (1991) *Learning Clinical Reasoning*. Williams & Wilkins, Baltimore

Kassirer, J., Moskowitz, A., Lau, J. and Pauker, S. (1987) Decision analysis: A progress report. *Annals of Internal Medicine*, 106, 275–291

Kolodner, J. and Kolodner, R. (1987) Using experience in clinical problem solving: Introduction and framework. *IEEE Transactions on Systems, Man, and Cybernetics*, 17, 420–431

Marek, K. (1989) Outcome measurement in nursing. *Journal of Quality Assurance*, 4, 1–9

Miller, G. (1956) The magical number seven, plus or minus two: some limits on our capacity to process information. *The Psychological Review*, 63, 81–97

Miller, M. and Malcolm, N. (1992) Critical thinking in the nursing curriculum. *Nursing & Health Care*, 11, 67–73

Naylor, M., Munro, B. and Brooten, D. (1991) Measuring the effectiveness of nursing practice. *Clinical Nurse Specialist*, 5, 210–215

Newell, A. and Simon, H. (1972) *Human Problem Solving*. Prentice-Hall, New Jersey

Nielsen, P. (1992) Quality of care: discovering a modified practice theory. *Journal of Nursing Care Quality*, 6, 63–76

Norman, G. (1988) Problem-solving, solving problems, and problem-based learning. *Medical Education*, 22, 279–286

Padrick, K., Tanner, C., Putzier, D. and Westfall, U. (1987) Hypothesis evaluation: a component of diagnostic reasoning. In *Classification of Nursing Diagnosis: Proceedings of the Seventh Conference* (ed. A. McClane). C. V. Mosby, Toronto, Canada, pp. 299–305

Parfitt, B. (1989) A practical approach to creative teaching: an experiment. *Journal of Advanced Nursing*, 14, 655–677

Petrucci, K. and Petrucci, P. (1991) Expert systems and nursing. *Nursing Economics*, 9, 188–190

Phillips, L. and Rempusheski, V. (1985) A decision-making model for diagnosing and intervening in elder abuse and neglect. *Nursing Research*, 34, 134–139

Putzier, D., Padrick, K., Westfall, U. and Tanner, C. (1985) Diagnostic reasoning in critical care nursing. *Heart and Lung*, 14, 430–436

Pyles, S. and Stern, P. (1983) Discovery of nursing gestalt in critical care nursing: the importance of the grey gorilla syndrome. *Image: The Journal of Nursing Scholarship*, 15, 51–57

Radwin, L. (1990) Research on diagnostic reasoning in nursing. *Nursing Diagnosis*, 1, 70–77

Redfern, S. and Norman, I. (1990) Measuring the quality of nursing care: a consideration of different approaches. *Journal of Advanced Nursing*, 15, 1260–1271

Rew, L. (1990) Intuition in critical care nursing practice. *Dimensions of Critical Care Nursing*, 9, 30–37

Rew, L. and Barrow, E. (1987) Intuition: A neglected hallmark of nursing knowledge. *Annals of Nursing Science*, 10, 49–62

Ryan, S. (1985) An expert system for nursing practice. *Journal of Medical Systems*, 9, 29–41

Sackett, D., Haynes, R. and Tugwell, P. (1985) *Clinical Epidemiology: A Basic Science for Clinical Medicine*. Little, Brown and Company, Boston, MA

Shamian, J. (1991) Effect of teaching decision analysis on student nurses' clinical intervention decision making. *Research in Nursing and Health*, 14, 59–66

Tanner, C. (1991) Curriculum revolution: the practice mandate. *Nursing and Health Care*, 427–430

Tanner, C. (1987) Teaching clinical judgement. In *Annual Review of Nursing Research* (eds J. Fitzpatrick and R. Tauton). Springer, New York, pp. 153–174

Tanner, C. (1983) Research on clinical judgement. In *Annual Review of Nursing Research* (ed. W. Holzemer). National League of Nursing, New York, pp. 3–39

Thiele, J. and Sloan, B. (1987) A survey of methods nurse educators employ to teach clinical judgement and decision making. In *Clinical Judgement and Decision Making: The Future With Nursing Diagnosis* (eds. K. Hannah, M. Reimer, W. Mills and S. Letourneau). John Wiley & Sons, New York, pp. 242–244

Tversky, A. and Kahneman, D. (1974) Judgement under uncertainty: Heuristics and biases. *Science*, 285, 1124–1131

Tversky, A. and Kahneman, D. (1977) Features of similarity. *Psychological Review*, 84, 327–351

Tversky, A. and Kahneman, D. (1981) The framing of decisions and the psychology of choice. *Science*, 211, 453–458

Wilkinson, J. (1992) *Nursing Process in Action*. Addison-Wesley Nursing, Redwood City, CA

6

Clinical reasoning in physiotherapy

Mark Jones, Gail Jensen and Jules Rothstein

Reform in health care is emerging as an important international, political and economic issue which will affect the relationship between the consumer and the provider of health care services. Consumers will expect greater accountability, effectiveness and efficiency from the provider and practitioners must have a broad understanding of not only disease, but also the determinants of health such as environment, socioeconomic conditions, cultural beliefs and human behaviour. There will be increasing emphasis on prevention and promotion of healthy lifestyles as well as involvement of patients/clients and families in the decision making process (Pew Health Commission, 1992). Physiotherapists, like other health practitioners, will be forced to handle the complex demands of this practice environment. Technical knowledge alone will be insufficient to solve the problem, as practitioners will also need to take 'wise action' in the face of uncertainty.

Clinical reasoning refers to the thought processes associated with a clinician's examination and management of a patient or client. Clinical reasoning is influenced by the therapist (e.g. needs and goals, values and beliefs, knowledge, cognitive, interpersonal and technical skills), the patient (e.g. values and beliefs, individual physical, psychological, social and cultural presentation), and the environment (e.g. resources, time, funding, and any externally imposed requirements). Physiotherapists work with a multitude of problem situations, many of which can be characterized by complexity, uniqueness and ambiguity. The goal of physiotherapists' reasoning is wise action. Wise action means making the best judgement in a specific context (Cervero, 1988).

The current focus on clinical reasoning is consistent with physiotherapy's continued growth as a profession. One of the key traits of a profession, autonomy, implies that the profession has a defined body of knowledge and has expertise in that domain. Professional expertise is not merely application of theoretical or research based knowledge in practice. Expertise evolves from professionals' use of critical analysis during and after their interaction with their patients, often in unclear or indeterminate situations (Schon, 1983; Kennedy, 1987; Cervero, 1988). For physiotherapists, expertise develops in part through clinical reasoning.

The growing interest in physiotherapy clinical reasoning is evident in the increasing representation of clinical reasoning theory papers and educational models in the physiotherapy literature aimed to facilitate clinical reasoning (e.g. Barr, 1977; May, 1977; May and Newman, 1980; Newman Henry, 1985; Wolf, 1985; Rothstein and Echternach, 1986; Dennis and May, 1987; Van der Sijde et al, 1987; Burnett and Pierson, 1988; Grant et al, 1988; Rose 1989a; Slaughter et al, 1989; Jones, 1989;

1992, 1994; Jones and Butler, 1991; Jones et al, 1994, Watts, 1989; Higgs, 1990; 1992a; 1992b; 1993; Shepard and Jensen, 1990; Terry and Higgs, 1993). However, physiotherapy research in clinical reasoning is still limited (e.g. Payton, 1985; Thomas-Edding, 1987; Jensen et al, 1990; 1992; May and Dennis, 1991; Christensen, 1993; Zvulun, 1993).

This chapter draws on physiotherapy research and theory in clinical reasoning, as well as findings and views outside of physiotherapy, to discuss the nature of clinical reasoning in physiotherapy. Educational issues pertaining to teaching clinical reasoning are not discussed here as this is covered in Sections 3 and 4 of this book. Future directions for physiotherapy with respect to clinical reasoning are dealt with in Chapter 27.

From problem-solving steps to cognition

As part of physiotherapy's professional awareness and maturing, efforts have been made to provide structured accounts of the clinical decision making steps taken by expert clinicians (e.g. May and Newman, 1980; Newman Henry, 1985; Wolf, 1985; Rothstein and Echternach, 1986; Echternach and Rothstein, 1989). As an example, Rothstein and Echternach (1986) proposed a conceptual model of clinical reasoning to logically guide therapists' evaluation and treatment planning activities. Their hypothesis-oriented model highlighted the following problem solving steps:

1. Collect initial data (e.g. interview, history, chart review, subjective examination)
2. Generate a problem statement and establish goals related to function and disability
3. Further data collection (e.g. physical examination
4. Generate working hypotheses about why goals are or cannot be met at the present time with testing criteria for each hypothesis
5. Plan re-evaluation methodology which includes examination of impairment and disability
6. Plan treatment strategy based on hypotheses
7. Plan tactics to implement strategy (i.e. specifics of treatment plan)
8. Implement tactics (i.e. treatment)
9. Reassessment (i.e. have goals been met?)
10. Continue or modify treatment or generate new hypotheses accordingly.

Support for the argument that physiotherapists go through the problem-solving steps as portrayed in the hypothesis-oriented algorithm by Rothstein and Echternach (1986) is available in a study by Payton (1985). Payton (1985) investigated the clinical reasoning of physiotherapists using the information processing methodology of retrospective stimulated recall. Ten expert physiotherapists (as nominated by one physical therapy academic faculty) were audio taped during a patient examination and the audio tape was then used to conduct a retrospective stimulated recall of the therapists' thoughts during the examination. The sequence of hypothesis formation and treatment planning was analysed. That is, the points were identified at which tentative and final hypotheses were formulated and plans were made. Payton (1985, pp. 926–927) demonstrated 'that a sample of skilled physical therapy clinicians go through essentially the same clinical reasoning process to generate physical therapy problem lists and treatment plans as some skilled physicians use to generate their problem lists and plans . . . physical therapists, like physicians, intermingled the steps of information gathering, problem list formation, and treatment planning'.

More recent discussions in the physiotherapy clinical reasoning literature have attempted to expand on the hypothesis-oriented algorithm through elaboration of the underlying cognition behind the various components of the problem solving process while highlighting the critical influences of knowledge, context and self monitoring, reflection or metacognitive skills (e.g. Higgs, 1990; 1992a; 1992b; Jensen et al, 1992; Jones, 1992; Jones et al, 1994). This is exemplified in Figure 6.1 which presents a model of the clinical reasoning process of physiotherapists as proposed by Jones (1992). This model is intended to provide a simple pictorial representation of clinical reasoning in physiotherapy. In all physiotherapy settings, the physiotherapist's reasoning begins with the initial data/cues obtained. For example, in a rehabilitation setting this may be a referral, case notes, observation of the patient in the waiting room as well as opening introductions

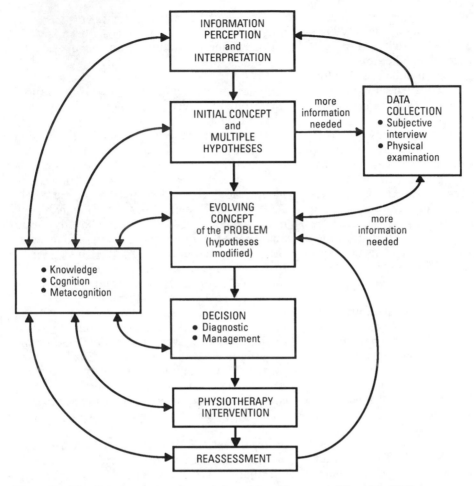

Figure 6.1   The clinical reasoning process (adapted from Barrows and Tamblyn, 1980)

and inquiries with the patient. This preliminary information will elicit a range of impressions or working interpretations. While typically not thought of as such, these can be considered hypotheses. The cognition involved in hypothesis generation includes a combination of specific data interpretations or inductions and the synthesis of multiple clues or deductions. In most settings the initial hypotheses will be quite broad such as 'looks like a back or hip problem' or 'looks like a major ambulation problem given the patient's deconditioned state and cognitive function'. Initial hypotheses may be physical, psychological or socially related with or without a 'diagnostic' implication.

All physiotherapists have an element of routine to their examination. Individual therapists will have identified through experience the categories of information which they have found to be particularly useful for problem identification and management decisions (e.g. site, behaviour and history of symptoms; family and social information; functional and structure specific tests of cognition, perception and the neuro-musculoskeletal system; ergonomic and environmental analysis; etc.). While a degree of routine commonly exists, specific inquiries and tests need to be tailored to each patient's unique presentation. Initial hypotheses will lead to certain inquiries and tests specific to that patient. This cognitive activity of hypothesis testing ideally includes the search for both supporting and negating evidence. The resulting data are then interpreted for their fit with previously obtained data and hypotheses considered. Even routine inquiries, tests and spontaneous information offered by the patient will be interpreted in the context of initial hypotheses. In this way the physiotherapist acquires an evolving understanding of the patient and the patient's problem. Initial hypotheses will be modified and new hypotheses considered. This hypothesis generation and testing process continues until sufficient information is obtained to make a diagnostic decision (i.e. identification of the source and underlying cause of the patient's impairments) and a management decision. The clinical reasoning process continues throughout the ongoing management. In particular, physiotherapy intervention serves as another test of hypotheses. Re-assessment either provides support for the hypotheses and chosen course of action or signals the need for hypothesis modification/generation or further data collection and problem clarification (e.g. additional physiotherapy examination or referral for other specialist consultation). At the micro level therapists are constantly reading patient responses and making in-treatment clinical decisions to modify and improvise their actions. At a macro level whole treatment sessions or even multiple treatments will be used to test management hypotheses.

The box to the left of Figure 6.1 highlights the strong relationship of the clinician's knowledge, cognition (e.g. data analysis and synthesis) and metacognition (i.e. awareness, self monitoring, reflective processes) with the process of clinical reasoning. Double headed arrows are used to convey that these factors influence all aspects of the clinical reasoning process and in turn are strengthened by clinical reasoning experience, particularly when clinicians think or reflect about what they do during and after a clinical encounter. Many clinicians, however, will be unaware of their use of this process. They may reason through a problem without recognizing the various aspects of their reasoning. They may also have reached a stage where a systematic process of reasoning is no longer used with many problems because past experience has enabled them to quickly identify problems and treatments. While awareness and understanding of one's own clinical reasoning is not essential to clinical practice, it is our view that by promoting awareness, reflection and critical appraisal, clinical reasoning can be enhanced.

An example of a type of hypothesis-directed inquiry used by therapists is seen in a study by Thomas-Edding (1987). In this study, 24 experienced (minimum of three years practical experience) and 24 novice (student) physiotherapists were videotaped during patient examinations. Each therapist was videotaped with two different simulated patients (one orthopaedic and one neurological). The analysis concentrated on quantification of the amount of time spent on various aspects of the evaluation process, and a qualitative description of the therapists' questions and comments made to the patient. The quantitative analysis revealed that experienced physiotherapists spent significantly more time with their patients. The qualitative analysis identified similarities between the experienced physiotherapist and the expert physicist or medical clinician. That is, while physiotherapy students appeared to conduct routine interviews, not specifically tailored to the individual patient, the experienced therapists attended to patient cues which then served to guide their subsequent data collection and interpretation. Also, rather than simply amassing information, the experienced therapists attempted to obtain a global picture of each condition.

Clinical reasoning models such as those proposed by Rothstein and Echternach (1986) and Jones (1992) need further investigation to establish their validity in relation to actual practice and to identify how clinical reasoning differs betwen expert (highly effective and efficient managers of patient problems) and non-expert clinicians. Chapter 1 in this book presents a spiral analogy as an attempt to further portray the integrated aspects of clinical reasoning which dynamically occur at varying process levels. The value of any conceptual model of clinical reasoning is to promote consideration, awareness and further exploration of the process's inherent elements and the significance such a process has for patient care. At a time when physiotherapy is still guilty of teaching and applying practice routines and protocols without adequate critical analysis and reflection, conceptual models of clinical reasoning make the less considered cognitive processes associated with problem-solving more accessible while challenging researchers, educators and clinicians to investigate, facilitate and strive to improve their own clinical reasoning.

Hypothetico-deductive reasoning or pattern recognition

Because the study of clinical reasoning in physiotherapy is a developing field of investigation, it is reasonable to turn to research and considerations in other similar professions in order to further discuss issues related to clinical reasoning that are equally relevant to physiotherapy. The physiotherapy research in clinical reasoning described provides some evidence that similarity exists, at least at a broad level, with clinical reasoning in medicine. That is, like medical clinicians, experienced physiotherapists do not simply collect patient data passively and follow non-specific treatment routines. Rather they actively reason through patient examination and treatment. Initial data collection elicits multiple hypotheses regarding the patient's problem(s) and treatment plans. Hypotheses are then tested through ongoing data collection (e.g. interview, physical examination, and treatment) and hypotheses are modified providing the therapist with an evolving understanding of the problem.

Consensus, however, has not been achieved within the medical literature regarding a single medical model of clinical reasoning (Feltovich and Barrows, 1984; Elstein et al, 1990; Groen and Patel, 1990). One of the models has portrayed clinical reasoning in medicine as a process of hypothetico-deductive reasoning (Elstein et al, 1978; Kassirer and Gorry, 1978; Barrows et al, 1978; 1982; Gale, 1982; Feltovich et al, 1984). In this model patient data elicit hypotheses which in turn are used to guide further inquiry. Initial hypotheses are then tested with on-going data collection. The seminal work of Elstein et al (1978) on medical problem solving revealed that both successful and unsuccessful diagnosticians utilized this process of hypothesis generation and testing.

Other authors have challenged this contention that clinical reasoning in medicine can be universally characterized as a hypothetico-deductive process (Berner, 1984; McGuire, 1984; Groen and Patel, 1985; 1990; Ridderikhoff, 1989; 1991). For example, Groen and Patel (1985) have suggested the clinical reasoning of experienced clinicians looks more like pattern recognition. Patel and colleagues (1986; 1989; 1990; 1991) demonstrated that accurate diagnosticians primarily used an inductive process of forward reasoning. Forward reasoning occurs when cues in the patient presentation serve to trigger a hypothesis or diagnosis. This is essentially a form of pattern recognition. Pattern recognition is based on the notion that the knowledge underlying clinical reasoning is stored in memory in the form of 'if . . . then . . . ' production rules (Greeno and Simon, 1986). That is, if certain features or conditions are present then certain diagnoses or management plans are elicited or recalled. The condition or 'if' of a production rule is a pattern of information that includes not only the features of the problem situation but also information held internally by the problem solver such as goals specific to that particular problem. Therefore when a problem is familiar, a set of rules can be accessed which will quickly lead to a solution. Forward reasoning is efficient, fast and dependent on a good knowledge base in the particular area of practice (Arocha et al, 1993).

Results from Patel et al's research (Patel and Groen, 1986; Patel et al, 1990; Patel and Groen, 1991) also demonstrated that clinicians used a combination of forward and backward reasoning in instances where diagnoses were incomplete or inaccurate. In backward reasoning, hypotheses elicit the re-interpretation of data against the hypotheses or the acquisition of new clarifying data. Hypothesis guided inquiry, where one reasons backward from hypothesis to data is equivalent to the hypothesis testing model described above. Arocha et al (1993) suggested backward reasoning occurs mainly when clinicians lack the knowledge to arrive at a solution based solely on pattern recognition of the presenting information. Backward reasoning is slow, cognitively demanding and generally more characteristic of the novice (Larkin et al, 1980; Arocha et al, 1993).

While the process of clinical reasoning in medicine is still being studied and clarified, it appears to involve a process of hypothesis generation followed by either hypothesis evaluation (e.g. hypothesis testing) and/or pattern recognition (Patel and Groen, 1986; 1991; Barrows and Feltovich, 1987). Whether hypothesis testing (i.e. backward reasoning) or pattern recognition (i.e. forward reasoning) is used will depend in part on the clinician's level of practical experience, knowledge and method of education as well as the nature of the clinical task itself (Arocha et al, 1993: Patel et al, 1991).

Clinical reasoning in physiotherapy should similarly involve a combination of hypothesis testing and pattern recognition. Pattern recognition is required to generate hypotheses, and hypothesis testing provides the means by which patterns are refined and proved reliable. But this may seem to over simplify what occurs when clinicians are faced with complex uncertain problem situations where physiotherapy management requires personal involvement (e.g. physical, emotional and social) in the patient's treatment. Problems often do not fit textbook presentations, and clinical rules of thumb do not always apply. Nor do all clinicians ascribe to the same rules. To better understand how clinical patterns are acquired and the nature of clinical patterns relevant to physiotherapy, key factors including knowledge, cognitive skills and context will be discussed further.

Key factors in clinical reasoning: considerations for physiotherapy

Clinical reasoning is influenced by factors relating to the specific task, the setting, the patient or client and the decision maker. May and Dennis provide an excellent discussion of these factors in Chapter 25. For purposes of this discussion we will only highlight certain critical aspects of those factors pertaining to the decision maker, including the knowledge base for decisions, the therapist's cognitive skills, and assessment of context.

Knowledge

Elstein et al (1978) found that clinical problem solving expertise varied greatly across cases and was dependent on clinicians' knowledge in a particular area. This highlighted the importance of clinicians' organization of knowledge more than the process of reasoning which has been continuously echoed throughout the literature (Barrows et al, 1978; 1982; Neufeld et al, 1981; Norman et al, 1982; Patel and Groen, 1986; 1991; Grant and Marsden, 1987; 1988; Cervero, 1988; Bordage et al, 1990; Bordage and Lemieux, 1991; Elstein et al, 1990; Schmidt and Boshuizen, 1993; Arocha et al, 1993). This view is exemplified by Custers et al (1993, p. 3) who stated 'for it is not the way problems are tackled, nor the thoroughness of

the investigation, nor the use of problem solving strategies, but the ability to activate the pertinent knowledge as a consequence of situational demands, which distinguishes experienced from inexperienced physicians'.

In physiotherapy, Hislop (1985, p. 29) concurred that 'clinical decisions are based on knowledge readily understood, readily recalled, and commonly encountered'. She goes on to caution that therapists must not allow the untold growth of knowledge to subvert our interest in patients themselves. We must be critical of knowledge sought and keep in perspective what we need to know versus what is nice, marginal or irrelevant to know (Hislop, 1985). One way to tackle this is to consider what knowledge physiotherapists use for their evaluation and management of patients. Physiotherapists utilize various forms of knowledge in their clinical reasoning. These include basic science and biomedical knowledge, clinical knowledge (often in the form of recognized clinical patterns and if/then rules of action), everyday knowledge about life and social interactions and tacit knowledge of the profession. Some aspects of knowledge as it relates to clinical reasoning will be discussed here. For a more detailed discussion of knowledge see Chapter 10.

Critical to any profession is a distinct, specialized, theoretically based body of knowledge (Goode, 1969; Houle, 1984) often labelled declarative knowledge (Ryle, 1949; Cervero, 1988). Declarative knowledge includes that which is known or believed. It provides the substance on which patterns are recognized, diagnoses are made and clinical if/then rules are based. That is, theory, facts and general principles provide clinicians with rules of thumb which guide interpretations, actions and explanations (Shepard and Jensen, 1990). This empirical and theoretical base of knowledge is derived out of research and practice experiences (Shulman and Sykes, 1986).

A growing body of medical literature suggests that biomedical knowledge is not explicitly utilized by practising clinicians involved in diagnosing a familiar case (e.g. Patel and Groen, 1986; Patel et al, 1990)(1). This may be, as Boshuizen and Schmidt (1992) have proposed (2) that with increasing clinical experience biomedical knowledge becomes encapsulated in

(1) See also Chapter 9.
(2) See also Chapter 2.

clinical knowledge. While physiotherapists' use of biomedical knowledge in clinical reasoning has not been investigated, anatomical, biomedical and pathophysiological knowledge is presumed to underlie therapists' clinical decisions (Harris and Dyrek, 1989; Schenkman and Butler, 1989). However the extent to which this knowledge is consciously considered or referred to in discussion may prove to vary with the level of expertise and case familiarity and is likely to be strongly affected by the practice philosophy of the individual therapist.

Within clinical practice declarative knowledge can be thought of as procedural knowledge (Ryle, 1949; Cervero, 1988). Procedural knowledge is not just the recall of information, but a transformation of information requiring critical analysis and deliberate action (Cervero, 1988). The clinician must be able to critically analyse or recognize the situation in order to arrive at and apply the appropriate 'if . . . then . . . ' guides to action. Cervero (1988) emphasized that both declarative (e.g. theoretical, biomedical) and procedural (e.g. clinical) knowledge are required for skilled performance and sound clinical reasoning. Important to our ability to characterize the clinical reasoning of physiotherapists is the contention that in any field, a major difference between experts and non-experts is that experts have far more procedural knowledge (Gagne, 1985; Cervero, 1988). Declarative knowledge initially provides the data to guide action. However with experience and repetition clinicians are able to perform without having to access declarative knowledge in familiar cases. Of educational importance, procedural knowledge is acquired predominantly through direct practical experience. That is, knowledge is made particularly meaningful and accessible when it is created or acquired in the context for which it must be used (Tulving and Thomson, 1973; Rumelhart and Ortony, 1977; Cervero, 1988; Schon, 1983; 1987; Shepard and Jensen, 1990).

Based on studies of architects, town planners, scientists, psychotherapists and organizational managers Schon (1983; 1987) contended that the use of research-based knowledge does not differentiate the expert from the non-expert. Instead Schon described three kinds of procedural knowledge that are inherent in professional expertise, that is 'knowing-in-action', 'reflection-in-action' and 'reflection-about-action'. Most spontaneous actions that professionals take are not elicited by a rule or plan that was consciously in the mind before acting (Cervero, 1988). Schon refers to this as 'knowing-in-action'. That is, the actions, recognitions, and judgements of professionals are often a function of their tacit knowledge. The tacit knowledge experts possess has also been labelled intuition (Benner, 1984). Intuition is the recognition of a situation, including the appropriate response or decision, when the features of that situation are embedded in the clinician's actions and reasoning and difficult to identify. This form of knowing is learned through experience. Not simply experience in years but experience which has included 'reflection-in-action' and 'reflection-about-action' undertaken in indeterminate or uncertain situations. 'Reflection-in-action' refers to thinking about what you are doing while you do it. That is, as the clinician encounters a problem, he or she engages in a process of critical analysis that allows for self-correction or adaptation of their practice. It is typically used in situations of uncertainty or when unexpected results are obtained. For example, in the midst of working through a difficult problem clinicians may ask themselves 'What is the key problem here? What are the salient features? What are the most likely explanations? How could I test these further?', etc. This 'reflective conversation' with the situation involves on the spot experiments or what could also be called hypothesis generation and testing. Reflection-about-action is a similar process that occurs retrospectively as the clinician thinks back about what happened in practice. Clinical reasoning that is reflective will eventually lead to recognition of patterns hidden within the ambiguity of the presentation or the acquisition of new patterns not previously appreciated.

Cognitive skills

Along with the different forms of knowledge associated with decision making, cognitive skills (e.g. data analysis and synthesis and inquiry strategies) are essential skills for professionals. Practitioners must be able to identify and solve problems that are often in ambiguous or uncertain situations (Barrows and Feltovich, 1987; Kennedy, 1987; Elstein et al, 1990). In physiotherapy there is a growing interest in students' awareness, learning and development of cognitive skills (e.g. Hislop, 1985;

Shepard and Jensen, 1990; Grant, 1992; Higgs, 1992a, 1992b; Jones, 1992, 1994; Jones, in press; Terry and Higgs, 1993). While clinical expertise has been linked more to the clinician's organization of knowledge than the process of clinical reasoning used (Elstein et al, 1978; Patel and Groen, 1991), cognitive skills and knowledge are interdependent. For example the inquiry strategy of hypothesis testing (including confirming and disconfirming strategies), plays a significant role in the acquisition of knowledge (Lawson et al, 1991). While the expert may not need to engage in hypothesis testing with all problems, it provides the means by which textbook clinical patterns can be tested, refined and new patterns can be learned (Barrows and Feltovich, 1987). Novices, who lack sufficient knowledge to recognize clinical patterns will rely on the slower hypothesis testing approach to work through a problem, where experienced clinicians are able to function more on pattern recognition. When confronted with a complex, unfamiliar problem, however, the expert, like the novice, will rely more on the hypothetico-deductive (i.e. hypothesis testing) method of clinical reasoning (Barrows and Feltovich, 1987; Patel and Groen, 1991).

Errors in clinical reasoning are frequently related to errors in cognition. Examples of these include overemphasis on findings which support an existing hypothesis, misinterpreting non-contributory information as confirming an existing hypothesis, ignoring findings which did not support a favoured hypothesis, and incorrect interpretations related to inappropriately applied inductive and deductive logic (Elstein et al, 1978; Ramsden, 1985; Jones, 1992). An example of a cognitive error in data analysis and synthesis was demonstrated by Norman et al (1992). These researchers illustrated how both expert and resident radiologists could be biased to alter their disease probability ratings and reports of symptomatic features identified in both normal and abnormal films when the history was manipulated to bias toward a positive result (3). Bordage and colleagues suggest that most diagnostic errors are not the result of inadequate medical knowledge as much as an inability to retrieve relevant knowledge already stored in memory (Bordage and Allen, 1982; Bordage and Zacks, 1984; Bordage et al, 1990;

Bordage and Lemieux, 1991). Cognitive errors may contribute to the development of poorly organized knowledge. Thus any consideration of clinical reasoning in physiotherapy must incorporate attention to cognitive skills.

Context

Another key factor to understanding the clinical reasoning of physiotherapists is the context in which the problem exists and is manifested by the patient or client. Context refers to the particular set of conditions and events which are associated with the development and maintenance of a problem and those aspects of the individual's life (e.g. physical, psychological and social) which are in turn affected by the problem. Most medical models of clinical reasoning have been criticized for not taking account of context from the patient's perspective, that is, for being too narrowly focused on diagnosis (Mishler, 1984; Mattingly, 1991). Mattingly (1991) has described clinical reasoning in medicine as applied science or scientific reasoning, where knowledge and theory are used to generalize and classify patients' signs and symptoms into known physiological processes and diagnostic patterns. She suggests it is this generalizability which is the power of theory-based reasoning. The reasoning is directed toward classification and application of the best means (e.g. treatment) to reach the end (e.g. good health). But this may not always be congruent with the patient's concerns.

While acknowledging the value of decisions involving cause and effect to expedient and effective medical treatment, it can be argued that this model of reasoning is inadequate to account for the clinical reasoning that occurs in clinicians whose task is personal (i.e. physical, emotional and social) involvement in the treatment itself as opposed to predominantly diagnosis. The variation of presentations within a diagnostic category is endless. Hence direct physical involvement in the patient's treatment requires sensitivity to the individual context of each patient's presentation. While procedural rules exist to provide a broad level of guidance in relation to procedural (e.g. reflex inhibiting postures to reduce hyper-reflexia, techniques to facilitate relaxed breathing), and

(3) For further discussion on this study and the implications it holds for clinical reasoning in light of categorization theory, the reader is referred to Chapter 11.

professional (e.g. ethics, confidentiality) aspects of intervention, these rules are incomplete and therapists must be able to adapt their responses to the unique presentations of each patient.

As opposed to diagnosis, Mattingly (1991, p. 983) suggested that the principal task of occupational therapists is to treat the patient's 'illness experience'. She defines illness experience as 'the meaning that a disability takes on for a particular patient, that is, how disease and diability enter the phenomenological world of each person' and suggests that 'clinical reasoning, taken in this sense, becomes applied phenomenology'. The individual meaning patients give to their disability will significantly influence emotions, expectations, goals, motivation and involvement in the treatment process. Mattingly (1991) provided the example of an activity such as toilet transfer where attention to the patient's 'illness experience' requires more than attending to the motor and cognitive skills inherent in the task. Treating a person requires attending to that person's feelings about losing control over this previously simple and private task.

Mattingly's criticisms of the applicability of the diagnostically-oriented medical model of clinical reasoning to occupational therapy, warrant consideration when discussing the clinical reasoning of physiotherapists which has been similarly compared to the medical model. Physiotherapy has only begun to formally theorize, research, and teach clinical reasoning in the last fifteen years. As part of the process of understanding clinical reasoning in physiotherapy, we must maintain a broad concept of what is involved.

The studies of Payton (1985) and Thomas-Edding (1987) demonstrated that physiotherapists utilized hypothesis-oriented inquiries in their clinical reasoning. It is interesting to note that experts spent more time with patients in the Thomas-Edding (1987) study. This is not consistent with the medical literature's accounts of an expert. Studies of experts in medicine have demonstrated that thoroughness in data gathering is not necessarily correlated with diagnostic accuracy (Marshall, 1977; Barrows et al, 1978; Norman et al, 1982; Norman et al, 1985). In the study of experienced physiotherapists, the greater use of time by experts may have resulted from the nature of physiotherapy practice which is less diagnosis driven than medicine. Therapists were focused on gathering

contextual or global data in the initial evaluation. While such information may not focus predominantly on diagnosis it may relate to management possibilities and thus it is essential information for a clinician whose personal involvement in the physical, 'hands on' treatment requires understanding of the patient and the problem for optimal management. Payton (1985) and Thomas-Edding (1987) did not set out to illuminate the full scope of physiotherapy clinical reasoning. Further insight into more phenomenological aspects of physiotherapy clinical reasoning however is available from recent research by Jensen and colleagues (1990; 1992).

Jensen et al (1990; 1992) used a qualitative research design to investigate differentiating features of master and novice physical therapists in orthopaedic settings. Their second study (Jensen et al, 1992) is particularly relevant to this discussion. In this study the sample group included eight physical therapists with varying levels of experience (2–13 years). These researchers collected data through onsite observation of each clinician with at least three patients, audio taped evaluation and treatment sessions, patient interviews, interviews with clinicians regarding perceptions of their own decision making and clinical skill, and reviews of patient records.

The results of this study support the notion that physiotherapy clinical reasoning is phenomenological. Jensen et al (1992) reported that master clinicians not only collected data related to pathology that helped validate or invalidate a diagnosis, but also gathered illness data which reflected the patient's perception of how the disease affected their lives. Therapists were seen to attend to both quantitative and phenomenological measures of improvement, the latter being illustrated by a therapist's statement: 'if the patients do not perceive they have been helped, they have not been helped' (Jensen et al, 1992, pp. 711–722). Master clinicians also reported designing their exercise interventions not only to fit with their evaluation data, but to fit the patient's environment as well.

Similar to the findings of Payton (1985) and Thomas-Edding (1987), Jensen et al (1992) found that master physiotherapy clinicians varied their examination and treatment according to the individual presentation of each patient. Judgement was not withheld until the evaluation was complete, but rather data were interpreted (e.g. hypotheses were formed) as it arrived. These data assisted in guiding further data collection (e.g. 'we found that experienced therapists consistently built their questions on the patient's responses . . . ') and all data were reported to be correlated. Acquisition of patient data was geared toward identifying the structure at fault, but information regarding the patient's environment, work and recreational activities was also obtained. Correlating data can be considered a form of hypothesis testing. While some information assisted in developing hypotheses related to diagnosis, other information was more useful to management considerations.

Therefore clinical reasoning in physiotherapy can be seen as both a hypothetico-deductive and a phenomenological process. That is, for physiotherapists to reach their own form of impairment-oriented diagnosis (Sahrman, 1988; Rose, 1989b; Dekker et al, 1993), they must engage in some form of diagnostic reasoning. In order to successfully interact with the patient or client in the management process however, physiotherapists must also attend to the individual's unique personal experience.

Is the hypothesis testing/pattern recognition model of medical clinical reasoning appropriate for the more context-oriented phenomenological approach physiotherapists use? We believe that hypothesis testing/pattern recognition (hypothetico-deductive reasoning) is as equally applicable to clinical reasoning which is focused on the individual's personal experience as it is to diagnostic reasoning. Taking a phenomenological approach to patients' problems requires attention to both diagnostically and non-diagnostically related cues and requires pattern recognition beyond diagnosis. In diagnostic reasoning clinical cues elicit hypotheses which are either suffcient alone to elicit recognition of a syndrome, or are tested through further data collection. Similarly, when attending to non-diagnostic aspects of a problem, physiotherapists must be able to recognize and interpret cues and inquire further to better understand the context of the individual's illness or dysfunction, but also to broadly test the hypothesis of the pattern suspected.

Because psychological and social aspects of the individual's illness or problem experience also form patterns, previous reflective experience in similar situations will lead the physiotherapist to certain responses and treatments. This would be an example of clinical knowledge which has been generated from thinking about or reflecting on practice. This is not to suggest that there is a discrete set of patterns requiring a similarly discrete set of responses. Rather, features of patients' or clients' presentation, including the meaning their problem(s) or health hold for them personally, are recognized by experts who respond appropriately on the basis of their clinical judgement. When these features can be made more explicit however, it enables less experienced therapists to learn more efficiently from their mentors. While new and unpredicted variations of presentations will always occur, by reflecting on the presenting cues and correlating the pattern with the management success, therapists learn new clinical patterns (diagnostic, psychological, social, cultural, management). That is, therapists who use a hypothesis testing approach to their reasoning will learn from their own experiences.

Clinical reasoning in physiotherapy: an evolving model

Based on our discussion we propose a model of clinical reasoning for physiotherapy that is broadly depicted as hypothetico-deductive, but which also emphasizes the importance of considering the context of the patient or client. Acquisition of expertise in physiotherapy evolves from the use of both theoretical and clinical knowledge combined in reflective experiences. In this way both diagnostic and non-diagnostic patterns are continually tested and refined as new patterns are acquired.

This broader approach, to attend to all aspects of the patient's impairment, is consistent with recent arguments for a broader consideration of physiotherapy diagnosis. Jette (1989) and Guccione (1991) have advocated that conceptual models representing physical, psychological, social, and cultural dimensions of health and illness are very applicable to physiotherapy practice. These models can assist therapists in developing a problem classification scheme that is more suitable to actual practice where therapists deal with patients' impairments and function.

Clinical knowledge accounts for the bulk of what expert clinicians know and provides the direction and relevance to the basic sciences and research. Hislop (1985, p. 34) made this point when she stated 'clinical science is the parent of today's basic science . . . Studies of physical disability or disordered motion cannot occur until the disorder is adequately described, the pain demarcated, or the motion pattern circumscribed'. This is not to demean the value of theoretical, research-based knowledge. Such academic knowledge appears to be important in 'the development of coherence in the explanation of clinical phenomena (4),' and also plays a role in increasing the range of diagnostic and management options available (Cervero, 1988). Theoretical knowledge allows connections to be made between clinical presentation and diagnosis, management and prognosis. For example, application of knowledge regarding neuropathology and pain mechanisms often provides clinicians with greater understanding of clinical presentations including management and prognostic implications. Thus, while theoretical knowledge requires clinical significance to be practical, it also provides a mechanism by which clinical knowledge can be re-shaped.

One of the challenges for physiotherapy in the future will be the integration of a developing body of theoretical knowledge with an evolving body of clinical knowledge. Harris (1993, p. 35) summarizes this situation well for professions.

> What is the appropriate relationship of reflective practice, and its elements of knowing-in-action and reflection-in-action . . . the applied arts and crafts of a profession . . . with the specialized bodies of knowledge associated with each profession? Reflective practice and the use of specialized bodies of knowledge are entirely complementary. Each is essential for professional practice, especially in interdeterminate zones of practice.

Rose (1989b, p. 536) proposed the fundamental objective of a physiotherapist 'is to either prevent or remediate dysfunctions that are primarily, but not exclusively, of the movement system'. This requires a reasoning process which attends to the physical, psychological and social aspects of an individual's problem. Clinical reasoning through some problems will appear to be pure diagnostic reasoning (i.e.

primarily directed toward identification of impairment). For example, a patient with an acute antalgic posture of the neck can often be successfully treated in one or two appointments. Here diagnostic reasoning is essential to correctly recognize the clinical syndrome and subsequently choose an effective treatment. The patient's personal life will often not be significantly affected and thus this is not a major issue in the therapist's reasoning. In other situations (e.g. cerebrovascular accident) the medical diagnosis is already determined but the physiotherapist must still identify the specific patient impairments and disabilities. The patient may be diagnosed as having had a right middle cerebral artery occlusion. While the neuroanatomy of the brain provides the broad pattern of presentation this disorder would manifest, it is insufficient to reveal the individual patient's perceptual, cognitive and motor capabilities. In addition to understanding the patient's physical impairments, successful management of this patient would also require attention to how the patient and the patient's family are personally affected and coping with the disability. Analogously, successful treatment of many orthopaedic problems requires attention to motivational and environmental factors to effect a lasting change (e.g. posture correction, etc.). That is, physiotherapy like other health professions, must attend to the patient's health needs or 'illness experience'.

If physiotherapists attend to both diagnostic and non-diagnostic clinical patterns, a relevant philosophical and pedagogical question is, should students and clinicians attempt to improve their clinical reasoning by seeking specific categories of clinical information when engaged in problem solving? Curriculum design theory would support such a strategy provided those with a vested interest (e.g. faculty, students, clinicians) agree on the relevance, validity and intended purpose of the information categories (Harris, 1993).

To date there has been no research to clarify the different types of hypotheses physiotherapists should or do use in their clinical reasoning. However one model that could provide useful directions was proposed by Jones (1992). With support from the stakeholders within his teaching environment, Jones (1992)

---

(4) Patel and Kaufman, Chapter 9.

suggested that inquiries and clinical decisions made in manual therapy could be broadly categorized into the following hypothesis categories:

- Source of the symptoms
- Contributing factors
- Precautions and contra-indications to physical examination and treatment
- Prognosis
- Management

Jones (1992) has proposed that identifying the most effective management in manual therapy requires reasoning about each of these hypothesis categories. The particular information sought in each patient case is unique to that patient's presentation. The reasoning behind the inquiries and physical tests are ultimately aimed at 'wise action'. The purpose is to identify and deliver the most effective management for that patient. Therapists recognize patient cues which in turn elicit hypotheses in one or more category. Clinical patterns exist within all of the hypothesis categories. As patient cues emerge and specific hypotheses are considered, the hypotheses should be tested for the remaining features of the pattern through further patient inquiry, physical tests and ultimately with the physiotherapy intervention.

These hypothesis categories are not proposed as a definitive list. They should always be re-evaluated for usefulness and representativeness of what experts actually do. These particular hypothesis categories have recently been modified to better reflect the reasoning and pattern recognition associated with the mechanisms of pain as seen by manual therapists (Jones et al, 1994; Butler, 1994). Other hypothesis categories might be more appropriate for different patient populations. Within the above characterization of hypothesis categories, psychological, social and environmental patterns are considered within the hypotheses pertaining to contributing factors, prognosis and management. This classification may seem inappropriate for therapists who deal with patient problems in which these variables feature more strongly. We do not believe the same hypothesis categories necessarily reflect the reasoning and evaluation/management priorities of all physiotherapists. We would encourage physiotherapists however, to consider the reasoning behind their inquiries, tests and

interventions. From this reasoning it should be possible to broadly identify categories of clinical judgements (i.e. hypotheses) which need to be made through the problem solving process. This provides a framework from which experts can be asked to expound on their clinical insight and provides a structure through which clinical patterns can be questioned and new patterns learned. Less experienced therapists can be assisted in their clinical reasoning. Rather than following routines or the latest trend, therapists can learn clinical reasoning. Routines may still be effective, but with a hypothesis testing approach they will always be tailored to the appropriate patient situation and continually tested for their effectiveness.

The increasing call for health professionals to consider not only physical, but also psychological, social, cultural and environmental factors in their practice requires the professional to have self-monitoring skills or metacognitive skills. Professionals need self-monitoring skills in order to plan, control, and evaluate problem solving knowledge and methods (Hassebrock et al, 1993). They are necessary to optimize the clinician's ability to learn from experience. But how do professionals acquire these skills? Schon (1983) proposes that the processes of reflection-in-action and reflection-about-action are central to clinicians' improved awareness of what they know and how they know it. This is critical if clinicians are going to learn from experience. That is some clinicians will learn little or nothing from their own patient experiences, instead relying on literature and continuing education to acquire new information. Other clinicians will continually revise and expand their clinical knowledge through their reflective approach to patient care. Use of conceptual models for clinical reasoning such as those proposed by Rothstein and Echternach (1986), Higgs (1990) and Jones (1992) is one strategy that may facilitate the development of therapists' metacognitive skills. They encourage physiotherapists to learn a logical approach to thinking through patient problems, that is, to learn clinical reasoning that is reflective.

Conclusion

While a growing interest in physiotherapy clinical reasoning exists amongst physiotherapy clinicians and educators, physiotherapy research in clinical reasoning is still limited. This chapter has presented conceptual models and described research from both within and outside physiotherapy. An evolving model of clinical reasoning in physiotherapy was put forward that is broadly depicted as hypothetico-deductive, with consideration being given to the patient's entire illness or problem experience. This is particularly important in a profession like physiotherapy where clinicians are personally (physically, professionally, emotionally and socially) involved in the treatment itself. Clinicians must attend to and search for cues, both diagnostic (i.e. source and cause of the patient's impairment), and non-diagnostic (e.g. psychological, social, and cultural aspects of the patient's problem) in order to arrive at management decisions that holistically attend to all relevant aspects of the individual's health. This requires a highly advanced organization of both theoretical and clinical knowledge and sound cognitive skills. In order to produce thinking therapists who have this phenomenological approach to patients, self-monitoring reflective skills are needed to complement a hypothetico-deductive method of clinical reasoning.

References

Arocha, J.F., Patel, V.L. and Patel, Y.C. (1993) Hypothesis generation and the coordination of theory and evidence in novice diagnostic reasoning. *Medical Decision Making*, **13**, 198–211

Barr, J.S. (1977) A problem-solving curriculum design in physical therapy. *Physical Therapy*, **57**, 262–270

Barrows, H.S. and Feltovich, P.J. (1987) The clinical reasoning process. *Medical Education*, **21**, 86–91

Barrows, H.S. and Tamblyn, R.M. (1980) *Problem-Based Learning: An Approach to Medical Education*. Springer, New York

Barrows, H.S., Feightner, J.W., Neufeld, V.R. and Norman, G.R. (1978) *Analysis of the Clinical Methods of Medical Students and Physicians*. Final report Ontario Department of Health, Hamilton, Ontario

Barrows, H.S., Norman, G.R., Neufeld, V.R. and Feightner, J.W. (1982) The clinical reasoning of randomly selected physicians in general medical practice. *Clinical and Investigative Medicine*, **5**, 49–55

Benner, P. (1984) *From Novice to Expert: Excellence and Power in Clinical Nursing Practice*. Addison-Wesley, Menlo Park, CA

Berner, E.S. (1984) Paradigms and problem-solving: a literature review. *Journal of Medical Education*, **59**, 625–633

Bordage G. and Allen, T. (1982) The etiology of diagnostic errors: process or content? An exploratory study. *Proceedings of the 21st Annual Conference of Research in Medical Education*. American Association of Medical Colleges, Washington, pp. 171–176

Bordage, G. and Lemieux, R. (1991) Semantic structures and diagnostic thinking of experts and novices. *Academic Medicine*, **66**, S70–S72

Bordage, G. and Zacks, R. (1984) The structure of medical knowledge in the memories of medical students and general practitioners: categories and prototypes. *Medical Education*, **18**, 406–416

Bordage, G., Grant, J. and Marsden, P. (1990) Quantitative assessment of diagnostic ability. *Medical Education*, **24**, 413–425

Boshuizen, H.P.A. and Schmidt, H.G. (1992) On the role of biomedical knowledge in clinical reasoning by experts, intermediates and novices. *Cognitive Science*, **16**, 153–184

Burnett, C.N. and Pierson, F.M. (1988) Developing problem-solving skills in the classroom. *Physical Therapy*, **68**, 1381–1385

Butler, D. (1994) The upper limb tension test revisited. In *Physical Therapy for the Cervical And Thoracic Spine* (ed. R. Grant) 2nd edn. Churchill Livingstone, New York, pp 217–244

Cervero, R.M. (1988) *Effective Continuing Education For Professionals*. Jossey-Bass, San Francisco

Christensen, N. (1993) Clinical pattern recognition in physiotherapists – a pilot study investigating the effect of different levels of clinical experience. Unpublished Master of Applied Science thesis, University of South Australia, Adelaide, South Australia

Custers, E., Boshuizen, H. and Schmidt, H. (1993) The influence of typicality of case descriptions on subjective disease probability estimations. Paper presented at the *Annual Meeting of the American Educational Research Association*. American Educational Research Association, Atlanta, April 12–16

Dekker, J., van Baar, M.E., Chr Curfs, E. and Kerssens, J.J. (1993) Diagnosis and treatment in physical therapy: an investigation of their relationship. *Physical Therapy*, **73**, 10–22

Dennis, J.K. and May, B.J. (1987) Practice in the year 2000: Expert decision making in physical therapy. In *Proceedings of the Tenth International Congress of the World Confederation of Physical Therapy*, World Confederation for Physical Therapy, May 17–22, Sydney, pp. 543–551

Echternach, J.L. and Rothstein, J.M. (1989) Hypothesis-oriented algorithms. *Physical Therapy*, **69**, 559–564

Elstein, A.S., Shulman, L.S. and Sprafka, S.A. (1990) Medical problem solving: A ten year retrospective. *Evaluation and the Health Professions*, **13**, 5–36

Elstein, A.S., Shulman, L.S. and Sprafka, S.S. (1978)

Medical Problem Solving: An Analysis of Clinical Reasoning. Harvard University Press, Cambridge, MA

Feltovich, P.J. and Barrows, H.S. (1984) Issues of generality in medical problem solving. In *Tutorials in Problem-Based Learning* (eds H.G. Schmidt and M.L. DeVolder). Van Gorcum, Assen/Maastricht, pp. 128–141

Feltovich, P.J., Johnson, P.E., Moller, J.H. and Swanson, D.B. (1984) LCS: The role and development of medical knowledge in diagnostic expertise. In *Readings in Medical Artificial Intelligence: The First Decade* (eds W.J. Clancey and E.H. Shortcliffe). Addison-Wesley, Reading, MA, pp. 275–319

Gagne, E.D. (1985) *The Cognitive Psychology of School Learning.* Little Brown, Boston

Gale, J. (1982) Some cognitive components of the diagnostic thinking process. *British Journal of Educational Psychology*, **52**, 64–76

Goode, W. (1969) The theoretical limits of professionalization. In *The Semi-Professions and Their Organization* (ed. A. Etzioni). Free Press, New York, pp. 266–313

Grant, J. and Marsden, P. (1987) The structure of memorized knowledge in students and clinicians: an explanation for diagnostic expertise. *Medical Education*, **21**, 92–98

Grant, J. and Marsden, P. (1988) Primary knowledge, medical education and consultant expertise. *Medical Education*, **22**, 173–179

Grant, R. (1992) Obsolescence or lifelong education: choices and challenges. *Physiotherapy*, **78**, 167–171

Grant, R., Jones, M.A. and Maitland, G.D. (1988) Clinical decision making in upper quadrant dysfunction. In *Physical Therapy of the Cervical and Thoracic Spine* (ed. R. Grant). Churchill Livingstone, New York, pp. 51–79

Greeno, J.G. and Simon, H.A. (1986) Problem solving and reasoning. In *Steven's Handbook of Experimental Psychology*, 2nd edn, Vol 2: *Learning and Cognition* (eds R.C. Atkinson, R. Hernstein, G. Lindsey and R.D. Luce). John Wiley and Sons, New York, NY, pp. 572–589

Groen, G.J. and Patel, V.L. (1985) Medical problem-solving: Some questionable assumptions. *Medical Education*, **19**, 95–100

Groen, G.J. and Patel, V.L. (1990) A view from medicine. In *Toward a Unified Theory of Problem Solving: Views from Content Domains* (ed. M. Smith). Lawrence Erlbaum Associates, Hillsdale, NJ, pp. 35–44

Guccione, A.A. (1991) Physical therapy diagnosis and the relationship between impairments and function. *Physical Therapy*, **71**, 499–504

Harris, B.A. and Dyrek, D.A. (1989) A model of orthopaedic dysfunction for clinical decision making in physical therapy practice. *Physical Therapy*, **69**, 548–553

Harris, I. (1993) New expectations for professional competence. In *Educating Professionals: Responding to New Expectations for Competence and Accountability* (eds L. Curry, J. Wergin et al). Jossey-Bass, San Francisco, CA, pp. 17–52

Hassebrock, F., Jonas, A.P. and Bauer, L. (1993)

Metacognitive aspects of medical problem solving. Paper presented to the *Annual Meeting of the American Educational Research Association.* American Educational Research Association, Atlanta

Higgs, J. (1990) Fostering the acquisition of clinical reasoning skills. *New Zealand Journal of Physiotherapy*, **18**, 13–17

Higgs, J. (1992a) Developing clinical reasoning competencies. *Physiotherapy*, **78**, 575–581

Higgs, J. (1992b) Developing knowledge: A process of construction mapping and review. *New Zealand Journal of Physiotherapy*, **20**, 23–30

Higgs, J. (1993) A program for developing clinical reasoning skills in graduate physiotherapists. *Medical Teacher*, **15**, 195–205

Hislop, H.J. (1985) Clinical decision making: Educational, data, and risk factors. In *Clinical Decision Making in Physical Therapy* (ed. S.L. Wolf). F.A. Davis, Philadelphia, pp. 25–60

Houle, C. (1984) *Continuing Learning in the Professions.* Jossey-Bass, San Francisco, CA, pp. 19–75

Jensen, G.M., Shepard, K.F. and Hack, L.M. (1990) The novice versus the experienced clinician: insights into the work of the physical therapist. *Physical Therapy*, **70**, 314–323

Jensen, G.M., Shepard, K.F. and Hack, L.M. (1992) Attribute dimensions that distinguish master and novice physical therapy clinicians in orthopedic settings. *Physical Therapy*, **72**, 711–722

Jette, A.M. (1989) Diagnosis and classification by physical therapists: A special communication. *Physical Therapy*, **69**, 967–969

Jones, M.A. (1989) Clinical reasoning in manipulative therapy education. Unpublished Master of Applied Science thesis, South Australian Institute of Technology, Adelaide, South Australia

Jones, M.A. (1992) Clinical reasoning in manual therapy. *Physical Therapy*, **72**, 875–884

Jones, M.A. (1994) Clinical reasoning process in manipulative therapy. In *Modern Manual Therapy, The Vertebral Column*, 2nd edn. (eds J. D. Boyling and N. Palastanga). Churchill Livingstone, London, England, pp. 471–489

Jones, M.A. and Butler, D. (1991) Clinical reasoning. In *Mobilization of the Nervous System* (ed. D. S. Butler). Churchill Livingstone, Melbourne, pp. 91–106

Jones, M.A., Christensen, N. and Carr, J. (1994) Clinical reasoning in upper quadrant dysfunction. In *Physical Therapy for the Cervical and Thoracic Spine* 2nd edn. (ed. R. Grant). Churchill Livingstone, New York, pp. 89–108

Kassirer, J.P. and Gorry, G.A. (1978) Clinical problem solving: A behavioral analysis. *Annals of Internal Medicine*, **89**, 245–255

Kennedy, M. (1987) Inexact sciences: Professional education and the development of expertise. In E. Rothkupf (ed.), *Review of Research in Education*, **14**, 133–168

Larkin, J.H., McDermott, J., Simon, D.P. and Simon, H.A. (1980) Expert and novice performance in solving physics problems. *Science*, **208**, 1335–1342

Lawson, A.E., McElrath, C.B., Burton, M.S., James, B.D., Doyle, R.P., Woodward, S.L., Kellerman, L. and Snyder, J.D. (1991) Hypothetico-deductive reasoning skill and concept acquisition: Testing a constructivist hypothesis. *Journal of Research in Science Teaching*, **28**, 953–970

Marshall, J. (1977) Assessment of problem-solving ability. *Medical Education*, **11**, 329–334

Mattingly, C. (1991) What is clinical reasoning? *The American Journal of Occupational Therapy*, **45**, 979–986

May, B.J. (1977) An integrated problem-solving curriculum design for physical therapy education. *Physical Therapy*, **57**, 807–813

May, B.J. and Dennis, J.K. (1991) Expert decision making in physical therapy: a survey of practitioners. *Physical Therapy*, **71**, 190–202

May, B.J. and Newman, J. (1980) Developing competence in problem solving: A behavioral model. *Physical Therapy*, **60**, 1140–1145

McGuire, C.H. (1984) Medical problem-solving: A critique of the literature. In *Proceedings of the 23rd Conference on Research in Medical Education*, Washington, pp. 3–12

Mishler, E. (1984) *The Discourse of Medicine: Dialectics of Medical Interviews*. Norwood, New Jersey

Neufeld, V.R., Norman, G.R., Feightner, J.W. and Barrows, H.S. (1981) Clinical problem-solving by medical students: a cross-sectional and longitudinal analysis. *Medical Education*, **15**, 315–322

Newman Henry, J. (1985) Identifying problems in clinical problem solving: Perceptions and interventions with non-problem-solving clinical behaviors. *Physical Therapy*, **65**, 1071–1074

Norman, G., Tugwell, P., Feightner, J.W., Muzzin, L.J. and Jacoby, L.L. (1985) Knowledge and clinical problem-solving. *Medical Education*, **19**, 344–356

Norman, G.R., Brooks, L.R., Coblentz, C.L. and Babcock, C.J. (1992) The correlation of feature identification and category judgments in diagnostic radiology. *Memory and Cognition*, **20**, 344–355

Norman, G.R., Tugwell, P. and Feightner, J.W. (1982) A comparison of resident performance on real and simulated patients. *Journal of Medical Education*, **57**, 708–715

Patel, V.L. and Groen, G.J. (1986) Knowledge-based solution strategies in medical reasoning. *Journal of Cognitive Science*, **10**, 91–108

Patel, V.L. and Groen, G.J. (1991) The general and specific nature of medical expertise: A critical look. In *Toward a General Theory of Expertise: Prospects and Limits* (eds A. Ericsson and J. Smith). Cambridge University Press, New York, NY, pp. 93–125

Patel, V.L., Evans, D.A. and Kaufmann, D.R. (1989) A cognitive framework for doctor–patient interaction. In *Cognitive Science in Medicine* (eds D. A. Evans and V. L. Patel). MIT Press, London, England, pp. 257–312

Patel, V.L., Groen, G.J. and Arocha, J.F. (1990) Medical expertise as a function of task difficulty. *Journal of Memory and Cognition*, **18**, 394–406

Patel, V.L., Groen, G.J. and Norman, G.R. (1991) Effects of conventional and problem-based medical curricula on problem solving. *Academic Medicine*, **66**, 380–389

Payton, O.D. (1985) Clinical reasoning process in physical therapy. *Physical Therapy*, **65**, 924–928

Pew Health Commission (1992) Executive Summary from the Pew Health Commission. 'Healthy America: Practitioners for 2005'. *Journal of Allied Health*, **Fall**, pp. 3–22

Ramsden, E.L. (1985) Basis for clinical decision making: Perception of the patient, the clinician's role, and responsibility. In: *Clinical Decision Making in Physical Therapy* (ed. S.L. Wolf) F.A. Davis, Philadelphia, pp. 25–60

Ridderikhoff, J. (1989) *Methods in Medicine: A Descriptive Study of Physicians' Behaviour*. Kluwer Academic Publishers, Dordrecht

Ridderikhoff, J. (1991) Medical problem solving: an exploration of strategies. *Medical Education*, **25**, 196–207

Rose, S.J. (ed.) (1989a) Clinical decision making in physical therapy. *Physical Therapy* (Special Issue), **69**

Rose, S.J. (1989b) Physical therapy diagnosis: Role and function. *Physical Therapy*, **69**, 535–537

Rothstein, J.M. and Echternach, J.L. (1986) Hypothesis-oriented algorithm for clinicians. A method for evaluation and treatment planning. *Physical Therapy*, **66**, 1388–1394

Rumelhart, D.E. and Ortony, E. (1977) The representation of knowledge in memory. In *Schooling and the Acquisition of Knowledge* (eds R.C. Anderson, R.J. Spiro and W.E. Montague). Lawrence Erlbaum Associates, Hillsdale, NJ, pp. 99–135

Ryle, G. (1949) *The Concept of the Mind*. The University of Chicago Press, Chicago, IL

Sahrman, S.A. (1988) Diagnosis by the physical therapist – a prerequisite for treatment: A special communication. *Physical Therapy*, **68**, 1703–1706

Schenkman, M. and Butler, R. B. (1989) A model for multi-system evaluation, interpretation, and treatment of individuals with neurologic dysfunction. *Physical Therapy*, **69**, 538–547

Schmidt, H.G. and Boshuizen, H.P.A. (1993) On acquiring expertise in medicine. *Educational Pyschology Review*, **5**, 205–221

Schon, D. (1983) *The Reflective Practitioner: How Professionals Think in Action*. Basic Books, New York, NY

Schon, D. (1987) *Educating the Reflective Practitioner*. Jossey-Bass, San Francisco, CA

Shepard, K.F. and Jensen, G.M. (1990) Physical therapist

curricula for the 1990s: Educating the reflective practitioner. *Physical Therapy*, **70**, 566–577

Shulman, L. and Sykes, G. (1986) *A National Board for Teaching? In Search of a Bold Standard: Report for Task Force on Teaching as a Profession.* Carnegie Forum on Education and the Economy, Washington, DC, May, pp. 1–13

Slaughter, D.S., Brown, D.S., Garder, D.L. and Perritt, L.J. (1989) Improving physical therapy students' clinical problem-solving skills: an analytical questioning model. *Physical Therapy*, **69**, 441–447

Terry, W. and Higgs, J. (1993) Educational programmes to develop clinical reasoning skills. *Australian Journal of Physiotherapy*, **39**, 47–51

Thomas-Edding, D. (1987) Clinical problem solving in physical therapy and its implications for curriculum development. In *Proceedings of the Tenth International Congress of the World Confederation for Physical Therapy*, World confederation for Physical Therapy, May 17–22, Sydney, Australia, pp. 100–104

Tulving, E. and Thomson, D.M. (1973) Encoding specificity and retrieval processes in episodic memory. *Psychology Review*, **80**, 352–373

Van der Sijde, P.C., Sellink, W.J.L. and Wurms, R.J. (1987) Developing audiovisuals for problem solving in physical therapy education. *Physical Therapy*, **67**, 554–557

Watts, N.T. (1989) Clinical decision analysis. *Physical Therapy*, **69**, 569–576

Wolf, S.L. (1985) *Clinical Decision Making in Physical Therapy.* F.A. Davis Company, Philadelphia

Zvulun, I. (1993) The development and preliminary testing of an assessment tool for clinical reasoning in physiotherapy. Unpublished Master of Applied Science thesis, University of South Australia, Adelaide, South Australia

7

Clinical reasoning in occupational therapy

Christine Chapparo and Judy Ranka

The nature and focus of occupational therapy today is complex and changing. Occupational therapy service provision has extended from medically based institutions to a variety of community, educational and social service agencies, and private practice. Demands of consumer groups, expectation of documentation, the need for accountability of services, and government intervention in service delivery have made an impact on every therapist. The explosion in technology and knowledge in occupational therapy itself, as well as in the sciences that support occupational therapy is overwhelming. Within this context occupational therapists have a mandate to develop and implement therapy programs aimed at promoting maximum levels of independence in life skills and optimal quality of life. The process of occupational therapy in this context consists of problem solving under conditions of uncertainty and change (Rogers and Masagatani, 1982; Schon, 1983).

The process of occupational therapy involves the therapist collecting, classifying and analysing information about client ability and life situation and then using these data to define client problems, goals and treatment focus (Rogers and Masagatani, 1982). The fundamental process involved in these activities is clinical reasoning.

However, many occupational therapists have raised concerns and questions about clinical reasoning. The questions include the following. What client cues do occupational therapists pay most attention to? What knowledge is required and used to meet the demands of

practice? What is the nature of thinking that takes place when occupational therapists develop responses to the problems they confront? What are the range of factors that are involved in making clinical judgements? Why are clinical decisions made the way they are?

Concern for the fallibility of clinical decisions (Rogers, 1983; Chapparo, 1993) has been related to the perceived inadequacies of academic programs in preparing students for the uncertainties they face in the workplace (Wittman, 1990; Cohn, 1991; Chapparo et al, 1992), the lack of adequate description and research about the thinking that guides occupational therapy practice (Rogers, 1983) and the lack of models of practice that adequately explain and give direction for diverse areas of occupational therapy practice (Keilhofner and Burke, 1977, 1983; Mosey, 1981; Grady et al, 1990).

The purpose of this chapter is to describe clinical reasoning in occupational therapy as it is portrayed by existing literature, scholars researching the area and occupational therapy clinicians themselves. Clinical reasoning will be examined from three perspectives. First, an historical perspective of the developing notions of clinical reasoning in occupational therapy will be outlined and parallels with the development of the profession will be drawn. Second, clinical reasoning will be described in terms of the various external and internal factors that impact on the process of reasoning and ultimately determine occupational therapy action. Third, clinical reasoning will be described from a process perspective, outlining current understanding of the process of thinking that results in clinical decision making in occupational therapy.

Clinical reasoning: an historical perspective

Throughout the development of the occupational therapy profession, elements of what is termed clinical reasoning have been referred to as treatment planning (Day, 1973; Trombly, 1988; Pelland, 1987), the evaluative process (Hemphill, 1982), clinical thinking (Line, 1969), a subset of the occupational therapy process, (Christiansen and Baum, 1991) and problem solving (Rogers and Masagatani, 1982; Hopkins and Tiffany, 1988). The clinical reasoning process has recently been described as 'a largely tacit, highly imagistic and deeply phenomenological mode of thinking' (Mattingly, 1991a, p. 979). Current descriptions and definitions of clinical reasoning have been influenced in part by the diverse nature and goals of occupational therapy practice as well as the philosophy of the profession itself. A brief review of the development of the profession illustrates how its history has influenced various reasoning strategies in current practice as well as the methods that have been employed for studying them.

Beliefs, values and humanism

Occupational therapy was founded on humanistic values (Meyer, 1922; Slagle, 1922; Hopkins, 1988; Yerxa, 1991). The view of occupation that was accepted by the profession early in its development centred around the relationship between health and the ability to organize the temporal, physical and social elements of daily living (Keilhofner and Burke, 1977, 1983; Breines, 1990). This view of occupation and occupational therapy treatment was highly influenced by theories of the Moral Treatment movement of the 18th and 19th centuries (Harvey-Krefting, 1985; Hopkins, 1988). The fundamental beliefs of that movement, as articulated by Pinel in 1801, acknowledged people's basic right to humane treatment (Pinel, 1948). From that set of beliefs, a client-centred philosophy evolved which served to unify the profession. The philosophy placed emphasis

on the rights of all people to develop the skills and habits required for a balanced, wholesome life (Shannon, 1977).

Following the tradition of pragmatism, early occupational therapy leaders subscribed to a belief in the unity of mind and body in action, and the profession was united in its philosophical approach to health through active occupation (Cohen, 1983; Breines, 1990). Fundamental to the creation of treatment principles was a thinking mode described by John Dewey, one of the early pragmatic theorists, whose work influenced the philosophical development of the profession. Dewey (1910, 1929) claimed that the actions of professionals depended on a unique mental analysis and interpretation of each situation encountered, with the purpose being to obtain an understanding of the significance and meaning in everyday life. The criteria for judging this significance, meaning and worth were practical, largely arbitrary, qualitative rather than quantitative, non-specialized and purposive (Stanage, 1987). Clinical reasoning of the time took the form of common sense inquiry and was structured around the goal of normalizing the activities and environments of clients who had problems in daily living.

The philosophy of practice and the thinking involved in structuring occupational therapy as described in the 1920s is echoed in today's views of clinical reasoning. For example, compare these two statements: 'An (occupational therapist) has to be guided by what she has been taught, but primarily by her own intelligent grasp of the situation' (Wigglesworth, 1923, p. 129), and 'The intentions and potentials of chronically disabled patients are difficult to discern, but a therapist of understanding will elicit them, and use them to help patients discover health within themselves.' (Rogers, 1983, p. 615).

The early pragmatic view of the subjective and individual reality of 'knowing' is mirrored, not only in contemporary occupational therapy practice, but in contemporary methods employed by the profession to study clinical reasoning. For example, Yerxa (1991, p. 201) writes: 'Persons are authors of their occupational behaviour simultaneously as biological, psychological, social, cultural and spiritual beings. Experiments that try to reduce occupation to a single cause–effect relationship lose sight of both the person and occupation and actually study something else'.

Science and reductionism

During its early years of development, occupational therapy quickly expanded its services to a variety of medically-based facilities, while managing to keep methodology and ideology focused on the client's performance in everyday occupations (Anderson and Bell, 1988). However, with an increased alliance to medical trends that focused on isolated cause and effect principles of illness, the holistic view of occupation ultimately came into conflict with the reductionistic paradigm of medicine from about the 1930s. This conflict profoundly and universally influenced the occupational therapy profession during the 1950s and 1960s to the point where authors have claimed that the field found itself in a 'period of crisis' using the Kuhnian terms of a paradigm shift (Keilhofner and Burke, 1977; Kuhn, 1970; Shannon, 1977).

During this time, therapists adapted their focus and actions to suit the changing philosophies of the medical contexts within which they worked. A significant shift occurred in the underlying principles of occupational therapy. Growing pressure from medicine for a more scientific rationale for practice (Licht, 1947) resulted in therapists reducing the focus of treatment to medically-related specialized areas where scientific explanations were possible (Keilhofner and Burke, 1983). Occupational therapists turned to kinesiologic, neurophysiological and psychodynamic explanations of human function and dysfunction (Keilhofner and Burke, 1977; Barris, 1984). The shift from a single theoretical concept based on occupation, to belief systems based on medical trends resulted in the development of two major paradigms from which many theoretical frameworks evolved. One maintained the original focus on the holistic, occupational nature of humans, the other focused on reductionist aspects of human inner mechanisms. The two were often in conflict with each other (Keilhofner and Burke, 1983).

During this period, the medical diagnosis permeated all aspects of occupational therapy clinical decision making. Formulation of the client's problem was in terms of the physical or psychiatric diagnosis rather than the occupational need (Spackman, 1968). Although occupational therapy's major objective was still to improve the independence of clients with disability (Jacob, 1964), forms of treatment began to focus on internal mechanisms. Clinical decision making became reductionistic as evidenced by examples of stated goals for treatment which were aimed at improving isolated units of function, such as particular physical or psychological attributes. The major occupational areas of work, play, sleep and rest as described by Meyer (1922) were reduced into separate compartments which became known as activities of daily living, employment, and leisure, and were assessed and treated separately. Consideration of rest, as well as the central concept of caring for self through a balanced sequence of activity found no place in the medical model and was discarded for many years. This type of reductionistic focus still persists in a number of current clinical reasoning practices (Eliason and Gohl-Giese, 1979; Bissel and Mailloux, 1981; Rogers and Masagatani, 1982; Keilhofner and Nelson, 1987; Trombly, 1988; Kleinman, 1988).

Elements of today's views of clinical reasoning were beginning to emerge in the literature and reflected the scientific influence of the time. Reilly (1960) for example proposed an early model of clinical reasoning for occupational therapy that was a type of critical–analytical thinking process. She described the elements of this process using the following formula: treatment plan equals the sum of the related raw data drawn from the data collecting instruments of observation, testing, interview and case history (Reilly, 1960; Day, 1973). During the 1970s this formula became formalized into the assessment and treatment planning part of the occupational therapy process which is still used and taught in the 1990s (Hopkins and Tiffany, 1988).

From Reilly's work, and in keeping with the adoption of more scientific modes of thinking, systems approaches were applied to clinical reasoning (Line, 1969; Harrison, 1972; Llorens, 1972). They were viewed as objective and logical problem solving strategies which were essentially linear in form. One exception is found in the work of Day (1973) who created a model to illustrate the arrangement, relationship and flow of the components of the treatment plan. The components were identified as problem identification, cause identification, treatment principle or assumption selection, activity selection and goal identification. All parts of the model flowed toward the goal as found in previous linear models. However, Day additionally hypothesized that the entry of each component was not necessarily in the linear sequence described. The model created depended on generating and testing a series of hypotheses about client problems and reactions to intervention. This circular view of generating alternate hypotheses, testing for validation of principles, assumptions or judgements formed, then returning to the problem is an early view of the cognitive aspect of clinical reasoning that forms a part of our understanding of clinical reasoning today (Rogers and Holm, 1991).

Theory development and conflict

Occupational therapy practice since the 1970s has been characterized by theoretical conflict as the profession universally re-examined its direction and focus. A number of theories, models and frames of reference have been proposed to explain the purpose of occupational therapy, with some emanating from other professions (Reed, 1984; Hopkins and Smith, 1988; Christiansen and Baum, 1991; Hagedorn, 1992). The result of this theoretical explosion, is contemporary practice wherein various frames of reference are valued by different and substantial segments of the profession.

If theories, models and frames of reference are indeed the 'tools of thinking', as suggested by Parham (1987), the impact of this theoretical diversity on clinical reasoning is clear. Each model or frame of reference directs the parameters and styles of reasoning that are determined by its implicit values, conceptual framework and scientific base. By adhering to a specific frame of reference, therapists follow a particular method of translating knowledge into action and are directed towards which techniques to use and which techniques to discard. This specialized style of reasoning and action has been supported and fostered by current trends in health care which has itself become divided into specialties over time. Occupational therapists in many instances have begun to refer to themselves as psychosocial therapists, physical disabilities therapists, hand therapists, or sensory integration therapists to designate the area of specialty (Schkade and Schultz, 1992). The existing pluralism appears to have defied attempts at synthesis (Lindquist et al, 1982; Katz, 1985) and

creates problems for those who seek an encompassing view of occupational therapy practice (American Occupational Therapy Association, 1979; Yerxa, 1979; Christiansen, 1990; Van Deusen, 1991). The present position is perhaps best explained by Henderson (1988, p. 569) who urges the profession to 'be unified in . . . (their) fundamental assumptions, but diverse in . . . (their) technical knowlege'.

In summary, the current nature of occupational therapy and the clinical reasoning processes that continue to form a basis for its identity, is founded in the history and humanistic philosophy that shaped the profession's beginning. Continuation of the profession's original belief in health through occupation is reflected in preoccupation with activity and 'doing' in contemporary clinical reasoning. The original belief in the client's right of choice and autonomy is reflected in current phenomenological approaches to clinical reasoning that strive to develop a picture of disorder as perceived by the client (Gillette and Mattingly, 1987; Mattingly, 1991b)

The continuing impact of the reductionist and analytic orientation of medicine on current clinical reasoning in occupational therapy is illustrated by the prominent place that diagnosis and disease are still given in the clinical reasoning process (Rogers and Masagatani, 1982; Mattingly, 1991a) and by the use of associated mechanistic reasoning strategies by many therapists (Barris, 1984; Keilhofner and Nelson, 1987). The influence of modes of scientific inquiry is reflected in a clinical reasoning style that involves systematic conceptualization and examination of clinical situations. Early scientific dogma has been tempered by the profession's emerging rejection of scientific dependency (Yerxa, 1991) and has resulted in modification of current concepts of clinical reasoning as being more than applied science (Mattingly, 1991a).

The most significant historical legacy to current occupational therapy practice has been the evolution of diversity. Contemporary clinical reasoning mirrors this. It is characterized by the use of multiple modes of reasoning that are employed simultaneously within one therapy session and are orchestrated by the skill of the therapist. In the 1990s, clinical reasoning is recognized as the core of occupational therapy practice. As a phenomenon for study, its contribution is in describing the commonalities and complexities of therapists' thinking. Its importance in defining the professional identity of occupational therapy is summed up by Pedretti (1982, p.12) who states, 'perhaps our real identity and uniqueness lies not as much in what we do, but in how we think'.

Factors involved in clinical reasoning

Four primary elements have consistently influenced therapist thinking throughout the history of the profession and continue to do so: the context within which therapy occurs, the client(s), theory, and the individuality of the therapist. These four elements and their interactions form many internal and external factors that have the potential to influence the way decisions are made by therapists. One way to describe these likely influences is to consider them as sources of motivation for decision making (Chapparo, 1993).

Organizational factors

The first of the possible sources of motivation for decision making is the impact of organizational influences over which therapists may have limited control. Elements of the external organizational context become important and powerful factors in establishing conditions (e.g. values of the organization) and constraints (e.g. policies, budget cuts) within which decision making occurs. However, therapists view themselves as autonomous individuals and reason according to their internalized values and theoretical perspectives. These reflect the sort of client–centred therapy that they feel should occur. Many times the theoretical perspective, or professional value held by the therapist may fail to account for the institutional conditions and in such situations these internal values and goals can come into direct conflict with organizational directions and limitations. The resulting dilemma for clinical reasoning is one of conflict between what therapists perceive should be done, what the client wants done and what the system will allow. Where there is a mismatch between the therapist's internal belief system and the external reality the result can be a limit of range of occupational therapy treatment options which are generated by the clinical reasoning process or decisions to implement treatment options that are not possible within the system.

In addition, therapists develop perceptions of the amount of control they have over their ability to carry out planned actions. This has a direct effect on their feelings of self-efficacy and on their behaviour (Schifter and Ajzen, 1985; Ajzen and Madden, 1986). Effective and creative problem solving requires the essential attributes of self-confidence and autonomy. If therapists have a tenuous sense of self-efficacy and control, then it is probable that they will have difficulty perceiving themselves as being active agents for facilitating change in their clients and this will influence their reasoning (Fidler, 1981). Therapy experiences, including the organizational elements of therapy also influence the practical knowledge the therapist develops. Such experiences are remembered by therapists as contextual patterns rather than decontextualized elements or rules (Schon, 1983; Gordon, 1988).

Client factors

The second source of motivation, client factors, is fundamental to the clinical reasoning process. A core tenet of occupational therapy is that treatment be in concert with the client's needs, goals, lifestyle and personal and cultural values (Rogers, 1983). Indeed, a salient criterion of an ethical action for occupational therapy is its agreement with the client's valued goals (Christiansen and Baum, 1991; Rogers, 1983). If therapists incorporate this professional value into their clinical reasoning, then making clinical decisions becomes not only a scientific or pragmatic issue, but an ethical issue.

Mattingly (1991b) and others (Rogers, 1983; Fleming, 1991b) describe one of the primary goals of clinical reasoning as determining the meaning of disability from the client's perspective. At least five types of knowledge about the client are required to establish a picture of this meaning (Mattingly,1991a). These are: knowledge of the client's motivations, desires and tolerances; knowledge of the environment and context within which client performance will occur; knowledge of the client's abilities and deficits; insight into the existing relationship with the client, its tacit rules and boundaries; and a predictive knowledge of client potential in the long term. Knowledge from all these factors becomes a dynamic information flow during the process of assessment and treatment, requiring that the therapist constantly review her/his understanding of how the client views (him)herself, how the client views therapy and the therapist, and what the client thinks should be done.

All these client factors are used by therapists in the reasoning process to create and update a conceptual model of the client (Rogers, 1983). Commonly, therapists use themselves as referents during this model creation (Sarbin et al, 1960; Rogers, 1983), thereby ascribing meaning to the client's individual situation according to their own criteria. Although this is viewed as a reasoning 'error' (Rogers, 1983), it is debatable to what extent therapists are able to uncouple their own values and perspectives to reach a full understanding of the client's situation. Rather, what is probable is that therapists develop an internal model of what they believe is the client's perspective and work from that belief system (Chapparo, 1993).

Theory factors

The third source of motivation for clinical decision making is the therapists' scientific knowledge about disease, human function and human occupation. Such knowledge is emphasized in literature which portrays occupational therapy clinical reasoning as the application of theory to practice (Parham, 1986, 1987; Pelland, 1987). Theory is purported to be useful because it gives direction for thinking, information about alternatives and expectations of function and deficits (Mattingly, 1991a). Professional knowledge has been described as applied theory whereby the process of 'naming' and 'framing' the problem occurs (Schon, 1983). This requires identifying and classifying abstract constructs according to some theory base (such as depression, motivation, occupational role, or cognitive ability). The identified construct becomes a cognitive mechanism that can facilitate the selection of strategies for assessment and treatment (Christiansen and Baum, 1991).

Theoretical knowledge alone, however, is insufficient to provide the basis for effective clinical reasoning. This is firstly because occupational therapy has a theory base that is incomplete and characterized by conflict. Secondly, therapists are required to make decisions in situations of uncertainty. Under these conditions, practical, intuitive knowledge is required. Such knowledge is tacit knowledge founded in experience of clinical events: a practical knowledge (Polanyi, 1958; Benner and Wrubel, 1982; Rogers, 1983; Gordon, 1988; Cohn, 1989; Mattingly, 1991a). Practical knowledge is integrated with theoretical knowledge to form a reasoning strategy that has been termed 'deliberative rationality' (Dreyfus and Dreyfus, 1986). When listening to therapists talk through their treatments this can be observed and conceptualized as a personal theory of why events occur in therapy (Chapparo, 1993).

Many therapists view decision making from a theoretical base as being 'objective', 'scientific' and value neutral. In fact, all theories themselves are value laden. Therapists choose theories because of their potential to explain client problems. For instance, occupational therapists working with children are likely to choose developmentally based theories. However, therapists also tend to choose to put into operation one theory over another because of the congruence between the values implicit in the theory and the personal/professional values of the therapist, rather than because of its scientific merit. Many issues arising in conflicts between therapists and other professionals do not relate to the logical soundness of the theoretical perspective, but the unspoken values embedded in the prescribed treatment approach (Parham, 1987).

Individual factors

The fourth source of motivation is individual factors which incorporate personal attitudes and values of the therapist. Individual factors can be conceptualized as occurring across two interrelated dimensions and culminating in ethical occupational therapy practice. First, at the most basic dimension, is our own personal value system: the fundamental beliefs and assumptions we have about oursleves, others and occupational therapy. Personal values can be internalized at several levels ranging from tentatively-held beliefs to strong convictions. The 'strength' with which a therapist adheres to a value can differ from person to person as well as from situation to situation (Hundert, 1987; Brockett, 1988). Personal values are important to clinical reasoning as they define the limits of acceptable behaviour for each individual therapist in any given clinical situation.

Each interpersonal interaction with a client is, for the therapist, a personal experience. Elements of the interaction – the self, personal relevance and feelings as well as cognition are stored for use in future decision making. Knowledge that results from those personal experiences and reflection on them becomes personal knowledge (Butt et al, 1982) and shapes what has been conceptualized as the architecture of self. For occupational therapists, personal interactions within the professional context result over time in the evolution of a personal form of professional knowledge that guides the way they think and act as occupational therapists (Butt et al, 1982; Fondiller, Rosage and Neuhaus, 1990).

A second dimension of ethical practice revolves around the question of to whom occupational therapists are responsible. Mirvits and Seashore (1979, p. 771) suggest that ethical dilemmas frequently develop 'not because roles are unclear but because they are clearly in conflict'. Individual therapists are responsible for resolving their own personal conflicts, addressing client needs and desires, working co-operatively with colleagues, serving the mission of the employing agency, contributing to the larger field of occupational therapy and promoting health in society. In responding to these multiple audiences, there is a search for balance and an ordering of priorities that becomes a part of the clinical reasoning process. For example one cannot assume that the personal code of ethics of even the most well-intentioned therapist will always coincide with those of the profession of occupational therapy as an institution when faced with conflict (Hundert, 1987). This is a particular problem that intrudes on the clinical reasoning of novice therapists. They have not been exposed to the struggle of conflicting values which results from 'problem cases' in the clinical situation and have not yet internalized many of the values of the profession. Part of the value of experience in problem solving goes beyond its contribution in terms of cognition and intuition. It involves the depth of an ethical approach to problem solving that is obtained through the evolution of a dynamic 'reflective equilibrium' over time as therapists struggle to solve ethical dilemmas within the clinical situation (Hundert, 1987).

Clearly, clinical reasoning in occupational therapy is a phenomenon involving balancing of a number of individual, theoretical and organizational factors. How therapists orchestrate these factors and which factors receive precedence in reasoning strategies is not yet clear.

Internal frame of reference

Clinical reasoning in occupational therapy can be conceptualized as being dependent on an individual's highly individualized, complex internal framework structure. The notion of an internal frame of reference is based on the work of Argyris, Schon, Ajzen and their colleagues (Argyris and Schon, 1976; Schon, 1983; Argyris et al, 1985; Ajzen and Madden, 1986; Schon, 1987). An internal frame of reference refers to a comprehensive view occupational therapists have of themselves, their situations, and their role within a clinical context. It is composed of theoretical elements, elements of understanding of the practical clinical situation and personal beliefs and values concerning what can and should be done in client-related circumstances (Chapparo, 1993). The framework is derived from theoretical and experiential learning, internalized values, perceptions of what relevant others (client and colleagues) think should occur and perceptions of contextual conditions such as the level of therapist autonomy permitted by the system. The internal frame of reference is a representational tool. It is used during the clinical reasoning process to order, categorize and simplify complex data in order to develop a plan for action for the given situation. Within this internal frame of reference, theoretical replication and application is associated with personal judgement: a practical wisdom. This occurs against a background of the sum of cultural and personal biases that inherently reside in each therapist and serve to colour and interpret clinical reality and ultimately, clinical reasoning (Chapparo, 1993).

Clinical reasoning: a multifaceted process

Considering the number of factors that impact on decisions therapists make, it is not surprising to find that scholars and researchers have hypothesized that multiple reasoning processes and strategies are used by occupational therapists. Modes of reasoning appear to relate to the area of practice, amount of therapist experience and stage of client treatment (Rogers and

Masagatani, 1982; Fleming, 1991a). It is possible that different reasoning modes exist relative to each of the factors found in the internal frame of reference (Chapparo, 1993) and that therapists shift from mode to mode during the course of therapy (Fleming, 1991a). This third section will explore how the various factors involved in clinical reasoning as described in the previous section are processed to form pictures of client problems, client potential, therapy action and outcome.

Clinical reasoning: an hypothetico-deductive process

Rogers and Holm (1991, p. 1045) assert that occupational therapy assessment involves not only the sensing and defining of client problems but also creation of a clinical image which represents a 'balanced view of occupational status' by reflecting both assets and deficits. They describe a process of diagnostic reasoning that culminates in a clinical image of the client regarding deficits in occupational role performance, occupational performance and the components of occupational performance (the 'occupational therapy diagnosis'). This process involves a progression from problem sensing to problem definition and problem resolution. Based on information processing approaches put forward in medical models of clinical reasoning (Elstein et al, 1978; Elstein and Bordage, 1979), Rogers and Holm (1991) outline a model of occupational therapy reasoning consisting of various cognitive operations identified as cue acquisition, hypothesis generation, cue interpretation and hypothesis evaluation.

As with earlier work (Rogers and Masagatani, 1982), Rogers and Holm's (1991) notion of diagnostic reasoning begins even before the therapist approaches a client. The 'problem sensing' stage results in decisions being made relative to information required to form an occupational diagnosis and within the context of the client's medical and occupational status. This stage of reasoning can be considered a 'pre-diagnostic interpretation' rather than an hypothesis (Gale and Marsden, 1982). The interpretation represents the therapist's interim, working and flexible identification of the general problem. The purpose of this interpretation is not limited to diagnosis. There also appears to be some judgement that occurs

about the need for further information in order to make clinical decisions. It is probable that therapists have individual ideas about how well defined the problem should be before 'hypothesis generation' can begin.

The view of clinical reasoning presented by Rogers and Holm (1991) is largely extrapolated from studies of clinicians other than occupational therapists. As they state, 'the validity of this approach rests on the generic nature of the diagnostic process' (Rogers and Holm, 1991, p. 1053). The cognitive processes discussed here become unique to occupational therapy when they are applied to occupational therapy concepts such as occupational role performance, occupational tasks and activities and component performance.

Fleming (1991a, b) and colleagues working on the American Occupational Therapy Association/American Occupational Therapy Foundation Clinical Reasoning Study referred to a type of reasoning process that incorporates the concepts outlined above and referred to it as procedural reasoning. She reports that experienced occupational therapists use these procedural reasoning strategies when thinking about the disease and deciding on treatment activities.

Information about the disorder is sought from the client using the best mode of communication possible. The following example from the practice area of psychiatry illustrates how an experienced therapist used an assessment mode other than language to determine the effects of thought disorder on a client and to determine the direction of treatment.

Steven was admitted after taking LSD which resulted in what looked like an acute psychotic episode. No one could get any sense out of him. He walked into my OT unit. He was talking nonsense and was unable to carry on a conversation with me. I could tell that he wanted to stay, so I asked him if he wanted to draw or paint. He painted six paintings in rapid succession. We didn't talk. I didn't ask him to talk about his paintings – he couldn't. When he had gone we looked at them. They were chaotic: lots of bright colours: highly detailed machinery parts and wheels painted in black on the colours: all the same. I got some understanding of the chaos inside his head. Based on the paintings, we (the team) decided to put him on a very structured, routinized program with OT for short periods involving activities that would not feed into the chaos. We set activities with definite boundaries. It was almost like putting him into a 'holding tank' until he was safe. After a few days he calmed down and I got him to do some more paintings to see the difference in his thought processes. They showed consistency, proportion, form: they were structured and calm. Steven was even able to start to talk about them. (Chapparo, 1993).

Using procedural reasoning modes, therapists engage in a dual search for problem definition and treatment selection. Mattingly (1991a) describes how experienced therapists generate two to four hypotheses regarding the cause and nature of functional problems and several more concerning possible direction for treatment. Among newer therapists, however, there is a tendency to generate fewer hypotheses. In this type of reasoning process, there appears to be no thought without inference. Inference in this context can be defined as the process of arriving at an idea of what is absent on the basis of what is at hand such as knowledge about the disorder, past experience with the client and established principles of treatment. The therapist uses this information to construct hypotheses about the nature of the problem through a process of critical reflection. The tendency of novice therapists is to jump to conclusions about the nature and direction of therapy without weighing the grounds on which the conclusion rests. The danger for experienced therapists is to place exclusive dependence on past experiences which have not been subjected to critical analysis. Without critical reflection, therapists forgo and cut short the act of inquiry. Critical reflection of knowledge is essential for effective procedural reasoning.

Characteristically, for occupational therapists, client problems are ill-structured problems. All information required for adequate reasoning is not available at the outset and the nature of the problems changes as assessment proceeds and treatment begins. The search for information by therapists is compounded by the fact that occupational therapy in many instances is not a well-known or well-defined profession in comparison to medicine, nursing or physiotherapy. Clients are not sure of the information occupational therapists are after. Both the occupational therapist and client work hard during initial reasoning stages to develop a reciprocal understanding of each other's roles. This perhaps becomes the initial stage of a process that structures an image of meaning for both the client and the therapist. While clients at this stage struggle to understand what occupational therapy is, what the therapist will do and what the outcome will be, therapists endeavour to develop an image of what disability and illness means from the client's perspective.

Clinical reasoning: a process of structuring meaning

When attempting to implement the full course of a therapy program that will potentially change life roles and functions for the client, occupational therapists are faced with profound problems of understanding. Specifically, this involves understanding the meaning of illness, disability and therefore therapy outcome from the client's perspective.

To understand the meaning of a situation means to make sense of the experience; to make an interpretation of it. In clinical reasoning processes, therapists use this interpretation to guide decision making or action. Clinical reasoning from this perspective can be defined partly as the process of making a new or revised interpretation of the meaning of illness or disability for each client seen. This interpretation leads to subsequent understanding, appreciation, and action. What therapists perceive and fail to perceive and what they think and fail to think in the interpretative process is powerfully influenced by sets of assumptions (internal frames of reference) that structure the way they interpret clinical experiences (Crepeau, 1991; Mezirow, 1991).

It is helpful to differentiate two dimensions of making meaning. Meaning schemes are sets of related and habitual expectations governing if–then relationships. Mattingly (1991b), cites Bruner (1990) in linking these meaning schemes to a paradigmatic mode of thinking. For example in occupational therapy, a therapist with experience in stroke rehabilitation expects to see signs of left hemiplegia when given referral notes on a client with diagnosis of right cerebrovascular accident. Meaning schemes are habitual, implicit rules for interpreting and are strongly linked to knowledge.

Meaning perspectives are made up of higher-order schemata, theories and beliefs. Meaning perspectives refer to the structure of assumptions and beliefs within which a new experience is interpreted. For example, occupational therapists make interpretations about clients based on values espoused by the notion of 'a helping profession', and their judgements are focused on client performance and satisfaction with occupational roles and tasks. Both meaning schemes and meaning perspectives selectively order and delimit clinical reasoning. They define therapists' expectations and affect the activity of perceiving, comprehending and remembering meaning within the context of communicating with clients (Berkson and Wettersten, 1984; Crepeau, 1991).

In occupational therapy, the process of clinical reasoning as a construction of intersubjective meaning involves understanding the meaning of what clients communicate (Crepeau, 1991; Fleming, 1991b). This process focuses on achieving coherence, rather than on exercising control over clients to improve performance (Crepeau, 1991). In occupational therapy this type of reasoning process is different from the hypothetico-deductive strategies found in procedural reasoning modes (Mattingly, 1991b; Heimstra, 1991).

Construction of meaning is a process where the occupational therapist attempts to understand what is meant by another person. It is less a matter of testing hypotheses than of searching, often intuitively, for themes and metaphors that can be used to fit unfamiliar client perspectives into a picture that is understandable to the therapist (Hammond, 1988; Heimstra, 1991; Fleming, 1991b; Chapparo, 1993). Fleming (1991b) refers to this process as interactive reasoning. She cites studies which demonstrate that occupational therapists engage in interactive reasoning for at least eight different reasons including: knowing the person as a person (Cohn, 1989); understanding disability from the client's point of view (Mattingly, 1991b); determining the success of a treatment session and communicating a sense of trust or hope (Langthaler, 1990).

Mattingly (1991b) describes how narrative thinking is central in providing therapists with a way to consider disability in phenomenological terms. She vividly describes two types of narrative thinking: one as a 'mode of talk'

that therapists use to shift disability from a physiological event to a personally meaningful one. The second type of narrative thinking involves the creation of images of the future for the client. The result of this type of thinking, as described by Mattingly, is purposeful occupational therapy that creates therapeutic activities which are meaningful to the client's life.

As with procedural reasoning, reflection is a critical part of this distinctive interaction reasoning process. Figure 7.1 illustrates the important role reflection plays in clinical reasoning and therapeutic action. All therapists reflect to some degree on the clinical decisions they make. It has already been described how therapists, during procedural reasoning strategies, reflect on knowledge stores in order to take the most appropriate therapeutic action. This could be termed 'thoughtful action'. However, reflection in the context of interactive modes of reasoning requires that therapists critically review sets of assumptions generated by their knowledge and beliefs to determine if they are viable for interpreting client meaning and to identify the reasons for and consequences of what they do from the client's perspective. The process through which this interpretation occurs in occupational therapy appears to involve a critical interpretative discourse with clients in order to validate meaning schemes and perspectives created (as per Crepeau, 1991; Mezirow, 1991).

Research on this area in occupational therapy suggests that therapists exhibit markedly different assumptions about what client perspectives are and how they can become 'known' (Fleming, 1991a), and therefore how judgements in the form of clinical reasoning can be made in the light of these assumptions. As with students, novice therapists believe they can know absolutely through concrete observation. They see their reasoning task as discovering the 'truth' or identifying some authority figure, who can explicate it (Chapparo et al, 1992). Therapists with experience usually accept that there are many problems for which there are no absolutely true answers. The task of clinical reasoning, as viewed by these occupational therapists is to construct a solution that is justifiable after consideration of all available information and all interpretations.

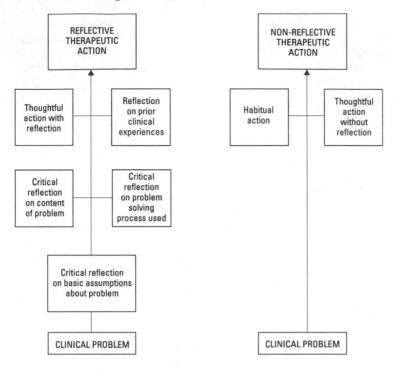

Figure 7.1   Reflection in clinical reasoning

Clinical reasoning: a process of ethical decision making

Despite evidence that personal values impact substantially on clinical reasoning processes in occupational therapy (Rogers and Holm, 1991; Haddad, 1988; Neuhaus, 1988; Fondiller et al, 1990; Mattingly, 1991b; Fleming 1991a; Chapparo, 1993), there exists no theoretical framework within which to conceptualize ethical problems in occupational therapy, to say nothing of how these problems are solved. A clinical problem becomes an ethical 'dilemma' when it seems that an occupational therapy treatment decision will violate the therapist's values. In the process of choosing a therapeutic action using the reasoning processes outlined above, occupational therapists are often forced to balance one value against another. While this process is typically unconscious it appears to drive cognitive aspects of clinical reasoning (e.g. making decisions or choices) at various points throughout the treatment program (Chapparo, 1993).

Most occupational therapy educators involved in discussion of ethical issues are struck by the simplicity of students' early articulations of their ethical positions. Discussions seem to revolve around 'always' and 'never' principles of right and wrong, and the evolution of more mature principles occurs as they struggle with issues related to problem cases (Hundert, 1987; Donelly, 1992). By comparison, experienced therapists are often differentiated from their less-experienced counterparts not only for their superior knowledge-based reasoning style but also for their wisdom in dealing with ethical issues. For occupational therapists, part of this wisdom comes from a continual process of weighing values associated with each alternative action. Each new problem becomes a moral experience and exposes a novel division of values conflicting around the facts of a client case. Each values dilemma a therapist faces contributes towards the clarification of the therapist's moral principles and the realignment of these principles with his/her moral experience.

Clinical reasoning: a process of imagery and integration

In her insightful description of clinical reasoning in occupational therapy, Fleming (1991a) proposes a reasoning theory of an occupational therapist with a 'three track mind'. After describing procedural and interactive reasoning strategies, Fleming goes on to propose that therapists use a process termed conditional reasoning to integrate the other two types of reasoning as well as to 'project an imagined future condition or situation for the person' (Fleming, 1991a, p. 1007). Fleming uses the term 'conditional' in three different ways. First, she argues, problems are interpreted and solutions are realized in relation to the whole person within their particular context. Second, therapists imagine how the present condition can be changed. Third, success or failure is determined by the level of client participation. As with other modes of reasoning, conditional reasoning is a multidimensional process involving complex and non-linear forms of thinking and reflection. This circular process results in the gradual modification of ideas and the development and implementation of a flexible therapy program. The notion of conditional reasoning lies not only in the ability of the therapist to engage the client in treatment, but also, very importantly, it necessitates that the therapist and client build 'a shared image of the person's future self' (Fleming, 1991a, p. 1012).

Conclusion

Clinical reasoning in occupational therapy, as in other health science professions, is a complex phenomenon that has only just begun to be described. Clinical reasoning in occupational therapy may be best described as the use of multiple reasoning strategies throughout the various phases of client management. Hypothetic-deductive modes of reasoning (including procedural reasoning as presented by Fleming (1991b)) are used when therapists think about client problems in terms of the disease and within the context of occupational performance. Interactive reasoning (Fleming, 1991a), involves developing an understanding of the meaning of existing problems from the client's perspective. It employs processes of narrative thinking (Mattingly, 1991b) and critical discourse with clients (Crepeau, 1991). Conditional reasoning (Fleming, 1991a) is a less definitive process by which occupational

therapists imagine the client in the future and in so doing, imagine the therapy outcome and the therapeutic action required to achieve that outcome. Underpining all these processes is a process of ethical reasoning and critical reflection.

Many external contextual factors act as motivating forces to clinical decisions made. Among them are, organizational structures and expectations, client needs and expectations, theoretical and scientific knowledge about disease and human occupations (Chapparo, 1993). Within the therapist's internal frame of reference, perceptions of these external factors are integrated with personal beliefs about such factors as perceived level of skill, personal knowledge, personal values and perceived level of control. From this internal frame of reference, images of clients and their problems are created as well as plans for therapeutic action which have time representations in the past, present and future, and which serve to direct clinical reasoning processes (Chapparo, 1993).

It is clear that current explanations and descriptions of clinical reasoning in occupational therapy are incomplete. Contemporary notions of clinical reasoning describe a highly individualistic mode of operation that is based in scientific knowledge and method, creative imagination, intuition, interpersonal skill and artistry operating within the frame of reference of the occupational therapy profession. As with any other skilled occupation, the difference between novice and expert is the degree of craftsmanship with which the therapist is able to arrive at the best clinical decisions. A description of clinical reasoning that best captures the complexity and breadth of processes and elements involved is that given by Rogers (1983, p. 615), who states:

The (occupational therapy) clinician functions as a scientist, ethicist, and artist. The scientific, ethical and artistic dimensions of clinical reasoning are inextricably entwined, and each strand is needed to strengthen the line of thought leading to understanding.
Without science, clinical inquiry is not systematic:
without ethics, it is not responsible;
without art, it is not convincing.

References

Ajzen, I. and Madden, T.J. (1986) Prediction of goal directed behaviour: Attitudes, intentions and perceived behavioural control. *Journal of Experimental Social Psychology*, **22**, 453–474

American Occupational Therapy Association (1979) *Commission on Practice: Uniform Terminology System for Reporting Occupational Therapy Services.* AOTA, Rockville, MD, AOTA

Anderson, B. and Bell, J. (1988) *Occupational Therapy: Its Place in Australia's History.* NSW Association of Occupational Therapists, Victoria

Argyris, A. and Schon, D. (1976) *Theory in Practice: Increasing Professional Effectiveness.* Jossey-Bass, San Francisco

Argyris, C., Putnam, R. and Smith, D.M. (1985) *Action Science: Concepts, Methods and Skills for Research and Intervention.* Jossey Bass, San Francisco

Barris, R. (1984) Toward an image of one's own: Sources of variation in the role of occupational therapists in psychosocial practice. *The Occupational Therapy Journal of Research*, **4**, 3–23

Benner, P. and Wrubel, J. (1982) Clinical knowledge development: The value of perceptual awareness. *Nurse Educator*, **7**, 11–17

Berkson, W. and Wettersten, J. (1984) *Learning From Error: Karl Popper's Psychology of Learning.* Open Court, La Salle, Ill

Bissel, J. and Mailloux, Z. (1981) The use of crafts in occupational therapy for the physically disabled. *American Journal of Occupational Therapy*, **35**, 369–374

Breines, E. (1990) Genesis of occupation: A philosophical model for therapy and theory. *Australian Occupational Therapy Journal*, **37**, 45–49

Brockett, R.G. (1988) *Ethical issues in adult education.* Teachers College, Columbia University, New York

Bruner, J. (1990) *Acts of Meaning.* University of Chicago Press, Chicago

Butt, R., Raymond, D. and Yamaguishi, L. (1982) Autobiographic praxis: Studying the formation of teacher's knowledge. *Journal of Curriculum Theorizing*, **7**, 87–164

Chapparo, C. (1993) Clinical reasoning: A model for occupational therapy in the practice area of neurology. Unpublished PhD Thesis. Macquarie University, Sydney

Chapparo, C., Ranka, J. and Hillman, A. (1992) *Curriculum Evaluation Project: The Practice Area of Physical Disabilities.* School of Occupational Therapy, The University of Sydney

Christiansen, C. (1990) The perils of plurality. *Occupational Therapy Journal of Research*, **11**, 259–265

Christiansen, C. and Baum, C. (1991) *Occupational Therapy: Overcoming Human Performance Deficits.* Slack, Thorofare, NJ

Cohen, S. (1983) The mental hygiene movement: The development of personality and the school: The medicalization of American education. *History of Education Quarterly*, **23**, 123–149

Cohn, E.S. (1989) Fieldworld education: Shaping a foundation for clinical reasoning. *American Journal of Occupational Therapy*, **43**, 240–244

Cohn, E.S. (1991) Clinical reasoning: Explicating complexity. *American Journal of Occupational Therapy*, **45**, 969–971

Crepeau, E.B. (1991) Achieving intersubjective understanding: Examples from an occupational therapy treatment session. *American Journal of Occupational Therapy*, **45**, 1016–1025

Day, D.J. (1973) A systems diagram for teaching treatment planning. *American Journal of Occupational Therapy*, **27**, 239–243

Dewey, J. (1910) *How We Think.* University of Chicago, Chicago

Dewey, J. (1929) *The Quest for Certainty: A Study of the Relation of Knowledge and Action.* G.P. Putnam's Sons, New York

Donelly, M. (1992) *Integration Issues in Occupational Therapy. Fourth Year Curriculum Hypotheticals.* School of Occupational Therapy, The University of Sydney, Sydney

Dreyfus, H. and Dreyfus, S. (1986) *Mind Over Machine: The Power of Human Intuition and Expertise in the Era of the Computer.* Free Press, New York

Eliason, M. and Gohl-Giese, A. (1979) A question of professional boundaries. *American Journal of Occupational Therapy*, **33**, 175–179

Elstein, A.S. and Bordage, G. (1979) Psychology of clinical reasoning. In *Health Psychology: A Handbook* (eds G. Stone, F. Cohen and N. Adler). Jossey Press, San Francisco

Elstein, A.S., Shulman, L.S. and Sprafka, S.A. (1978) *Medical Problem Solving: An Analysis of Clinical Reasoning.* Harvard University Press, Cambridge, MA

Fidler, G. (1981) From crafts to competence. *American Journal of Occupational Therapy*, **35**, 567–573

Fleming, M.H. (1991a) The therapist with the three track mind. *American Journal of Occupational Therapy*, **45**, 1007–1014

Fleming, M.H. (1991b) Clinical reasoning in medicine compared with clinical reasoning in occupational therapy. *American Journal of Occupational Therapy*, **45**, 988–996

Fondiller, E.D., Rosage, L.J. and Neuhaus, B.E. (1990) Values influencing clinical reasoning in occupational therapy: An exploratory study. *Occupational Therapy Journal of Research*, **10**, 41–54

Gale, J. and Marsden, P. (1982) Clinical problem solving: the beginning of the process. *Medical Education*, **16**, 22–26

Gillette, N. and Mattingly, C. (1987) Clinical reasoning in

occupational therapy. *American Journal of Occupational Therapy*, **41**, 399–400

Gordon, D. (1988) Clinical science and clinical expertise: Changing boundaries between art and science in medicine. In *Biomedicine Examined* (eds M. Lock and D. R. Gordon). Kluwer Academic Publishers, pp. 257–295

Grady, A., Guilfoyle, E. and Moore, J. (1990) *Children Adapt*, 2nd edn. Slack, Thorofare, New Jersey

Haddad, A.M. (1988) Teaching ethical analysis in occupational therapy. *American Journal of Occupational Therapy*, **42**, 300–304

Hagedorn, R. (1992) *Occupational Therapy: Foundations for Practice. Models, Frames of Reference and Core Skills.* Churchill Livingstone, London

Hammond, K.H. (1988) Judgement and decision making in dynamic tasks. *Information and Decision Technologies*, **14**, 3–13

Harrison, E. (1972) Interdisciplinary barriers to the application of systems engineering. *American Journal of Occupational Therapy*, **26**, 225–233

Harvey-Krefting, L. (1985) The concept of work in occupational therapy: A historical review. *American Journal of Occupational Therapy*, **39**, 301–307

Heimstra, R. (1991) Translating personal values and philosophy into practical action. In *Ethical Issues in Adult Education* (ed. R.G. Brockett). Teachers College, Columbia University, New York

Hemphill, B.J. (1982) The evaluative process. In *The Evaluative Process in Psychiatric Occupational Therapy*, (ed. B. J. Hemphill). Charles Slack, Thorofare, NJ

Henderson, A. (1988) 1988 Eleanor Clarke Slagle Lecture. Occupational therapy knowledge: From practice to theory. *American Journal of Occupational Therapy*, **42**, 567–576

Hopkins, H.L. (1988) An historical perspective on occupational therapy. In *Willard and Spackman's Occupational Therapy*, 7th edn. (eds H.L. Hopkins and H.D. Smith). J. B. Lippincott, Philadelphia, pp. 16–37

Hopkins, H.L. and Smith, H. D. (eds) (1988) *Willard and Spackman's Occupational Therapy*, 7th edn. Lippincott, Philadelphia

Hopkins, H.L. and Tiffany, E.G. (1988) Occupational therapy – a problem-solving process. In *Willard and Spackman's Occupational Therapy*, 7th edn (eds H.L. Hopkins and H.D. Smith). J.B. Lippincott, Philadelphia, pp. 102–111

Hundert, E.M. (1987) A model for ethical problem solving in medicine, with practical applications. *American Journal of Psychiatry*, **144**, 839–846

Jacob, F. (1964) Occupational therapy in a psychiatric unit in a general hospital. *Australian Journal of Occupational Therapy*, **11**, 10–16

Katz, N. (1985) Occupational therapy's domain of concern: Reconsidered. *American Journal of Occupational Therapy*, **39**, 518–524

Keilhofner, G. and Burke, J. (1977) Occupational therapy after 60 years: An account of changing identity and knowledge. *American Journal of Occupational Therapy*, **31**, 675–689

Keilhofner, G. and Burke, J. (1983) The evolution of knowledge in occupational therapy: Past, present and future. In *Health Through Occupation* (ed. G. Keilhofner). F.A. Davis, Philadelphia

Keilhofner, G. and Nelson, C. (1987) The nature and implications of shifting patterns of practice in physical disabilities occupational therapy. *Occupational Therapy in Health Care*, **3**, 187–198

Kleinman, A. (1988) *The Illness Narratives: Suffering, Healing and the Human Condition.* Basic Books, New York

Kuhn, T. (1970) *The Structure of Scientific Revolutions*, 2nd edn. University of Chicago Press, Chicago

Langthaler, M. (1990) *The Components of Therapeutic Relationship in Occupational Therapy.* Unpublished Master's Thesis, Tufts University, Medford, Massachusetts

Licht, S. (1947) The objectives of occupational therapy. *Occupational Therapy Rehabilitation*, **28**, 17–22

Lindquist, J.E., Mack, W. and Parham, L.D. (1982) A synthesis of occupational behaviour and sensory integration concepts in theory and practice, Part 1, Theory and practice. *American Journal of Occupational Therapy*, **36**, 365–374

Line, J. (1969) Case method as a scientific form of clinical thinking. *American Journal of Occupational Therapy*, **23**, 308–313

Llorens, L. (1972) Problem-solving the role of occupational therapy in a new environment. *American Journal of Occupational Therapy*, **26**, 234–238

Mattingly, C. (1991a) What is clinical reasoning? *American Journal of Occupational Therapy*, **45**, 979–986

Mattingly, C. (1991b) The narrative nature of clinical reasoning. *American Journal of Occupational Therapy*, **45**, 998–1005

Meyer, A. (1922) The philosophy of occupational therapy. *Archives of Occupational Therapy*, **1**, 1–10

Mezirow, J. (1991) How critical reflection triggers transformative learning. In *Fostering Critical Reflection in Adulthood* (ed. J. Mezirow). Jossey-Bass, San Francisco

Mirvits, P.H. and Seashore, S.E. (1979) Being ethical in organizational research. *American Psychologist*, **34**, 766–780

Mosey, A. (1981) *Occupational Therapy. Configuration of a Profession.* Raven Press, New York

Neuhaus, B.E. (1988) Ethical considerations in clinical reasoning: The impact of technology and cost containment. *American Journal of Occupational Therapy*, **42**, 288–292

Parham, D. (1986) Applying theory to practice. In *Proceedings: Occupational Therapy Education: Target 2000.* American Occupational Therapy Association, Rockville, Maryland, pp. 119–122

Parham D. (1987) Toward professionalism: The reflective therapist. *American Journal of Occupational Therapy*, **41**, 555–561

Pedretti, L.W. (1982) *The Compatibility of Current Treatment Methods in Physical Disabilities with the Philosophical Case of Occupational Therapy*. San Jose University, San Jose (unpublished)

Pelland, M.J. (1987) A conceptual model for the instruction and supervision of treatment planning. *American Journal of Occupational Therapy*, **41**, 351–359

Pinel, P. (1948) Medical philosophical treatise on mental alienation. In *Occupational Therapy Source Book* (ed. S. Licht). Williams and Wilkins, Baltimore, p. 19

Polanyi, M. (1958) *Personal Knowledge*. Routledge and Kegan Paul, London

Reed, K.L. (1984) *Models of Practice in Occupational Therapy*. Williams and Wilkins, Baltimore

Reilly, M. (1960) Research potentiality of occupational therapy. *American Journal of Occupational Therapy*, **14**, 206–209

Rogers, J.C. (1983) Eleanor Clarke Slagle Lectureship – 1983: Clinical reasoning: The ethics, science and art. *American Journal of Occupational Therapy*, **37**, 601–616

Rogers, J.C. and Holm, M. (1991) Occupational therapy diagnostic reasoning: A component of clinical reasoning. *American Journal of Occupational Therapy*, **45**, 1045–1053

Rogers, J.C. and Masagatani, G. (1982) Clinical reasoning of occupational therapists during the initial assessment of physically disabled patients. *Occupational Therapy Journal of Research*, **2**, 195–219

Sarbin, T.R., Taft, R. and Bailey, D.E. (1960) *Clinical Inference and Cognitive Theory*. Holt, Rinehart and Winston, New YorkSchifter, D.E. and Ajzen, I. (1985) Intention, perceived control and weight loss: An application of the theory of planned behaviour. *Journal of Personality and Social Psychology*, **49**, 843–851

Schkade, J.K. and Schultz, S. (1992) Occupational adaptations: Toward a holistic approach for contemporary practice, Part 1. *American Journal of Occupational Therapy*, **46**, 829–837

Schon, D.A. (1983) *The Reflective Practitioner: How Professionals Think in Action*. Basic Books, New York

Schon, D.A. (1987) *Educating the Reflective Practitioner: Toward a New Design for Teaching and Learning in the Professions*. Jossey-Bass, San Francisco

Shannon, P. (1977) The derailment of occupational therapy. *American Journal of Occupational Therapy*, **31**, 229–234

Slagle, A.C. (1922) Training aids for mental patients. *Occupational Therapy and Rehabilitation*, **1**, 11–14

Spackman, C. (1968) A history of the practice of occupational therapy for restoration of physical function: 1917–1967. *American Journal of Occupational Therapy*, **22**, 67–76

Stanage, S.M. (1987) *Adult Education and Phenomenological Research: New Directions for Theory, Practice and Research*. Kreiger Pub. Co., Florida

Trombly, C.A. (1988) *Occupational Therapy for Physical Dysfunction*, 3rd edn. Williams and Wilkins, Baltimore

Van Deusen, J. (1991) The issue is. Can we delimit the discipline of occupational therapy? *American Journal of Occupational Therapy*, **44**, 175–176

Wigglesworth, M. (1923) Round table on training courses. *Archives of Occupational Therapy*, **2**, 119–131

Wittman, P.P. (1990) The disparity between educational preparation and the expectations of practice. *American Journal of Occupational Therapy*, **44**, 1130–1131

Yerxa, E.J. (1979) The philosophical base of occupational therapy. In *Occupational Therapy: 2001 A.D.* American Occupational Therapy Association, Rockville, Maryland, pp. 26–30

Yerxa, E.J. (1991) Seeking a relevant, ethical and realistic way of knowing for occupational therapy. *American Journal of Occupational Therapy*, **45**, 199–204

Section Three

Dimensions of teaching clinical reasoning

8

Teaching clinical reasoning in health science curricula

Kathryn Refshauge and Joy Higgs

The fundamental assumptions underlying this text are firstly that clinical reasoning is an essential part of health science curricula and secondly that it can be 'taught', or rather that teachers can facilitate the process of the development of clinical reasoning ability. Accepting these assumptions raises several issues for teachers, including the need to understand the nature of clinical reasoning and how it develops and the question of how teachers can help students develop clinical reasoning ability. This chapter will address these issues.

The importance of clinical reasoning

The term health professional implies a qualified health care provider who demonstrates professional autonomy, competence and accountability (Higgs, 1993a). Medicine has long held this title. The other health disciplines have emerged to professional status over many years of serious endeavour and commitment, discarding a technical and directed role to achieve professional autonomy. Professional status incorporates the responsibility to make independent and accountable clinical decisions. Demand is increasing for quality care and accountability, from consumers, from society, from within the health professions themselves, from health care authorities, and where relevant, from registration bodies (Higgs, 1990).

Clinical decisions need to be made within the complex, uncertain and subjective context of people living in varying conditions of health and illness. Kassirer and Kopelman (1991, p. vii) describe this as caring for patients who present 'problems that might be confusing and contradictory, characterized by imperfect, inconsistent, or even inaccurate information'. In addition to dealing with this complex clinical information, health professionals are expected to deal effectively with an increasing body of scientific knowledge. It is apparent then, that to meet the expectations of society and earn the right to act as autonomous health care providers, health professionals need to be skilled in making clinical decisions. Indeed, the ability to make sound clinical judgements could be described as the most important factor in effective clinical practice. The importance placed upon clinical reasoning by the health professions is evident in the increasing acceptance of explicit teaching of clinical reasoning in health science curricula (Elstein, 1981; Margolis et al, 1982; Neame et al, 1985; Tanner, 1987; Burnett and Pierson, 1988; Higgs, 1990; Kassirer and Kopelman, 1991; Rogers et al, 1991; Schwartz, 1991).

The nature of clinical reasoning and its development

Tanner (1987, p. 155) argues that the teaching of clinical reasoning should be based on '(a) an understanding of how competent individuals proceed in determining what observations to make, in identifying health problems from those observations, and in deciding on appropriate actions; and (b) an understanding of the progression of such competence, from beginning level to the development of expertise' (1). This poses a dilemma for the teacher since there is no universally accepted model, explanation or interpretation of clinical reasoning or its development and the question of whether all clinicians use a single general reasoning process is unresolved (Gale and Marsden, 1982). Ongoing research and developments occurring in this field will continue to deepen our understanding of clinical reasoning.

At this stage, however, teachers are faced with the question 'which model should I encourage my students to emulate?'. The choice could be hypothetico-deductive reasoning (Elstein et al, 1978; Jones, 1992), pattern recognition (Scadding, 1967; Barrows and Feltovich, 1987), problem solving (Bashook, 1976; Payton, 1985), the phenomenological model adopted in occupational therapy (Mattingly, 1991), models of backward reasoning and forward reasoning (Ridderikhoff, 1989; Patel and Groen, 1991), models as in nursing which emphasize intuition (Benner and Tanner, 1987; Rew and Barrow, 1987) or a combined model (2).

Since no one model is ideal in all circumstances and the very process of clinical reasoning is inextricably linked to the unique knowledge base of the professional discipline (and indeed to the individual clinician), then it follows that clinical reasoning needs to be taught in context. Thus, the teacher's choice of clinical reasoning model for a given program of study needs to take into consideration such factors as the conceptual framework of the health science discipline in question (e.g. nursing), the specific learning environment or curricular context and the stage of development of the learner(s). For instance, practice in the use of the hypothetico-deductive reasoning model may be highly desirable for undergraduate medical students who are learning how to collect and process a multitude of clinical data and make diagnostic and treatment decisions. By comparison, exploration of the phenomenological model may be best suited to occupational therapy students learning within a 'wellness' framework rather than a traditional medical

model. And, for a group of postgraduate physiotherapy students (for instance) with a wealth of clinical expertise, examination of clinical reasoning using a pattern recognition model may enable these students to critique their prior learning, deepen their knowledge bases and gain a greater understanding of, and expertise in the use of clinical reasoning strategies.

A number of fundamental characteristics of the complex phenomenon of clinical reasoning do appear to be commonly supported in emerging research, models and theories. The importance of the clinician's knowledge as both the underpinning of reasoning and an integral part of the clinical reasoning process, providing essential ongoing input for comparison with, or supplementation for clinical data being collected, is widely accepted. Investigations into the characteristics of expert clinicians have strongly supported the link between the presence of a rich, well-organized and relevant knowledge base and reasoning expertise (Norman, 1985; Bordage and Lemieux, 1986; Patel et al, 1986; Grant and Marsden, 1987; Gilhooly, 1988; Grant et al, 1988; Norman, 1988).

Educators are also accepting the importance of knowledge in clinical reasoning ability. To deal with the knowledge explosion of the last few decades, many education programs adopted the goal of developing problem solving skills in their students with an attendant diminishing emphasis on knowledge acquisition (Norman, 1990). These programs failed to recognize that effective problem solving or reasoning requires a large store of relevant knowledge. They were also based on the assumption that such skills are generalizable and could be transferred to clinical reasoning. Recent findings, such as the work of Browning et al (1988) who tested the correlation between general problem solving test scores and clinical performance measures and found no correlation between the two, have challenged this assumption. Grant (1991) argues that the emphasis on problem solving skills as the key to lifelong learning was 'illusory'. She proposes that greater emphasis should be placed on the self-reliance of learners in acquiring knowledge, and that problem solving is simply part of

---

(1) Both of these issues are discussed at length in Sections 1 and 2 of this text. Refer particularly to Chapters 1 and 2.

(2) As presented in Chapter 1.

the broader notion of reflective inquiry, as described by Schon (1988).

The nature of clinically-relevant knowledge is another relevant factor, with growing credence being given to knowledge which is gained through experience, through construction of ideas by the clinician and through creative cognitive processes, as well as 'knowledge of the field' which is learned (3). Also, the contextual-specificity of knowledge is recognized, Candy (1988) argues that functioning autonomously as an expert in a field requires 'subject-matter autonomy'. Professions build up a form of 'professional logic' which incorporates a way of interpreting information that is unique to that profession, usually based on empirical evidence, experience and clinical wisdom.

The concept of clinical reasoning as an active and dynamic process of structuring and interpreting information has been supported by research into the process of clinical reasoning (Gale and Marsden, 1982). That is, the idea that clinicians passively receive information then process these data to make decisions, as implied in early problem solving models, has largely been discarded. This is not to say, however, that clinicians are conscious of all of the information they receive. Indeed, one of the important goals of clinical reasoning education should be to help clinicians be more aware of received data, of their own knowledge and of their processes of reasoning. To achieve this goal, learners in clinical reasoning programs need to develop their metacognitive abilities.

Finally, there is growing argument (Jones and Butler, 1991; Higgs, 1992) that clinical reasoning as a concept and process is much greater than making decisions relating to diagnosis. Reasoning and decision making occurs throughout the clinician's interaction with the client and ideally involves the client's input into decision making in such activities as determining appropriate courses of data collection, determining the reliability, importance and relevance of data collected, identifying diagnoses or patients' problems and concerns, planning intervention or patient self-management strategies, evaluating outcomes and pursuing ongoing management.

Incorporation of the generally accepted activities or features of clinical reasoning (as discussed above) into health science teaching programs is recommended. In addition, the authors would argue that in the absence of a commonly accepted model of clinical reasoning, it is desirable for learners to develop their own understanding of the clinical reasoning process and of how they reason as the first step in facilitating improved clinical reasoning. This can be accomplished through exploration of how others describe or have investigated clinical reasoning, examination of the differences between reasoning in novices and experts, reflection on their own reasoning and discussions with other students.

In undertaking this exploration students are also incorporating into their understanding of clinical reasoning their unique and evolving knowledge bases (comprising theoretical, research, experiential and personal knowledge), their learning and thinking approaches and the sets of values, beliefs and attitudes against which they compare new information and make decisions. Each of these factors influences students' clinical reasoning behaviour. For instance, if new knowledge or ideas are incongruent with their belief system, individuals may reject the new information. In addition, people lean towards a confirmatory bias, where they tend to accept information that supports their beliefs, and reject or ignore information that conflicts with their beliefs (Elstein et al, 1978). To enhance the reasoning of health professionals, it is incumbent upon both the teacher and the learner to explore the values or belief systems of the students, to ensure that they explore new ideas and process information in more appropriate ways.

Issues in teaching clinical reasoning

Curriculum framework and design

Clinical competence requires the application of sound knowledge through clinical reasoning and decision making in the clinical context. For this reason most health science educators have embraced the concept of teaching clinical

---

(3) Refer to Chapter 10 for a more detailed discussion of the nature of knowledge, and Chapter 2 for a discussion of the role of biomedical knowledge in clinical reasoning.

reasoning, and have incorporated it into their curricula.

Clinical reasoning may be taught as a separate subject within a curriculum or as an integral aspect of all areas/subjects within the curriculum. The first option has the advantage of drawing attention to this skill rather than diffusing it among the various other learning goals of the curriculum. More time can be spent in refining individual students' clinical reasoning skills, or in identifying and addressing deficiencies in their knowledge and reasoning abilities. The more general approach has the potential advantages of reinforcing reasoning and the integration of knowledge in all areas of learning, and promoting transfer of learning from classroom to clinical settings.

Shepard and Jensen (1990) refer to explicit and implicit curricula, the latter indicating the messages received by students as to the importance of many aspects of their learning program which are not clearly articulated in formal curriculum documents. Both of these forms of curricula reinforce and direct students' learning. These authors emphasize the importance of using both the explicit and implicit curricula to promote reflection in learning and the development of reflective knowledge and skills which can help learners (and clinicians) to deal with what Schon (1987) labels 'the indeterminate zones of practice' or the uncertainty, uniqueness and value conflicts which characterize human situations. What is needed with these situations is a 'reflective practitioner' or one who incorporates reflection into clinical reasoning practices.

Mismatches between implicit and explicit curricula cause confusion and non-optimal learning. It is important, therefore, for teachers to avoid what has been described as a discrepancy between 'espoused theory' vs 'theory-in-use' (Bowden, 1988). In studying this practice in a number of university programs Bowden (1988, p. 257) found that teachers wanted their students to possess qualities such as 'problem-solving ability in their profession, lateral thinking, insight, integrity, perspective, self-motivation, ability to "self-learn", and an understanding of the structure of (relevant) knowledge'. (Such outcomes would be desirable in a clinical reasoning course.) However, when investigating why students did not achieve these outcomes, Bowden identified that a mismatch had occurred between

espoused theory (and its intended outcomes) and the way the students were actually taught and assessed. The challenge for the educator then, is to select an educational philosophy or conceptual framework which is appropriate for the subject to be taught and to authentically adopt this 'espoused theory' in practice.

We would argue that the ideal choice of educational philosophy and framework for clinical reasoning programs is adult learning. This is because both clinical reasoning and adult learning involve an inseparable link between the individual's knowledge base and his or her cognitive (learning or reasoning) processes, an ability to seek information and knowledge as required (to learn or to make clinical decisions), a capacity to engage in self-monitoring, evaluation and development and responsibility for decisions taken.

According to Finger (1990) adult learning provides a means of achieving transformation of the learner and his or her situation since this approach helps the learner find a 'way out' of a problem situation. Adoption of this approach, therefore, would enable the student to learn through the experience of solving his or her learning problems while at the same time learning about clinical reasoning or the transformation of clinical problems into solutions. The notion of 'changing students' conceptions of aspects of the world around them' is regarded by Ramsden and his colleagues as 'the core of education' (Ramsden, 1988a, p. vii). Education can be enhanced, argues Ramsden (1988b), by understanding how students are thinking and learning, by helping students learn to understand how subject experts see relevant phenomena and by enabling students to change their conceptions of these phenomena.

The principles and practice of adult learning come closest to this goal. In adult learning students need to take an active part in the learning process, the teacher and learner are engaged in interdependent learning (Griffith, 1987) and learning is directed towards growth of the learner. Table 8.1 (Terry and Higgs, 1993) provides an overview of environmental conditions which promote adult learning, teaching decisions the educator and learner need to make to engage successfully in adult learning and the characteristic behaviours of effective adult learners. These provide a guide for teachers wishing to adopt this approach.

Table 8.1   Adult learning conditions and behaviours

Environmental conditions	Decision making/management factors	Adult learning behaviours
Motivation	Shared goals	Problem solving
Acceptance of learner as person	Shared management	Interaction with teacher and other
Freedom/autonomy	Mutual decision making/planning	learners
Individuality	Shared resource acquisition	Active participation in learning
Emphasis on abilities/experience	Learner involvement in learning needs,	Self-correction
Student-centred learning	diagnosis and evaluation	Interdependence
Resource rich environment	Learner direction in posing questions/	Critical reflection
Mutual respect/trust	seeking answers	Progressive mastery
Teacher support/facilitation	Effective communication	Active seeking of meaning
Learning via experience relevant to	Choice in participation	Individual pacing
learner	Collaborative facilitation	Empowered self-direction
Praxis – integrating reflection, theory,	Ongoing review by teacher and learners	Internal drive/motivation
practice, experience	Learner identification of community	Reciprocal learning
Interaction between learners	goals and needs as part of own	Experiential learning
Effective/appropriate group dynamics	learning context	
Security/support	Learner acceptance of responsibility	

From Terry and Higgs (1993).

Teaching knowledge that is purposeful and requires deep learning

As previously discussed, health professionals today need to be capable of performing competently in an autonomous, professional capacity, of maintaining this competence, and of generating knowledge throughout their careers. They also need to be able to respond to the changing health care needs of the community (Cox, 1988; Foreman, 1986). Effective reasoning and decision-making abilities can enhance the likelihood of an individual successfully achieving these outcomes. As suggested, continued knowledge acquisition is of fundamental importance for effective reasoning by accountable health professionals. Further, success in the above behaviours requires the ability to acquire knowledge using a deep learning approach.

Research in the area of student learning (Entwistle and Ramsden, 1983) has identified that contexts/curricula which foster deep learning are characterized by freedom in learning, less formality, good teaching input, a good social climate and clear goals. Surface or rote learning approaches are more likely to occur where there are heavy workloads. Curriculum planning therefore needs to ensure that learning environments are created that will foster deep learning. Table 8.2 (from Ramsden, 1988b, p. 19) presents an overview of deep and surface approaches to learning. A comparison between Tables 8.1 and 8.2 and the above discussions on adult and deep learning indicates the similarity between these two learning approaches and the conditions which foster them.

Table 8.2   Deep and surface approaches to learning

Deep approach *Intention to understand*	Surface approach *Intention to complete task requirements*
Focus on 'what is signified' (e.g. the author's argument)	Focus on the 'signs' (e.g. the text itself)
Relate and distinguish new ideas and previous knowledge	Focus on discrete elements
Relate concepts to everyday experience	Memorize information and procedures for assessments
Relate and distinguish evidence and argument	Unreflectively associate concepts and facts
Organize and structure content	Fail to distinguish principles from evidence, new
Internal emphasis: 'A window through which aspects of	information from old
reality become visible, and more intelligible' (Entwistle	Treat task as an external imposition
and Marton, 1984)	External emphasis: demands of assessments, knowledge cut
	off from everyday reality

From Ramsden (1988b).

The learning environment

The above discussion emphasizes the importance of the learning environment. According to Ramsden (1985) the effects of learning environments can be best understood if they are thought of as operating at several levels:

(a) At the level of the learning task. Here relevance of the task to the student promotes intrinsic motivation and a deep (or meaning-oriented) approach to learning. Alternatively, extrinsic motivation increases the likelihood of surface learning.

(b) At the teacher level. Here, teacher attitude, enthusiasm, concern for helping students understand and ability to appreciate students' learning difficulties all influence students' approaches and attitudes to studying.

(c) At the department or course level. In particular the forms of assessment used at this level have a strong influence on approaches to studying, with many courses encouraging a surface approach to learning through the use of assessment methods which reward reproductive answers.

(d) At the institution level. Differences in institutional values and purposes can also influence students' learning.

In planning a learning program the teacher needs to consider the environmental influences and constraints at each of these levels and also the opportunities which different learning environments provide. In problem-based learning curricula many environmental levels may be well co-ordinated to reinforce the learning of clinical problem solving skills and knowledge throughout the students' learning experiences. Norman and Schmidt (1992), educators from the renowned problem-based learning institutions of McMaster University and the University of Limburg, Maastricht, respectively, have conducted a review of problem-based learning. They concluded that while there may be minimal differences in the overall knowledge or competence of students educated via problem-based learning or conventional curricula, that problem-based learning curricula promote better retention of knowledge, interest in learning and development of self-directed learning skills. They stress the advantage this mode of curriculum provides in allowing students to learn knowledge and problem-solving skills in the context of clinical problems and emphasize the importance of immediate corrective feedback.

More conventional curricula are frequently divided into a 'pre-clinical' component (or rather an on-campus program which is likely to include the teaching of clinical as well as pre-clinical skills and knowledge) and a subsequent or interwoven 'clinical' or 'fieldwork' component. Clinical reasoning can be explored either in the classroom, or in the clinic.

In the classroom students can learn from mistakes, explore alternative treatment decisions, change their minds and examine many detailed aspects of knowledge use and evaluation in the absence of both time constraints and the potential negative effects on patients which can occur in the clinical context. The classroom setting also allows for discussion of students' thinking and the potential effects their decisions may have, and encourages feedback from both peers and teachers. However, attention must be devoted to transfer of these skills from the classroom to the clinical context. To enhance transfer into the clinical setting, it is essential that clinical educators develop a clear understanding of the process of teaching clinical reasoning that is consistent with classroom teaching. They need to create time to facilitate the students' reasoning and use of knowledge, and to provide feedback on these areas as well as on technical skills.

On campus pre-clinical teaching in health science curricula commonly addresses the basic and applied sciences (e.g. anatomy, physiology and biomechanics) and the medical sciences (e.g. pathology) which form an essential part of the clinician's knowledge base. In addition, students learn health science subjects such as the study of occupational performance, paediatric nursing, obstetrics and musculoskeletal physiotherapy. In these clinical subjects, in particular, structured learning activities can be implemented which are aimed at promoting the development of clinical reasoning skills and the integration of knowledge students have gained from life experiences as well as knowledge developed throughout their curriculum. Such learning activities can include small group learning tutorials, peer teaching, cognitive mapping, role play, verbalizing interpretation of patient data in simulated clinical settings, and experts discussing their interpretation of a problem. Peer teaching is another useful used method of fostering the development and evaluation of knowledge. Communicating thoughts, arguments and rationales requires the student to understand and organize what they know and how they use knowledge. Experience in peer teaching (Higgs, 1990) has shown that when learners are attempting to create learning experiences for others, they learn a great deal about the nature of their own knowledge, the breadth of this knowledge, the cognitive links they make, and the value and validity of their knowledge.

As well as developing reasoning skills and knowledge in the classroom students need to test the application of this knowledge in appropriate contexts. Clinical education provides this context. During clinical placements much of the daily activity of health science students relates to clinical problem solving since students are continually seeking, absorbing, interpreting, evaluating and summarizing clinical information and making clinical decisions on the basis of this information (Whelan, 1988). Experiences during clinical education promote an understanding of patients' conditions and needs as well as the students' own abilities in meeting these needs.

The reality of the clinical setting has many advantages even though it provides constraints to the exploration of clinical reasoning in action, such as potential dangers to the patient and time pressures. Holmes (1975) proposed that clinical education is vital for students to gain confidence in handling patients, develop their clinical/technical skills and acquire skills in decision making. The clinical setting also provides the complex context and conditions students will face in practice (e.g. the consequences of their actions, the variability and personalities of patients). Several groups of health personnel have been found to reason better in real treatment situations than in simulated situations (Dennis and May, 1987; Gale and Marsden, 1982). Practice broadens experience, and therefore enhances performance. It has also been found (Norman, 1990) that the context in which learning occurs has a profound effect on the student's ability to recall learning, with recall occurring best in situations similar to that in which it was learned. Finally, the role of patients in teaching and providing feedback is a further advantage of clinical settings. It is necessary, therefore, that health science curricula actively utilize both classroom and clinical settings for this purpose.

Processing learning experiences

Regardless of the learning environment the key factor to students' learning is their experiences and the way they learn from these. Learning through experience is what people do throughout their lives. It has been described as 'simultaneously an educational philosophy, a range of methodologies, and a framework for being, seeing, thinking and acting, on individual and collective levels. It involves the active transformation and integration of different forms of experience. These processes lead to new understandings, and the development of a wide range of capabilities' (McGill and Weil, 1989, p. 245). Boud (1993, p. 35) describes the key contributing elements of experience as a basis for learning as follows:

- experience is the foundation of, and stimulus for learning
- the effects of prior experience influence all learning
- learners actively construct their own experience
- learning is a holistic process which has affective, cognitive and conative features
- learning is socially and culturally constructed
- learning occurs in a socio-emotional context.

It is important to remember that simply participating in learning activities is not enough to generate learning or new knowledge. Many learners are not fully aware of the interactions in which they are participating or in the full potential of their social, psychological and material environment as a source of learning (Boud and Walker, 1990). Learning experiences need to be processed through reflection, by attempting to make sense of the experience, and by relating this experience to previous learning.

Reflection is an important element in promoting deep, meaningful learning (Engel, 1991). Opportunities need to be created before, during and after learning activities (Boud, 1988; Boud and Walker, 1991) to promote reflection and thereby foster learning, and to develop students' ability to perform as 'reflective' (and thus effective) practitioners

(Schon, 1987). Reflection can be promoted, for instance, by encouraging the use of a diary for reflecting on learning activities, scheduling appropriate breaks between classes, and encouraging group activities.

Related to active reflection as a means of enhancing learning, are the skills of self-evaluation and metacognition (or reflective self-awareness). Metacognition, as described by Flavell (1976), refers to awareness of one's cognitive processes and the exertion of control over them. These behaviours are desirable attributes of health science professionals who are endeavouring to process information in order to make sound clinical decisions and who are seeking to improve their knowledge base and clinical reasoning expertise.

Research has identified the value of metacognition in helping learners develop learning and problem-solving skills (Biggs and Telfer, 1987). In developing a greater awareness of their cognition individuals are better able to perform these mental processes. This argument supports the use of learning activities which prompt students to use, articulate, critique and review their clinical reasoning. In doing this students are able to raise their awareness of their thinking and develop an enhanced capacity for responsible self-direction and decision making.

Assessment and feedback

A further consideration in the quest to promote deep learning, is the provision of feedback. The nature of feedback on the learner's performance is known to be important in influencing learning in various ways (Gagne, 1974; Romiszowski, 1981; 1984), such as in encouraging either surface or deep learning. When students are only enlightened as to their errors and omissions, surface learning will be achieved. On the other hand, feedback can promote deep learning by discussing with students their understanding of issues, use of knowledge, or evaluation of information.

Closely linked with feedback is assessment of students. What and how students learn is also influenced by what they are assessed upon and how they are assessed (Rowntree, 1977;

Dahlgren, 1978; Elton, 1982; Thomas and Bain, 1982; Newble and Jaeger, 1983; Ramsden, 1984). Studies by Marton and Saljo (1976) and Ramsden (1984) have demonstrated that it is easier to encourage students to adopt a surface (or rote learning) approach than a deep (or meaningful) learning approach, and that the learning approach can be strongly influenced by the choice of assessment methods. It has been demonstrated that deep learning is fostered through assessment which rewards understanding, such as essay writing, as opposed to examinations based on recall of information (Watkins, 1984; Eizenberg, 1986).

As discussed earlier, students seek messages from the curriculum (e.g. from stated goals, learning activities and assessment) to guide their learning. Students' perceptions of these messages and of conflicts between them can result in their adopting learning behaviours contrary to those intended by the teachers. In particular, learning behaviour and outcomes are influenced by the learner's perception of the demands of assessment (Ramsden, 1984). In designing and conducting assessment procedures, therefore, the nature of the assessment process and how it is presented to, and perceived by the learners is important. The method of assessment also needs to be reliable and valid, for the behaviour being assessed, e.g. understanding, recall, evaluation. (4)

There needs to be consistency between the goals of learning, the activities used, the feedback given, and the assessment procedures implemented. If deep learning is desired to enhance the value as well as the breadth of the learner's knowledge, then learning activities, feedback and assessment procedures must all be consistently aimed at encouraging deep learning.

The role of the teacher and learner in adult learning programs

Health sciences education is a process of socialization into the professional role. Previous discussion has identified the parallel responsibilities of the learner and the autonomous clinician for their decisions and actions. In adult learning environments which seek to foster

(4) Further discussion on student assessment is found in Chapter 13.

deep learning, there is a dual emphasis on the teacher creating a climate which Rogers (1983) labels 'responsible freedom' and on the learners accepting both the privileges and responsibilities this entails. To succeed in this environment students need to develop higher learning skills including self-direction, critical self-appraisal and metacognition, to actively participate in both the learning activities provided and in the management of their learning and to seek help, guidance and feedback when appropriate.

An important factor to remember in planning for this creative, interdependent and dual (teacher and learner) managed learning environment is that not all learners will enter the current learning program with these advanced learning skills. The concept of 'learner task maturity' has been developed (Higgs, 1993b) to represent the idea of the level of readiness and ability to the learner to deal with demands of a specific learning task at a given time. This construct was developed to reflect the willingness and ability of learners to play a responsible and self-directed role in a given learning situation, and their ability to respond flexibly and appropriately to the demands of the learning situation.

The role of the teacher is to assess the learner's task maturity for the given learning situation and to create a learning system in which the learner can achieve optimal learning experiences and outcomes. Where the learner's task maturity is low, for instance due to unfamiliarity with the learning task or environment or due to limited advanced learning abilities, then a more structured learning program is appropriate. However, the emphasis on liberation of the student to experience, to learn and to develop as a learner (and in this case as a clinical reasoner) is central. Where the learner's task maturity is high, the learner and teacher can act as co-manager in the resultant 'liberating (learning) program system' (Higgs, 1993b).

Related questions in teaching clinical reasoning

The previous section has dealt with central educational issues associated with teaching clinical reasoning. This section will deal with a number of specific related questions associated with clinical reasoning, which the educator should address in planning a clinical reasoning learning program.

Communicating and justifying decisions

The demands of accountability which accompany the increased autonomy of health professionals require effective communication and justification of clinical decisions to many sectors of society, including government bodies, other members of the health care team and clients and their families. In addition to behaving in a competent, ethical and professional manner, clinicians need to be able to explain, clearly and credibly, the scientific and therapeutic basis for their actions and the expected outcomes, within the context of the individual client's needs, wishes and situation. Students can learn to communicate and justify their decisions effectively through clinical reasoning learning activities such as verbalizing their interpretation of patient data, and justifying their choice of intervention.

Involving the client

In the same way that the roles and responsibilities of health professionals are changing, so are clients' choices, rights and responsibilities in relation to their own health. Payton et al (1990) advocate client involvement in decision making which pertains to the management of their health and well-being. They argue that this process of client participation is based on the 'recognition of the values of self-determination and the worth of the individual' (p. ix). Based on their understanding of their clients' rights and responsibilities, students and graduate clinicians need to develop their own guidelines for when and how much involvement the client should have in reasoning and decision making. Mutual decision making and two-way communication require skills in negotiation as well as explaining. The clinical setting is a highly appropriate context in which to refine these skills under the guidance of clinical educators.

Utilizing protocols

Health professionals frequently use protocols as a part of the process of data collection. Although protocols imply rigid routines and lack of variation in response to individuals or to situations, they may also be regarded as scanning activities as described by Barrows and Tamblyn (1980). Scanning activities aim to identify cues requiring further investigation. They can assist in ensuring that adequate data are collected, thereby avoiding premature closure of hypothesis generation.

Pedantic and unthinking use of data collection routines can be time-wasting and can also result in a plethora of confusing, and perhaps irrelevant data causing difficulty in data analysis, particularly for the novice. The skilled clinician may choose to use data collection routines strategically. It is therefore appropriate to encourage students to explore the value of using protocols as a basis for comprehensive and efficient data collection and to help them learn how to use them strategically when or if desirable.

Conclusion

Clinical reasoning teaching is widely regarded as an essential part of health science curricula. It provides a framework for integrating students' learning, for preparing them for their role as autonomous, responsible health care professionals and for helping students deal with the complex and variable elements of clinical practice. By making clinical reasoning a conscious and strategic part of their clinical practice, student and graduate clinicians are encouraged to examine and express their opinions and ideas and to develop a greater awareness of how they reason and how their knowledge values and beliefs influence their clinical reasoning.

The challenge faced by health science educators of enhancing skills in clinical reasoning can be met by addressing four key elements: a comprehensive, valid and well-organized knowledge base; reasoning skills (i.e. cognitive, evaluative and metacognitive skills); a values and belief system; and clinical skills and clinical experience. This chapter has presented adult learning as an ideal framework for the development of these clinical reasoning skills and for fostering deep and lifelong learning. The learners' active participation in creating and managing their own learning experiences and in deriving meaning for them is at the core of this learning approach.

References

Barrows, H.S. and Feltovich, P.J. (1987) The clinical reasoning process. *Medical Education*, **21**, 86–91

Barrows, H.S. and Tamblyn, R.M. (1980) *Problem-Based Learning – An Approach to Medical Education*. Springer Publishing Company, New York

Bashook, P.G. (1976) A conceptual framework for measuring clinical problem-solving. *Journal of Medical Education*, **51**, 109–114

Benner, P. and Tanner, C. (1987) Clinical judgment: How expert nurses use intuition. *American Journal of Nursing*, January, 23–31

Biggs, J.B. and Telfer, R. (1987) *The Process of Learning* (2nd edn.). Prentice Hall, Sydney

Bordage, G. and Lemieux, M. (1986) Some cognitive characteristics of medical students with and without diagnostic reasoning difficulties. In *Proceedings of the 25th Annual Conference of Research in Medical Education of the American Association of Medical Colleges*. American Association of Medical Colleges, New Orleans, Louisiana, 185–190

Boud, D. (1988) How to help students learn from experience. In *The Medical Teacher* (eds K. Cox and C.E. Ewan) (2nd edn.). Churchill Livingstone, Edinburgh, pp. 68–73

Boud, D. (1993) Experience as the base for learning. *Higher Education Research and Development*, **12**, 33–44

Boud, D. and Walker, D. (1990) making the most of experience. *Studies in Higher Education*, **12**, 61–80

Boud, D. and Walker, D. (1991) *Experience and Learning: Reflection at Work*. Deakin University Press, Geelong, Victoria

Bowden, J. (1988) Achieving change in teaching practices. In *Improving Learning: New Perspectives* (ed. P. Ramsden). Kogan Page Ltd, London, pp. 255–267

Browning, C., Thomas, S. and Oates, J. (1988) Clinical decision making and clinical performance. Paper presented at the *2nd International Health Sciences Education Conference*. Cumberland College of Health Sciences, Sydney

Burnett, C.N. and Pierson, F.M. (1988) Developing problem-solving skills in the classroom. *Physical Therapy*, **68**, 1381–1385

Candy, P. (1988) On the attainment of subject-matter autonomy. In *Developing Student Autonomy* (ed. D. Boud) (2nd edn.). Kogan Page Ltd, London, pp. 59–76

Cox, K. (1988) Professional and educational context of medical education. In *The Medical Teacher* (eds K. Cox and C.E. Ewan) (2nd edn.). Churchill Livingstone, Edinburgh, pp. 4–8

Dahlgren, L.O. (1978) Qualitative differences in conceptions of basic principles in economics. Paper read at the *Fourth International Conference on Higher Education*, University of Lancaster, 1978

Dennis, J.K. and May, B.J. (1987) Practice in the year 2000: expert decision making in physical therapy. In *Proceedings of the 10th International Congress of the World Confederation of Physical Therapy* (Sydney, 1987). Australian Physiotherapy Association, Sydney, pp. 543–551

Eizenberg, N. (1986) Applying student learning research to practice. In *Student Learning: Research into Practice – The Marysville Symposium* (ed. J.A. Bowden). Centre for Study of Higher Education, The University of Melbourne, Parkville, pp. 21–60

Elstein, A.S. (1981) Educational programs in medical decision making. *Medical Decision Making*, **1**, 70–73

Elstein, A.S., Shulman, L.S. and Sprafka, S.A. (1978) *Medical Problem Solving: An Analysis of Clinical Reasoning*. Harvard University Press, Cambridge, Massachusetts

Elton, L.R.B. (1982) Assessment for learning. In *Professionalism and Flexibility in Learning* (ed. D. Bligh). SRHE, Guildford

Engel, C.E. (1991) Not just a method but a way of learning. In *The Challenge of Problem Based Learning* (eds. D. Boud and G. Feletti). Kogan Page, London, pp. 23–33

Entwistle, N.J. and Marton, F. (1984) Changing conceptions of learning and research. In *The Experience of Learning* (eds. F. Marton, D. Hounsell and N. Entwistle). Scottish Academic Press, Edinburgh

Entwistle, N.J. and Ramsden, P. (1983) *Understanding Student Learning*. Croom Helm, London

Finger, M. (1990) Does adult education need a philosophy? Reflections about the function of adult learning in today's society. *Studies in Higher Education*, **12**, 81–98

Flavell, J.H. (1976) Metacognitive aspects of problem solving. In *The Nature of Intelligence* (ed. L. B. Resnick). Lawrence Erlbaum, Hillsdale, New Jersey

Foreman, S. (1986) The changing medical care system: Some implications for medical education. *Journal of Medical Education*, **61**, 11–21

Gagne, R.M. (1974) *Principles of Instructional Design*. Holt, Rinehart and Winston, New York

Gale, J. and Marsden, P. (1982) Clinical problem solving: the beginning of the process. *Medical Education*, **16**, 22–26

Gilhooly, K.J. (1988) *Thinking: Directed, Undirected and Creative* (2nd edn.). Academic Press, New York

Grant, J. and Marsden, P. (1987) The structure of memorized knowledge in students and clinicians: an explanation for diagnostic expertise. *Medical Education*, **21**, 92–98

Grant, R. (1991) Obsolescence or lifelong education: Choices and challenges. In *Proceedings of the World Confederation for Physical Therapy 11th International Congress*. World Confederation for Physical Therapy, London 1991, pp. 145–149

Grant, R., Jones, M. and Maitland, G. (1988) Clinical decision making in upper quadrant dysfunction. In *Clinics in Physical Therapy – Physical Therapy of the Cervical and Thoracic Spine* (ed. R. Grant). Churchill Livingstone, New York, pp. 51–79

Griffith, G. (1987) Images of interdependence: Authority and power in teaching/learning. In *Appreciating Adults Learning: From the Learners' Perspective* (eds D. Boud and V. Griffin). Kogan Page Ltd, London, pp. 51–63

Higgs, J. (1990) Fostering the acquisition of clinical reasoning skills. *New Zealand Journal of Physiotherapy*, **18**, 13–17

Higgs, J. (1992) Developing clinical reasoning competencies. *Physiotherapy*, **78**, 575–581

Higgs, J. (1993a) Physiotherapy, professionalism and self-directed learning. *Journal of the Singapore Physiotherapy Association*, **14**, 8–11

Higgs, J. (1993b) The teacher in self-directed learning: manager or co-manager? In *Learner Managed Learning* (ed. N.J. Graves). World Education Fellowship, Leeds, pp. 122–131

Holmes, B. (1975) The compleat physiotherapist. *Physiotherapy Canada*, **27**, 90–91

Jones, M.A. (1992) Clinical reasoning in manual therapy. *Physical Therapy*, **72**, 875–884

Jones, M.A. and Butler, D.S. (1991) Clinical reasoning. In *Mobilisation of the Nervous System* (ed. D. S. Butler). Churchill Livingstone, Melbourne, pp. 91–106

Kassirer, J.P. and Kopelman, R.I. (1991) *Learning Clinical Reasoning*. Williams and Wilkins, Baltimore

Margolis, C.Z., Barnoon, S. and Barak, N. (1982) A required course in decision-making for preclinical medical students. *Journal of Medical Education*, **57**, 184–190

Marton, F. and Saljo, R. (1976) On qualitative differences in learning, II – Outcome as a function of the learner's conception of the task. *British Journal of Educational Psychology*, **46**, 115–127

Mattingly, C. (1991) The narrative nature of clinical reasoning. *The American Journal of Occupational Therapy*, **45**, 998–1005

McGill, I. and Weil, S.W. (1989) Continuing the dialogue: New possibilities for experiential learning. In *Making Sense of Experiential Learning: Diversity in Theory and Practice* (eds S.W. Weil and I. McGill). The Society for Research into Higher Education and Open University Press, Milton Keynes, pp. 245–272

Neame, R.L.B., Mitchell, K.R., Feletti, G.I. and McIntosh, J. (1985) Problem-solving in undergraduate medical students. *Medical Decision Making*, **5**, 312–324

Newble, D.I. and Jaeger, K. (1983) The effect of assessments and examinations on the learning of medical students. *Medical Education*, **17**, 165–171

Norman, G.R. (1985) Objective measurement of clinical performance. *Medical Education*, **19**, 43–47

Norman, G.R. (1988) Problem-solving skills, solving problems and problem-based learning. *Medical Education*, **22**, 279–286

Norman, G.R. (1990) Editorial: problem-solving skills and

problem-based learning. *Physiotherapy Theory and Practice*, **6**, 53–54

Norman, G.R. and Schmidt, H.G. (1992) The psychologcial basis of problem-based learning: A review of the evidence. *Academic Medicine*, **67**, 557–565

Patel, V.L. and Groen, G.J. (1991) The general and specific nature of medical expertise: a critical look. In *Toward A General Theory Of Expertise: Prospects and Limits* (eds A. Ericsson and J. Smith). Cambridge University Press, New York, pp. 93–125

Patel, V.L., Groen, G.J. and Frederiksen, C.H. (1986) Differences between medical students and doctors in memory for clinical cases. *Medical Education*, **20**, 3–9

Payton, O.D. (1985) Clinical reasoning process in physical therapy. *Physical Therapy*, **65**, 924–928

Payton, O.D., Nelson, C.E. and Ozer, M.N. (1990) *Patient Participation in Program Planning: A Manual for Therapists*. F.A. Davis, Philadelphia

Ramsden, P. (1984) The context of learning. In *The Experience of Learning* (eds F. Marton, D. Hounsell and N. Entwistle). Scottish Academic Press, Edinburgh

Ramsden, P. (1985) Student learning research: Retrospect and prospect. *Higher Education Research and Development*, **4**, 51–70

Ramsden, P. (1988a) Preface. In *Improving Learning: New Perspectives* (ed. P. Ramsden). Kogan Page, London, pp. vii–ix

Ramsden, P. (1988b) Studying learning: Improving teaching. In *Improving Learning: New Perspectives* (ed. P. Ramsden). Kogan Page, London, pp. 13–31

Rew, L. and Barrow, E. (1987) Intuition: a neglected hallmark of nursing knowledge. *Advances in Nursing Science*, **10**, 49–62

Ridderikhoff, J. (1989) *Methods in Medicine: A Descriptive Study of Physicians' Behaviour*. Kluwer Academic Publishers, Dordrecht.

Rogers, C.R. (1983) *Freedom to Learn for the 80's*. Charles E. Merrill Publishing, Ohio

Rogers, J.C., Swee, D.E. and Ullian, J.A. (1991) Teaching medical decision making and students' clinical problem solving skills. *Medical Teacher*, **13**, 157–164

Romiszowski, A.J. (1981) *Designing Instructional Systems: Decision-making in Course Planning and Curriculum Design*. Kogan Page, London

Romiszowski, A.J. (1984) *Producing Instructional Systems: Lesson Planning for Individualized and Group Learning Activities*. Kogan Page, London

Rowntree, D. (1977) *Assessing Students*. Harper and Row, London

Scadding, J.G. (1967) Diagnosis: The clinician and the computer. *The Lancet*, **1**, 877–882

Schon, D.A. (1987) *Educating the Reflective Practitioner*. Jossey-Bass, San Francisco

Schon, D.A. (1988) From technical rationality to reflection-in-action. In *Professional Judgement* (eds J. Dowie and A. Elstein). Cambridge University Press, Cambridge, pp. 60–77

Schwartz, K.B. (1991) Clinical reasoning and new ideas on intelligence: implications for teaching and learning. *The American Journal of Occupational Therapy*, **45**, 1033–1037

Shepard, K.F. and Jensen, G.M. (1990) Physical therapist curricula for the 1990s: educating the reflective practitioner. *Physical Therapy*, **70**, 566–573

Tanner, C.A. (1987) Teaching clinical judgement. *Annual Review of Nursing Research*, **5**, 153–173

Terry, W. and Higgs, J. (1993) Educational programmes to develop clinical reasoning skills. *Australian Journal of Physiotherapy*, **39**, 47–51

Thomas, P.R. and Bain, J.D. (1982) Consistency in learning strategies. *Higher Education*, **11**, 249–259

Watkins, D. (1984) Student perceptions of factors influencing tertiary learning. *Higher Education Research and Development*, **3**, 33–50

Whelan, G. (1988) Improving medical students' clinical-problem-solving. In *Improving Learning: New Perspectives* (ed. P. Ramsden). Kogan Page, London, pp. 199–214

9

Clinical reasoning and biomedical knowledge: implications for teaching

Vimla L. Patel and David R. Kaufman

We are entering a period of time in which health science curricula world-wide are undergoing dramatic transformations and experiencing significant structural changes. These changes are likely to shape the practice of the health sciences for decades to come. The role of biomedical knowledge in clinical medicine is one of the focal issues in this transformation. Basic science knowledge reflects a subset of biomedical knowledge, although at points in the chapter the two terms are used interchangeably. There are many competing views and assumptions concerning the role of biomedical knowledge and its proper place in a health science curriculum. In this chapter, we consider some of these arguments in the context of empirical evidence from cognitive studies in medicine.

The role of basic science knowledge is a subject of considerable debate in medical education. It is generally accepted that basic science or biomedical knowledge provides a foundation upon which clinical knowledge can be built. However, its precise role in medical reasoning is controversial (Clancy, 1988; Patel et al, 1989a). Biomedical knowledge has undergone a dramatic transformation over the past couple of decades. This has presented unique and formidable challenges to medical education. There is considerable uncertainty concerning the relationship between basic science conceptual knowledge of subject matter and the practice of physicians (e.g. Dawson-Saunders et al, 1990).

In recent years, there has been a dramatic increase in the volume of medical knowledge, especially in cellular and molecular biology (Friedman and Purcell, 1983). Medical schools have typically responded by adding the new content to existing courses, increasing the number of classroom lectures and assigning more textbook readings (Stritter and Mattern, 1983). This has resulted in a dramatic decrease in laboratory time and small group teaching during the preclinical years. The basic science courses are increasingly taught by Ph.D. research scientists from diverse departments (e.g. anatomy) with minimal background in clinical medicine. There is also a lack of coordination between the different basic science departments affiliated with each medical school.

The future role of basic science knowledge

There have been increasing expressions of dissatisfaction with basic science teaching in medicine. It has been argued that substantial parts of the basic science in medical schools are irrelevant to the future needs of practitioners, and that the biomedical concepts are presented at a time when students are not prepared to grasp their significance (Neame, 1984). This argument could be extended to cover other health science disciplines as well. Furthermore, the method of presenting information in a didactic lecture format and with text readings that do not usually include clinical reasoning exercises encourages passivity and rote learning. This inhibits the development of understanding. Neame (1984) argues that preclinical courses fail to achieve their objectives of imparting useful and relevant knowledge to the future clinical practitioner. In addition, the primary evaluations of students are based on multiple choice examinations that emphasize recall of factual information rather than conceptual understanding and integration of concepts.

Serious concerns have been raised about whether future health science practitioners will require the kinds of scientific training that their predecessors had received. One of the arguments suggests that technical innovations, in particular the computer, will render much of basic science training unnecessary. Cavazos (1984) expresses this point of view very clearly:

> Medical education should not be designed to develop scientists nor students who are encyclopedias of scientific trivia, no matter how vital that trivia might be in pursuit of pure science. We have no need to teach medical students vast quantities of information which results in memorization when such information can be computer-stored and retrieved in seconds. We do have a need to graduate ethical and compassionate students with high level skills in data analysis and independent critical thinking (Cavazos, 1984, p. 763).

This quote underscores a particular cynicism towards the teaching of basic knowledge and the view that the training of medical scientists and humane medical practitioners are competing goals. The proposal offered by Cavazos, which very likely captures the sentiment of some medical educators, demonstrates a significant misunderstanding about the nature of knowledge acquisition. The view expressed equates understanding with the accumulation of facts and since computers can store facts better than humans, why not take advantage of it. He fails to appreciate that storing information is not the same as structuring useful and accessible knowledge (Cruess et al, 1985). Even if a practitioner could access information that effortlessly, it would be of relatively little value if he or she did not have some prior knowledge to interpret this information. In our view it is unlikely that ethical, compassionate, and highly skilled technicians would be a suitable replacement for today's clinical practitioners.

The issue of technological change and its relationship to a scientific foundation for medical practitioners is a source of considerable debate. The issue is whether technological innovation will require that physicians master an ever expanding body of scientific knowledge or the future technology will render such knowledge superfluous. According to Prokop (1992), there are clear historical trends that are likely to continue. New discoveries in science will continue to provide physicians with increasingly powerful investigative tools with which to see the workings of the human body and through which to prevent disease. When we consider the historical precedents, it seems likely that the best clinical judgement will require a broader understanding of both biology and medicine than ever before (Prokop, 1992).

Epistemological and curricular issues

Medical knowledge consists of two types of knowledge: clinical knowledge, including knowledge of disease entities and associated findings; and basic science knowledge, incorporating subject matter such as biochemistry, anatomy, and physiology. Basic science or biomedical knowledge is supposed to provide a scientific foundation for clinical reasoning.

It had been widely accepted that biomedical and clinical knowledge could be seamlessly integrated into a coherent knowledge structure that supported all cognitive aspects of medical practice, such as diagnostic and therapeutic reasoning (Feinstein, 1973). From this perspective, clinical and biomedical knowledge become intricately intertwined providing medical practice with a sound scientific basis. These assumptions have increasingly been called into question (Neame, 1984; Patel et al, 1989a).

Since the Flexner (1910) report at the beginning of this century, medical schools have made a strong commitment to this epistemological framework. The medical curricula at most medical schools are partitioned into preclinical courses which predominantly teach the basic sciences during the first and second years of medical school. The remaining two years of medical school and further postgraduate training consists of clinical courses and practicums.

The content of a basic curriculum covers a great expanse of knowledge in a relatively short period of time. To illustrate the depth and breadth of content coverage, Figure 9.1 presents a partial model of the biomedical science courses taught in the medical school of McGill University, which has a conventional medical curriculum. Medical students are required to take courses in six major biomedical domains during their first 18 months of medical school. The physiology courses are taught for a total of 205 hours, more than any of the other core courses. We can further partition the physiology course into major subsections. Figure 9.1 illustrates only six of the subsections. Cardiovascular physiology is the subject matter that receives the most amount of time within the physiology courses; it is taught over 28 hours. This course covers a range of complex topics, such as cardiac output and cellular hemodynamics. Each of these topics receives at most a few hours of lecture time. In these brief periods of time, a lecturer must, at minimum, cover the basic concepts in each topic, explain its relationship to other parts of the system (and the course) and provide some demonstration of its relevance in a clinical context.

As discussed previously, the purpose of basic science teaching is to provide a scientific foundation for tasks of clinical practice, such as diagnosis and therapeutics. Medical problem solving can be characterized as ill-structured, in the sense that the initial states, the definite goal state, and the necessary constraints are unknown at the beginning of the problem solving process. In a diagnostic situation, the problem space of potential findings and associated diagnoses is enormous. The problem space becomes defined through the imposition of a set of plausible constraints, that facilitate the application of specific decision strategies (Pople, 1982). For example, a physician when faced with a multi-system problem such as hypokalemic periodic paralysis associated with hyperthyroidism may need to confirm the more common disorder of hyperthyroidism before solving the more vexing problem of hypokalemia. Once this is confirmed, there are a set of constraints in place such that there are classes of disorders that co-occur with hyperthyroidism and there are a set of symptoms that have not yet been accounted for by this disorder and are consistent with hypokalemic periodic paralysis. As expertise develops, the disease knowledge of a clinician becomes more dependent on clinical experience and clinical problem solving is increasingly guided by the use of exemplars and analogy, and becomes less dependent on a functional understanding of the system in question.

Biomedical knowledge by comparison is of a qualitatively different nature embodying elements of causal mechanisms and characterizing patterns of perturbation in function and structure. Schaffner (1986) characterizes biomedical science as a *series of overlapping interlevel*

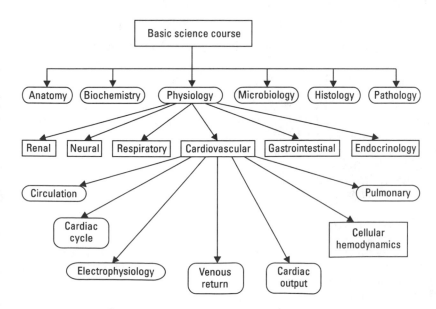

Figure 9.1 A partial model of basic science courses in the medical curriculum at McGill University

temporal models. Temporal models include collections of entities that undergo a process of change and can be represented as a sequence of events. For example, acute left ventricular failure can produce a disequilibrium in which the output of blood on the right side of the heart temporarily exceeds the output of the left side of the heart. The process by which the output from the left and right sides of the heart equilibrates can be understood in terms of a sequence of events in which there is a change in the pressure–volume relationships in different segments of the circulatory system which will affect the flow dynamics and restore the equilibrium over repeated cardiac cycles. In the physical sciences, time is usually embodied in differential equations. The explicit temporal sequence is of considerably greater significance in biomedical theories (Schaffner, 1980). The term interlevel refers to the fact that entities grouped within a biomedical theory are at different levels of aggregation.

This multi-levelled knowledge can be arranged in a hierarchical schema of scientific sources. Blois (1988) illustrates the interlevel reasoning process in the context of Wilson's disease, which is a central nervous system disorder caused by a metabolic defect in which the body cannot properly eliminate copper from the blood. At each higher level in the hierarchy, there are newly emergent properties not entirely predictable from lower levels. He identifies seven levels of hierarchy in Wilson's disease, from the atomic level findings such as decreased serum copper to 'patient as a whole' abnormalities such as malaise and labile affect. Each new level has different conceptual entities and a unique language of description. The lower-level abnormalities are revealed by laboratory tests and the higher-level attributes come from patients' reports and physical examinations. Each higher level introduces a greater degree of inexactness in ascribing causality. For example, it is difficult to precisely account for the patient's altered emotional states. This problem is rather atypical. Few diseases can be traced across aggregate levels in this manner. However, biomedical research is increasingly building these vertical connections that provide medical science with a deeper understanding of biomedical disorders. The example serves to highlight the challenge of synthesizing information from different levels of aggregation.

It should be noted that not all biomedical disciplines can be characterized by having explicitly causal or temporal components. In particular, anatomy and histology are predominantly concerned with aspects of structure. At the clinical level, models of disease are commonly described in terms of associations between clinical findings and diagnoses.

The focus of the instructional approach for the biomedical curriculum is necessarily on the extensive coverage of a broad corpus of knowledge as opposed to in-depth conceptual understanding. Each domain and even each subdomain represents a unique ontology with distinct conceptual entities and relations between entities. The volume of information in any one of these disciplines or subdisciplines is now so large that it cannot be completely mastered even by a full-time graduate student pursuing doctoral studies for five years (Prokop, 1992). It is unreasonable to expect that medical students can master five or more fields in the first 18 months of medical school. The degree of conceptual integration, from a horizontal perspective (across subject domains) and vertical perspective (in terms of the depth within subject matters) is immense. In our view it is not tenable, given a finite time frame and finite psychological resources, to coordinate these multiple sources of knowledge and harmonize all biomedical knowledge with a clinical body of knowledge of disease entities and associated findings.

Research in clinical reasoning

In this section, we review some of the pertinent research in medical reasoning. The focus is on research that addresses the role of basic science knowledge in clinical medicine. Studies in medical clinical reasoning encompass different domains of knowledge (e.g. cardiology and radiology) and a wide range of performance tasks.

Lesgold et al (1988) investigated the abilities of radiologists, at different levels of training and expertise, to interpret chest X-ray pictures and provide a diagnosis. The results revealed that the experts were able to initially detect a general pattern of disease. This resulted in a gross anatomical localization and served to constrain the possible interpretations. Novices had greater difficulty focusing in on the important structures and were more likely to maintain inappropriate interpretations despite discrepant findings in the patient history. The authors concluded that the knowledge that underlies expertise in radiology includes the mental representation of anatomy, a theory of anatomical perturbation, and the constructive capacity to transform the visual image into a three-dimensional representation. The less expert subjects had greater difficulty in building and maintaining a rich anatomical representation of the patient.

Norman et al (1989) compared subjects' performance at various levels of expertise in tasks that required them to diagnose and sort dermatological slides according to the type of skin lesion present. The results indicated that experts were more accurate in their diagnoses and took significantly less time to respond than did novices. The sorting task revealed that each group sorted the slides according to different category types. Expert dermatologists grouped the slides into superordinate categories, for example 'viral infections', which reflected the underlying pathophysiological structure. Novices tended to classify lesions according to their surface features, for example 'scaly lesions'. The implication is that experts' knowledge is organized around domain principles, which facilitate the rapid recognition of significant problem features. This is referred to as domain knowledge.

Clinical reasoning strategies and expertise

In recent years, a considerable amount of research has been undertaken comparing the comprehension and problem solving of experts, intermediates, and novices in domains of knowledge, such as chess (Charness, 1991) and physics (Chi et al, 1981). The picture that emerges from this research is that experts use a quite different pattern of reasoning from that used by novices or intermediates and organize their knowledge differently. Three important aspects are that experts (a) have a greater ability to organize information into semantically meaningful, interrelated chunks, (b) do not process irrelevant information and (c) in routine situations, tend to use highly specific knowledge-based problem solving strategies (Ericsson and Smith, 1991). The use of knowledge-based strategies has given rise to an important distinction between data-driven

strategy (forward reasoning) in which hypotheses are generated from data, and hypothesis-driven strategy (backward reasoning) in which one reasons backward from a hypothesis and attempts to find data that elucidate it. Forward reasoning is based on the domain knowledge and thus is highly error-prone in the absence of adequate domain knowledge. Backward reasoning is slower and may make heavy demands on working memory (because one has to keep track of such things as goals and hypotheses). It is most likely to be used when domain knowledge is inadequate.

In experiments with expert physicians, clinicians showed little tendency to use basic science in explaining cases, whereas medical researchers showed preference for detailed, basic scientific explanations, without developing clinical descriptions (Patel et al, 1989a). In medicine, the pathophysiological explanation task has been used to examine clinical reasoning (Feltovich and Barrows, 1984; Patel and Groen, 1986). Pathophysiology refers to the physiology of disordered function. This task requires subjects to explain the causal pattern underlying a set of clinical symptoms. Protocols from this task can be used to investigate the ability of clinicians to apply basic science concepts in diagnosing a clinical problem. In one study (Patel and Groen, 1986), expert practitioners (cardiologists) were asked to solve problems within their domain of expertise. Their explanations of the underlying pathophysiology of the cases, whether correctly or incorrectly diagnosed, made virtually no use of basic science knowledge. In another study (Patel et al, 1990b), cardiologists and endocrinologists were asked to read both endocrinology and cardiology cases, recall case information, and explain the underlying pathophysiology of the problems. Subjects, thus, were operating both within and outside their domains of expertise. The clinicians did not appeal to principles from basic biomedical science, even when they were working outside their own domain of expertise; rather, they relied on clinical associations and classifications to formulate solutions. The results suggest that basic science does not contribute directly to reasoning in clinical problem solving for experienced clinicians.

However, it should be noted that biomedical information was used by practitioners when the task was difficult or when they were uncertain about their diagnosis (Joseph and Patel, 1990; Patel et al, 1990b). In these cases, biomedical information was used in a backward-directed causal reasoning manner. This provided some kind of coherence to the explanation of clinical cues that could not be easily accounted for by the primary diagnostic hypothesis that was being considered.

Basic science in students' explanations of clinical cases

We developed a series of experiments in our laboratory designed to elucidate the precise role of basic science in clinical reasoning (Patel et al, 1988; Patel et al, 1990a; Patel et al, 1991b). Our purpose was to determine to what extent basic sciences and clinical knowledge are complementary. One study made use of a standard paradigm in research relating comprehension to clinical reasoning. The authors presented medical students at McGill University with basic science material immediately prior to presenting a clinical case (Patel et al, 1988). Such a procedure is designed to maximize the likelihood that subjects will use related information from separate knowledge sources. Specifically, we prepared a clinical text on acute bacterial endocarditis and three related basic science texts on the physiology of fever, hemodynamics, and microcirculation. Subjects were grouped according to their level of medical school training: students in their first year of medical school; second-year medical students who had completed all basic medical sciences, but had not begun any clinical work; and final-year medical students three months before graduation. The subjects were asked to read the four texts, recall in writing what they had read, and then explain the clinical problem in terms of the basic science texts. In our analysis, we coded subjects' statements into propositions and relations among propositions to establish, as precisely as possible, what information and inferences subjects employed in performing their tasks. This type of analysis follows a well-developed paradigm in cognitive science for the interpretation of verbal data.

In general, subjects' recall of the basic science texts was poor, indicating a lack of well-developed knowledge structures in which to organize this information. Recall of the clinical text appeared to be a function of clinical experience, but there was no similar correlation

between basic science and experience. In the explanation of the problem, the second-year students made extensive use of basic science knowledge. Fourth-year students gave explanations that resembled those of expert physicians outside their domain of specialization, except that the students made more extensive use of basic science information than we find in experts' explanations. It is interesting to note that their greater use of basic science actually resulted in more consistent inferences. Our results can be interpreted as indicating that basic science knowledge is used differently by the three groups of subjects.

In a second experiment, using the same number of subjects at similar levels of training, we asked for recall and explanation of cases when basic science information was provided after the clinical problem (Patel et al, 1990a). We can characterize reasoning as a two-stage process: diagnostic reasoning is characterized by inference from observation to hypothesis; and predictive reasoning is characterized by inference from hypothesis to observations. The fourth-year students were able to use basic science information in a highly effective manner, thus facilitating both diagnostic and predictive reasoning. The second-year students were also able to use this information effectively, but diagnostic reasoning was not facilitated. The first-year students were not able to use basic science information any more effectively when it was given after the clinical problem than when it was given before the clinical problem. The results suggest that reasoning toward a diagnosis from the facts of a case is frustrated by attempting to use basic science knowledge unless the student has already developed a strong diagnostic hypothesis. Thus, the addition of basic science knowledge seems to improve the accuracy of diagnoses offered by final-year medical students, but does not improve the accuracy of diagnoses by first- and second-year students. The most straightforward explanation is that final-year students, who have had some clinical experience, rely on clinically relevant features in a case to classify the diagnosis (if broadly) and make selective predictions of features that are susceptible to analysis in terms of the basic science facts they have read (Patel et al, 1989a). This tendency of clinical solutions to subordinate basic scientific ones, and for basic science not to support the clinical organization of facts in a case, was evident among expert physicians as discussed earlier.

Arocha et al (1993) presented medical trainees with cases where they had to generate an initial hypothesis and then were presented evidence disconfirming the initial suggestion. In a manner similar to expert physicians, the novices in this study used little basic science information during the diagnostic process. The strategy that the subjects followed was more like a search through a space of findings based on the weighting of these findings against the possible diagnostic hypothesis they were entertaining at the time. Recourse to pathophysiological information only happened in special situations when the problem solving process broke down, and the subjects had to tie 'loose ends' or 'unaccounted information' in the case. The results of this study are consistent with previously described findings as most students did not use basic science information to evaluate competing diagnoses. These results are also consistent with other reported findings that suggest that unprompted use of biomedical concepts in clinical reasoning decreases as a function of expertise (Boshuizen et al, 1988).

Reasoning and biomedical knowledge in different medical curricula

Patel et al (1991a; 1993) attempted to replicate the above studies in an established problem-based learning (PBL) medical school at McMaster University. The Medical School at McGill University has what is usually called a conventional curriculum (CC).

Employing the same methods and procedures used in the studies described earlier, students at three equivalent levels of training were tested in the McMaster medical curriculum. The results showed that when basic science information was provided *before* the clinical problem, there was a lack of integration of basic science into the clinical context in both schools. This resulted in (a) lack of global coherence in their knowledge structures, (b) errors of scientific fact, and (c) disruption of the process of diagnostic reasoning.

When basic science was given *after* the clinical problem, there was integration of basic science into the clinical context in both schools. It is concluded that clinical problems cannot be easily embedded into a basic science context, but basic science can be more naturally embedded within a clinical context. However, this phenomenon is observed as a short term effect in the undergraduate medical curricula; the long term effects of this kind of an integration process are not known.

It is our belief that when one is attempting to learn two unknown domains, it is better to learn one well, in such a way that it is used as an 'anchor' for the new domain. We also know that basic science knowledge has a causal underlying structure that can be remembered as a story, and clinical knowledge has a classificatory structure of patient signs and symptoms. In our opinion, basic science knowledge would make a better 'anchor' than clinical knowledge. Our earlier finding that basic science cannot be easily integrated into clinical structure, and the suggestion that basic science form a better anchor, gives rise to a paradox. It appears that one may need to make a compromise such that there is some core basic science taught at the beginning of the curriculum followed by an early introduction of clinical problems, where early basic science will produce some form of anchor and early clinical problems will provide the structure support.

The results of our study (Patel et al, 1991a; 1993) suggest that in the conventional curriculum, (a) basic science and clinical knowledge are generally kept separate, (b) clinical reasoning may not require basic science knowledge, (c) basic science is spontaneously used only when students get into difficulty with the patient problem, and (d) basic science serves to generate globally coherent explanations of the patient problem with connections between various components of the clinical problem. It is proposed that in a conventional curriculum, the clinical aspect of the problem is viewed as separate from the biomedical science aspect, the two having different functions.

In this PBL curriculum, basic science and clinical knowledge are spontaneously integrated. However, this integration results in students' inability to decontextualize the problem, i.e. the basic science is so tightly tied to the clinical context that students appear to be unable to detach basic science even when the clinical situations demand it. In addition, a greater number of elaborations are made when students 'think' about problem features using basic science and clinical information. However, these greater elaborations result in fragmentation of knowledge structures resulting in the lack of global coherence (various parts of the problem are not connected). Finally, within PBL such elaborations result in factual errors that persist from first-year students' responses to the final year. These differences could conceivably be due to the emphasis on detailed causal reasoning and elaboration, since this might be assumed to generate more load on working memory.

Progressions in understanding of biomedical concepts

In the preceding studies, we examined the role of basic science knowledge in a clinical context. Evidence emerged to suggest that the biomedical concepts were not, in and of themselves, well understood by most students. In this section, we focus on a study related to students' understanding of important biomedical concepts.

Our investigations of medical problem solving indicate that biomedical knowledge is not used optimally in clinical contexts (Patel et al, 1989b). These research findings suggest that basic science is used differentially in different tasks and in different medical domains, that experts and novices differ in their use of basic science and that, in many instances, basic science knowledge may actually interfere with clinical reasoning. The evidence also suggests that students possess substantial inert knowledge that frustrates their ability to apply specific biomedical concepts to clinical problem solving tasks. As discussed previously, the problems appear to be at least equally pervasive in problem-based medical schools with integrated curricula. The results also suggest that when used appropriately biomedical knowledge can facilitate explanation (Patel et al, 1989b).

Patel et al (1991b) examined medical students' understanding of complex biomedical concepts in the domain of cardio-pulmonary physiology. In particular, the study focused on the concepts related to ventilation/perfusion matching. The concept of ventilation/perfusion matching is a fundamental concept, whose understanding is integral to diverse domains of medicine. It has applications in both diagnostic and therapeutic contexts. It was found that students at the end of first year of the medical school exhibited significant misconceptions in reasoning about ventilation/perfusion matching in the context of a clinical problem.

Specifically, students had considerable difficulty in conceptualizing the cardio-pulmonary system as a closed mechanistic system. Students' explanations revealed that they reason about each lung as if it were semi-autonomous and did not impose constraints on the other lung's functioning. It was also observed that students were not able to map clinical findings onto pathophysiological manifestations. This can partly be explained by the fact that the pulmonary physiology course that preceded the study did not make these relationships sufficiently explicit.

The results of this study are consistent with other research (cf. Patel et al, 1989a) that indicates that students' oversimplified representations of biomedical phenomena fail to support clinical reasoning. Feltovich et al's (1989) research in the related domain of congestive heart failure documented widespread misconceptions in students' understanding about the structure and function of the cardiovascular system. Congestive heart failure is a syndrome in which the heart's effectiveness as a pump can diminish greatly and as a result the rate of blood flow slows dramatically. The misconception that was expressed by over 60% of first and second year medical students in a study, and by some medical practitioners, suggests that heart failure is caused by the heart getting too big, which in turn stretches the cardiac muscle fibres. The force of contraction is determined by *mechanical/anatomical* factors and activational factors (energetic). The primary cause of congestive heart failure is activational, whereas the misconception emphasized the mechanical overstretching as the cause for heart failure. These authors describe in detail the various components of the knowledge and the sources of learning and instruction that contribute to the overall misconception.

This study represented the first experiment in a research program designed to characterize students' and physicians' understanding of significant biomedical concepts and their utilization in clinical contexts. More recently we conducted a detailed study (Kaufman et al, 1992) to characterize students' and physicians' understanding of biomedical concepts in the domain of cardiovascular physiology. In the experiment, subjects were presented with questions and problems pertaining to the concepts of *cardiac output*, *venous return*, and the mechanical properties of the cardiovascular and circulatory system. The stimulus material included several areas of questions and problems such as: basic physiology (e.g. explain the effects of an increase in preload on stroke volume); applied physiology (e.g. extreme exercise); pathophysiology (e.g. the hemodynamic effects of hemorrhage); medical disorders (e.g. congestive heart failure) and brief clinical problems. This afforded us an opportunity to investigate subjects' reasoning within and across levels in the hierarchical chain of biomedicine. The first links in the chain are the physical principles related to the dynamics and statics of the storage and flow of fluids through tubes. In particular, a basic understanding of pressure–volume and pressure–flow relationships is essential to understanding this subject matter.

The results of our study indicate a wide range of conceptual errors and errors of analysis, in subjects at different levels of expertise. These errors were prominent in different sections of the study but tended to carry over into other sections. Overall, there was an evident increase in conceptual understanding with levels of training. The students who were tested at the very beginning of medical school began their learning with preconceptions that were not commensurate with the assimilation of new knowledge. For instance, one subject was lacking in basic physical science knowledge and had difficulties reasoning about pressure gradients.

There were particular misconceptions that would appear to be a function of formal learning. For example, a misconception was manifested in the responses of six subjects, including two fourth year students and two cardiology residents. It was related to a confounding of venous resistance and venous compliance. The notion is that since an increase in venous resistance is associated with a decrease in compliance, then the net effect of resistance would be to increase venous return. If one considers the meaning of resistance, which all of these subjects clearly understood, then it appears quite counterintuitive that resistance can facilitate (as opposed to impede) blood flow. This would suggest that this misconception is a function of formal learning rather than acquired through experience.

The more advanced subjects in our study, including the senior students and physicians experienced more difficulty in responding to the basic physiology than they did applying the very same concepts in more clinically-oriented problems. On several occasions, the physicians would use clinical analogies to explain physiological processes (for example, using aortic stenosis to account for the effects of afterload on end-systolic pressure). More often than not the analogies did not successfully result in correct explanations. However, when provided with pathophysiological conditions or medical disorders requiring pathophysiological explanations (e.g. congestive heart failure), the physicians were able to draw on their clinical knowledge to great effect. The distance in the hierarchy (e.g. from physical science to pathophysiology) had a considerable effect on the likelihood of successful transfer of knowledge.

Most subjects at each level of training exhibited a strong cardiocentric bias. That is, they tended to construct explanations using concepts related to cardiac function, without any due consideration of the factors that affect venous return. This bias was evident even in response to clinical problems. One's understanding of these basic science concepts could have implications for particular therapeutic practices, such as fluid management, where decisions have to be made that take into account factors that affect both the peripheral circuit (vessels of the cardiovascular system) and cardiac function.

Biomedical knowledge and clinical science: two different worlds?

In this chapter, we have considered epistemological and curricular issues related to the role of basic science knowledge in clinical medicine, discussed empirical studies related to the use of biomedical knowledge in clinical reasoning contexts, and considered studies that examined students' and physicians' understanding of biomedical concepts. What inferences can we make concerning the role of basic science knowledge in clinical practice? We will consider two theoretical hypotheses.

Schmidt and Boshuizen (1992) proposed a learning mechanism, *knowledge encapsulation*, for explaining how biomedical knowledge becomes subsumed under clinical knowledge as a function of training. Knowledge encapsulation is a learning process which involves the subsumption of biomedical propositions, concepts and their interrelations in an associative net, under a small number of higher level clinical propositions with the same explanatory power. These authors suggest that through the exposure to clinical training, biomedical knowledge becomes encapsulated and integrated into clinical knowledge. They cite a wide range of clinical reasoning and recall studies which purportedly support this kind of learning process. Of particular importance is the well-documented finding that with increasing levels of expertise, physicians produce explanations at higher levels of generality, using fewer and fewer biomedical concepts while producing consistently accurate responses (Patel et al, 1989b).

In our view, the notion of knowledge encapsulation represents an idealized perspective on the integration of basic science in clinical knowledge. The reasons for our scepticism are rooted in several sources. Basic science knowledge plays a different role in different clinical domains. For example, clinical expertise in perceptual domains such as dermatology and radiology, necessitates a relatively robust model of anatomical structures, which is the primary source of knowledge for diagnostic classification. In other domains, such as cardiology and endocrinology, basic science knowledge has a more distant relationship with clinical knowledge. Furthermore, the misconceptions evident in physicians' biomedical explanations would argue against well-developed encapsulated knowledge structures where basic science knowledge could easily be retrieved and applied when necessary.

As discussed previously, biomedical knowledge represents a complex multi-levelled hierarchical structure. Given what we know about epistemology of basic science knowledge and what we know about the nature of basic science curricula, then it is not tenable to develop such 'neatly-packaged' knowledge structures. Our contention is that neither conventional nor problem-based curricula could foster this kind of learning process. There is a successful integration of basic science knowledge into clinical structure with PBL curriculum. However, it has also created the problem of students' inability to decontextualize it once it is integrated (Patel et al, 1993). This problem should be attended to if one assumes that relevant basic science knowledge is naturally embedded into clinical knowledge. Indeed, this appears to be a basic assumption of the clinical rationale for medical education. On the other hand, the biomedical sciences have a structure that is quite different from the clinical sciences. If this is the case, then one would expect clinicians to exhibit an inability to decontextualize basic science knowledge learned in a clinical context.

It is our view that the results of research into medical clinical reasoning are consistent with the idea that clinical medicine and the biomedical science constitute two distinct and not completely compatible 'worlds', with distinct modes of reasoning and quite different ways of structuring knowledge (Patel et al, 1989a). Clinical knowledge is based on a complex taxonomy which relates disease symptoms to underlying pathology. In contrast, the biomedical sciences are based on general principles defining chains of causal mechanisms. Thus, learning to explain how a set of symptoms is consistent with a diagnosis may be very different from learning how to explain what causes a disease.

Perhaps the key role played by basic science may not be in facilitating clinical reasoning per se, but in facilitating explanation and coherent communication (Patel et al, 1989a; 1989b). Physicians do not commonly offer basic science explanations when they are reasonably sure of their diagnoses. However in times of uncertainty, physicians do resort to scientific explanations which are coherent, even if inaccurate. We also see this in medical students when they attempt to integrate knowledge across domains. Basic science provides a powerful means of connecting disparate phenomena and of generating explanations that, if still inaccurate, are much more coherent. The critical observation, then, is that well-organized, coherent information is easier to remember than disjointed collections of facts. Thus, the ability to explain something, even idiosyncratically to oneself, is necessary if information is to be communicated effectively and retained in memory for further analysis and, more importantly, for learning.

It is argued, then, that the role of basic science, besides providing the concepts and vocabulary required to formulate clinical problems, is to create a basis for establishing and assessing coherence in the explanation of biomedical phenomena. Basic science does not provide the axioms, the analogies, or the abstractions required to support clinical problem solving. Rather, it provides the principles that make it possible to organize observations that defy ready clinical classification and analysis. We also contend that, because clinical reasoning demands the co-ordination of multiple tasks and goals, the ability to organize and communicate observations is an absolute prerequisite for medical expertise.

We have proposed that basic science knowledge is a valuable tool in the development of coherence in the explanation of clinical phenomena. This role of basic science is underappreciated by the general medical and educational communities. In response to the proposal that the teaching of basic science and clinical knowledge should be completely merged, Trelstad (1991) argues that 'basic science is a unique and special activity that when melded into a clinical environment, will only be diluted in focus and quality' (p. 1186). This suggestion echoes the concerns and issues raised in this chapter. While we believe that teaching of basic science in context is important, it is not sufficient for promoting the robust transfer of usable knowledge. The 'two world hypothesis' implies that each body of knowledge be given special status in the medical curriculum and that the correspondences between the two worlds need to be developed.

A common finding in research into scientific domains is the inherent difficulty students have in transferring knowledge across contexts and the failure of instruction to promote robust transferable knowledge. This is readily apparent in the lack of utility within clinical contexts of basic science knowledge, as it is commonly taught. Salomon and Perkins (1989) propose a useful distinction for characterizing different kinds of transfer and the relative time points at which transfer occurs. *Forward-reaching transfer* occurs when one abstracts basic elements in anticipation for later application. This type of transfer would be expected when one is acquiring basic science knowledge in a classroom setting. *Backward-reaching transfer* is required when one faces a new situation and deliberately searches for relevant knowledge already acquired. This kind of transfer is exemplified in situations when one is engaged in a clinical reasoning task and needs to abstract particular principles to explain a complex problem. The challenge for medical schools is to present concepts in diverse contexts and make the relationships between the specific and general aspects explicit. This entails striking the right balance between presenting information in applied contexts (e.g. as illustrated by a clinical problem),

yet allowing students to derive the appropriate abstractions and generalizations to further develop their models of conceptual understanding. This would enhance the opportunities for promoting forward-reaching and backward-reaching transfer and thus facilitating the role of basic science knowledge as a valuable resource for developing coherent explanations in a clinical reasoning context.

Acknowledgements

The work for the preparation and writing of this chapter was supported by Social Sciences and Humanities Research Council of Canada (SSHRC 410-92-1535). We thank André Kushniruk for providing helpful comments and Susan St.-Pierre for formatting the final copy of the manuscript.

References

Arocha, J.F., Patel, V.L. and Patel, Y.C. (1993) Hypothesis generation and the coordination of theory and evidence in novice diagnostic reasoning. *Medical Decision Making,* **13**, 198–211

Blois, M.S. (1988) Medicine and the nature of vertical reasoning. *New England Journal of Medicine,* **318**, 847–851

Boshuizen, H.P.A., Schmidt, H.G. and Coughlin, L.D. (1988) On the application of medical basic science in clinical reasoning: Implications for structural knowledge differences between experts and novices. In *Proceedings of the Tenth Annual Conference of the Cognitive Science Society* (eds V.L. Patel and G.J. Groen). Lawrence Erlbaum Associates, Hillsdale, NJ, pp. 517–523

Cavazos, L.F. (1984) Basic science studies: Their purpose in medical education. *Journal of Medical Education,* **59**, 763

Charness, N. (1991) Expertise in chess: The balance between knowledge and search. In *Toward a General Theory of Expertise: Prospects and Limits* (eds A. Ericsson and J. Smith). Cambridge University Press, New York, pp. 39–63

Chi, M.T.H., Feltovich, P.J. and Glaser, R. (1981) Categorization and representation of physics problems by experts and novices. *Cognitive Science,* **5**, 121–152

Clancey, W.J. (1988) Acquiring, representing and evaluating a competence model of diagnostic strategy. In *The Nature of Expertise* (eds M.T.H. Chi, R. Glaser and M. Farr). Lawrence Erlbaum Associates, Hillsdale, NJ, pp. 343–418

Cruess, R.L., Patel, V.L. and Groen, G.J. (1985) Basic science studies. (Response to the Editorial Comments). *Journal of Medical Education,* **60**, 208

Dawson-Saunders, B., Feltovich, P.J., Coulson, R.L. and Steward, D. (1990) A survey of medical school teachers to identify basic biomedical concepts medical students should understand. *Academic Medicine*, 7, 448–454

Ericsson, A. and Smith, J. (eds) (1991) *Toward a General Theory of Expertise: Prospects and Limits*. Cambridge University Press, New York

Feinstein, A.R. (1973) An analysis of diagnostic reasoning: The domain and disorders of clinical macrobiology. *Yale Journal of Biology and Medicine*, 46, 264–283

Feltovich, P.J. and Barrows, H.A. (1984) Issues of generality in medical problem solving. In *Tutorials In Problem Based Learning* (eds H.G. Schmidt and M.L. De Volder). van Gorcum, Assen, Holland, pp. 128–142

Feltovich, P.J., Spiro, R. and Coulson, R.L. (1989) The nature of conceptual understanding in biomedicine: The deep structure of complex ideas and the development of misconceptions. In *Cognitive Science in Medicine: Biomedical Modeling* (eds D.A. Evans and V.L. Patel). The MIT Press, Cambridge, MA, pp. 113–172

Flexner, A. (1910) *Medical Education In The United States And Canada*. Bulletin Number Four, Carnegie Foundation for the Advancement of Teaching, New York

Friedman, C.F. and Purcell, E.F. (1983) *The New Biology and Medical Education: Merging the Biological Information, and Cognitive Sciences*. Josiah Macy Jr. Foundation, New York

Joseph, G.-M. and Patel, V.L. (1990) Domain knowledge and hypothesis generation in diagnostic reasoning. *Medical Decision Making*, 10, 31–46

Kaufman, D.R., Patel, V.L. and Magder, S.A. (1992) *Development of Conceptual Understanding of Biomedical Concepts*. Technical Report # CME92-CS4. Centre for Medical Education, McGill University, Montreal, Quebec

Lesgold, A.M., Rubinson, H., Feltovich, P.J., Glaser, R., Klopfer, D. and Wang, Y. (1988) Expertise in a complex skill: Diagnosing X-ray pictures. In *The Nature of Expertise* (eds M.T.H. Chi, R. Glaser and M.J. Farr). Lawrence Erlbaum Associates, Hillsdale, NJ, pp. 311–342

Neame, R.L.B. (1984) The preclinical course of study: help or hindrance. *Journal of Medical Education*, 59, 699–707

Norman, G., Brooks, L.R., Rosenthal, D., Allen, S.W. and Muzzin, L.J. (1989) The development of expertise in dermatology. *Archives of Dermatology*, 125, 1063–1068

Patel, V.L. and Groen, G.J. (1986) Knowledge-based solution strategies in medical reasoning. *Cognitive Science*, 10, 91–116

Patel, V.L., Groen, G.J. and Scott, H.S. (1988) Biomedical knowledge in explanations of clinical problems by medical students. *Medical Education*, 22, 398–406

Patel, V.L., Evans, D.A. and Groen, G.J. (1989a) On reconciling basic science and clinical reasoning. *Teaching and Learning in Medicine: An International Journal*, 1, 116–121

Patel, V.L., Evans, D.A. and Groen, G.J. (1989b) Biomedical knowledge and clinical reasoning. In *Cognitive Science in Medicine: Biomedical Modeling* (eds D.A. Evans and V.L. Patel). The MIT Press, Cambridge, MA, pp. 49–108

Patel, V.L., Evans, D.A. and Kaufman, D.R. (1990a) Reasoning strategies and use of biomedical knowledge by students. *Medical Education*, 24, 129–136

Patel, V.L., Groen, G.J. and Arocha J.F. (1990b) Medical expertise as a function of task difficulty. *Memory and Cognition*, 18, 394–406

Patel, V.L., Groen, G.J. and Norman, G.R. (1991a) Effects of conventional and problem-based medical curricula on problem solving. *Academic Medicine*, 66, 380–389

Patel, V.L., Kaufman, D.R. and Magder, S. (1991b) Causal reasoning about complex physiological concepts by medical students. *International Journal of Science Education*, 13, 171–185

Patel, V.L., Groen, G.J. and Norman, G.R. (1993) Reasoning and instruction in medical curricula. *Cognition and Instruction*, 10 (4), 335–378

Pople, H.E. (1982) Heuristic methods for imposing structure on ill-structured problems: The structuring of medical diagnostics. In *Artificial Intelligence in Medicine* (ed. P. Szolovitz). Western Press, Boulder, CO, pp. 119–190

Prokop, D.J. (1992) Basic science and clinical practice: How much will a physician need to know? In *Medical Education in Transition* (eds R.Q. Marston and R.M. Jones). The Robert Wood Johnson Foundation, Princeton, NJ, pp. 51–57

Salomon, G. and Perkins, D.N. (1989) Rocky roads to transfer: Rethinking mechanism of a neglected phenomenon. *Educational Psychologist*, 24, 113–143

Schaffner, K.F. (1980) Theory structure in the biomedical sciences. *The Journal of Medicine and Philosophy*, 5, 57–97

Schaffner, K.F. (1986) Exemplar reasoning about biological models and diseases: A relation between the philosophy of medicine and philosophy of science. *Journal of Medicine and Philosophy*, 11, 63–80

Schmidt, H.G. and Boshuizen, H.P.A. (1992) Encapsulation of biomedical knowledge. In *Advanced Models of Cognition for Medical Training and Practice* (eds D. A. Evans and V.L. Patel). NATO ASI. Series F: Computer and Systems Sciences, Vol 97. Springer-Verlag, Heidelberg, Germany, pp. 265–282

Stritter, F.T. and Mattern, W.D. (1983) Thoughts about the medical school curriculum. In *The New Biology and Medical Education: Merging the Biological Information, and Cognitive Sciences* (eds C.P. Friedman and E.F. Purcell). Josiah Macy Jr. Foundation, New York, pp. 228–235

Trelstad, R.L. (1991) The nation's medical curriculum in transition: Progression or retrogression? Reactions to the Robert Wood Johnson Foundation Commission on Medical Education. *Human Pathology*, 22, 1183–1186

10

Propositional, professional and personal knowledge in clinical reasoning

Joy Higgs and Angie Titchen

Reason is light in darkness . . . Be wise – let Reason, not Impulse, be your guide. Yet be mindful that even if Reason be at your side, she is helpless without the aid of Knowledge. (Kahlil Gibran, translated by Ferris, 1962a, p. 54)

Knowledge is a fundamental element in the definition and operation of a profession. Firstly, the body of knowledge of a profession is a key to delineating and describing the profession, and the generation of knowledge *by* the profession is a charter of being a profession. Secondly, knowledge is essential for reasoning and decision making, which lie at the centre of professional practice. In the health professions, clinical reasoning provides the vehicle for knowledge use in clinical practice as well as for knowledge generation through clinical practice. Thus, knowledge and clinical reasoning are interdependent phenomena.

This chapter will examine the phenomenon of knowledge from several perspectives. The first section will consider the nature of knowledge and approaches or paradigms that can be adopted to generate knowledge. From this background, types of knowledge and ways of using knowledge will be examined, including the use of knowledge in clinical rea-

soning. Teaching implications concerning the place of knowledge in clinical reasoning will be mentioned briefly throughout the chapter and will be explored in greater depth in Chapter 26 (1).

The study of knowledge occupies the branch of philosophy termed epistemology. Three important themes have been identified from the wealth of epistemological literature examined in this chapter. These themes are the manner in which knowledge is developed (e.g. through experience or the use of scientific method), the contextual or subject relevance of the approach to knowing and the verification or grounding of claims of knowledge. For instance, viewpoints differ on whether knowledge claims may be deemed to be verified if they are independent of the knower and/or if they are dependent upon the reality of the individual. In relation to the relevance of the approach to the context, Skinner (1985, p. 6) describes the recent decades as being characterized by 'upheavals and transformations that have served to restructure the human sciences (including) . . . the widespread reaction against the assumption that the natural sciences offer an adequate or even a relevant model for the practice of the social disciplines'.

(1) The reader is also referred to Chapters 2 and 9 of this text. In Chapter 2 Boshuizen and Schmidt present a model of developing clinical reasoning expertise based on the acquisition and encapsulation of science and clinical knowledge. In Chapter 9 Patel and Kaufman discuss the importance of biomedical knowledge in understanding clinical phenomena and in the process of clinical reasoning.

The nature of knowledge

What is knowledge?

The term 'knowledge' is itself a value-laden term. It implies an awareness which is judged to reach some standard (generally set by the particular type of epistemology adopted by the person judging this awareness). Barnett (1990, p. 41) argues that the search for an agreed set of criteria 'which absolutely separate legitimate from non-legitimate knowledge is bound to fail-ure'. However, he concludes that it is possible to deal with knowledge and knowledge claims, using a flexible framework which comprises the four key elements apparently common to all knowledge-oriented activities, i.e. social interaction, personal commitment, the develop-ment of the mind, and value implications of knowledge.

In this chapter we present a similar perspec-tive. We propose a view of knowledge in which both personal and public validation are sought, both propositional (theoretical/scientific) and non-propositional knowledge are accorded validity, and where knowledge is regarded as a dynamic phenomenon undergoing constant change and testing. 'Knowledge (of the indivi-dual)' is defined as *an awareness of the individual which has current conviction for the individual, gained through the testing of acquired or self-generated understanding.* The individual's claims to knowledge, therefore, need to be accompanied by a personal commitment to that claim. And knowledge claims, particularly in relation to professional and propositional knowledge in the health sciences, need to be subject to testing through such processes as scrutiny by others, reflection, concrete experi-ence or active experimentation. A related term 'knowledge (of the field)' refers to *knowledge claims by a particular group which currently has general acceptance within the field, disci-pline or paradigm in question.* Again such knowledge claims imply the need for both con-viction and testing.

This interpretation of knowledge is largely based on a constructivist perspective which con-tends that all knowledge is 'a deliberate con-struction of human beings striving to know about nature and experience' (Gowin, 1981, p. 27). The key elements of this definition are that knowledge is constructed not discovered, that individuals create unique constructions or inter-pretations of nature and of their own experi-ences, and that knowledge is the product of a dynamic and indeed difficult process of know-ing, or striving to understand. In such striving, the individual's depth and certainty of knowl-edge grows. In addition, what is being learned and the relationships between elements of such knowledge are tested and refined, both against the individual's own prior knowledge and experience, and also against external knowl-edge (including the knowledge and experiences of others and the established knowledge of the field).

The argument that learners construct their knowledge from experience lends support to a number of educational strategies. These include: the adoption of educational approaches which provide opportunities for students to experience and construct their own reality (e.g. through experiential learning); fos-tering the use of metacognition to help students to learn to conceptualize, test and construct their knowledge; recognizing learners' levels of expertise in knowledge construction; and pro-viding learning strategies to foster development of their expertise (Tinkler, 1993).

Knowledge validation: conviction, truth and evidence

To examine the question of knowledge valida-tion we will examine the notions of conviction, truth and evidence. These terms have been the subject of much debate. Thompson (1972), for instance, raises the question of whether knowl-edge, belief and opinion are distinct categories with differing levels of guarantee and truth. Similarly, Gowin (1981) presents theory, facts, assertions and assumptions as elements of knowledge which vary in their functions and intensities in any specific set of knowledge claims.

To know something is to have a conviction about the validity of what is claimed to be known. Thus knowledge (or the product of knowing) involves an understanding about something which carries with it a high level of conviction. By comparison, an individual may be able to remember information, data or facts but not be convinced of their validity.

The knowledge base of an individual is a personal matter. Therefore, the truth of knowl-edge is the individual's truth in the same way that a person has conviction in his or her beliefs. In his *personal construct theory* Kelly presents the view 'that there is no objective, absolute truth and that events are only meaningful in relation to the ways that are constructed by the individual' (Cohen and Manion, 1985, p. 315). Kelly argues that individuals act in accordance with their perceptions and interpretations of their environment, in terms of their existing mental structures.

As well as personal truth, knowledge has truth if it is deemed or judged to have intersubjective acceptance. However, since the human mind and judgement are required to determine this correspondence, then knowledge cannot be said to be unquestionably impersonal. Reid (1986, p. 34) asserts that the truth of knowledge is 'not ultimately the conformity of statement with fact – which is impersonal and formal, and exclusive to the knowledge which can be expressed in linguistic statements – but the *adequacy* of the cognitive grasp of its objects by (a) personal living mind'. According to Reid (1986, p. 31) the 'prevailing and dominant view of what knowledge is, is that it is sufficiently grounded in factual–perceptual and/or conceptual evidence'. He argues that this constraint of knowledge in its dependence upon propositional truth, limits acceptance and appreciation of non-propositional forms of knowledge. We share this concern in relation to the health care field, particularly, where personal knowledge plays a large part in identifying individual needs and understanding individual behaviour.

The nature of the evidence which validates knowledge is an important element of knowledge interpretation. In particular, it is important to note, that as well as being individually constructed, reality and knowledge are socially constructed. That is, reality exists because we give meaning to it (Berger and Luckmann, 1985). Thus, the individual's perceptions of reality, truth and knowledge have subjective dimensions or interpretations, as well as objective dimensions (reflecting the 'world out there'). What is termed 'objective reality', although it is a socially constructed interpretation of the world out there, gains an objective character or is seen as evidence, due to its testing in the public domain and because it 'transcends the domain of subjective or private experience' (Wildemeersch, 1989, p. 63). Kleinig (1982) argues that the social context in which knowledge is generated and tested promotes a particular focusing of attention by the individual. He contends that recognition of these social (context) determinants of knowledge is important to free individuals to reflect upon and question accepted elements and patterns/categories of knowledge and also accepted ways of structuring understanding (e.g. science, religion, psychology). They can then directly scrutinize, or seek to know, the reality which 'accepted' forms of knowledge supposedly reflect, and seek to interpret and structure their own understanding in ways which are meaningful to them. In the health care field, for instance, the competing messages of the medical model and the wellness model need to be considered when individuals are attempting to set their own directions and priorities for practice.

Despite the importance of knowledge validation it is essential to also see knowledge as a developing or dynamic phenomenon. Perkins (1986, p. xiii), for instance, presents the concept of 'active knowledge that one thinks critically and creatively about and with, not just passive knowledge that does little but await the final exam'. Similarly, Kleinig (1982, p. 152) argues 'the knowing subject must continually reflect on and test what is presented to it'. Ayer (1956, p. 222) takes the argument further by contending that when seeking to verify knowledge claims we should take scepticism of these claims seriously since this will enable us to learn 'to distinguish the different levels at which our claims to knowledge stand'. Thus knowing is a continual process of generating, refining and understanding knowledge. This is well illustrated in the words of the Taoist philosopher Nan Ch'uan: 'stay free of concepts and certainties because they confine and limit' (Grigg, 1990, p. xx). In Taoism, the word *knowing* is used infrequently. '*Knowing* has a connotation of boundless certainty, somewhat like *overstanding*. The universe is never *overstood*. *Know* at least suggests temporal limitations. Understanding has a softer, more yielding . . . quality, less of an overbearing sense' (Grigg, 1990, p. xx). We would argue that clinicians need to develop an appreciation of the reliability of their knowledge; to be able to defend their knowledge, but at the same time, acknowledge that much of the range and depth of their knowledge has conditional certainty in terms of contextual relevance and durability.

Approaches to generating knowledge

Research paradigms

Research paradigms provide a means of generating knowledge. The term paradigm is used in science, to describe the model in which a community of scientists generate knowledge. Within a paradigm, assumptions, problems, research strategies, criteria and techniques are shared and taken for granted by the community. Three paradigms will be considered: the empirico-analytical paradigm, the interpretive paradigm and the critical research paradigm, which stem from the philosophical stances of positivism, idealism and realism, respectively.

The empirico-analytical paradigm

The scientific method (as adopted in the natural sciences) belongs to the empirico-analytical paradigm. It is based on 'logical positivism' or 'logical empiricism' philosophy. This approach was postulated by a group of philosophers named the 'Vienna Circle' and has dominated the philosophy of science from the 1920s to the 1960s (Manley, 1991). The scientific paradigm or empiricist model of knowledge relies on observation and experiment in the empirical world, resulting in generalizations about the content and events of the world, which can be used to predict future experience (Moore, 1982). Knowledge is discovered (i.e. universal and external truths are grasped) and justified on the basis of empirical processes which are reductionist, value neutral, quantifiable, objective and operationalizable. Only statements publicly verifiable by sense data are valid.

The empirico-analytical paradigm provides the basis for the medical model. In some areas of medicine, particularly those dealing with biological aspects of human functioning, the grounding of knowledge of the field in experimental reasearch is strongly supported. For instance, the International Conference on Exercise, Fitness and Health in Toronto 1988 produced the following consensus statement about the current status of knowledge of the field: 'Knowledge was considered as firm and generally accepted if the data were from large or multiple randomized studies with clear-cut results and a low statistical risk of errors. In some cases, data from small or few randomized studies were also used, particularly if trends were consistent across studies. Other types of evidence, including correlational data and studies with inconsistent results, were generally not used in developing the consensus statement' (Bouchard et al, 1990, p. 4). Sackett (1989) similarly, argues that *rules of evidence* should apply when clinicians determine the clinical management of patients, and provides five grades or levels of evidence ranging from large randomized trials with low error risk to case series with no controls. He argues that non-experimental evidence based on the experiences of seasoned clinicians tends to overestimate efficacy since such experiences are associated with an over-emphasis on favourable treatment outcome recollections, the universal tendency for regression toward the mean of unusual results and the absence of blind judgement in evaluating clinical practice outcomes.

In many of the other health professions, it is being questioned whether the medical model and its underlying paradigm is a sufficient, or indeed preferred, model for the health sciences. The medical model is increasingly being regarded as inappropriate for the study of people by other health professions and for holistic care which balances both biological and behavioural aspects of human functioning. This questioning is evident in nursing (Kidd and Morrison, 1988; Holmes, 1990; Doering, 1992; Watson, 1990), in physiotherapy (Schmoll, 1987; Shepard, 1987; Parry, 1991; Richardson, 1992) and in occupational therapy (Reilly, 1960; Breines, 1990; Cohen, 1983; Mattingly, 1991). Practitioners in these fields are identifying a dissonance between the philosophical bases for practice and research (Holmes, 1990; Manley, 1991). There is a greater emphasis in nursing and occupational therapy in particular, on the humanistic movement and on knowledge generated within the interpretive and critical paradigms. Humanistic psychology has derived much of its theoretical support from the existential–phenomenological approach to understanding of human events (Holmes, 1990). In this approach knowledge relates to the individual's consciousness and feelings arising from his/her experiences (Kneller, 1958) and where knowledge is generated through a search for meaning, beliefs and values, and through looking for wholes and relationships with other wholes. This way of knowing is different to that in the medical model where facts are described and phenomena are reduced to component parts to describe, explain and predict how these parts work, when and where.

Criticisms of the empirico-analytical paradigm in relation to the human sciences (including the health sciences) are numerous. The most influential of these criticisms came from Thomas Kuhn in his classic study *The Structure of Scientific Revolutions* (1970). He argues that 'normal science' fails to live up to its (Popperian) ideal of a rational pursuit of knowledge because our paradigms filter the way we access, interpret and test data. Skinner (1985, p. 10) interprets Kuhn's conclusion as follows: 'there *are* no facts independent of our theories about them, and in consequence no one way of viewing, classifying and explaining the world that all rational persons are obliged to accept'.

The empirico-analytical paradigm relies on the 'fundamentally misconceived' argument that 'all successful explanations must conform to the same deductive model' and fails to recognize that 'the explanation of human behaviour and the explanation of natural events are logically distinct undertakings' (Skinner, 1985, p. 6). Psychologists argue that the normative presuppositions of positivism and the desire to analyse behaviour by causal laws fails to recognize the individual's ability to choose and to act strategically, rather than simply responsively (Skinner, 1985). Similarly, Habermas (1974) argues that in trying to model the social sciences on the natural sciences, 'positivism' fails to recognize one of the significant features which makes us human, i.e. the capacity for 'self-reflection' or 'reflexivity' and the consequent ability to change our future (in Giddens, 1985). Another argument is provided by Polanyi (1958) who contends that 'logical positivism and all the current structure of science cannot save us from the fact that all knowledge is uncertain, involves risk, and is grasped and comprehended only through the deep, personal commitment of a disciplined search' (cited in Rogers, 1983, p. 278).

This personal search for knowledge and the concept of subjectivity and individuality of knowledge is inherent in existentialist philosophy. According to existentialism, knowledge which is objective and systematized can only be hypothetical, not decisive. 'Neither purely rationalistic nor purely empirical views are capable of internalizing human experience . . . (rather) existentialist knowledge . . . originates in, and

is composed of, what exists in the individual's consciousness and feelings as a results of his experiences . . . likewise, the validity of knowledge is determined by its value to the individual.' (Kneller, 1958, pp. 58, 59). The notion of learning from experience links existentialism to the interpretive paradigm.

The scientific method is also criticized for its rejection of the effects of the nature and uniqueness of the contexts in which human beings exist (Manley, 1991). This criticism is particularly significant in relation to human behaviour and to the generation of knowledge and understanding which results from individual experiences. Boud and Walker (1991, p. 13) argue 'What (individuals) . . . bring to the situation has an important influence on what is experienced and how its is experienced. (They) . . . possess a personal foundation of experience, a way of being present in the world, which profoundly influences the way in which that world is experienced and which particularly influences the intellectual and emotional content of the experiences and the meanings that are attributed to it', i.e. the individual's personal foundation of knowledge.

The interpretive paradigm

We will now discuss a number of alternative approaches and research methodologies which are rooted in the interpretive paradigm, and which are considered to be more suitable for the generation of empirical knowledge in the human sciences. These derivatives include: hermeneutics, constructivism, phenomenology, grounded theory and ethnography.

Skinner (1985, p. 6) argues that 'from many different directions the cry has . . . gone up for ,the development of a hermeneutic approach to the human sciences, an approach that will do justice to the claim that the explanation of human action must always include – and perhaps even take the form of – an attempt to recover and interpret the meanings of social actions from the point of view of the agents performing them'. Hermeneutics refers to the theory of interpretation. Writing in this tradition, Gadamer (1975) contends that to understand human behaviour we need to seek to understand the reasons behind that behaviour. He also states that understanding is a holistic process seeking the relationship of the individual phenomenon to our conception of the totality in question. Since the health and well being of individuals involves understanding human behaviour, it is evident that hermeneutics has much to offer the search for knowledge in this field.

Constructivist philosophy is 'concerned with how people individually make sense of their worlds and how they create personal systems of meaning that guide them throughout their lives' (Candy, 1991, p. xv). In comparison to the objectivist view of knowledge as 'something external to be "mastered"' the constructivist approach views knowledge as 'an internal construction or an attempt to impose meaning and significance on events and ideas. . . . (A) corollary of this is that because no two people have had identical experiences, each person constructs a more-or-less idiosyncratic explanatory system: a unique map of the topography that we call reality' (Candy, 1991, p. 251). This view of knowledge has significant implications for teaching clinical reasoning. In particular, it is desirable to help learners explore their knowledge and challenge the content and organization of their knowledge maps.

Various qualitative research methodologies have become increasingly adopted by the health sciences since they provide valuable and relevant methods for exploration of human behaviour and experiences. Knowledge gained from such research has an important role to play in clinical reasoning. In grounded theory research, the social psychology of symbolic interactionism, which focuses on the acting individual, rather than the social system, provides the framework for research. The researcher 'intentionally becomes immersed in the world of the research subjects' (Bowers, 1988, p. 43). Ethnography provides a description of a phenomenon from a given societal or cultural focus (Omery, 1988). Phenomenological research (Heidegger, 1962; Schutz, 1962) provides another valuable alternative. It strives 'to understand and describe lived experiences' (Swanson-Kauffman and Schonwald, 1988, p. 97). These interpretive methodologies offer fruitful ways to study day to day experiences and practice in ways which retain experiential and contextual integrity (Rabinow and Sullivan, 1979; Benner, 1984; MacLeod, 1990; Brown and McIntyre, 1993). They do not look for cause–effect relationships or use the experimental method; rather they look at the whole and take account of the context of the situation, the timings, the subjective meanings and intentions within the particular situation. The implication here, for teaching and learning, is that educational strategies should be designed to retain experiential and contextual integrity and wholeness. They should also seek to uncover the meanings and significant aspects of the situation from the perspective of the actor.

The critical paradigm

The critical paradigm advocates becoming aware of how our thinking is socially and historically constructed and how this limits our actions, in order to challenge these learned restrictions, compulsions or dictates of habit (Freire, 1970; Kemmis, 1985; Mezirow, 1990). This tradition of generating emancipatory knowledge was established in the early nineteenth century in German universities. In this epistemology, knowledge is not grasped or discovered but is acquired through critical debate. 'What counts as knowledge is negotiated through a discourse allowing a critique and counter-critique by participants subscribing to the conventions of a shared form of life' (Barnett, 1990, p. 138). Emancipatory knowledge promotes understanding about how to transform current structures, relationships and conditions which constrain development and reform. The emancipatory tradition also focuses on the development of the individual, assuming that the process of becoming an adult requires critical thinking, reflecting upon the assumptions which underlie ideas and actions, and considering alternative ways of thinking (Brookfield, 1987). The continuous development of the individual is described by Mezirow (1981) as 'perspective transformation'. He uses the term 'transformation learning' to mean 'the process of learning through critical self-reflection, which results in the reformulation of a meaning perspective to allow a more inclusive, discriminating, and integrative understanding of one's experience' and a greater capacity to act on these insights (Mezirow, 1990, p. xvi). Emancipatory knowledge would be used in clinical reasoning to seek solutions to problems that seem inevitable due to seemingly unchangeable organizational structures, relations and social conditions. Educational strategies would seek to facilitate critical self-reflection upon one's knowledge and how it is used and transformed through action, and would foster critical debate of the ideas of self and others.

Ways of knowing

In addition to exploring research paradigms to identify methods of generating knowledge, it is valuable to consider other fields of study, particularly education, which have examined a broader concept: 'ways of knowing'. A great deal has been written on the type (or categories) of knowledge which result from the different paths to knowledge and on the relative legitimacy, credibility and value of these different ways of knowing. Four distinct frameworks for categorizing ways of knowing will be examined.

Habermas (1972) proposes a framework of technical, practical and emancipatory interests. These classifications of knowledge are derived from the three different scientific paradigms within which knowledge is generated. Technical knowledge is associated with the empirico-analytical paradigm, practical knowledge with the interpretive paradigm and emancipatory knowledge with the critical paradigm. These three kinds of knowledge are all empirical; however, in medicine and the health care professions, technical knowledge is more valued than both practical and emancipatory knowledge (Carper, 1978; Schon, 1983; Aldridge, 1991).

Reason and Heron (1986) describe another framework comprising three ways of knowing: gaining knowledge through direct encounter with persons, places or things (i.e. experiential knowledge), gaining knowledge related to skills or competencies through activity (i.e. practical knowledge) and gaining knowledge about things through conversation (and reading, etc.) (i.e. propositional knowledge). In discussing Reason and Heron's model, Bawden (1991) argues that, in order to make best use of the various ways of knowing, it is necessary to understand them and know how to choose and use them appropriately.

Carper (1978) produced a landmark paper on the structure of the domain of nursing knowledge. She identified four fundamental patterns of knowing: empirics (science); aesthetics (art); personal knowledge; and ethics (moral knowledge), and proposed that none of them alone should be considered sufficient or mutually exclusive. *The empirical pattern of knowing* is 'factual, descriptive and ultimately aimed at developing abstract and theoretical explanations. It is exemplary, discursively formulated and publicly verifiable' (Carper, 1978, p. 15). The empirical pattern of knowing has long been the predominant and most valued pattern in the professions and has come to be seen as the only valid and reliable knowledge because of the personal and idiosyncratic nature of the other patterns.

In the *aesthetic pattern of knowing*, knowledge is generated through subjective acquaintance, the direct feeling of experience, and is often not amenable to discourse. Such knowing focuses on the significance of behaviour, the uniqueness of the particular situation and a variety in modes of perceiving reality. This knowing gives the clinician greater choice in the design and delivery of patient care. In addition, the resulting increased sensitivity and awareness of the variety of subjective experiences will make clinical reasoning more complex and difficult.

Carper's third fundamental pattern of knowing is that of *personal knowledge* which she considers to be the most problematic and difficult to learn and teach. Personal knowledge is about knowing, encountering and actualizing oneself, not knowing *about* oneself, but knowing oneself. This knowing is situated within a relationship with another human being and within confronting him/her as a person. The therapeutic use of self means rejecting the approach to the patient as to an object and means engaging in a personal relationship. Personal knowledge can also overcome the limitations of the general laws and abstractions of empirical knowledge which cannot describe and encompass the uniqueness of the individual, encountered as a person. Personal knowledge 'can be broadly characterized as subjective, concrete and existential. It is concerned with the kind of knowing that promotes wholeness and integrity in the personal encounter, the achievement of engagement rather than detachment' (Carper, 1978, p. 20).

The fundamental pattern of knowing which Carper calls *ethics* focuses on issues of obligation, or on what ought to be done. Knowledge of ethical codes will not provide all the answers to moral dilemmas or remove the necessity for having to make moral choices in health care. Everyday decision making by health professionals in their choices of goals and actions is based on normative judgements. Sometimes the principles and norms which underpin these choices are in conflict. For example, a common goal is to achieve or maintain a patient's independence and responsibility for him or herself. However, valuing independence may be at the expense of helping the person to adjust to a situation where physical or social dependence is necessary. Building on Carper's (1978) work, Sarter (1988) adds a fifth way of knowing called 'intellectual/interpretive', which includes gaining knowledge through philosophical analysis, metaphysical analysis or hermeneutics.

A fourth framework of ways of knowing is provided by Kolb (1984) who regards learning as being a holistic process of adapting to the world, rather than an isolated classroom activity. He argues that new knowledge is generated through confrontation among four modes of experiential learning: concrete experience, reflective observations, abstract conceptualization and active experimentation. To make sense of learning experiences, the learner needs abilities in each of these four areas. Knowledge is gained through *prehension* or 'grasping or taking hold of experience in the world' either through comprehension (conceptual interpretation or symbolic representation) or apprehension (i.e. learning through tangible, immediate experiences). Alternatively, knowledge is generated through *transformation* of the grasped knowledge either through intention (internal reflection) or extension (active external manipulation of the external world).

From the above discussion, it can be concluded that there are many ways of knowing or paths to knowledge and that some paths are more suitable to the variability and complexity of the human sciences, and thus to the study and practice of clinical reasoning. We have seen that knowledge is generated not only through research, but also through direct encounter, engagement and activity. Restricting oneself to any single paradigm or way of knowing can result in a limitation to the range of knowledge and the depth of understanding which can be applied to a given problem situation. Schon (1987, p. 13) concludes that professional practice requires a combination of the different paradigms. He argues that, 'in the terrain of professional practice, applied science and research-based technique occupy a critically important though limited territory,

bounded on several sides by artistry' which is 'an exercise in intelligence, a kind of knowing (that is) . . . inherent in the practice of professionals'.

For effective clinical reasoning, we consider that health professionals rely upon the scientific knowledge of human behaviour and body responses in health and illness, the aesthetic perception of significant human experiences, a personal understanding of the uniqueness of the self and others and the ability to make decisions within concrete situations involving particular moral judgements. Each way of knowing, therefore, has a place in the education of health science students and in the practice of clinical reasoning.

Types of knowledge

In Western philosophy, knowledge has been commonly classified into two categories: propositional knowledge (or 'knowing that') and non-propositional knowledge (or 'knowing how') (Polanyi, 1958; Kuhn, 1970). In Table 10.1 the terms used in the literature are located within these two knowledge categories. Propositional knowledge is derived through research and scholarship, with an attempt to generalize findings. Non-propositional knowledge is derived primarily through practice, without an attempt to generalize. In this chapter we are presenting three overlapping and interactive types of knowledge. We are using the labels 'propositional knowledge' to refer to knowledge which has been ratified or supported by the field; 'professional craft knowledge' which incorporates 'knowing how' and tacit knowledge of the profession, and 'personal knowledge' or knowledge which is tied to the individual's reality or experience. These are illustrated in Figure 10.1.

A hierarchical relationship has grown up between propositional and non-propositional knowledge, with the former having a higher status. Schon (1983) states that in the early 20th century, professions sought to gain prestige by establishing their schools in universities. This led to the adoption of a model of practice where professional activity consisted of instrumental problem-solving, made rigorous by the use of scientific theory and technique. The physician's diagnosis and treatment of disease became one of the prototypes of a science-

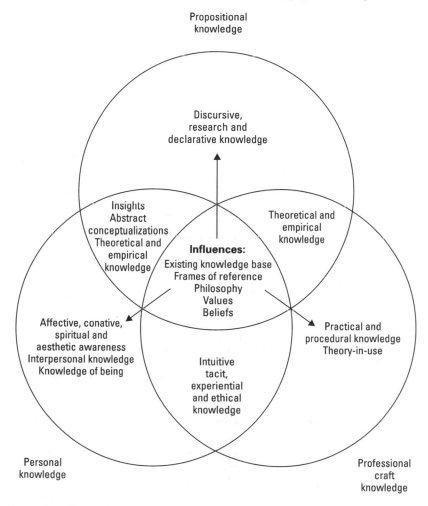

Figure 10.1 Types of knowledge and internal influences on knowledge generation

based technical practice where craft and artistry were supplanted and considered to have no place in rigorous practice (Schon, 1983). Research was carried out within the predominant empirico-analytical paradigm and the substance and structure of medical knowledge (i.e. technical knowledge), thus generated, became the foundation for organizing knowledge and methods of practice in the health professions. More recently, as these professions sought admission to higher education, propositional knowledge became more valued than non-propositional knowledge. It may be that the lower status of the latter (combined with its often tacit nature) is the reason why it has not been explored extensively in research and education (Eraut, 1985).

We support Barnett's (1990) argument that modern society is unreasonably dominated by the cognitive framework of science, to the extent that other forms of knowledge are downgraded and not even regarded as real knowledge. He argues that in a world where problems are not discrete nor solutions definite, we need knowledge beyond science.

Propositional–public knowledge

The term 'propositional knowledge' encompasses book knowledge and the presentation of the abstract, logical and formal relationships between concepts or constructs, and formal statements concerning interactional and causal relationships between events (Benner, 1984). Heron (1981) states that: 'the outcome of

Table 10.1 Propositional and non-propositional knowledge

Propositional knowledge, i.e. 'knowing that'	Non-propositional knowledge, i.e. 'knowing how to do something'
Empirically derived through research	Empirically derived primarily through practice/experience

Alternative terms
  Empirical knowledge (Carper, 1978)
	Alternative terms
	  Professional artistry (Schon, 1983, 1987)
	  Professional craft knowledge (Brown and McIntyre, 1993; Titchen, 1993)
	  Procedural knowledge (Biggs and Telfer, 1987) or 'theory-in-use'

Related terms
  Discursive knowledge
  Declarative knowledge	

Types of propositional knowledge (Habermas, 1972)
  Technical knowledge
  Practical knowledge
  Emancipatory knowledge
	Types of non-propositional knowledge
	  Experiential knowledge (Reason and Heron, 1986; Kolb, 1984)
	  Practical knowledge (Benner, 1984; Reason and Heron, 1986)
	  Aesthetic, personal and ethical knowledge (Carper, 1978)
	  Intuitive knowledge (Agan, 1987; Rew and Barrow, 1987; Benner, 1984; McCormack, 1992)

research is stated in propositions, which claim to be assertions of facts or truths, a contribution to the corpus of knowledge statements . . . (A proposition) is a statement about the world. It does not constitute the world; is not part of, or found in, the world' (Heron, 1981, p. 27). Propositional knowledge can be generated in any research paradigm, whether empirico-analytical, interpretive or critical. Related terms are *discursive knowledge* (i.e. rational knowledge resulting from discourse) and *declarative knowledge* (i.e. 'knowing about a topic so that one may declare that knowledge; an aspect of espoused knowledge' (Biggs and Telfer, 1987, p. 543).

Professional craft knowledge

According to Schon (1987, p. 10) in recent years there has been an increasing concern raised about the growing gap between research-based (propositional) knowledge taught in professional schools and the practical knowledge and 'actual competencies required of practitioners in the field'. This gap can be attributed in part to the knowledge explosion, to the rapid change in the nature and demands of the context in which the professionals are acting, and to the very uncertainty of the professional workplace. Health science schools need to prepare students to develop the knowledge and skills to work in these contexts. Schon (1987) argues that in order to deal with the crisis of

professional knowledge and education we need to recognize that outstanding practitioners do not have more professional knowledge but more 'wisdom', 'talent', 'intuition' or 'artistry'. And, we need to assimilate such knowledge into the dominant model of (propositional) professional knowledge and to give this artistic knowledge recognition in an environment which supports the hegemony of scientific knowledge.

Procedural (Biggs and Telfer, 1987) or practical (Heron, 1981; Benner, 1984) knowledge encompasses practical expertise and skills. It guides everyday activities of caring for patients and underpins the practitioner's rapid and fluent response to a situation. Short-term, taken-for-granted goals are achieved by strategies which take account of, and show sensitivity to, a multiplicity of situation variables. The practitioner reacts to the whole situation and makes highly skilled judgements without being conscious of a deliberate way of acting. Such knowledge is often tacit in nature and may remain hidden if practitioners do not reflect upon or document their everyday practice. Benner (1984) suggests that practical knowledge has remained tacit in nursing because it is so much taken-for-granted and seen as so obvious and ordinary that it is rarely articulated. Thus much of the knowledge a practitioner uses in problem-solving and in making clinical judgements is tacit and individual (Polanyi, 1958; Carroll, 1988). However, recent research is bringing such knowledge into the public domain (e.g. Benner, 1984; MacLeod, 1990; Lawler, 1991) thus transforming it into propositional knowledge.

Heron (1981) sees evidence of practical knowledge in a skill, knack or proficiency whether it is physical and/or mental. He distinguishes it from experiential knowledge, which he sees as a fundamental kind of knowing of an entity of some kind (person, place or thing), which results from sustained interaction and acquaintance. Similarly, Burnard (1987) states that experiential knowledge is necessarily personal and idiosyncratic. We see experiential knowledge as a necessary, but not sufficient, condition for acquiring practical knowledge in any given context.

The ability of health practitioners to interpret incomplete and ambiguous data and to identify implications which are not directly deducible from explicit data depends upon clinical knowledge or judgement which can be likened to intuitive knowledge (as described by Agan, 1987; Rew and Barrow, 1987; McCormack, 1992). Benner (1984) defines intuitive knowledge as 'understanding without a rationale' and as consisting of perceptual awareness which does not rely on consciously identifiable environmental cues. She found, for example, that nurses were able to read a patient's face and discern global, subtle changes before there were any documentable changes in vital signs. Such intuitive (clinical) knowledge is based on experience and imagination. It is built upon previous knowledge and understanding as well as creative ideas. As such, it can be best labelled a 'learned awareness or contextual receptivity' as compared to the more innate idea of intuition as 'inherent intuitiveness' which is a more individual and idiosyncratic phemonenon. Clinical intuition or clinical judgement is compatible with analytical clinical reasoning and is often used in a complementary manner (Benner and Tanner, 1987). The depth of clinical judgement or intuition demonstrated by an expert clinician is, we argue, born of a wealth of personal experience of clinical practice in combination with a processing of prior learning. This notion of a growing depth of knowledge relates to Boshuizen and Schmidt's (1992) model of developing expertise in clinical reasoning which involves the encapsulation of scientific and clinical knowledge.

Recently, an alternative term or metaphor, 'professional craft knowledge', has been introduced which combines these different types of non-propositional knowledge (Brown and McIntyre, 1993; Titchen, 1993). In this chapter we use this metaphor to mean knowledge which in large measure is intuitive (clinical) knowledge and which includes the cognitive, but not the psychomotor aspects of practical knowledge and experiential knowledge as described here. We use the term 'professional craft knowledge' because it is rhetorically useful in that it gives a sense of the aesthetic and of knowing what and when, as well as how. Titchen (1993) includes personal knowledge in her description of professional craft knowledge, but to examine each of these in more detail in this chapter, we have made a distinction between professional craft knowledge and personal knowledge.

Personal knowledge

We have presented propositional knowledge as being public, objective knowledge of the field and knowledge of the external world, and professional craft knowledge as knowledge within the professional domain which has both public and individual forms. Professional craft knowledge relates more to theory-in-use and non-declarative forms of knowledge (e.g. tacit knowledge and intuition). In addition we have identified a third category of knowledge which has particular relevance to clinical reasoning in the health professions: personal knowledge. *Personal knowledge is defined here as the unique frame of reference and knowledge of self which is central to the individual's sense of self.* It is the result of the individual's personal experiences and reflections on these experiences (Butt et al, 1982).

In developing this definition we have incorporated and extended Carper's (1978) concept of personal knowledge as knowing oneself. At the same time, we recognize that knowledge of self is the core of personal knowledge and wisdom. This core idea is illustrated in writings from eastern philosophy, for example, Gibran (translated by Ferris, 1962b, p. 58) writes 'the essence of wisdom is . . . self-knowledge' and Lao Tzu (translated by Grigg, 1990, p. 65) contends that 'knowing self is called wisdom'. We would argue that an individual's knowledge base has a personal foundation, since it is constructed and tested within the individual's frame of reference which comprises the individual's value systems, prior learning and current knowledge convictions. We also suggest that the individual has a store of personal knowledge into which other knowledge becomes incorporated, or which becomes revised as a result of the individual's developments in knowing. Wylde (1989, p. 115) explains this journey to knowing as follows: 'I have learnt that it is only possible to use something I have read or heard, if that "something" connects with my own experiencing'.

The individual's internal frame of reference and store of personal knowledge shapes the architecture of the self and the individual's construction of reality, and creates what could be termed the individual's unique personal intentionality (Butt, 1985). Weiser (1987) uses the term consciousness to refer to the 'primary frames of meaning with which we interpret our own life and the world'. The individual's behaviour is highly influenced by his/her frame of reference. Within this frame of reference, scientific knowledge and professional knowledge are translated into decisions for practice which are influenced by the individual's convictions and judgements about the worth of this knowledge and its relevance to the current situation. New knowledge is compared with the individual's existing system of beliefs and values. If new knowledge or ideas are incongruent with their belief system, individuals may reject the new information. Barnett (1990) also argues that the generation of knowledge by the individual is a developmental process which occurs within a value system and that these values provide an important influence on the knowledge which develops. This argument is developed by Reid (1986, p. xii) who contends that:

> In the long history of Western culture, and in our educational curricula, 'knowledge' has been identified with its discursive propositional forms, and the curriculum (has) not only been hugely dominated by them, but dominated largely to the exclusion of non-discursive knowledge and understanding, implying a separation of thinking and knowledge and understanding, implying a separation of thinking and feeling. This divisiveness is, on any liberal view of education as concerned with whole persons, disastrously destructive. It is destructive in that the capaci-

ties for feeling and understanding required for the development of non-discursive awareness remain undeveloped and so wither and become atrophied.

Within the health professions, this argument has particular significance since it is the well-being of the whole person which lies at the heart of health care. Clinicians need to develop a personal knowledge base, including a depth of self-understanding which will enable them to understand complex human desires for dignity, independence and support, to appreciate the needs and frames of reference of their patients or clients, to learn to cope with pain, frailty and human endeavour and to learn to deal with ethical dilemmas within the clinical situation. According to Hundert (1987) this is achieved through the development of a dynamic 'reflective equilibrium'. Personal knowledge needs to incorporate affective (feelings), conative (purposefulness, will) and spiritual elements of self, to look beyond the limits of cognition. The philosopher Gibran, for instance, argues 'and what is word knowledge but a shadow of wordless knowledge?' (Gibran, 1926, p. 103). Ranjan (1992) supports a greater emphasis on spirituality in learning involving 'going beyond the senses of the body to the light of the heart and letting Being be our teacher . . . Seeing in each circumstance, crisis or relationship an opportunity and a challenge to access deeper and richer resources within ourselves . . . (to) move from fragmented knowledge to wisdom' (Ranjan, 1992, p. 80).

In considering personal knowledge and its place in clinical reasoning, we encourage educators to adopt an approach which values and focuses on personal experience and which does not diminish or lose the 'humanness' of a relationship. Self-evaluation and an understanding of the need to test and re-test knowledge to justify knowledge claims needs to be promoted. We suggest that there should be a recognition and valuing of a variety of ways of knowing including reflection, conceptualization, experimentation and experience, and that students' development of self-knowledge as both person and professional should be nurtured. Students need to be helped to adopt various roles in the client/patient/professional relationship, and to examine how their own beliefs, values, perceptions and interpretations of their environment influence their clinical reasoning.

From the distinctions made between propositional and non-propositional knowledge comes the goal of 'enhancing the knowledge creation capacity of individuals and professional communities' (Eraut, 1985, p. 117) by: recognizing that much professional expertise lies outside the higher education system; fostering knowledge exchange between higher education and the professions; ensuring that students are taught by practising health professionals as well as by academics; and incorporating skills of knowledge generation and self-directed learning into curricula (*see also* Higgs and Boud, 1991).

Knowledge and clinical reasoning

An important aspect of the development of higher cognitive skills and clinical reasoning ability is the ability to construct and use knowledge. The construction of knowledge requires the individual to process experience and to develop a representation of reality. This could be described as developing constructs which help to explain or interpret reality, or engaging in mental abstraction and interpretations based on experience.

Nickerson et al (1985) argue that knowledge and thinking are interdependent, since the development of knowledge requires thinking and thinking can be defined as the ability to apply knowledge. These authors identify two key features of expertise: 'the ability to manage one's intellectual resources and to use whatever domain-specific knowledge one has most efficiently' and the presence of a wealth of domain-specific knowledge (Nickerson et al, 1985, p. 68). The importance of domain-specific knowledge in problem-solving expertise is widely supported (Greeno, 1980; Hayes, 1981; Bordage and Lemieux, 1986; Grant and Marsden, 1987; Norman, 1988). Baron and Sternberg (1987, p. 28), however, argue that 'although domain-specific knowledge is essential to good thinking within a domain, it is not sufficient to assure that good thinking will occur'. As well as relevant knowledge, skills in cognition (critical, creative, reflective and dialectical thinking) and metacognition are essential for effective thinking and problem solving. Similarly, Alexander and Judy (1988) conclude that 'there are at any rate two undisputed findings from cognitive research over the last twenty years. One is that those who know more about a particular domain generally understand and remember better; the other is that those who regulate and monitor their cognitive processing (i.e. use metacognition) during task performance do better' (cited in Radford, 1991, p. 10).

Metacognition refers to being aware of one's own cognitive processes and exerting control over these processes (Flavell, 1976). Metacognitive skills can be thought of as cognitive skills that are necessary for the management of knowledge and other cognitive skills (Biggs, 1988). Biggs (1986, p. 143) argues that 'high quality human performance inevitably requires metacognitive as well as cognitive components. To perform well, one needs to be aware not only of the knowledge and algorithms required for the task, but of one's own motives and resources, the contextual constraints, and to plan strategically on that knowledge'. By becoming more metacognitive about their learning, students are more able to adopt deep and strategic approaches to learning which are important to achieve meaningful learning and success in tertiary education. The development of metacognitive skills has also been shown to enhance problem solving (Biggs and Telfer, 1987).

Apart from investigations into the relationship between knowledge and clinical reasoning ability, recent research has also focused on the structure of knowledge. Glaser (1984, p. 97), for instance, has found that problem solving ability is enhanced by 'the possession and utilization of an organized body of (relevant) conceptual and procedural knowledge'. To support this contention Glaser provides evidence from several fields: from studies in developmental psychology (Chase and Simon, 1973; Chi, 1978; Siegler and Richards, 1982); in novice/expert problem solving (Larkin et al, 1980; Lesgold et al, 1981; Chi et al, 1982) and from the investigation of aptitude and intelligence (Pellegrino and Glaser, 1982).

According to Rumelhart and Ortony (1977, p. 99) people 'process and reprocess information, imposing on it and producing from it knowledge which has structure' and a human memory system which is 'a vast repository of such knowledge'. The value of the individual's existing cognitive structure to their cognition and generation of knowledge was supported by Ausubel (1977, p. 94) who stressed the importance of 'the availability in cognitive structure of specifically relevant anchoring ideas'.

Knowledge structure also refers to the individual's 'meaning perspective' or a 'structure of assumptions that constitutes a frame of reference for interpreting the meaning of an experience' (Mezirow, 1990, p. xvi). The accumulated propositional, professional and personal knowledge of the individual constitutes his/her unique knowledge base. Thus, such knowledge bases have contextual influences generated by the societal, professional, paradigmatic and experiential situations in which the individual's knowledge was generated. The relevance of the individual's knowledge base to the task in hand is also very important (Feltovich et al, 1984).

To analyse this notion of knowledge structures, it is valuable to turn to the study of schemata (i.e. abstractions or representations of previous experience). 'Schema theory attempts to describe how acquired knowledge is organized and represented and how such cognitive structures facilitate the use of knowledge in particular ways' (Glaser, 1984, p. 100). Schemata are particularly valuable in that they provide background knowledge (often tacit knowledge) which helps people interpret new information. New events are labelled 'instantiations' (2) of these schemata (Howard, 1987). And, as new instances are interpreted, the prior knowledge constructions or schemata are tested. The process of categorization also provides a means (and theory) for the structuring of knowledge (3). Medin (1989, p. 1469) describes the importance of categorization by saying that 'clinicians need some way to bring their knowledge and experience to bear on the problem under consideration, and that requires the appreciation of some similarity or relationship between the current situation and what has gone before'.

In medical research a number of findings have linked knowledge structure to expertise in clinical reasoning. Schmidt et al (1990, p. 611) present a theory of the development of expertise in which it is argued that expertise is

based on cognitive structures that describe the features of prototypical or even actual patients. These cognitive structures, referred to as 'illness scripts' contain relatively little knowledge about pathophysiological causes of symptoms and complaints, but a wealth of clinically relevant information (4). Similarly, Grant and Marsden (1988) have found that expertise is based on knowledge structured from individual experience rather than the common core of knowledge taught at medical school. Patel and Groen (1986) ascribe expertise to the presence of a knowledge base containing reasoning rules.

From the notion of schemata and knowledge organization, the importance of prior knowledge and the significance of domain-specific knowledge, the teacher can derive several valuable guides to the teaching of clinical knowledge and clinical reasoning. These include teaching clinical reasoning skills within the relevant discipline-specific domain and encouraging students to explore their knowledge, its validity and its structure, in the light of their clinical experience and the established knowledge of the field. It is also valuable to encourage students to develop their ability to generate and use clinical knowledge in the clinic as well as in the classroom.

Conclusion

To provide a valid and functional basis for clinical reasoning in health care, an individual's knowledge base needs to comprise propositional, professional and personal knowledge. Propositional knowledge in the health fields, due to continual changes in health and illness phenomena and related sciences and technologies will continue to face rapid growth as well as rapid obsolescence. Ongoing research and theoretical development conducted within the three research paradigms is required, particularly in developing professions. Professional craft knowledge possibly provides a deeper and more practical basis for coping with the uncertainties of health care contexts. At the same time, such knowledge is faced with demands for verifica-

---

(2) For further discussion on the notion of instantiations refer to Chapter 2.

(3) The process of categorization and its importance to clinical reasoning is discussed in Chapter 11.

(4) Refer to Chapter 2 for further discussion of this theory.

tion and accountability. Methods of making such knowledge accessible and available for public scrutiny need to be found. Personal knowledge is a vital element in the ability to deal with the interpersonal, ethical, emotional and spiritual aspects of human interactions and the clinician's own choices and dilemmas. Each of these three areas of knowledge needs to work in harmony to provide the depth of understanding which is needed to underpin effective clinical reasoning.

In constructing their knowledge bases, individuals endeavour to make sense of their experiences. An important aspect of this process of knowledge generation is understanding the nature of knowledge and the different ways of developing knowledge, and learning how to adopt an approach to knowing which is appropriate to the context in question. Clinicians need to seek continually to enrich their knowledge bases in each of the three knowledge areas and to test the knowledge acquired. The acquisition of such a knowledge base will enhance the clinician's expertise in clinical reasoning.

We have argued that since propositional, professional and personal knowledge each have a valid and important place in clinical reasoning, curricula should foster the development of each and give each appropriate recognition. This process includes recognizing the importance of well-tested knowledge of the field as a guide to such interventions as medication prescription, the importance of professional craft knowledge in making decisions related to intervention choices, and the real value of personal knowledge in enhancing human interactions. We argue that inattention to personal and professional craft knowledge in professional curricula could limit the development of students' clinical reasoning skills. It is therefore essential for health professional educators to look carefully at the nature of knowledge to guide teaching and curriculum development. It is also important to challenge the traditional notion that knowledge is only generated through research, and to promote the equally valuable notion that practitioners generate knowledge through their practice and through their own personal search for meaning (Schon, 1983; Eraut, 1985; Elliott, 1991; Higgs, 1992; Titchen and Binnie, 1993).

References

Agan, R.D. (1987) Intuitive knowing as a dimension of nursing. *Advances in Nursing Science*, **10**, 63–70

Aldridge, D. (1991) Aesthetics and the individual in the practice of medical research: discussion paper. *Journal of the Royal Society of Medicine*, **84**, 147–150

Alexander, P.A. and Judy, J.E. (1988) The interaction of domain-specific and strategic knowledge in academic performance. *Review of Educational Research*, **58**, 375–404

Ausubel, D.P. (1977) Cognitive structure and transfer. In *How Students Learn* (eds N. Entwistle and D. Hounsell). Institute for Research and Development in Post-Compulsory Education, University of Lancaster, Lancaster, pp. 93–103.

Ayer, A.J. (1956) *The Problem Of Knowledge*. Penguin Books, London

Barnett, R. (1990) *The Idea of Higher Education*. The Society for Research into Higher Education and Open University Press, Buckingham

Baron, J.B. and Sternberg, R.J. (1987) *Teaching Thinking Skills: Theory and Practice*. W. H. Freeman and Co, New York

Bawden, R. (1991) Toward a praxis of situation improving. In *The Challenge of Problem Based Learning* (eds D. Boud and G. Feletti). Kogan Page, London, pp. 308–314

Benner, P. (1984) *From Novice to Expert: Excellence and Power in Clinical Nursing Practice*. Addison-Wesley, London

Benner, P. and Tanner, C. (1987) Clinical judgment: how expert nurses use intuition. *American Journal of Nursing*, **87**, 23–31

Berger, P. and Luckmann, T. (1985) *The Social Construction of Reality*. Penguin, Harmondsworth

Biggs, J. (1988) The role of metacognition in enhancing learning. *Australian Journal of Education*, **32**, 127–138

Biggs, J.B. (1986) Enhancing learning skills: the role of metacognition. In *Student Learning: Research Into Practice – The Marysville Symposium* (ed. J.A. Bowden). Centre for the Study of Higher Education, The University of Melbourne, Parkville, pp. 131–148

Biggs, J.B. and Telfer, R. (1987) *The Process of Learning*. Prentice-Hall, Sydney

Bordage, G. and Lemieux, M. (1986) Some cognitive characteristics of medical students with and without diagnostic reasoning difficulties. In *Proceedings of the 25th Annual Conference of Research in Medical Education of the American Association of Medical Colleges*. American Association of Medical Colleges, New Orleans, pp. 185–190

Boshuizen, H.P.A. and Schmidt, H.G. (1992) On the role of biomedical knowledge in clinical reasoning by experts, intermediates and novices. *Cognitive Science*, **16**, 153–184

Bouchard, C., Shephard, R.J., Stephens, T., Sutton, J.R. and McPherson, B.D. (1990) *Exercise, Fitness and*

Health: A Consensus of Current Knowledge. Human Kinetics Books, Champaign, Illinois

Boud, D. and Walker, D. (1991) *Experience and Learning: Reflection at Work*. Deakin University Press, Geelong, Victoria

Bowers, B.J. (1988) Grounded theory. In *Paths to Knowledge: Innovative Research Methods For Nursing* (ed. B. Sarter). National League for Nursing, New York, pp. 33–60

Breines, E. (1990) Genesis of occupation: A philosophical model for therapy and theory. *Australian Occupational Therapy Journal*, **37**, 45–49

Brookfield, S.D. (1987) *Developing Critical Thinkers*. Open University Press, Milton Keynes

Brown, S. and McIntyre, D. (1993) *Making Sense of Teaching*. Open University Press, Milton Keynes

Burnard, P. (1987) Towards an epistemological basis for experiential learning in nurse education. *Journal of Advanced Nursing*, **12**, 189–193

Butt, R. (1985) Curriculum: Metatheoretical horizons and emancipatory action. *Journal of Curriculum Theorizing*, **6**, 7–21

Butt, R., Raymond, D. and Yamaguishi, L. (1982) Autobiographic praxis: Studying the formation of teacher's knowledge. *Journal of Curriculum Theorizing*, **7**, 87–164

Candy, P.C. (1991) *Self-direction for Lifelong Learning*. Jossey-Bass, San Francisco

Carper, B.A. (1978) Fundamental patterns of knowing. *Advances in Nursing Science*, **1**, 13–23

Carroll, E. (1988) The role of tacit knowledge in problem solving in the clinical setting. *Nurse Education Today*, **8**, 140–147

Chase, W.G. and Simon, H.A. (1973) The mind's eye in chess. In *Visual Information Processing* (ed. W. G. Chase). Academic Press, New York, pp. 215–281

Chi, M.T.H. (1978) Knowledge structures and memory development. In *Children's Thinking: What Develops?* (ed. R. Siegler). Erlbaum, Hillsdale, New Jersey, pp. 73–96

Chi, M.T.H., Glaser, R. and Rees, E. (1982) Expertise in problem solving. In *Advances in the Psychology of Human Intelligence*, Volume 1 (ed. R. Sternberg). Erlbaum, Hillsdale, New Jersey, pp. 7–75

Cohen, L. and Manion, L. (1985) *Research Methods in Education*, 2nd edn. Croom Helm, London

Cohen, S. (1983) The mental hygiene movement: The development of personality and the school: The medicalization of American education. *History of Education Quarterly*, **23**, 123–149

Doering, L. (1992) Power and knowledge in nursing: a feminist poststructuralist view. *Advances in Nursing Science*, **14**, 24–33

Elliott, J. (1991) *Action Research for Educational Change*. Open University Press, Milton Keynes

Eraut, M. (1985) Knowledge creation and knowledge use in professional contexts. *Studies in Higher Education*, **10**, 117–133

Feltovich, P.J., Johnson, P.E., Moller, J.H. and Swanson, D. B. (1984) LCS: The role and development of medical knowledge in diagnostic expertise. In *Readings in Medical Artificial Intelligence: The First Decade* (eds W.J. Clancey and E.H. Shortliffe). Addison-Wesley, Reading, pp. 275–319

Ferris, A.R. (Translator) (1962a) *A Second Treasury of Kahlil Gibran*. Castle Books, New Jersey

Ferris, A.R. (Translator) (1962b) *Spiritual Sayings of Kahlil Gibran*. Citadel Press, Secaucus, New Jersey

Flavell, J.H. (1976) Metacognition aspects of problem solving. In *The Nature of Intelligence* (ed. L.B. Resnick). Lawrence Erlbaum, Hillsdale, New Jersey

Freire, P. (1970) *Cultural Action for Freedom*. Harvard Educational Review, Massachusetts

Gadamer, H.G. (1975) Hermeneutics and social science. *Cultural Hermeneutics*, **2**, 312

Gibran, K. (1926) *The Prophet*. Heinemann, London

Giddens, A. (1985) Jurgen Habermas. In *The Return of Grand Theory in the Human Sciences* (ed. Q. Skinner). Cambridge University Press, Cambridge, pp. 121–140

Glaser, R. (1984) Education and thinking: the role of knowledge. *American Psychologist*, **39**, 93–104

Gowin, D.B. (1981) *Educating*. Cornell University Press, Ithaca, New York

Grant, J. and Marsden, P. (1987) The structure of memorized knowledge in students and clinicians: an explanation for diagnostic expertise. *Medical Education*, **21**, 92–98

Grant, J. and Marsden, P. (1988) Primary knowledge, medical education and consultant expertise. *Medical Education*, **22**, 173–179

Greeno, J.G. (1980) Trends in the theory of knowledge for problem solving. In *Problem Solving and Education: Issues in Teaching and Research* (eds D.T. Tuma and R. Reif). Lawrence Erlbaum Associates, Hillsdale, New Jersey, pp. 9–23

Grigg, R. (1990) *The Tao of Being*. Wildwood House, Hants, England

Habermas, J. (1972) *Knowledge and Human Interest*. Heinemann, London

Habermas, J. (1974) *Theory and Practice* (translated by J. Viertel). Heinemann, London

Hayes, J.R. (1981) *The Complete Problem Solver*. Franklin Institute Press, Philadelphia

Heidegger, M. (1962). *Being and Time*. Harper and Row, New York

Heron, J. (1981) Philosophcal basis for a new paradigm. In *Human Inquiry: A Sourcebook of New Paradigm Research* (eds P. Reason and J. Rowan). John Wiley & Sons, Chichester, pp. 19–35

Higgs, J. (1992) Developing knowledge: a process of construction, mapping and review. *New Zealand Journal of Physiotherapy*, **20**, 23–30

Higgs, J. and Boud, D. (1991) Self-directed learning as part of the mainstream of physiotherapy education. *The Australian Journal of Physiotherapy*, **37**, 245–251

Holmes, C.A. (1990) Alternatives to natural science foundations for nursing. *International Journal of Nursing Studies*, **27**, 187–198

Howard, R.W. (1987) *Concepts and Schemata: An Introduction*. Cassell Education, London

Hundert, E.M. (1987) A model for ethical problem solving in medicine, with practical applications. *American Journal of Psychiatry*, **144**, 839–849

Kemmis, S. (1985) Action research and the politics of reflection. In *Reflection: Turning Experience Into Learning* (eds D. Boud, R. Keogh and D. Walker). Kogan Page, London, pp. 139–163

Kidd, P. and Morrison, E.F. (1988) The progression of knowledge in nursing: a search for meaning. *IMAGE: Journal of Nursing Scholarship*, **20**, 222–224

Kleinig, J. (1982) *Philosophical Issues in Education*. Routledge, London

Kneller, G.F. (1958) *Existentialism and Education*. Science Editions, John Wiley and Sons, New York

Kolb, D.A. (1984) *Experiential Learning: Experience as the Source of Learning and Development*. Prentice-Hall, Englewood Cliffs

Kuhn, T.S. (1970) *The Structure of Scientific Revolutions*, 2nd edn. University of Chicago Press, Chicago

Larkin, J., McDermott, J., Simon, D.P. and Simon, H.A. (1980) Expert and novice performance in solving physics problems. *Science*, **208**, 1335–1342

Lawler, J. (1991) *Behind the Screens: Nursing, Somology and the Problem of the Body*. Churchill Livingstone

Lesgold, A.M., Feltovich, P.J., Glaser, R. and Wang, Y. (1981) *The Acquisition of Perceptual Diagnostic Skill in Radiology* (Tech. Rep. PDS-1). Learning Research and Development Center, University of Pittsburgh, Pittsburgh

MacLeod, M. (1990) Experience in everyday nursing practice: A study of 'experienced' ward sisters. Doctoral Thesis, University of Edinburgh, Edinburgh

Manley, K. (1991) Knowledge for nursing practice. In *Nursing: A Knowledge Base for Practice* (eds A. Perry and M. Jolley). Edward Arnold, London, pp. 1–27

Mattingly, C. (1991) The narrative nature of clinical reasoning. *American Journal of Occupational Therapy*, **45**, 998–1005

McCormack, B. (1992) Intuition: concept analysis and application to curriculum development. 1. Concept analysis. *Journal of Clinical Nursing*, **1**, 339–344

Medin, D.L. (1989) Concepts and conceptual structure. *American Psychologist*, **44**, 1469–1481

Mezirow, J. (1981) A critical theory of adult learning and education. *Adult Education*, **32**, 3–24

Mezirow, J. (1990) Preface. In *Fostering Critical Reflection in Adulthood: A Guide to Transformative and Emancipatory Learning* (eds J. Mezirow and Associates). Jossey-Bass, San Francisco, pp. xiii–xxi

Moore, T.W. (1982) *Philosophy of Education: An Introduction*. Routledge and Kegan Paul, London

Nickerson, R.S., Perkins, D.N. and Smith, E.E. (1985) *The Teaching of Thinking*. Lawrence Erlbaum Associates, Hillsdale, New Jersey

Norman, G.R. (1988) Problem-solving skills, solving problems, and problem-based learning.. *Medical Education*, **22**, 279–286

Omery, A. (1988) Ethnography. In *Paths to Knowledge: Innovative Research Methods for Nursing* (ed. B. Sarter). National League for Nursing, New York, pp. 17–32

Parry, A. (1991) Physiotherapy and methods of inquiry: conflict and reconciliation. *Physiotherapy*, **77**, 435–438

Patel, V.L. and Groen, G.J. (1986) Knowledge based solution strategies in medical reasoning. *Cognitive Science*, **10**, 91–116

Pellegrino, J.W. and Glaser, R. (1982) Analyzing aptitudes for learning: Inductive reasoning. In *Advances in Instructional Psychology*, Volume 2 (ed. R. Glaser). Erlbaum, Hillsdale, New Jersey, pp. 269–345

Perkins, D.N. (1986) *Knowledge as Design*. Lawrence Erlbaum, Hillsdale, New Jersey

Polanyi, M. (1958) *Personal Knowledge: Towards a Post-Critical Philosophy*. Routledge and Kegan Paul, London

Rabinow, P. and Sullivan, M. (1979). *Interpretive Social Science*. University of California Press, Berkeley

Radford, J. (1991) Teaching and learning: A selective review. In *Helping Students to Learn: Teaching, Counselling, Research* (eds K. Raaheim, J. Wankowski and J. Radford). The Society for Research into Higher Education and Open University Press, Buckingham, pp. 1–15

Ranjan, (1992) Silent learning: Experience as a way of knowledge. In *Empowerment Through Experiential Learning: Explorations of Good Practice* (eds J. Mulligan and C. Griffin). Kogan Page, London, pp. 76–81

Reason, P. and Heron, J. (1986) Research with people: the paradigm of cooperative experiential enquiry. *Person-Centred Review*, **1**, 457–476

Reid, L.A. (1986) *Ways of Understanding and Education*. Heinemann Educational Books, London

Reilly, M. (1960) Research potentiality of occupational therapy. *American Journal of Occupational Therapy*, **14**, 206–209

Rew, L. and Barrow, E.M. (1987) Intuition: a neglected hallmark of nursing knowledge. *Advances in Nursing Science*, **10**, 49–62

Richardson, B. (1992) Professional education and professional practice: Do they match? *Physiotherapy*, **78**, 23–26

Rogers, C.R. (1983) *Freedom to Learn for the 80's*. Charles E. Merrill, Ohio

Rumelhart, D.E. and Ortony, A. (1977) The representation of knowledge in memory. In *Schooling and the Acquisition of Knowledge* (eds R.C. Anderson, R.J. Spiro and W.E. Montague). Lawrence Erlbaum, Hillsdale, New Jersey, pp. 99–135

Sackett, D.L. (1989) Rules of evidence and clinical recommendations on the use of antithrombotic agents. *Chest*, **95**, S2–S4

Sarter, B. (ed.) (1988) *Paths to Knowledge: Innovative Research Methods for Nursing*. National League for Nursing, New York

Schmidt, H.G., Norman, G.R. and Boshuizen, H.P.A. (1990) A cognitive perspective on medical expertise: theory and implications. *Academic Medicine*, **65**, 611–621

Schmoll, B.J. (1987) Ethnographic inquiry in clinical settings. *Physical Therapy*, **67**, 1895–1897

Schon, D.A. (1983) *The Reflective Practitioner: How Professionals Think in Action*. Temple Smith, London

Schon, D.A. (1987) *Educating the Reflective Practitioner*. Jossey-Bass, San Francisco

Schutz, A. (1962) *Collected Papers*, Volumes 1–3. Kluwer Academic, The Netherlands

Shepard, K.F. (1987) Qualitative and quantitative research in clinical practice. *Physical Therapy*, **67**, 1891–1894

Siegler, R.S. and Richards, D.D. (1982) The development of intelligence. In *Handbook of Human Intelligence* (ed. R. J. Sternberg). Cambridge University Press, Cambridge

Skinner, Q. (1985) Introduction: The return of grand theory. In *The Return of Grand Theory in the Human Sciences* (ed. Q. Skinner). Cambridge University Press, Cambridge, pp. 1–20

Swanson-Kauffman, K. and Schonwald, E. (1988) Phenomenology. In *Paths to Knowledge: Innovative Research Methods for Nursing* (ed. B. Sarter). National League for Nursing, New York, pp. 97–110

Thompson, K. (1972) *Education and Philosophy*. Basil Blackwell, Oxford

Tinkler, D.E. (1993) A 'constructivist' theory of acquisition, and its implications for learner-managed-learning. In *Learner Managed Learning* (ed. N.J. Graves). World Education Fellowship, Leeds, pp. 132–148

Titchen, A. (1993) Engaging with the whole person as a person: Professional craft knowledge in patient-centred nursing. Paper presented at a seminar on *Patient-centred Health Care*, Green College, Oxford, 22–23 April, 1993. National Institute for Nursing, Oxford

Titchen, A. and Binnie, A. (1993) A unified action research strategy in nursing. *Educational Action Research*, **1**, 25–33

Watson, J. (1990) Caring knowledge and informed moral passion. *Advances in Nursing Science*, **13**, 15–24

Weiser, J. (1987) Learning from the perspective of growth of consciousness. In *Appreciating Adults' Learning: From the Learners' Perspective*. Kogan Page, London, pp. 99–111

Wildemeersch, D. (1989) The principal meaning of dialogue for the construction and transformation of reality. In *Making Sense of Experiential Learning: Diversity in Theory and Practice* (ed. S. W. Weil and I. McGill). The Society for Research into Higher Education and Open University Press, Milton Keynes, pp. 60–69

Wylde, J. (1989) Coming to know: A personal knowledge. In *Making Sense of Experiential Learning: Diversity in Theory and Practice* (ed. S. W. Weil and I. McGill). The Society for Research into Higher Education and Open University Press, Milton Keynes, pp. 114–115

11

Parallels between the process of clinical reasoning and categorization

Brett K. Hayes and Roger D. Adams

Over the past two decades the application of concepts and methods from cognitive psychology has provided a useful framework for the study of clinical decision making (1). This chapter continues this theme by exploring the relevance to clinical decision making of theory and research from what has, to date, been a somewhat neglected area of study, namely, human categorization. In particular, the chapter will examine the applicability of 'categorization' as a descriptor for many of the cognitive processes involved in clinical diagnosis and treatment planning. We will then briefly review three competing models of categorization and discuss their implications for the understanding of clinical reasoning and the teaching of clinical reasoning skills. Finally, the way in which categorization processes evolve with clinical experience will be explored.

What is categorization and why is it important?

Categorization occurs whenever we treat two or more distinguishable objects or events equivalently (Mervis and Rosch, 1981). Categorization processes can be seen to operate routinely in everyday life when we decide that some object is a member of a familiar category such as *dog*, *cat* or *bird* or when, in the practice of a health profession, a clinically-relevant decision is made. For example, in radiology, a clinician might view an X-ray of a lung and, on the basis of the visual features that she or he observes, make a preliminary diagnosis such as atelectasis (collapsed lung), multiple tumour or pathology free. Similarly, in sports physiotherapy, the clinician will take a history, watch an injured athlete's gait, manually examine the injured limb, and subsequently may make a diagnosis of hamstring rupture, ACL tear or no structural damage. Whenever a diagnostic label is assigned to a particular patient, categorization can be said to have taken place.

In general terms, the ability of human beings to categorize is extremely useful because it allows us to make sense of the almost infinite variety of stimuli in the world and to go beyond the information contained in a particular case or instance. Moreover, the diagnosis of a case allows the clinician to draw inferences about other clinical features that are likely to be present in that case, the typical clinical course of the condition and, hence, guides the selection of appropriate treatment strategies.

Recent research in cognitive psychology has taught us much about how people learn and use categories in everyday life (see Medin, 1989; Mervis and Rosch, 1981; Smith and Medin, 1981 for reviews) and there is a growing awareness that many of the issues examined in such research have considerable relevance to the understanding of clinical reasoning (cf. Papa

---

(1) Refer to chapters by Boshuizen and Schmidt, Patel and Arocha and Patel and Kaufman.

et al, 1990; Norman et al, 1992a; Schmidt et al, 1990). Our aim is to identify and review some of this evidence and to explore how it can guide approaches to the teaching of clinical reasoning. Before we proceed, however, we need to deal with two issues relating to the scope of application of categorization theory to clinical domains.

The first relates to just which clinical disciplines can benefit from a better understanding of categorization processes. Some in the clinical literature (e.g. Norman et al, 1992b) have suggested that the parallels between categorization processes and the processes involved in diagnosis may be limited to fields such as radiology, dermatology, and pathology where the rapid and simultaneous processing of perceptual cues is important in clinical judgements. Basic categorization processes are seen as less important in primary care or internal medicine in which self-reported data about a patient's history, their physical condition and the results of laboratory tests must be gathered over an extended period of time, analysed and integrated before a diagnosis can be made. We believe that this exclusive emphasis on the 'pattern recognition' component of categorization is unwarranted and overly conservative in its estimation of the relevance of categorization theory. Categorization, while often involving the recognition of perceptual patterns, should be regarded as a type of schema abstraction (cf. Medin and Ross, 1992) in which we decide the meaning of objects, events or cases and how we should behave towards them. Hence, categorization theory has proved useful in the analysis of how people come to apply categorical labels to complex stimuli such as personality profiles and biographical descriptions (e.g. Lingle et al, 1983), elaborate semantic concepts (e.g. Lakoff, 1986) and psychiatric diagnoses (Cantor et al, 1980; Horowitz et al, 1981). There seems no good reason, therefore, why categorization research cannot also provide useful insights into the complex clinical decisions associated with fields such as internal medicine, nursing, occupational therapy and physiotherapy where social, emotional and environmental, as well as physical cues, are important parts of a patient's presentation.

A second important issue relates to the components of the therapeutic process in which categorization might operate. The clearest parallel with everyday object categorization is in the assignment of a diagnostic label to a presenting patient and indeed the main focus of this chapter will be on the role that categorization plays in diagnosis. One should not assume, however, that this is the only way that categorization affects clinical reasoning. Categorization also operates whenever we decide on a particular treatment regimen for an individual or when we judge a case to have a poor, fair or good prognosis. To illustrate, let us say that we have two treatments available, treatment A and treatment B. Even if we eschew the use of diagnostic labels we are unlikely to treat every individual case as completely unique. In choosing a treatment for a given patient we will be guided by the degree to which that person is similar to previous patients who had responded well to treatment A rather than treatment B or vice versa. Of course, when we draw on our experience in this way we are categorizing. Categorization can, therefore, be seen to exert a pervasive influence on a variety of aspects of the process of assessment and treatment of health problems.

Models of category acquisition and representation

One of the reasons why a familiarity with the categorization literature is useful for those interested in clinical reasoning is that much of this research has been concerned with how novel categories are learned or acquired as a result of experience with individual instances or case examples. Interest has been centred on the parameters that affect category acquisition, how categories are stored in memory and how acquired category knowledge guides the classification of both familiar and novel instances. Clearly, a better understanding of such processes may inform approaches to the teaching of diagnostic and other pattern recognition skills and provide insights into how the perception of a case may change with increasing case experience or expertise. To this end we will begin with a brief review of the major models and findings in the area of category learning.

Classical and prototype models of category learning

Until about two decades ago most models of human category learning assumed that natural categories were represented in memory as sets of 'defining' features that are both necessary and sufficient for category membership (e.g. Bruner et al, 1956). That is, it was believed that all members of the category share some common feature or properties, that all instances are equally good members of a category and that the boundaries between categories are distinct. To illustrate the clinical implications of this approach consider a common diagnostic category such as influenza which might be defined formally as 'an acute infectious disease due to influenza virus. Infection is of the upper respiratory tract with general constitutional symptoms of fever, malaise, and muscular aches' (Critchley, 1978, p. 886). The classical view would make the highly questionable predictions that all of these definitional features should be present in each and every case of influenza and that this symptom set does not overlap with other diagnostic categories.

Both clinical intuition and a wealth of research into everyday human categorization (e.g. Rosch, 1975; Smith and Medin, 1981) suggest that this 'classical' theory of category structure is incorrect. Instead, most researchers studying clinical diagnosis (e.g. Komaroff, 1979; Bursztajn et al, 1981) now assume that the clinical features that a person observes are only related in a probabilistic way to categorical labels. Although certain clinical features may be correlated strongly with the presence of a particular condition, in most cases no single clinical sign or symptom is thought to be both necessary and sufficient for the diagnosis of a particular disease. Like the object categories examined by Rosch (1975), diagnostic categories can be said to have an 'internal structure', with some individual cases or instances judged to be more typical of the disease category as a whole than others. Hence, medical students and doctors judge conditions such as ulcerative colitis and duodenal ulcers as better examples of the general diagnostic category 'gastrointestinal disorders' than problems such as oesophageal spasm (Bordage and Zacks, 1984).

The rejection of the classical model has led to the search for alternative ways of explaining the process of human categorization. One of the most influential of such approaches is the view that through exposure to category members one comes to abstract the central tendency of these exemplars (e.g. Posner and Keele, 1968). This 'prototype' representation would contain the features that are most frequently associated with category members and is thought to be used as a basis for categorization decisions. A novel instance is classified as a member of that category whose prototype it most closely resembles. In a diagnostic context it would be argued that as a result of exposure to a variety of cases which share a common underlying pathology a clinician abstracts and stores a summary of the characteristic symptoms, signs or 'features' of that condition. Future diagnoses involving this condition would involve a comparison between the features of the presenting case and those of the stored diagnostic prototype or schema.

Early evidence that people do abstract prototypes during the course of category learning came from studies such as Posner and Keele's (1968) who trained adult subjects to classify small sets of random dot patterns into a number of alternative categories. Each item was presented individually, the subject made a classification judgement and was given corrective feedback. Importantly, the prototype of each category, which was formed from the statistical average of the category members, was not presented during this training period. Upon learning to classify correctly each of the training items, subjects proceeded to a test phase in which they were presented with training instances, novel category items and the prototypes of each of the training categories. The prototypes, which had not been encountered previously, were classified more accurately and quickly than any other new pattern and as accurately as the training instances. Posner and Keele (1968) and many other researchers since that time (e.g. Homa, 1984) believed that this finding showed that people routinely form prototypes when they are learning a novel category and that these play an important part in their subsequent classification decisions.

Bordage and Zacks (1984) have investigated the use of prototype representations in medical students' and general practitioners' knowledge of physical diseases. They first obtained ratings of how typical a set of individual diseases were of a number of general categories of medical disorder (e.g. respiratory disorders, endocrine disorders, infections, neoplasms, dispnoea) and asked their subjects to list diseases that belonged to each category. Highly typical and atypical diseases were then presented in a semantic verification procedure in which subjects had to make speeded decisions about the truth (e.g. 'diabetes mellitus is a kind of endocrine disorder') or falsity (e.g. 'otitis media is a kind of gastrointestinal disorder') of a number of statements. Both doctors and students responded more quickly and with fewer errors to the statements involving 'typical' diseases than they did for the 'atypical' disorders.

It would be wrong of course to think that prototype abstraction was the only categorization process involved in clinical decision making. Information about the central tendency of previously experienced cases is just one of the many factors that contribute to the assignment of a diagnosis to a patient. Just as important in many ways is knowledge of the degree to which individual cases vary around the central tendency or prototype. Some diseases (e.g. inguinal hernia) might be said to have 'low variability' because their clinical presentation tends to be quite similar across cases. Other disorders such as bowel cancer manifest themselves in very different ways in different individuals. A skilled clinician relies on his or her knowledge of such clinical variability in arriving at a diagnosis.

To find solid empirical evidence regarding the learning and use of information about category variability we need only return to Posner and Keele's (1968) seminal work. In the training phase of their category-learning study they systematically manipulated the within-category variability of the sets of visual patterns presented to subjects. The low variability sets contained items that were very similar to one another and to the category prototype, the high variability condition contained both highly typical and atypical items, and the moderate condition was made up of items with an intermediate level of variability. The level of variation in the training items was found to have a significant effect on the subsequent transfer test, with subjects trained on moderately variable items classifying more test patterns correctly than either of the other two groups. This result has since been replicated and extended with demonstrations that knowl-

edge of property-variability within a category may in some cases be the primary basis for categorization decisions (e.g. Rips, 1989) and that training with instances that vary in their typicality leads to better retention of category properties over extended periods of time (Homa and Vosburgh, 1976).

In the disease or injury diagnosis context these findings are significant in two ways. First, they confirm our earlier assertion that object categorization, like clinical diagnosis, involves consideration of both the central tendency (i.e. most typical) of category features as well as the range of variability in these features which exists in the category. More importantly the findings of researchers such as Posner and Keele (1968) point to an important principle that may guide future studies of diagnostic training. Such research indicates that if we wish to equip clinicians to accurately diagnose a range of cases that share the same underlying pathology then we need to train them with cases that vary considerably in the typicality of their clinical signs and symptoms. The presentation of only 'typical' cases of a particular condition will result in a rather narrow and error-prone diagnostic schema.

Although we suspect that many clinical training programs already incorporate this advice, to our knowledge no controlled training study has yet tested the hypothesis. The category learning procedure used by Posner and Keele (1968) and many others subsequently (e.g. Medin and Schaffer, 1978) could, however, be easily adapted for this purpose. One would begin by presenting trainee clinicians with cases belonging to a number of illness or injury categories. By obtaining normative ratings of the typicality of each case relative to the category as a whole, one would also be able to manipulate the degree of within-category variability in the training sets. When the trainees had learned to classify the training items they could be presented with old, novel and prototypical cases and their accuracy in diagnosis of each of these case types compared.

Exemplar approaches to categorization

Even if we assume that people learning categories routinely store information about both prototypes and category variability many would argue that we still underestimate the complexity of human categorization processes. Many influential models of categorization assume that category learning is actually a process of storage of the memory traces of individual category members or exemplars. Categorization, therefore, is seen to involve a comparison of a novel instance to some or all of the known exemplars of the category (see Brooks, 1987; Medin and Ross, 1989; Medin and Schaffer, 1978 for a detailed discussion of such models). In a diagnostic context, this model would predict that disease and injury categories are represented by the individual cases that a clinician has encountered in the past, and the diagnosis of a new case will be determined by its similarity to past cases of particular illness or injury states.

Exemplar models have little trouble in explaining people's sensitivity to variability within a category (Smith and Medin, 1981). In direct comparisons of prototype and exemplar models in laboratory-based category learning experiments, the latter have also tended to be more successful (e.g. Brooks, 1987; Medin and Ross, 1989).

Brooks et al (1991) have provided a clear demonstration of the influence of knowledge of prior instances in the diagnosis of skin disorders. Medical residents and experienced physicians first rated how typical a number of photographs of dermatological lesions were of their respective diagnostic categories. This exposure to concrete examples was found to facilitate the accuracy of the subsequent diagnosis of cases involving perceptually similar lesions, but not dissimilar cases belonging to the same diagnostic category or cases belonging to an alternative category. This effect was found to persist even when a 2-week delay between the initial and test cases was introduced and was not affected by instructions to diagnose on the basis of 'first impressions' or to give careful consideration to alternative diagnoses.

Hence, exposure to concrete prior examples of diagnostic categories can and does influence diagnostic classification, even in clinicians with ample experience of the clinical features of the conditions under consideration. It remains to be shown that such facilitative effects can be found in less 'perceptual' diagnostic domains. Nevertheless, this effect, which was of the order of 10 to 20 per cent improvement in diagnostic accuracy over cases that did not resemble

the old instances, is a compelling argument in favour of great consideration of the role of exemplar effects in clinical diagnosis.

A further reason for the serious examination of exemplar-based categorization models in the analysis of diagnosis is the fact that such models are better than prototype models at explaining the learning of feature correlations. Although at some early stage of training clinicians learn about each of the individual signs and symptoms of a disorder many would argue that diagnosis and other important clinical judgements are strongly influenced by the detection of significant clusters of clinical features that tend to co-occur across cases (Schwartz and Griffin, 1986). An analogous process can be seen to occur in everyday categorization where, with sufficient experience, we develop a sensitivity to co-variation between features. Thus, for example, in the course of learning about members of the category 'bird' one comes to expect that if a particular member of this category is large it will not sing or if it is small we would predict it makes its nest in trees.

Exemplar models of categorization, in general, have been shown to give better accounts of feature correlation learning than models which assume that only prototype information is stored (e.g. Medin and Schaffer, 1978; Medin and Ross, 1989). The applied implication of this finding is that an exemplar- or case-based approach to training should be the preferred method for teaching students about significant correlations between clinical features. Indirect support for this thesis was found in a recent study by Wattenmaker (1991) who examined ways of facilitating people's sensitivity to feature correlations in artificial categories composed of sets of fictitious biographical descriptions. Each of these categories contained some feature pairs which always appeared together. Subjects were first trained with instructions that emphasized the memorization of each individual instance or which encouraged them to look for the features that were shared between category members. Those given the exemplar-based training performed far better in a subsequent task in which the same subjects were presented with pairs of correlated features and asked to choose the category to which these feature pairs belonged.

The implication of this finding for the teaching of clinical reasoning skills seems clear. If we wish trainee clinicians to become sensitive to relationships between the clinical features of a disorder then a system that emphasizes the careful analysis of individual cases is to be preferred to one that focuses simply on the common typical features of the diagnostic class.

Which categorization model best fits the clinical context?

We have seen that exemplar approaches to clinical reasoning have some advantages over models which assume that most decisions are based on a consideration of only the prototypical features of a disorder. But surely an extreme exemplar-based account of clinical categorization, in which only individual case examples are stored, is equally misleading. After all, most clinical training courses begin the teaching of diagnosis with a description of the typical clinical features of a problem. Moreover, the implication that skilled diagnosis involves greater reliance on analogy to previously experienced cases seems to run contrary to previous findings that medical experts are distinguished by their 'chunking' of diagnostic features into abstract, higher order units (e.g. Norman et al, 1979; Lesgold et al, 1988).

A growing number of researchers are now coming to emphasize the flexibility of human categorization acknowledging that for most categories, people have access to category-wide generalizations as well as the specific details of previous exemplars (cf. Brooks, 1987; Hayes and Taplin, 1993; Homa, 1984; Medin and Ross, 1989). Which of these two sources of information has the greatest influence on categorization decisions seems to depend upon the specific structure of the category learning situation. One factor that influences the use of prototype knowledge, namely within-category variation, has already been discussed. A second factor, the size of the category being learned, has also been established as an important determinant of the use of prototype and exemplar information. When a person's experience is limited to only a few category instances, as is the case for the novice clinician, their classification decisions are likely to be strongly influenced by the idiosyncratic features of these cases (Homa et al, 1981). As the number of exemplars that have to be learned increases, people come to rely more on knowledge of prototypical features in assigning cate-

gory membership. Other factors that have been shown to modulate the use of exemplar- or prototype-based strategies of categorization are the number of times that a particular case is repeated during training (Homa et al, 1991), the number of categories to be learned (Homa and Chambliss, 1975), the delay between initial exposure to category members and subsequent classification tasks (Homa, 1984), and the level of corrective feedback given to subjects about category membership decisions (Homa and Cultice, 1984).

In drawing out the implications of these findings for medical diagnosis we are reminded of the comments made by Norman et al (1992b) in their review of the literature on expertise in radiology and dermatology. These authors noted that one of the failings of research in this area is the absence of detailed studies examining task factors that may influence the use of perceptual and reasoning strategies in the diagnostic process. The human categorization literature reviewed above indicates that such task factors are indeed important in determining the approach to, and effectiveness of, diagnosis, and identifies a number of specific factors that are well worth investigating in a clinical setting.

The effects of expertise

In addition to acquiring a better grasp of the prototypical features of a variety of diseases (e.g. Homa et al, 1981), increasing clinical experience may lead to more subtle and complex changes in the conceptual structure of clinicians. Comparisons of expert and novice clinicians have shown that experts possess more differentiated and flexible diagnostic categories than novices (e.g. Feltovich et al, 1984) as well as being better able to perceive the abstract similarities between conditions that have very different clinical features (Murphy and Wright, 1984). The importance of such knowledge of the complex relationships between different disorders was further illustrated in a study by Pauker et al (1976). They observed that in taking patient histories, expert doctors not only generated a hypothetical diagnosis more quickly than students but were also able to call to mind more alternative diagnostic categories that plausibly explained the clinical features of a presenting case (e.g. they noted that a case of multiple pulmonary emboli could be mistaken for cardiomyopathy). This rather complex pattern of results is consistent with the growing recognition in the wider categorization literature that, with experience, category knowledge moves beyond a consideration of prototypical features or the details of particular instances. Expert categorizers also develop heuristics, rules of plausible reasoning, and theories about the links between different categories that guide their inferences (Murphy and Medin, 1985).

The effects that such complex knowledge frameworks can have on category learning has been demonstrated using a category-sorting procedure by Medin et al (1987). University undergraduates were asked to sort eight instances of fictitious diseases into two 'sensible' groups of equal size. The set was structured so that it could be divided by attending to either of two pairs of correlated category features. Although in terms of the objective category structure either feature pair was an equally valid way of sorting the categories, subjects showed a strong tendency to sort on the basis of feature pairs for which they could see a plausible causal link (e.g. earache and dizziness) rather that feature pairs that were seen as less closely connected (e.g. itchiness and weight gain). Hence, the subjects' prior knowledge of the causal relationships between certain symptoms had a profound effect on their learning of feature relationships in a novel category.

The influence that such complex cognitive strategies have on the encoding of clinical features during radiological diagnosis has been investigated by Norman and his colleagues (Norman et al, 1992a). These researchers first provided expert and resident radiologists with X-ray films accompanied by a clinical history that led them to expect that the cases were either normal or showed signs of bronchiolitis. After reading the history the clinicians were asked to list all symptomatic features present in the X-ray and to estimate the probability of disease. When they were biased to expect a positive result from the patient history the expert and novice radiologists gave higher disease probability ratings and found significantly more symptomatic features in both abnormal and normal films than when the case history was normal. This latter result is startling in many ways since it shows that the bias created by the patient histories was strong enough to

lead even experienced radiologists to report clinical signs which in the normal slides were not actually present.

Norman et al (1992a) concluded that hypotheses and expectations formed very early in the diagnostic process can directly affect the search for, and encoding of, clinical features and subsequent diagnosis. While this is almost certainly true in some cases the evidence from the object categorization literature suggests that the relationship between one's expectations about a patient based on background history and the search for clinical features may actually be far more complex (cf. Murphy and Medin, 1985; Medin, 1989). Wisniewski and Medin (1991) examined the interaction between 'top-down' information such as a person's prior expectations or hypotheses about category assignment and 'bottom-up' information such as the presence or absence of particular features in a visual category-learning task. They found evidence for a bidirectional interaction between these two types of information. As in the Norman et al (1992a) study people's different expectations led them to selectively attend to different features in generating category membership rules, to treat the same visual features in different ways and to encode particular combinations of features into higher-order chunks. Significantly, however, when subjects were given further information about the accuracy of their category assignments, particularly when they were given negative feedback, they changed their categorization strategies. Some subjects shifted their interpretation of specific visual features while others changed their criteria for category membership or shifted their focus to consider features that they had previously ignored.

Such results indicate that while 'top-down' expectations may guide initial feature search in diagnosis, there is an ongoing interaction between expectations and data such that clinical information which strongly contradicts one's initial hypotheses may change one's expectations and diagnostic strategies for future cases. This process is illustrated in Figure 11.1. The figure highlights a number of aspects of the process of clinical diagnosis that warrant further investigation. Following Norman et al (1992a) further research is needed to understand exactly how a clinician's initial hypotheses or any other information which biases his or her expectations about a

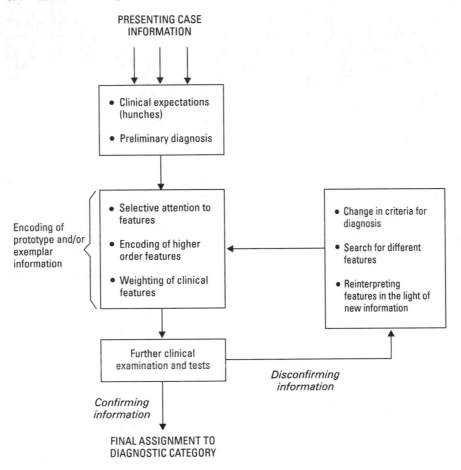

Figure 11.1   A model of clinical diagnosis based upon contemporary categorization research

particular case affects the search for clinical signs and symptoms. Similarly, we need a better grasp of how clinicians shift their diagnostic strategies when they receive information which disconfirms their original hypotheses about a case and the best way to present this negative feedback to them (see Schwartz and Griffin, 1986 for some suggestions regarding how such research should proceed). Finally, the way in which clinical expertise alters and tunes both the 'top down' expectations about a patient's condition as well as the actual clinical information which is deemed significant for diagnosis need to be investigated more thoroughly.

Conclusions

The pioneering work of Bordage and Zacks (1984), and of Norman, Brooks and their col-

leagues has already succeeded in demonstrating the usefulness of theoretical models and methods from the human categorization literature in the exploration of the clinical reasoning process. Our purpose here was to clarify and extend this theoretical framework and to highlight the many areas of clinical decision making that could benefit from an approach that sees such decisions as complex categorization tasks. In particular, categorization theory informs the debate about how diagnostic categories might be represented in memory, indicates the significant task variables that may mediate the use of different diagnostic strategies and provides guide-lines for how clinical training could be structured to enhance sensitivity to the co-occurrence of significant clinical features. Categorization research concerning the effects of one's 'top down' knowledge on feature encoding is also a fertile source of hypotheses about the way in which prior knowledge of a patient or diagnostic expectations influence feature search and how this process might change with clinical expertise.

Acknowledgement

The preparation of this paper was supported by a University of Sydney, Faculty of Health Sciences Grant to the authors.

References

Bordage, G. and Zacks, R. (1984) The structure of medical knowledge in the memories of medical students and general practitioners: Categories and prototypes. *Medical Education*, **18**, 406–416

Brooks, L.R. (1987) Decentralised control of categorization: The role of prior processing episodes. In *Concepts and Conceptual Development: Ecological and Intellectual Factors in Categorization* (ed. U. Neisser). Cambridge University Press, Cambridge, pp. 141–174

Brooks, L.R., Norman, G.R. and Allen, S.W. (1991) Role of specific similarity in a medical diagnosis task. *Journal of Experimental Psychology: General*, **120**, 278–287

Bruner, J.S., Goodnow, J. and Austin, G. (1956) *A Study of Thinking*. Wiley, New York

Bursztajn, H., Feinbloom, R.I., Hamm, R.M. and Brodsky, A. (1981) *Medical Choices, Medical Chances*. Delacorte Press, New York

Cantor, N., Smith, E.E., French, R. and Mezzich, J. (1980) Psychiatric diagnoses as prototype categorization. *Journal of Abnormal Psychology*, **89**, 181–193

Critchley, M. (ed.) (1978) *Butterworth's Medical Dictionary*, 2nd edn. Butterworth-Heinemann, Oxford

Feltovich, P.J., Johnson, P.E., Moller, J.H. and Swanson, D. B. (1984) LCS: The role and development of medical knowledge in diagnostic expertise. In *Readings in Medical Artificial Intelligence: The First Decade* (eds W.J. Clancey and E.H. Shortliffe). Addison-Wesley, Reading, MA

Hayes, B.K. and Taplin, J.E. (1993) Developmental differences in the use of prototype and exemplar-specific information. *Journal of Experimental Child Psychology*, **55**, 329–352

Homa, D. (1984) On the nature of categories. In *The Psychology of Learning and Motivation*. Vol 18 (ed. G.T. Bower). Academic Press, New York, pp. 49–94

Homa, D. and Chambliss, D. (1975) The relative contributions of common and distinctive information on the abstraction of ill-defined categories. *Journal of Experimental Psychology: Human Learning and Memory*, **104**, 351–359

Homa, D. and Cultice, J. (1984) Role of feedback, category size, and stimulus distortion on the acquisition and utilization of ill-defined categories. *Journal of Experimental Psychology: Learning, Memory and Cognition*, **10**, 83–94

Homa, D., Dunbar, S. and Nohre, L. (1991) Instance frequency, categorization, and the modulating effect of experience. *Journal of Experimental Psychology: Learning, Memory, and Cognition*, **17**, 444–458

Homa, D., Sterling, S. and Trepel, L. (1981) Limitations of exemplar-based generalization and the abstraction of categorical information. *Journal of Experimental Psychology: Human Learning and Memory*, **7**, 418–439

Homa, D. and Vosburgh, R. (1976) Category breadth and the abstraction of prototypical information. *Journal of Experimental Psychology: Human Learning and Memory*, **2**, 322–330

Horowitz, L., Wright, J.C., Lowenstein, E. and Parad, H. (1981) The prototype as a construct in abnormal psychology: 1. A method for deriving prototypes. *Journal of Abnormal Psychology*, **90**, 568–574

Komaroff, A.L. (1979) The variability and inaccuracy of medical data. *Proceedings of the IEEE*, **67**, 1196–1207

Lakoff, G. (1986) *Women, Fire and Dangerous Things: What Categories Tell us About the Nature of Thought*. Chicago University Press, Chicago

Lesgold, A.M., Rubinson, H., Feltovich, P., Glaser, R., Klopfer, D. and Wang, Y. (1988) Expertise in a complex skill: Diagnosing x-ray pictures. In *The Nature of Expertise* (eds M.T.H. Chi, R. Glaser and M. Farr). Erlbaum, Hillsdale, NJ, pp. 322–351

Lingle, J.H., Altom, M.W. and Medin, D.L. (1983) Of cabbages and kings: Assessing the extensibility of natural object concept models to social things. In *Handbook of Social Cognition* (eds R. Wyer, T. Srull and J. Hartwick). Erlbaum, Hillsdale, NJ, pp. 71–116

Medin, D.L. (1989) Concepts and conceptual structure. *American Psychologist*, **44**, 1469–1481

Medin, D. and Ross, B. (1989) The specific character of abstract thought: Categorization, problem-solving and induction. In *Advances in the Psychology of Human Intelligence*. Vol 5 (ed. R. Sternberg). Academic Press, San Diego, CA, pp. 189–223

Medin, D. and Ross, B. (1992) *Cognitive Psychology*. Harcourt, Brace and Jovanovich, Orlando, FL

Medin, D.L. and Schaffer, M.M. (1978) Context theory of classification learning. *Psychological Review*, **85**, 207–238

Medin, D.L., Wattenmaker, W.D. and Hampson, S.E. (1987) Family resemblance, conceptual cohesiveness and category construction. *Cognitive Psychology*, **18**, 158–194

Mervis, C.B. and Rosch, E. (1981) Categorization of natural objects. *Annual Review of Psychology*, **32**, 89–115

Murphy, G.L. and Medin, D.L. (1985) The role of theories in conceptual coherence. *Psychological Review*, **92**, 289–316

Murphy, G.L. and Wright, J.C. (1984) Changes in conceptual structure with expertise: Differences between real-world experts and novices. *Journal of Experimental*

Psychology: Learning, Memory and Cognition, **10**, 144–155

Norman, G.R., Brooks, L.R., Coblentz, C.L. and Babcock, C.J. (1992a) The correlation of feature identification and category judgments in diagnostic radiology. *Memory and Cognition*, **20**, 344–355

Norman, G.R., Coblentz, C.L., Brooks, L.R. and Babcock, C.J. (1992b) Expertise in visual diagnosis: A review of the literature. *Academic Medicine*, **67**, S78–S83

Norman, G.R., Jacoby, L.L., Feightner, J.W. and Campbell, E.J.M. (1979) *Proceedings of the 18th Annual Conference on Research in Medical Education*, **18**, 163–168

Papa, F.J., Shores, J.H. and Meyer, S. (1990) Effects of pattern matching, pattern discrimination, and experience in the development of diagnostic expertise. *Academic Medicine*, **65**, S21–S22

Pauker, S.G., Gorry, G.A., Kassirer, J.P. and Schwartz, W.B. (1976) Towards the simulation of clinical cognition: Taking the present illness by computer. *The American Journal of Medicine*, **60**, 981–996

Posner, M.I. and Keele, S.W. (1968) On the genesis of abstract ideas. *Journal of Experimental Psychology*, **77**, 353–363

Rips, L.J. (1989) Similarity, typicality, and categorization. In *Similarity, Analogy, and Thought* (eds S. Vosniadou and A. Ortony). Cambridge University Press, New York, pp. 21–60

Rosch, E. (1975) Cognitive representations of semantic categories. *Journal of Experimental Psychology: General*, **104**, 192–233

Schmidt, H.G., Norman, G.R. and Boshuizen, H.P.A. (1990) A cognitive perspective on medical expertise: Theory and implications. *Academic Medicine*, **65**, 611–621

Schwartz, S. and Griffin, T. (1986) *Medical Thinking: The Psychology of Medical Judgment and Decision Making*. Springer-Verlag, New York, NY

Smith, E.E. and Medin, D.L. (1981) *Categories and Concepts*. Harvard University Press, Cambridge, MA

Wattenmaker, W.D. (1991) Learning modes, feature correlations, and memory-based categorization. *Journal of Experimental Psychology: Learning, Memory and Cognition*, **17**, 908–923

Wisniewski, E.J. and Medin, D.L. (1991) Harpoons and long sticks: the interaction of theory and similarity in rule induction. In *Concept Formation: Knowledge and Experience in Unsupervised Learning* (eds D.H. Fisher, M.J. Pazzani and P. Langley). Morgan Kaufman, San Mateo, CA, pp. 237–278

12

Educational technology in the teaching of clinical reasoning and access to knowledge resources

Allan Christie and Mark Jones

Clinical reasoning is a cognitive process which is difficult to explain, demonstrate and assess. Therefore teaching clinical reasoning requires educational methods which make the internal process more accessible. Clinical reasoning is also closely associated with knowledge. Thus learning clinical reasoning requires educational experiences which promote active integration of both cognitive processes and the associated knowledge into learners' existing knowledge structures. Educational activities using technology can be designed to achieve similar learning goals to more traditional classroom or small group educational programs, while offering additional advantages with respect to reduced costs, increased accessibility and improved content selection.

Clinical reasoning is becoming more cognitively demanding as the body of knowledge within respective health professions continues to grow. Educational technology in the form of knowledge resources can assist clinicians in their reasoning by providing support systems for clinical decision making and by providing greater access to the collective knowledge of the profession.

Technology is an umbrella term which may be defined as 'the totality of the means employed to provide objects necessary for human support'. Our approach to the use of technology in education is that it must be a

tool to support the education process and not direct it. It is not the technology that is important, but rather what it allows the learner to achieve with respect to the attainment of knowledge and the development of problem solving skills. Ready access to information, and ensuring that the learner is an active participant in the learning process, are two important components of facilitating clinical reasoning. Computer-based educational technologies have much to offer with respect to these factors and, in addition, they allow students to learn at their own pace and in their own time. The students are able to revisit the same information repeatedly; this has clear applicability to remedial learning which, in turn, can assist mastering a particular topic or concept.

For these reasons, computer assisted learning technologies will be the focus of this chapter. Educational technology which can be used for the development of clinical reasoning skills will be reviewed with consideration given to the educational needs addressed by this technology and the applicability of experiential learning theory to this mode of education. Specific examples of computer assisted learning will then be presented. Lastly, computer-based knowledge resources will be described together with examples of multimedia databases and networked resources currently available.

Educational technology and the development of clinical reasoning skills

Educational needs in the teaching of clinical reasoning: why use computers?

When the use of educational technology for supporting or replacing more traditional teaching methods is raised, the first question often asked is 'How can computers be used in teaching . . . ?'. Approaching the use of technology in education from this perspective ignores the underlying pedagogical problem and dooms any computer-based education project to failure. The first questions to ask are 'What is the educational problem?' and, more importantly, 'Why is it a problem?'.

Consideration of the problems involved in teaching clinical reasoning skills raises several issues. It is important to provide a greater range of patient problems than can normally be found in the clinical setting at any particular time. That is, patient problems encountered by students are largely 'luck of the draw'. There is no assurance that students will have the opportunity to experience the full range of problems they are expected to recognize and manage, and no assurance that the complexity of the problems they do encounter will be appropriate for their stage of learning. Further, clinical supervision is relatively expensive and this resource must be used as efficiently as possible. Attendance at, or participation in, a learning activity will not guarantee that learning occurs. Students must be actively involved in the learning process and new information must be meaningfully integrated into their existing knowledge structures.

Educational technology, specifically interactive computer technology, provides an excellent means of supplementing existing efforts to teach clinical reasoning and to facilitate the acquisition of knowledge. For example, when self-instructional interactive computer activities are designed to present real life clinical scenarios, students' cognitive processes such as hypothesis generation, hypothesis testing and problem formulation/re-formulation can be prompted. This form of active participation assists in activating students' existing knowledge while varying forms of feedback and resource direction enable integration of new information into the development of new knowledge structures. Experiential learning theory provides a useful basis on which interactive learning programs to facilitate the development of clinical reasoning and acquisition of knowledge can be created.

Applicability of experiential learning theory to computer assisted learning

Kolb (1984) describes the learning cycle as proceeding from concrete experience to observations and reflections, through the formulation of abstract concepts and generalizations to the testing of the implications of these concepts in new experiences. When students are involved in the concrete experience of examining and treating a patient, they draw upon existing knowledge as they observe and interpret patient cues. The specific generation of hypotheses, and the associated data collection needed to support or refute them, parallels the formation of abstract concepts and generalizations (e.g. hypotheses) outlined in Kolb's experiential learning cycle. Although hypothesis generation is relatively automatic for an expert, students must reflect on the clinical cues presented to them and interpret that information in the light of their existing knowledge. Kolb's cycle finishes with ideas being tested in new experiences which, in turn, initiates the opportunity for further learning as a new cycle commences. Similarly, students must test their hypotheses within the full presentation of a single patient as well as across presentations of different patients. Within the examination and management of a single patient, hypotheses (e.g. diagnostic and therapeutic) are tested through ongoing examination, management and re-assessment; across a number of patients, the consistency of the patterns recognized is also being continually tested. Thus clinical reasoning is an experiential learning activity, and computer assisted learning programs designed to enable all elements of the learning cycle to occur will assist in the development of clinical reasoning skills.

Examples of computer assisted learning

Computer technology is available to provide both direct and indirect assistance to the development of clinical reasoning skills. Direct assistance is available through interactive computer-based education since this enables students to develop and practise clinical reasoning while interacting with the computer programs.

Indirect assistance is available through decision support systems and electronic information systems; help on deciding further action is provided by the former while databases, discussion groups and other resources are provided by the latter.

Interactive computer assisted learning

Computer assisted learning techniques cover many different formats such as drill and practice, tutorial, simulation, games and tests. All address issues of learning at various cognitive levels and with varying capabilities of addressing clinical reasoning process skills and knowledge. An interactive program is one in which the learner is actively involved in responding in either a qualitative or quantitative manner to allow the instruction to continue (Cohen, 1984). Pressing the 'Enter' key on the computer keyboard in order to see another screen of information is not interaction. Rather, interactive computer programs involve the learner in seeking information, answering questions and making decisions.

In the traditional clinical setting, it is often very difficult to provide suitable patients for students to develop and apply their clinical reasoning skills. These difficulties arise because of time constraints placed on 'hands-on' clinical practice in an already full curriculum, the cost of clinical supervision, and the somewhat random nature of patient selection that is available. A cost-effective way to supplement actual clinical supervision is provided by the use of computer-generated patient simulations. Simulation in general has the advantage of providing situations or systems which would otherwise be too expensive, too time-consuming, too dangerous, or unavailable. A prototype of today's computer-based patient problem simulations is the patient-management problem (PMP) originally pioneered as an evaluation tool in medical education (Rimoldi, 1955; 1961; McGuire and Babbott, 1967). McGuire and Babbott (1967) identified five characteristics of clinical simulations which provided the basis of computer-generated patient simulations. They were: 1) information is presented in terms that a patient or referring physician would use, not as a summary of pertinent information; 2) a series of sequential interdependent decisions represents various stages in the diagnostic workup and management; 3) results of decisions are presented in a realistic form; 4) harmful or ineffectual decisions cannot be retracted; and 5) an allowance for different medical approaches with appropriate responses for each approach is made.

Various formats of the PMP have since been developed to simulate clinician–patient interaction for both learning and assessment purposes (Rosenblatt and Gaponoff, 1984). Although the credibility of the PMP as an assessment tool has been questioned (see Chapter 13), simulated clinical encounters do provide an excellent experiential means by which knowledge and reasoning can be enhanced (Henry and Holzemer, 1993). This is especially the case if alternative techniques are not available.

Innovative examples of patient simulation programs can be found in the work of Hon (1982) and Edwards and Hannah (1985) who developed a self-training system in cardiopulmonary resuscitation (CPR). In this system, a life-size mannequin with electronic sensors embedded at strategic locations was linked to a computer and an interactive videodisc system. A videodisc is an LP-sized optical disc (somewhat analogous to an oversized audio compact disc) that stores an analogue (continuous) audio–video signal on a metal surface which is covered with a smooth plastic coating. The interactive component of the videodisc system is provided by the computer program that provides the instructional material and controls the videodisc player. It was found that instruction using the videodisc system was as effective as traditional CPR instruction. However, the use of the interactive videodisc system also helped to address issues involving instructor attrition, variability of instructor standards, and the delivery of CPR instruction to people with limited access to traditional courses.

This CPR simulation is an example of traditional computer assisted instruction (CAI) which tends to be quite rigid with pre-defined knowledge structures and often limited explanations available to the students. This is not surprising with CAI having its roots in programmed learning with its behaviouristic underpinnings (as per Skinner, 1968). Although simulation programs attempt to address higher cognitive levels associated with experiential learning, they can also be somewhat restrictive with respect to the range of permissible responses from users. For example, there may be certain limits to user responses for the program to continue, or decisions made with respect to a particular clinical scenario may lock the user into following a pre-defined path through the case presentation.

While the focus of the CPR computer simulation system is primarily directed towards knowledge and motor skill acquisition, programs can also be designed to concentrate on inquiry, hypothesis generation and hypothesis testing aspects of clinical reasoning. An example of a patient simulation program where clinical reasoning is emphasized is the interactive videodisc called 'Community Health Nursing – The Initial Home Visit' described by Hawkins in 1988 (pers. comm.). In this case, through a scenario of nursing a client with urinary incontinence, knowledge is tested, interpersonal relationship skills are explored, nursing care plans are developed and clinical reasoning through client assessment and management is facilitated. A natural language interface is used in this program for student responses; this adds realism to the learning experience. Whenever the situation calls for a response from users, a special input screen appears automatically and users can type in what they want to say, indicate whether what was typed is a question or comment and to whom (e.g. patient or relative) the question or comment is addressed. This provides the opportunity for unconstrained user input followed by appropriate 'intelligent' responses from the program. It allows users to follow various paths through the simulation and, therefore, allows them to follow their own path of reasoning. The program provides access to four clients in an initial home visit scenario. In addition, after the visit has been completed the user needs to know how to produce a report containing the nursing diagnosis, its justifications, and a care plan. Three basic knowledge and skill areas are involved: 1) how to establish a helping relationship with the client; 2) knowledge of types, causes and treatments of urinary incontinence; and 3) reasoning through client assessment and management. Tutorial assistance is available throughout the program. This provides comments about the user input and permits users to see and hear video segments of an experienced community health nurse working in a similar scenario. Topics such as making a good start, setting the envir-

onment, developing the relationship, 'completing the circle', and problem assessment are covered by these video segments. This videodisc is used in a number of ways, as a motivational aid to learning, as an evaluation exercise, and as an instructional tool where users learn how to integrate acquired skills and apply the knowledge in a realistic situation.

This simulation is a good example of an Intelligent Computer Assisted Instruction (ICAI) program which is adaptable to different situations (Aegerter et al, 1992). Such programs are able to provide a realistic learning environment whereby students can practise clinical reasoning process skills, and receive immediate feedback on relevant knowledge issues. The use of artificial intelligence methods that attempt to mimic or duplicate the functions of the human brain allows for the creation of programs which contain knowledge of the field being studied. This explicit coding of knowledge makes ICAI programs adaptable to different learning situations where the focus can be placed on clinical reasoning process skills rather than knowledge acquisition.

A program such as CBX (Computer-Based Clinical-Simulation Examination) developed by the National Board of Medical Examiners is another example of these systems being applied in the medical field (Clyman and Orr, 1990). CBX allows candidates to manage patients through simulated time with minimal interference by testing cues. As the candidate manages the case, the patient's condition changes as a result of both the underlying problem and the candidate's management decisions. The system is very open-ended in that approximately 8500 terms are recognized and this, coupled with simulated timing for actions, provides an extremely rich source of data about candidate performance.

Decision-support systems

Indirect assistance to the development of clinical reasoning skills is available through expert systems that provide decision support capabilities (Delitto et al, 1989). Shortliffe (1987) defined a clinical decision support system as any computer program that deals with clinical data or medical knowledge and which performs one or more of the following tasks: information management, attention focusing, and patient-specific consultation.

The information management category refers primarily to hospital information systems that permit the storage and retrieval of patient data but generally do not assist professionals in the use of the data to solve specific clinical problems. Interpretation is left to the individual.

Attention-focusing systems examine data for abnormal values or combinations of values, such as pharmaceutical applications which warn of adverse drug interactions. Focusing is the principle underlying the use of computer-generated reminders to increase compliance with predefined protocols of care.

The task of patient-specific consultation refers to what are commonly known as expert systems used in clinical diagnosis and therapy planning. Expert systems refer to knowledge-based structures that can contain protocols for eliciting input from the user and large databases with decision rules or algorithms to weight the information obtained. That is, they use the knowledge provided by their creators to enter, organize, and summarize data. The outputs from these systems are often patient classifications or diagnoses with suggested treatment strategies. However, making the final diagnosis for the patient's problems remains a uniquely human task. Some systems which are beginning to be introduced into nursing practice to support the process of clinical decision making include COMMES (Creighton OnLine Multiple Modular Expert System) (Petrucci and Petrucci, 1991), CANDI (Computer Aided Nursing Diagnosis and Intervention) (Roth et al, 1989), and ARKS (A Research-Knowledge System) (Graves, 1990). In the CANDI system there are two levels of inquiry: *screening* questions and *in-depth* questions. Each screening question may branch to one or more in-depth questions. The net result is a fairly complete assessment guide.

A criticism of expert systems is that they tend to restrict thinking by fostering tunnel vision. This is a reflection on their implementation rather than the capabilities of the tool itself. The elicitation of knowledge from experts, the engineering of that knowledge into the structure required by the specific expert system tool, and the integration of the final expert system into a total decision support system are extremely difficult, costly and time consuming tasks. It is easier to isolate a single area of concern and provide a tool to address that problem while

'holding all other factors constant'. This forces users themselves to provide the breadth of vision so often lacking. If expert systems are regarded as aids to clinical decision making rather than usurping that process, then the judgement of the clinician can be integrated with the decision-enhancing responses of information-based systems. The feedback obtained from decision-support systems provides clear opportunity for the knowledge acquisition which is so integral to clinical reasoning. Other examples of clinical decision support systems include classic systems such as MYCIN (Shortliffe, 1975 cited by Heathfield and Wyatt, 1993) and INTERNIST (Miller et al, 1982) and more modern systems such as HELP (Health Evaluation through Logical Processing).

Alerting (i.e. the automatic notification of appropriate personnel of a time-critical or action-orientated decision) is used extensively in the HELP system. The use of alerts has resulted in a reduction in physician and nursing errors in patient management, increased compliance with predefined standards of care, decreased length of stay, and time spent in life-threatening situations. The HELP system also provides support for improving management decisions, an example of which is given in Table 12.1. Recommended changes in FIO_2 (fraction inspired oxygen), and suggested times for drawing next blood gases based on laboratory and clinical data, are provided by the HELP system.

Clearly, the clinical decision-making process is far too complicated to be totally 'computerized', and these systems should be seen as simply tools for assisting clinicians towards their own diagnoses and management decisions.

Computer-based knowledge resources

Information processing theory assumes that human problem solvers are constrained by limitations of memory (Newell and Simon, 1972). A practitioner's clinical reasoning skills in a particular domain are closely related to the availability of knowledge in the specific domain as well as the practitioner's amount of case experience (Elstein et al, 1978; Cervero 1988; Aegerter et al, 1992; Custers et al, 1993).

Table 12.1   Example of a management decision output from HELP

HELP test W603 2111465
HELP management decisions

Date	Time	
26 Sep	05:20	Alternating mode 4 hour wait with 0 hours and 55 minutes remaining. Draw arterial blood gas (ABG) at 6:15 hours
26 Sep	06:09	Decrease membrane lung fraction of oxygen ($FmlO_2$) by 0.10 from 1.00 to 0.90. Draw ABG in 15 minutes
26 Sep	06:35	Reduce FIO_2 by 10%, from 70% to 60%. Draw ABG in 15 minutes
26 Sep	07:09	Continue to monitor and draw an ABG at 8:40; FIO_2 decrease at 6:40, with 1 hour and 31 minutes remaining in 2 hour wait
26 Sep	08:43	Decrease membrane lung fraction of oxygen ($FmlO_2$) by 0.10 from 0.90 to 0.80. Draw an ABG in 15 minutes
26 Sep	09:10	Continue to monitor and draw an ABG at 10:46 $FmlO_2$. Decrease at 8:46 with 1 hour and 36 minutes remaining in 2 hour wait

From Pryor and Clayton (1991) cited by Hannan (1993)

Interactive educational programs using patient simulation were discussed previously with respect to their use to facilitate clinical reasoning and knowledge development. Interactive programs can also be designed with greater focus on knowledge acquisition which is both necessary for, and a byproduct of, effective clinical reasoning. Two important ways to achieve this are through the use of computer-based education packages, which can provide interactive learning experiences that focus on knowledge acquisition, and through information retrieval systems provided by access to local databases and networked resources.

Increasingly, computer-based education packages are being developed incorporating high quality visual images (photographic-quality resolution), motion video and sound that add to the fidelity of information that is provided to students (Christie, 1990). These various media types are collectively referred to as 'multimedia' and the hype surrounding this term in computer publications and advertising carries with it the risk of adopting this technology as an end in itself. Indeed, the use of multimedia enables information to be conveyed as a meaningful representation of actual events in clinical practice. However, the educational value of these programs can be compromised if aspects of instructional design and good educational planning are absent from the development process.

There are many examples of multimedia programs intended to assist students in the acquisition of knowledge. Mangione et al (1992) developed a program for use in the teaching of pulmonary auscultation. In this program animation, digitized pictures and sounds recorded from actual patients are used to teach medical students how to correctly interpret auscultation findings. The program reviewed all breath sounds, adventitious lung sounds, and transmitted voice sounds. Among other features are the review of the pathogenesis of the various sounds, their physical characteristics, their roentgenologic equivalents, and their mechanisms of production and transmission. Such a program can provide teaching material which can be reviewed repeatedly without putting heavy demands on the time of faculty members. Instead of involving students in reasoning through a patient case as occurs in the interactive computer-based patient simulations, the focus of these programs is generally on recognition and interpretation of patient information necessary for problem solving. Further examples of multimedia programs providing discipline-specific information in the areas of Medical Laboratory Science, Medical Radiations, Occupational Therapy and Physiotherapy have recently been completed and have been put together as a Health Sciences Multimedia CD-ROM (Compact Disc – Read Only Memory) by the first author. The Medical Radiations module is illustrative of the type of material included on this CD-ROM; the topic of ultrasonography is presented and students are asked to interpret ultrasound scans for various pathological conditions.

Knowledge in the form of multimedia databases and interactive programs provides a vast resource of easily accessible information for both students and clinicians. Until recently many multimedia databases and interactive programs have used the videodisc for its high quality audio and video properties. A videodisc has 54 000 uniquely identified frames with each frame representing a slide image or one frame in a video image. There are three separate broadcast video formats (PAL, NTSC and SECAM) used around the world and this initially caused compatibility problems as a PAL formatted videodisc could not be played in a NTSC videodisc player for instance. However, this issue has been overcome somewhat with dual format (PAL and NTSC) videodisc players (e.g. Sony LV 3600D) now being widely available. A major advantage of videodisc technology is that the player can be easily controlled by computer and this, coupled with the player's rapid random access capability, makes it extremely useful for database searches and interactive programs. Images taken from the videodisc can be displayed on the computer screen, and sized according to the instructional need.

An example of videodisc technology is the PAL format 'Orthopaedics' videodisc program developed by the first author (Christie, 1987; 1988). The videodisc contains 1981 slides and 34 motion segments. Nine of these segments cover various aspects of traction whilst others cover topics from knee arthroscopy and removal of a long-leg plaster, to getting a patient with a total hip replacement out of bed and crutch/frame walking. The software is currently being rewritten using Asymetrix ToolBook, a software development tool, to take advantage of the graphical user interface of the Microsoft Windows environment which runs on DOS-based computers. Essentially what is provided is a simple menu interface through which the learner can access textual information on a particular topic. However, the text is augmented by relevant 'thumb-nail' images and if the learner wishes to view the still frame or video, clicking on the 'thumb-nail' image will result in an enlarged window overlaying the text in which the still frame or video is played. In this way the learner is able to read, see and hear information thereby maximizing the 'reality' of the situation. Many other examples of the use of interactive videodisc in health sciences teaching are available (Blackman et al, 1985; Baker and Ziviani, 1986; Barker, 1988).

There are also many videodiscs commercially available that provide collections of high qual-

ity visual images. For instance, there is the UK National Medical Slide Bank with approximately 12 000 images showing the visual manifestations of a wide range of diseases, as well as aspects of medical treatment and health-care practice. The Bristol Biomedical Videodisc Project has 24 000 still frames of medical, dental and veterinary images and a videodisc entitled 'The Skeletal Radiology: the Bare Bones Teaching Collection' has over 650 individual cases. The National Libraries of Medicine in North America also has a large catalogue of videodiscs that may be purchased (Waterfield, 1993).

One of the greatest strengths of videodisc (i.e. the analogue broadcast quality video images) is increasingly becoming one of its greatest weaknesses as digital video technology evolves. The conversion of all media types (text, graphics, video, sound) to digital information provides a number of benefits. There is no need for expensive peripheral devices (e.g. videodisc or videotape players); there is no need for specialized add-in cards for the computer to connect to the video player; and there is no need to be concerned with the various video formats worldwide. Unfortunately, there is a down side. A plethora of digital formats for text, graphic, video and sound currently exist which can limit their use. There is readily available conversion software to change one media format to another. However, choosing the appropriate software package and determining the correct file format to use are not trivial tasks.

The digitization of video and related media types has sparked a tremendous growth in the market for CD-ROM players. CD-ROMs are similar in size to audio CDs and have a storage capacity of approximately 650 Mb (megabytes). This enables the storage of large amounts of textual information (250 000 A4 pages). However, when developing applications that combine still and moving video with sound, textual information and computer graphics, its limits are soon reached. Uncompressed full-screen full-motion digital video requires approximately 25 to 30 Mb per second (1 Mb per frame). However, compressed video playing in a small window on the computer screen is adequate for many purposes and in this case is often less than 1 Mb per second of digital video.

The compact size and relative robustness of the CD-ROM, combined with the ability to produce CD-ROMs 'in-house', indicates that the current popularity of CD-ROM is just a harbinger of things to come in the very near future. Some CD-ROM titles that are presently available have been catalogued by Waterfield (1993) and include:

- Anatomist: Human anatomy work in text and pictures
- Biological age: Multimedia dentistry and paediatrics
- Cancer on disk (1988): Articles and supplements from *Cancer* 1988
- Paediatric Infectious Disease (1985–1990)
- Paediatrics on disk (1983–1990): Collected issues of the *Journal of Pediatrics*
- Primary cancers of the skin: Histopathological reference covering all forms of the melanoma
- Renal tumours of children: covering onset and identification

Networking

To this point the use of education technology in providing access to a practical body of knowledge has been limited to resources (computer disks, peripheral devices such as CD-ROM player) that have a physical presence. With the burgeoning use of computer networks over the last five years, vast amounts of information and access to experts worldwide in related fields of interest are now readily available. World-wide access is provided by the Internet (a collection of thousands of interconnected computer networks), which is used by approximately one million people daily. Computer mediated communication is now a common activity with the use of electronic mail, internet relay chat, electronic news groups and electronic discussion groups providing avenues for the discussion and dissemination of information on virtually any topic. To illustrate the utility of computer mediated communications in providing information and expert advice, a recent dialogue from the Medical Decision Making List is paraphrased (the email addresses and names of the people posting to this list have been removed). In this example a member of the discussion list is asking for suitable references related to the issue of over- and under-treatment. Within a short period of time two responses are posted to the discussion list from members who work in Cardiac Surgery/Cardiology, Cedars-Sinai,

Los Angeles and the Bureau of Health Economics, New York State Department of Health. The paraphrased dialogue follows:

Sender: smdm-1@dartcms1.dartmouth.edu
Subject: Looking for references – over & under treatment.
I think most of us would agree that 'outcomes research' or health services research studies have frequently found that treatments of questionable efficacy often catch on and are overused, while at other times, effective treatments are neglected or underused. Thus, some patients are either overtreated or undertreated. If you concur with the general proposition, I am looking for some readable articles which review the literature on this issue. The intended audience would be first- and second-year residents in internal medicine, possibly expanding later to medical students. I'd like to be able to provide these readers with a reasonable introduction to the field, and while new articles on this topic appear regularly, I am looking now for a good introduction and review. Could be either a review article, or a chapter in a yearbook or textbook. Suggestions are most welcome.
[name deleted]
University of Illinois at Chicago
College of Medicine

Subject: Re: References
Lots of them are available and can be obtained by searching Medline for 'appropriateness', 'variability in care'. Also search under R Brook, Barbara McNeal, David Pryor. The biggest problem is the definition of over and undertreatment
[name deleted]
Cardiac Surgery/Cardiology
Cedars-Sinai, LA

Subject: Re: References
I would recommend a recent article by Charles Phelps which might provide a good introduction to the methods used in studying appropriateness. The references contained therein may also prove useful for further reading of specific studies. The citation is:
Phelps CE. The methodologic foundations of studies of the appropriateness of medical care. N Eng J Med 1993; 329:1241-45
I hope this is helpful.
[name deleted]
Bureau of Health Economics
NYS Department of Health

As demonstrated in the above example, the collegial nature of Internet communications makes this an excellent resource for individuals or groups seeking assistance or knowledge about any topic. In our particular case, this would be clinical reasoning.

Other resources relevant to the Health Sciences are available on the Internet. For instance, there is a copyrighted document entitled *Health Science Resources on Bitnet/ Internet* and compiled approximately five times a year by Lee Hancock of the University of Kansas Medical Center that may be retrieved using a program called File Transfer Protocol (FTP). A convention exists on the Internet that computers around the world can make particular directories available to anyone for retrieving files simply by logging into the computer using the log in name of 'anonymous' and the person's email address. In the case of the Health Sciences Resources document, a person can use anonymous FTP to ftp.sura.net and, in the directory \pub\nic, retrieve the document 'medical.resources.xxx' where xxx is the date of the release. This document is quite comprehensive detailing numerous discussion lists (see Table 12.2 below for a sample), FTP sites, electronic newsletters, data archives (e.g. BIOSIS, CancerNet, GENBANK), online medical libraries and so on.

Other examples of world-wide resources that have some applicability to the teaching of clinical decision making, particularly in relation to knowledge acquisition, include the following:

- A collection of medical education related software that may be obtained using anonymous FTP to FTP.UCI.EDU. This medical education software repository is provided as a service by the University of California, Irvine. The Centre for Biomedical Informatics of the State University of Campinas, Brazil, also provides an anonymous-access FTP node (CCSUN.UNICAMP.BR or 143.106.1.5) under the subdirectory pub/medicine for public domain medical software.

- A collection of physiotherapy-related resources is also available. It was written and researched by Frank Braun from Stockton University and is available from the PHYSIO discussion group (MAILBASE@MAILBASE.AC.UK) as 'net-resources-1.txt'.

- There are a number of sources of AIDS information on the Internet:
  Gopher: selway.umt.edu 700 in the directories:
  Internet health-related information/ Computer Software and Information Databases/AIDS Information, and
  Internet health-related information/US Federal Agency Information/AIDS Related Info (NIAID).

In an increasingly digital world, knowledge resources are proliferating at an incredible rate.

Table 12.2 A sample of health sciences related discussion lists

List name	Server	Description
BACKS-L	UVMVM.UVM.EDU	Research on low back pain, disability
BIOMCH-L	NIC.SURFNET.NL	Biomechanics and Movement Science
BRAIN-L	VM1.MCGILL.CA	Mind–Brain Discussion Group
C+HEALTH	IUBVM.UCS.INDIANA.EDU	C+Health is intended to promote sharing of information, experiences, concerns, and advice about computers and health
NRSING-L	NIC.UMASS.EDU	Nursing Informatics List
PBLIST	UTHSCSA.EDU	The PBLIST list exists to promote discussion of problem-based learning (PBL) in health sciences education
PHYSIO	MAILBASE@MAILBASE.AC.UK	Discussion list for physiotherapists
SMDM-L	DARTCMS1.DARTMOUTH.EDU	An electronic bulletin board service for members of the Society for Medical Decision Making and others interested in the theory and practice of decision making
STROKE-L	UKCC.UKY.EDU	Cerebrovascular accident. The purpose of the Stroke List is to share information and opinions, ideas and inquiries that relate to the topic of stroke

The few examples provided here simply serve to indicate the breadth of resources available. Indeed, the amount of information available through computer networks can be overwhelming and information literacy skills need to be honed to take advantage of this resource.

Conclusion

Throughout this chapter the authors have attempted to demonstrate how the appropriate use of technology in its various forms (interactive programs, multimedia databases, videodisc, CD-ROM, and networked resources) can assist in the teaching and learning of clinical reasoning. By actively involving students in the learning process, new information can be meaningfully integrated into students' existing knowledge structures. Computer-based patient problem simulations enable process skills (e.g. hypothesis generation and testing, planning, hypothesis reformulation) to be highlighted in addition to the knowledge acquisition promoted through such activities. Decision-support systems provide information that enhances clinical decision making; through this process the opportunity also exists for knowledge acquisition on the part of the clinician. Knowledge resources abound in the health sciences area. Multimedia databases are becoming common-place and the staggering amount of information available through computer networks threatens knowledge acquisition unless students develop skills to search efficiently these online information resources.

When used as an adjunct to classroom and clinical supervision, computer assisted learning technology can assist overcoming the cost and time constraints that increasingly burden our educational programs while enhancing our ability to facilitate the clinical reasoning ability of our students.

Acknowledgement

We wish to thank Barrie Bowden, Lecturer, School of Computer and Information Science, University of South Australia for his review and suggestions in the development of this chapter.

References

Aegerter, P., Auvert, B., Gilbos, V. et al (1992) An intelligent computer-assisted instruction system designed for rural health workers in developing countries. *Methods of Information in Medicine*, **31**, 193-203.

Baker, J. and Ziviani, J. (1986) Interactive videodisc: two bites at the cherry. In *Proceedings of the 4th Annual Computer Assisted Learning in Tertiary Education Conference*, ASCILITE, Dec. 1–3, Adelaide, South Australia, 38– 45

Barker, S.P. (1988) Comparison of effectiveness of interactive videodisc versus lecture–demonstration instruction. *Physical Therapy*, **68**, 699-703

Blackman, J.A., Albanese, M.A., Huntley, J.S. and Lough, L.K. (1985) Use of computer–videodisc system to train medical students in developmental disabilities. *Medical Teacher*, **7**, 89-97

Cervero, R.M. (1988) *Effective Continuing Education for Professionals.* Jossey-Bass, San Francisco

Christie, A.D. (1987) The use of interactive videodisc in the teaching of orthopaedics in physiotherapy. In *Proceedings of the 5th Annual Computer Assisted Learning in Tertiary Education Conference*, ASCILITE, Nov. 30th–Dec. 2nd, Sydney, New South Wales, 164–169

Christie, A.D. (1988) Evaluation of an educational innovation–interactive videodisc in the health sciences. In *Proceedings of the 6th Annual Computer Assisted Learning in Tertiary Education Conference*, ASCILITE, Dec. 4th–7th, Canberra, 47–63

Christie, A.D. (1990) The use of interactive videodisc in the teaching of orthopaedics in physiotherapy. *Medical Teacher*, **12**, 175–180

Clyman, S.G and Orr N.A. (1990) Status report on the NBME's computer-based testing. *Academic Medicine*, **65**, 235–241

Cohen, V.B. (1984) Interactive features in the design of videodisc materials. *Educational Technology*, **24**, 16–20

Custers, E., Boshuizen, H. and Schmidt, H. (1993) The influence of typicality of case descriptions on subjective disease probability estimations. Paper presented at the Annual Meeting of the American Educational Research Association, American Educational Research Association, Atlanta, April 12–16

Delitto, A., Shulman, A.D. and Rose, S.J. (1989) On developing expert-based decision-support systems in physical therapy: the NIOSH low back atlas. *Physical Therapy*, **69**, 554–558

Edwards, M.J.A. and Hannah, K.J. (1985) An examination of the use of interactive videodisc cardiopulmonary resuscitation instruction of the lay community. *Computers in Nursing*, **3**, 250–252

Elstein, A.S., Shulman, L.S. and Sprafka, S.S. (1978) *Medical Problem Solving: An Analysis of Clinical Reasoning.* Cambridge, MA: Harvard University Press

Graves, J.R. (1990) A research-knowledge system (ARKS)

for storing, managing, and modeling knowledge from the scientific literature. *Advances in Nursing Science*, **13**, 34–45

Hannan, T. (1993) Computerised clinical decision support – mechanisms and benefits. *Fellowship Affairs*, **12**, 17–18, 30

Heathfield, H.A. and Wyatt, J. (1993) Philosophies for the design and development of clinical decision-support systems. *Methods of Information in Medicine*, **32**, 1–8

Henry, S.B. and Holzemer, W.L. (1993) The relationship between performance on computer-based clinical simulations and two written methods of evaluation: cognitive examination and self-evaluation of expertise. *Computers in Nursing*, **11**, 29–34

Hon, D. (1982) Interactive training in cardiopulmonary resuscitation. *Byte*, **7**, 108–138

Kolb, D.A. (1984) *Experiential Learning: Experience as the Source of Learning and Development*. Prentice-Hall Inc., New Jersey

Mangione, S., Nieman, L.Z. and Gracely, E.J. (1992) Computer-aided learning and assessment. *Academic Medicine* , **67**, S63–S67

McGuire, C.H. and Babbott, D. (1967) Simulation technique in the measurement of problem-solving skills. *Journal of Educational Measurement*, **4**, 1–10

Miller, R.A., Pople, H.E. Jr and Myers, J.D. (1982) INTERNIST-1, an experimental computer-based diagnostic consultant for general internal medicine. *New England Journal of Medicine*, **307**, 468–476

Newell, A. and Simon, H. (1972) *Human Problem Solving*. Prentice-Hall, New Jersey

Petrucci, K.E. and Petrucci, P.R. (1991) Nursing and technology. *Nursing Economics*, **9**, 188–190

Pryor, T.A. and Clayton, P.D. (1991) Decision support systems for clinical medicine. Tutorial 11. 15th Annual Symposium on Computer Applications in Medical Care (cited by Hannan) (1993)

Rimoldi, H.J.A. (1955) A technique for the study of problem solving. *Educational and Psychological Measurement*, **15**, 450–461

Rimoldi, H.J.A. (1961) The test of diagnostic skills. *Journal of Medical Education*, **36**, 73–79

Rosenblatt, R.A. and Gaponoff, M. (1984) The microcomputer as a vehicle for continuing medical education. *Journal of Family Practice*, **18**, 629–632

Roth, K., DiStefano, J.J. and Chang, B.L. (1989) CANDI – development of the automated nursing assessment tool. *Computers in Nursing*, **7**, 222–227

Shortliffe, E.H. (1987) Computer programs to support clinical decision-making. *Journal of American Medical Association*, **258**, 61–66

Skinner, B.F. (1968) *The Technology of Teaching*. Appleton-Century-Crofts, New York

Waterfield, M. (1993) Learning materials: computer-assisted learning. *Journal of Audiovisual Media in Medicine*, **16**, 87–90

13

Assessing clinical reasoning

David Newble, Cees van der Vleuten and Geoffrey Norman

The term 'clinical reasoning' is used in varying ways by different authors as will be apparent when reading this book. In this chapter we will use it as a component of clinical competence which, in other publications, might be referred to as 'clinical problem-solving'. Our interest in its assessment reflects a wider concern with methods of assessment of both clinical competence and on-the-job clinical performance.

Clinical reasoning can be viewed as one of three components which comprise clinical competence, the others being 'relevant knowledge' and 'relevant skills' see Figure 13.1. The latter includes interpersonal, clinical and technical skills. Clinical reasoning can broadly be considered to be the intellectual activity which synthesizes information obtained from the clinical situation, integrates it with previous knowledge and experience, and uses it for making diagnostic and management decisions. Each component of competence is influenced by a range of attitudinal aspects which are difficult to define and even more difficult to consider in any assessment procedure.

For assessment and test development purposes, these three components are often considered separately so that specific tests are devised to assess knowledge (e.g. multiple choice tests), clinical skills (e.g. an objective structured clinical examination) or clinical reasoning (e.g. patient management problems). In fact, these components are likely to be highly inter-related (Norman et al, 1985).

Historical perspective

In the 1960s and 1970s there was considerable interest in the development of methods which assessed 'clinical problem-solving skills'. This came, partly, from a concern to test at a greater depth than could be achieved with objective Multiple Choice Question (MCQ) type tests and partly from an interest in the research being done at this time on the clinical reasoning process. The main thrust was to simulate on paper, and later by computer, the process by which a doctor took a history, obtained information from the physical examination and made diagnostic, investigational and management decisions.

The pioneering work in this field was done by Rimoldi (1961) who devised a method to investigate the diagnostic ability of medical students. It consisted of a deck of cards each containing a question relating to history taking, a physical examination feature or a laboratory investigation pertinent to a patient problem. The answer to each was on the back of the card. He recorded the number of cards used and the order in which they were selected as the students attempted to diagnose the problem. He showed differences in the performance of students of varying seniorities as compared to practising clinicians. He concluded that such a method could be used to measure objectively students' diagnostic skill and to train them in clinical reasoning. This technique was adapted by Helfer and Slater

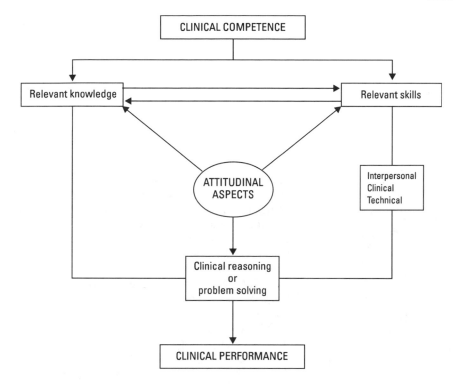

Figure 13.1 Components of clinical competence

(1971) and called the Diagnostic Management Problem.

A slightly more sophisticated method was developed at the University of Illinois and called the Patient Management Problem (PMP) (McGuire and Babbott, 1967). A typical PMP begins with a variable amount of information about the patient and identifies the doctor–patient setting. The student is then requested to collect further data sequentially in either a linear or branching fashion. A variety of technical devices are available (e.g. tabs, invisible ink, compounds which can be erased) to obscure the data until selected. After collecting the history and examination data, ostensibly in the manner and order that would have pertained in the live patient situation, the student may be allowed to select investigations and/or make diagnostic and management decisions. The pathway of the student is compared to that of an expert or criterion group and composite scores are determined for such things as thoroughness, efficiency and proficiency.

By 1974, eighteen varieties of PMP could be identified (Galofre, 1974). PMPs became widely used for certification purposes being accepted

more on the basis of their perceived fidelity than their psychometric properties. They were seen as a more valid measure of problem solving ability than other paper-and-pencil tests, with the advantage of being objectively scored.

Alternative approaches were also explored at this time. These included the Sequential Management Problem (SMP) (Berner et al, 1974) and the Modified Essay Question (MEQ) (Hodgkin and Knox, 1975). Each of these introduces into the simulation varying amounts of sequential data and feedback. Student answers are written-in rather than selected from a fixed list of options, overcoming to some extent the cueing problem associated with most PMP formats (see below).

The SMP commences with a case vignette and students are asked to write down what additional data they require. These responses are collected and the complete set of appropriate data for the first section of the simulation, as determined by a criterion group, is provided. The students then request further information or are asked to interpret the data and make diagnostic or management decisions. Each case will have a number of sections which the students answer sequentially. The SMP has not been used widely, probably because of the practical difficulties involved in collecting each section before the next is made available. Because of this, little information has been published on the reliability and validity of the SMP (Neufeld and Norman, 1985).

The MEQ, on the other hand, has been used quite extensively by the medical profession in some parts of the world both for in-course assessments and for the certification of competence. This reflects, in part, their relative ease of construction as compared to PMPs (Feletti, 1980). A typical MEQ once again begins with a case vignette. Students are asked to respond to questions in a short essay format. New information is provided sequentially which relates to differing and evolving circumstances of the same case. Some skill is required to avoid providing cues to earlier or subsequent sections of the MEQ. Few studies are available of the reliability and validity of this method but it has face validity, appears to be acceptable and is practicable (Feletti, 1980; Neufeld and Norman, 1985).

Patient management problems

Despite initial enthusiasm and widespread use there have been growing concerns about the credibility of PMPs, whether presented in the written or computer-based format. These concerns relate partly to some technical and psychometric limitations and partly to research which raises doubt as to whether they are truly measures of problem-solving. Some of these concerns are discussed below.

Cueing

One technical problem with PMPs, which was recognized early, was that of cueing. For scoring purposes, PMPs provide a predetermined, and usually limited, selection of responses from which to choose. Having these lists provides a prompt to the examinee which improves performance and distorts clinical problem-solving behaviour (McCarthy, 1966; Goran et al, 1973; Norman and Feightner, 1981; Newble et al, 1982). Great ingenuity has been shown in trying to minimize this effect but it remains largely unsolved at this time.

Scoring

Scoring has been the major technical difficulty associated with PMPs. The development of a score is usually one which involves a panel of experts who decide, by consensus, on the acceptable pathway through the problem and on the weight (positive and negative) which should be given to the options in each section of the simulation. The students' scores are compared to those of the expert panel and computed into composite scores such as proficiency, efficiency, thoroughness, and overall competence. Many forms of this weighted scoring system of varying complexity have been developed. However, correlations between methods are high (Bligh, 1980; Norman and Feightner, 1981; Norcini et al, 1983).

In fact, this high correlation could have been anticipated. Numerous studies in a wide number of domains have shown that virtually all weighting schemes, regardless of complexity, have very high correlations with simple counts of items (Wainer, 1976). Since most PMPs consist of large numbers of history-based items, physical examination findings and routine laboratory tests, nearly all scores reduce to a measure of thoroughness of data gathering, a measure which has been shown to be unrelated to diagnostic accuracy (Norman et al, 1985). It is apparent that experts may follow many pathways through a problem, and moreover, experts take many shortcuts since they can more optimally use information than novices. The net result is that true expert performance on a PMP is frequently penalized (Marshall, 1977).

Confidence in PMPs has been further undermined by research comparing performance on PMPs of experienced clinicians with less experienced clinicians or students. In some studies, students have been shown to score higher than qualified doctors (Newble et al, 1982). The conventional scoring systems may over-reward thoroughness which again may lead to higher scores for less competent and less efficient problem solvers (Marshal, 1977). Despite efforts to deal with the problems associated with scoring no satisfactory solution has been achieved (Swanson et al, 1987).

Content or case specificity

Research has demonstrated consistently that performance on one PMP is a very poor predictor of performance on another PMP. For a number of studies these correlations across problems was of the order 0.1–0.3 (Norman et al, 1985). This appears to undermine one of the original hypotheses underlying the development of problem solving simulations, i.e. that they are measuring problem solving ability. If this was so, correlations between PMPs ought to be high since those who are better problem solvers, either as a result of native intelligence or learned skills, should exhibit superior performance across a wide range of problems, independent of specific content knowledge. The explanation of this phenomenon is referred to variously as 'content specificity' or 'case-specificity'. Interestingly, this is not a finding peculiar to PMPs but is seen for other methods which assess aspects of clinical competence and performance, including oral examinations (Swanson, 1987), vignette-based written tests (De Graaf et al, 1987; Page et al, 1990), chart audits (Erviti et al, 1980), performance-based tests (Van der Vleuten and Swanson, 1990) and computer-based simulations (Swanson et al, 1987).

Given these limitations, doubt has been cast on the value of the PMP and, indeed, for any format which involves extensive and lengthy testing with relatively few cases. Some authors have suggested they should not be used for decision making purposes until their validity has been more clearly established (Swanson et al, 1987). However, the experience with PMPs has alerted us to our limited understanding of the nature of clinical reasoning. Among other things, it has stimulated research of a more fundamental nature into the cognitive functioning of medical students amd doctors.

New concepts of clinical reasoning

In the 1970s and 1980s several studies showed that expert clinicians performed little better than less experienced doctors on a variety of simulations of clinical problem solving (Neufeld and Norman, 1985). This phenomenon occurred not only with PMPs but also with problems presented by real and standardized patients (Schmidt et al, 1990). These studies challenged the paradigms underlying previous test development. Knowledge gained from cognitive psychological research into the nature of clinical reasoning and of

the differences between experts and novices is now providing new insights which promise to redirect test development (Norman et al, 1989; Schmidt et al, 1990). This chapter is not the place to review these psychological developments. More detailed discussions are contained in Chapters 2, 4, 9 and 11. However, a brief abstraction of this work here may be of value to test developers.

Current understanding would suggest that problem solving ability is not a separate skill or entity which grows with training and experience and cannot be measured independent of relevant content knowledge. In other words, it has not generally been possible to establish that a person who is good at solving problems in one type of situation is predictably superior at solving problems in other types of situation. For example chess grandmasters are only exceptional at solving chess problems (De Groot, 1965; Chase and Simon, 1973). Thus, problem solving ability appears to be highly dependent on knowledge, not just the amount of knowledge but also its specificity and the way it is structured, stored, accessed and retrieved. This is not to say that knowledge alone is sufficient for efficient and effective clinical reasoning. Higher order control processes also play an integral role (Bransford et al, 1986). These two components have been researched and discussed in great depth and from several different disciplinary perspectives, which makes generalization difficult and the terminology confusing for the uninitiated (Bransford et al, 1986; Elstein et al, 1990; Schmidt et al, 1990). A simplified model is presented in Figure 13.2. We have chosen higher order control processes as a relatively neutral term to include a wide range of intellectual strategies which may be brought to bear as problems are being solved. A flavour of the other terms used by writers in this aspect of problem solving can be gained from the following: metacognition; executive thinking; categorization; rehearsal, organization and re-organization; chunking; debugging; the deep approach; hypothetico-deductive thinking.

Organized knowledge is seen by some as the key to successful problem solving. It is the specificity of the knowledge and how it is structured and retrieved in relation to the problem that determines success and expertise (Norman et al, 1989). One such theory proposes that knowledge is structured in various ways or levels (Bordage and Lemieux, 1991). Novices

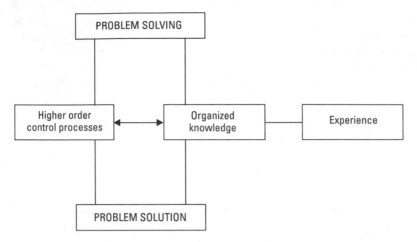

Figure 13.2   Aspects of problem solving

tend to have low or dispersed levels of knowledge. As experience grows knowledge is elaborated and compiled into complex structures and schemata. This is heavily influenced by the context in which the experience was attained.

An alternative theory of knowledge organization proposes three different kinds of information relevant to solving clinical problems. The most elementary is knowledge of disease processes and causal relationships, the basic science of medicine. At a later level, students acquire 'illness scripts' which are quite literal list-like structures relating signs and symptoms to disease prototypes (Feltovich and Barrows, 1984). At the highest level of functioning, the expert uses a sophisticated form of pattern recognition characterized by speed and efficient use of information (Schmidt et al, 1990; Brooks et al, 1991). It is theorized that this latter representation is drawn, to a large degree, from direct experience with patients and that pattern recognition is, in fact, recognition at a holistic level of the similarity between the present patient and previous patients. Some studies have experimentally demonstrated some features of this process. For example, recent experience has demonstrated that similar appearing dermatologic lesions can influence diagnostic accuracy and expert radiologists have been shown to recognize chest lesions using a process which is apparently only loosely related to the presence or absence of specific signs (Brooks et al, 1991). In fact, in the latter case, a biasing history can change not only the likelihood of diagnosis but also the judgement of the presence or absence of

specific signs (Norman et al, 1992). Seeing a vivid example of a clinical problem as much as several weeks earlier can change diagnostic judgements on other cases which match only on age, sex and chief complaint (Van Rossum et al, 1989).

This is not to indicate that all expert clinical reasoning is by pattern recognition. It is hypothesized that, when experts find themselves in a position where clear analogies are not present and the problem is difficult, they may revert to more analytical methods and, in rare circumstances, may analyse the problem with basic principles available to the beginning medical student.

According to this theory, it is evident that effective clinical reasoning may follow one of several routes. If the problem is one with which the person has had considerable previous experience then the problem is probably recognized very early by a pattern recognition process. Little active thinking is required and there is a rapid resolution of the problem. In fact, the problem is not really a problem any more for that person. On the other hand, if the situation does present a problem for that person, more systematic intellectual activities must be brought into play, either a formal testing of hypotheses through accumulation and weighting of specific data, or causal reasoning at the level of basic disease mechanisms. An individual will demonstrate a range of approaches, both within and across problems, depending on that person's previous experience and exposure to problems of a similar nature.

To the extent that this view is correct, it is evident why early attempts to assess clinical reasoning were doomed. We cannot consider a generic process. Instead, we must contemplate the evaluation of several qualitatively different strategies. Some, like pattern recognition, are very efficient and, in fact, may be all over in seconds. These strategies will defy any attempts at measurement of the process. Some, like causal reasoning, are focused on detailed reasoning about mechanisms and are little concerned with data acquisition. As a result, they are inadequately captured by a focus on observable behaviours like history taking and physical examination. These issues have serious implications for assessment.

New developments

It is not very encouraging, but probably close to the truth, to say that we have no method of assessing clinical reasoning which stands up to critical scrutiny. On the other hand, we are at the cutting edge of test development which makes this an exciting area in which to work. Given that much success has been achieved in improving the methods of assessing knowledge and skills it is likely that there will be a major assault on assessing clinical reasoning over the next few years.

The research referred to in the previous section is likely to form the basis for much of this new development. Preliminary attempts are being made to transpose the experimental laboratory instruments of the psychologists into practical methods of testing competence (Norman, 1989). Others are attempting to modify current test methods to take into account these new concepts (Case et al, 1991).

Taking the model of problem solving (Figure 13.2) as a guide we could approach assessment in one of several ways. We could ignore the reasoning process entirely and focus assessment on the problem solution or 'outcome'. This would entail presenting the student with an appropriate range of problems in a high fidelity format and concentrating on the quality of the problem solution in terms of the diagnosis or the management plan. This might be a logical, and even desirable, approach in the post-graduate era but has less attraction in the undergraduate phase where information on the intermediate stages of problem-solving would

be of interest from a teaching as well as from an assessment point-of-view. Such a 'process' approach would attempt to measure aspects of higher order control processes and aspects of the organized knowledge/experience, that is, both its presence and its utilization.

Some progress is being made in developing measures for some aspects of the clinical reasoning process though most must still be regarded as experimental. For example, several workers have explored methods similar to those used in the classic studies of the problem solving skills of chess grand masters (De Groot, 1965; Chase and Simon, 1973) with chess scenarios replaced by clinical case protocols. In one exploratory study, Newble and Raymond (1992) showed a rising trend in the ability to recall medical case-based material associated with increasing medical expertise. This trend was not evident for the recall of non-medical material. In another study, Schmidt and Boshuizen (1993) showed that severely restricting the reading time of exposure to clinical material allowed differences in recall relating to expertise to emerge. The demands on memory can also be altered by adjusting the complexity of the task. For instance, Norman et al (1989) showed that the use of fluid and electrolyte problems, combined with instructions to solve the problem and then recall the data, led to large differences in recall related to expertise. While such studies provide some support for the validity of the previously described concepts as a basis for understanding the clinical reasoning processes of medical practitioners they are unlikely to be of great value as forms of assessment. Speeded 'recall of data' tests might well be good discriminators but it is hard to imagine them being acceptable for routine use.

Other workers have been seeking more practical ways of exploiting the relationship of expertise to the organized knowledge base and clinical experience. Case et al (1988) have devised a 'pattern recognition test' in which students are presented with a series of brief case scenarios based on a single chief complaint (e.g. shortness of breath) and must select the most appropriate diagnosis from a long menu of potential diagnoses (see Table 13.1). Such a format, if proved to be valid, would be attractive due to its adaptability for machine scoring and computer analysis.

An alternative approach is to present students with less familiar amd more complex

Table 13.1   Example of long menu extended-matching question

Theme:	*Shortness of breath*	
Options:	A. Anaemia	K. Lung cancer
	B. Aortic stenosis	L. Metabolic acidosis
	C. Aspiration pneumonia	M. Mitral insufficiency
	D. Asthma	N. Mitral stenosis
	E. Bacterial pneumonia	O. Myocardial infarction
	F. Chronic obstructive pulmonary disease	P. Pneumocystis carinii
	G. Congestive heart failure	Q. Pneumothorax
	H. Hypertrophic outlet obstructive	R. Primary pulmonary hypertension
	cardiomyopathy	S. Pulmonary embolism
	I. Hyperventilation	T. Pulmonary fibrosis-silicosis
	J. Laryngeal spasm	

Lead in: For each patient with shortness of breath, select the most likely diagnosis.

1. A 55-year-old woman who smokes has had a chronically productive cough and progressive shortness of breath for 5 years
2. A 64-year-old woman has had shortness of breath, a temperature to 101.5 °F, purulent sputum, and pleuritic chest pain on the left for 3 days
3. A . . . .
4. A . . . .
etc.

scenarios which might require some deductive reasoning as well as pattern recognition. That such an approach may have merit has been demonstrated by Norman et al (1994). They showed that the use of complex written clinical situations containing a minimum of clinical information and laboratory data could clearly differentiate between first year residents, second year residents and specialists with diagnostic accuracy being 25%, 50% and 91% respectively. They also showed that the experts were more likely to use physiological concepts to explain abnormal patterns of laboratory data and were less likely to rely on pattern recognition in these complex and atypical situations.

It is a little more difficult to conjecture how one might measure higher order control processes. The research methods used by Patel and Groen (1991), with propositional networks and characterization of forward and backward reasoning, are an attempt in this direction. Another similar approach has been to concentrate on the underlying reasoning process as the student tries to understand the pathophysiological mechanisms involved in the problem. The focus is more on the process than the outcome of the problem-solving activity (Jean et al, 1993; Des Marchais et al, 1993). However, such methods are too labour intensive as yet for routine applications.

Irrespective of the approaches and methods that will eventuate from these research efforts, several things have become clear. The first is that the assessment must be anchored in case-based material presented in a way that will induce and sample clinical reasoning activities. Simply testing the recall of factual material is no longer tenable. The second is that laboriously taking a student through the full data gathering and investigational phase of a real or simulated clinical case is an inefficient approach when the concern is to evaluate clinical reasoning skills. This is because of the content specificity problem and the consequent need to present students with large numbers of cases before satisfactory levels of test reliability can be achieved. For example, it has been shown that up to 8 hours of testing time may be required to achieve reliable assessments with PMPs because of this problem (Norcini et al, 1985).

Such studies have triggered a search for more 'cost-effective' methods. One possible way of doing this emerged from the first Cambridge Conference (Norman et al, 1985). The idea was based on the premise that any single case contained a lot of 'deadwood' from a clinical reasoning perspective. For example, in one case the critical challenge might be in eliciting and interpreting elements within the history with little further being added by the physical examination and laboratory investigations. In another case situation the challenge might be in the appropriate selection and interpretation of laboratory results. In other words, it may be possible to focus the problem solving stimulus.

The concept of the 'Cambridge Case' has not been fully explored. However, one concrete outcome has been the 'key feature' approach developed for the Medical Council of Canada certification examinations as an alternative to PMPs (Bordage and Page, 1987). In this procedure, clinical situations, as presenting in actual practice, are produced as a written case scenario. The 'key features' are identified on the basis of those elements critical to the resolution of the problem. Questions aimed at the 'key features' are then devised and may be posed in a variety of formats (e.g. short answer, MCQs or selection from longer menus of options). Such an approach allows a sample of 40–50 cases to be administered in the same time as that required to administer 12–15 PMPs. This should considerably enhance reliability (by sampling case situations more widely) though its validity as a test of clinical reasoning has yet to be proved.

Implications and advice for the teacher

As has become evident from this review, our success in developing valid measures of clinical reasoning for student assessment and research has been limited. If this is the disheartening reality, what should we as educators do in day-to-day practice? Should we discard whatever we are currently using and wait for better times? Or are there some guidelines that could be concluded from the findings so far which would allow us to proceed with some forms of assessment of clinical reasoning, albeit with caution.

Unfortunately there are no fixed answers to these questions and any recommendations must depend on the particular context of the testing situation. For instance, the answer may be quite different for tests which are to be used in undergraduate courses largely for formative purposes compared to those which are to be used for major postgraduate certifying examinations where high levels of reliability are demanded. Similarly measures of clinical reasoning used in research may adopt specific strategies, such as the use of very difficult cases, to clearly identify a group of expert problem solvers.

There are several key points we would wish to make. First, it is hard to imagine a credible assessment of clinical competence which does not attempt to evaluate clinical reasoning skills. An assessment using less-than-perfect instruments is preferable to no assessment at all of this component. This is an issue of validity which must apply to the whole assessment procedure.

A second compelling argument not to discard our imperfect instruments is the very direct and powerful relationship between assessment and student learning. Academic success is largely defined by examination performance and academic success is what students are seeking. Thus, students will devote much of their energy to identifying and studying for what they believe will be in their examination (Newble and Entwistle, 1986). This impact of examinations on student learning will often be greater than that of the training program and is sometimes referred to as 'consequential validity'. Students may, in reality, be pursuing a program which is quite different to that which the teacher believes they are following – an effect called the 'hidden curriculum'. The implication of this is that such effects must be seen as inevitable, if not desirable. The only answer is to ensure a good match, at least in the student's mind, between the assessment procedures and the expected outcomes of the course. A failure to do so may have serious consequences as evident in the case study reported by Newble and Jaeger (1983). The bottom line is that if the imperfect instruments of clinical reasoning which are currently available are the best we have we should probably continue to use them until better ones have been developed.

If this is to be our recommendation we must, as a third point, emphasize that every effort should be made to reduce the known problems associated with our current test methods. A few suggestions are:

1. Develop assessment tasks around real-life clinical scenarios which are representative of the problem situations that students will be expected to deal with at the conclusion of the course. Such tasks may be presented in simple written form (MCQ, short answer); in more complex written form (MEQ, 'key features' approach); as written or computer-

based simulations; in structured oral form; or by appropriate questioning about real or simulated patients. For assessing clinical reasoning, the method may actually be of less importance than we are intuitively inclined to believe.

2. Concentrate on the content within the tasks. It must be of a complexity which ensures that the problem solving process is induced. It should require the student to retrieve relevant information amd apply it to make a diagnosis, make decisions about management and so on within the particular situation or context. It should not be possible to answer the question by simple recall of knowledge. A useful guide might be that the question posed could not be answered without the contextual information.

3. The focus of the assessment should reflect the expected level of expertise of the students. At lower levels (e.g. junior undergraduates) the focus should be more on the process of clinical reasoning and should reward thoroughness. At higher levels of expertise outcome and efficiency should be rewarded.

4. Where written tests are used, cueing effects should be avoided or minimized. This can be done simply by using open-ended questions and accepting the burden of marking. This should not overstrain resources for the assessment of relatively small numbers of candidates (e.g. in medical schools) but can be a major difficulty for large national examinations with a cast of thousands. An alternative becomes the more innovative objective test formats such as those using long menus of options or the pattern recognition items.

5. Where direct observational methods are used it is important to find out what is going on in the students' minds as they tackle the problem solving task. This can be accomplished by asking the student to verbalize his or her thought process during or after the patient encounter, by the use of probing questions by the assessor or via a post-encounter written assessment. These procedures should focus on hypothesis generation, diagnosis and decision making.

6. Scoring systems should be kept simple. Most systems which have attempted to weight components differentially produce similar outcomes. Simple counts, limited pathways, simple decision rules for aggregating scores and avoidance of lengthy answers are all strategies to be recommended.

7. Deal with the content-specificity problem. This requires sampling widely from as many problems or cases as possible. It is wiser to sample less within a single problem in favour of sampling more problems. If this can be combined with the 'Cambridge Case' or 'key features' concept so much the better. This will maximize both efficiency and the clinical reasoning value per problem or case.

8. Avoid long unfolding cases with multiple pathways. While conceptually attractive, and perhaps being very valuable in a teaching situation, they are difficult to construct and administer, and a nightmare to score.

9. Control other known sources of error. Inadequate sampling (content specificity) seems to be the major source of error in testing aspects of clinical competence, including clinical reasoning. Nevertheless, other factors should be controlled. The most evident of these will be errors associated with marking and rating. Training of examiners for their roles and introducing structure into any rating or marking task can considerably improve reliability. As a general principle more is to be gained by having examiners score a single task or question for all candidates than score across a range of tasks or questions for a limited group of candidates. This effectively allows the effect of hawks and doves to even out. In an oral or viva situation, greater gains and reliability will be achieved by having single examiners assess students on two separate tasks rather than a pair of examiners assess students on only one task.

As a final comment, we would encourage experimentation. There is no one single best method of assessing clinical reasoning. Opportunities abound for creative activity and for teachers to contribute to the development of more valid and reliable test procedures.

References

Berner, E.S., Hamilton, L.A. and Best, W.R. (1974) A new approach to evaluating problem solving in medical students. *Journal of Medical Education*, **49**, 666–672

Bligh, T.J. (1980) Written simulation scoring: A comparison

of nine systems. Presented at the American Educational Research Association Annual Meeting, American Eductional Research Association, New York

Bordage, G. and Lemieux, M. (1991) Semantic structures and diagnostic thinking of experts and novices. *Academic Medicine*, **66**, S70-S72

Bordage, G. and Page, G. (1987) An alternative approach to PMP's: The 'key features' concept. In *Further Developments in Assessing Clinical Competence* (eds I. R. Hart and R.M. Harden) Can-Heal Publications, Montreal, pp. 59–72

Bransford, J., Sherwood, R., Vye, N. and Rieser, J. (1986) Teaching thinking and problem solving. *American Psychologist*, **41**, 1078-1089

Brooks, L.R., Norman, G.R. and Allen, S.W. (1991) The role of specific similarity in a medical diagnostic task. *Journal of Experimental Psychology: General*, **120**, 278–287

Case, S.M., Swanson, D.B. and Stillman, P.S. (1988) Evaluating diagnostic pattern recognition: The psychometric characteristics of a new item format. In *Proceedings of the 27th Conference on Research in Medical Education*, Association of American Medical Colleges, Washington, pp. 3–8

Case, S., Swanson, D.B. and Van der Vleuten, C. (1991) Strategies for student assessment. In *The Challenge of Problem-Based Learning* (eds D. Boud and G. Feletti), Kogan Page, London, pp. 260–273

Chase, W.G. and Simon, H.A. (1973) Perception in chess. *Cognitive Psychology*, **4**, 55-81

De Graaf, E., Post, G. and Drop, M. (1987) Validation of a new measure of clinical problem-solving. *Medical Education*, **21**, 213–218

De Groot, A. (1965) *Thought and Choice in Chess*. Mouton, The Hague

Des Marchais, J.E., Dumais, B. and Vu, N.V. (1993) An attempt at measuring ability to analyze problems in the Sherbrooke problem-based curriculum: A preliminary study. In *Problem-Based Learning as an Educational Strategy*, (eds P. Bouhuijs, H. Schmidt, and R. Berkel). Network Publications, Maastricht, pp. 239–248

Elstein, A.S., Shulman, L.S. and Sprafka, S.A. (1990) Medical problem solving: A ten year retrospective. *Evaluation and the Health Professions*, **13**, 5–36

Erviti, V., Templeton, B., Bunce, J. and Burg, F. (1980) The relationship of pediatric resident recording behaviour across medical conditions. *Medical Care*, **18**, 1020–1031

Feletti, G.I. (1980) Reliability and validity studies on modified essay questions. *Journal of Medical Education*, **55**, 933–941

Feltovich, P.J. and Barrows, H.S. (1984) Issues of generality in medical problem solving. In *Tutorials in Problem Based Learning: A New Direction in Teaching the Health Professions* (eds H.G. Schmidt and M.L. de Volder). Van Gorcum, Assen, Holland, pp. 128–142

Galofre, A. (1974) *A Review of Written Paper Management Simulations*. Center for Educational Development, University of Illinois, Chicago

Goran, M.J., Williamson, J.W. amd Gonnella, J.S. (1973) The validity of patient management problems. *Journal of Medical Education*, **48**, 171–177

Helfer, R.E. and Slater, C.H. (1971) Measuring the process of solving clinical diagnostic problems. *British Journal of Medical Education*, **5**, 48–52

Hodgkin, K. and Knox, J.D.E. (1975) *Problem Centred Learning: The Modified Essay Question in Medical Education*. Churchill Livingstone, Edinburgh

Jean, P., des Marchais, J.E. and Delorne, P. (1993) *Apprendre a Enseigner Les Sciences de Sante*. Internal report, University of Montreal, Montreal

Marshall, J. (1977) Assessment of problem-solving ability. *Medical Education*, **11**, 329–334

McCarthy, W.H. (1966) An assessment of the effect of cueing items in objective examinations. *Journal of Medical Education*, **41**, 263–266

McGuire, C.H. and Babbott, D. (1967) Simulation technique in the measurement of problem solving skills. *Journal of Educational Measurement*, **4**, 1–10

Neufeld, V.R. and Norman, G.R. (1985) *Assessing Clinical Competence*, Springer, New York

Newble, D.I., Hoare, J. and Baxter, A. (1982) Patient management problems: Issues of validity. *Medical Education*, **16**, 137–142

Newble, D.I. and Jaeger, K. (1983) The effect of assessments and examinations on the learning of medical students. *Medical Education*, **17**, 165–171

Newble, D.I. and Entwistle, N.J. (1986) Learning styles and approaches: Implications for medical education. *Medical Education*, **20**, 162-175

Newble, D.I. and Raymond, G.A. (1992) Clinical memory as a potential measure of clinical problem solving ability. In *Approaches to the Assessment of Clinical Competence, Part 1*. (eds R. M. Harden, I. R. Hart and H. Mulholland). Centre for Medical Education, Dundee, pp. 347–351

Norcini, J.J., Swanson, D.B., Webster, G.D. and Grosso, L. J. (1983) A comparison of several methods of scoring patient management problems. In *Proceedings of the 22nd Annual Conference on Research in Medical Education*, Association of American Medical Colleges, Washington, pp. 41–46

Norcini, J.J., Swanson, D.B., Grosso, L J., Shea, J. and Webster, G.D. (1985) Reliability, validity and efficiency of multiple choice questions and patient management item formats in the assessment of physician competence. *Medical Education*, **19**, 238–247

Norman, G.R. (1989) Reliability and construct validity of some cognitive methods of clinical reasoning. *Teaching and Learning in Medicine*, **1**, 194–199

Norman, G.R. and Feightner, J.W. (1981) A comparison of behaviour on simulated patients and patient management problems. *Journal of Medical Education*, **55**, 529–537

Norman, G., Bordage, G., Curry, L. et al (1985) A review of recent innovations in assessment. In *Directions in Clinical Assessment. Report of the First Cambridge Conference* (ed. R.E. Wakeford), Cambridge University School of Clinical Medicine, Cambridge, pp. 9–27

Norman, G., Allery, L., Berkson, L. et al (1989) The psychology of clinical reasoning: Implications for assessment. Paper from the Fourth Cambridge Conference, Cambridge University School of Clinical Medicine, Cambridge

Norman, G.R., Brooks, L.R. and Allen, S.W. (1989) Recall by experts and novices as a record of processing attention. *Journal of Experimental Psychology: Learning, Memory and Cognition*, 5, 1166–1174

Norman, G.R., Brooks, L.R., Coblentz, C.K. and Babcook, C. J. (1992) The correlation of feature identification and category judgments on diagnostic radiology. *Memory and Cognition*, 20, 344–355

Norman, G.R., Trott, A.D., Brooks, L.P. and Smith, E.R.M. (1994) Cognitive differences in clinical reasoning related to postgraduate training. *Teaching and Learning in Medicine*, 6, 114–120

Page, G., Bordage, G., Harasym, P., Bowmer, I. and Swanson, D. (1990) A revision of the Medical Council of Canada's qualifying examination: Pilot test results. In *Teaching and Assessing Clinical Competence* (eds W. Bender, R.J. Hiemstra, A.J.J. Scherpbier and R.P. Zwierstra). BoekWerk Publications, Groningen, pp. 403–407

Patel, V.L. and Groen, G.J. (1991) The general and specific nature of medical expertise: A critical look. In *Toward a General Theory of Expertise: Prospects and Limits* (eds A. Ericsson and J. Smith). Cambridge University Press, Cambridge, pp. 93–125

Rimoldi, H.J.A. (1961) The test of diagnostic skills. *Journal of Medical Education*, 36, 73–79

Schmidt, H.G., Norman, G.R. and Boshuizen, H.P.A. (1990) A cognitive perspective on medical expertise: Theory and implications. *Academic Medicine*, 65, 611–621

Schmidt, H.G. and Boshuizen H.P.A. (1993) On the origin of 'intermediate effects' in clinical case recall. *Memory and Cognition*, 22, 338–351

Swanson, D.B. (1987) A measurement framework for performance-based tests. In *Further Developments in Assessing Clinical Competence* (eds I.R. Hart and R.M. Harden). Can-Heal Publications, Montreal, pp. 13-45.

Swanson, D.B., Norcini, J.J. and Grosso, L.J. (1987) Assessment of clinical competence: Written and computer-based simulations. *Assessment and Evaluation in Higher Education*, 12, 220–246

Van Rossum, H.J.M., Briet, E., Bender, W. and Meinders, A.E. (1989) The transfer effect of one single patient demonstration on diagnostic judgement of medical students: Both better and worse. In *Teaching and Assessing Clinical Competence* (eds W. Bender, R.J. Hiemstra, A.J.J. Scherpbier and R.P. Zwierstra). BoekWerk Publications, Groningen, pp. 435–440

Van der Vleuten, C. and Swanson, D.B. (1990) Assessment of clinical skills with standardized patients: State of the art. *Teaching and Learning in Medicine*, 2, 58–76

Wainer, H. (1976) Estimating coefficients in linear models: It don't make no nevermind. *Psychological Bulletin*, 83, 213–217

14

Self-monitoring of clinical reasoning behaviours: promoting professional growth

Doris L. Carnevali

Clinical reasoning is a complex set of cognitive skills involving the use of existing knowledge and the acquisition and processing of information. It is used to make accurate, specific judgements, diagnoses and prognoses about a person's or family's health status and situation and to plan for rational, appropriate and individualized treatment or care.

Achievement of expertise in clinical reasoning is a personal process. Others can offer knowledge, guidance, and role models, but the accuracy, precision, and efficiency associated with expertise in clinical reasoning must be developed by the individual clinician. Thus, it becomes a personal responsibility to consistently:

- gain and systematically store discipline-specific knowledge and clinical experience on an ongoing basis
- achieve a working knowledge of the processes involved in clinical reasoning and critically practise those skills in varying clinical situations
- engage in self-evaluation and reflection on evaluation sought from others as a means of maintaining excellence and ongoing professional growth.

Ongoing self-evaluation of one's clinical reasoning tends to become an increasingly difficult professional task. As the clinician continues to make clinical judgements many times each day, over time the process becomes an automatic, unconscious activity (Benner, 1984; Schmidt et al, 1990; Squire et al, 1992). In the busy, demanding world of health care this is a normal and necessary evolution. Automaticity however, can have both advantages and disadvantages. Early, accurate sensing of the existence of a clinical problem and being able to take action without having to laboriously and consciously engage in the clinical reasoning process can be life saving. On the other hand, patterns of thinking and observing can become so habituated that needed flexibility and innovative approaches are no longer used and clinical judgements can become less accurate (Dawson and Arkes, 1987).

This latter possibility points up the need to periodically examine one's clinical reasoning behaviour. It is possible to seek awareness of one's cognitive activities, either during the process of cognition or through recall, and then to engage in self-analysis (Carnevali and Thomas, 1993). It is also possible to ask colleagues to critique one's judgements and the reported clinical reasoning that supports them, in order to gain fresh eyes with which to view one's practice. However, this will happen only if the clinician recognizes and values the need for recurring evaluation of clinical reasoning as a professional responsibility.

Attaining command of the complex mental and physical skills associated with expert clinical reasoning tends to be a slow, ongoing process resulting from integration of a growing body of theoretical and clinical knowledge and experience (Schmidt et al, 1990). Having a knowledge base related to the clinical reasoning process itself is a basic foundation.

Artistry and expertise is gained by repeated use of the skills in varying situations, and by systematically storing new experiences and knowledge for ease of retrieval.

Expertise in the clinical reasoning process involves several components including:

- understanding what is currently known of memory systems and the diagnostic reasoning processes used
- systematically storing one's theoretical and clinical knowledge base in long term memory, to facilitate its access for clinical judgement and decision making activities
- building a growing body of clinical experiences involving a variety of clinical phenomena, situations and treatments, and storing them for ease of retrieval
- gaining expertise in discipline-specific data acquisition and the use of one's cognitive processes in varying clinical situations and care settings.

This chapter will offer some guidelines and clinical exercises that can be used to improve clinical reasoning. The areas to be addressed are: gaining working knowledge associated with memory as it is used in clinical reasoning and in the organization of knowledge for use in making clinical judgements and treatment decisions, and developing skills in information processing as it is used in making clinical judgements.

Use of memory in clinical reasoning

Three forms of memory are currently thought to be involved in clinical reasoning. These are sensory, working (or short term) and long term memory (Ashcraft, 1989; Baddeley, 1990). Each form of memory has particular capacities and limitations and each serves particular functions in clinical reasoning. The clinician's knowledge and clinical experience need to be stored with these capacities and limitations in mind so that each type of memory can be used most effectively (Carnevali and Thomas, 1993). In addition, the clinical reasoning process itself must utilize strategies that acknowledge and accommodate both the richness and constraints of memory.

Sensory memory

Sensory memory is the entry point to the memory system and holds incoming stimuli for 0.5–3.0 seconds (Ashcraft, 1989). It is here that incoming stimuli from the clinical situation are either translated into mental representations for transmission to working memory; or they are lost (Coltheart, 1983) (refer to Figure 14.1).

Effective use of sensory memory for clinical reasoning depends upon having working knowledge of:

- Significant cues associated with clinical phenomena within one's discipline-specific domain, that should be noticed and attended to. This includes not only the clear, obvious stimuli, but also those that are subtle, disguised, or ambiguous as well as those that are extraneous or should not be present.
- The discipline-specific language used to transform stimuli into mental information.

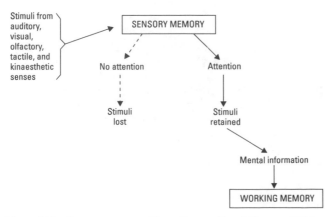

Figure 14.1   Sensory memory. From Carnevali and Thomas (1993) with permission

This is the initial identification or interpretation of sensory stimuli. In the cognitive science literature, this assignment of descriptors to incoming stimuli is called encoding (Ashcraft, 1989; Baddeley, 1990).

Students in any health care field learn from lectures, reading, and clinical experiences about salient risk factors and recognition features (or cues) associated with specific phenomena. They also learn the language or images used to describe them. This knowledge can be stored in such a way as to affect the initial cognitive processes of seeking, giving attention to, and labelling stimuli coming into sensory memory. With ongoing patient (and family) encounters, thoughtful clinicians can modify, sharpen, and refine their skills in initially noticing and encoding significant stimuli entering sensory memory.

SENSORY MEMORY EXERCISES

1. As you listen to lectures and read about clinical phenomena in your health care field, identify specifically the associated risk factors and manifestations one should seek, notice, and label. Make note of cues that should not be present. Identify words or images that are used to represent the norms and variations in these stimuli. Identify the range of clinical situations and settings in which these phenomena and stimuli might be encountered and the variety of ways such data might be sought or present themselves.
2. Engage in a patient encounter. Try to be aware of the incoming stimuli you notice and the initial words or images you use to transform stimuli into mental representations.
3. Ask a colleague, teacher, or mentor (in your own health care field and eventually in other health care fields), to join you in engaging in a clinical encounter and repeat Exercise 2. Compare what each of you noticed and the initial descriptors you used. Analyse the differences in clinical reasoning and judgements that could arise from these differences. Accept the differences without trying to modify them.
4. Recall clinical situations in which you failed to notice significant stimuli or used incorrect or too general words or images to represent them. Consider the kinds of clinical judgements that could result from failing to attend to incoming stimuli or ineffectively labelling them.

Working memory

Incoming stimuli that have been transformed into mental information move from sensory memory to working memory which is the next component of the memory system used in clinical reasoning. Working memory can be likened to a processing centre or the workroom of the memory system that temporarily takes in and uses mental information from both sensory memory and long term memory (Ashcraft, 1989; Waldorp, 1987; Salame and Baddeley, 1982) (refer to Figure 14.2).

Working memory is required to accomplish a tremendous workload during clinical reasoning. Despite this extensive workload, working memory has major limitations and constraints including the following:

- restricted duration (i.e. 15–20 seconds unless mental rehearsal or other processing takes place)
- a capacity of only 5–9 chunks of information at any time (Miller, 1956). A chunk is a cluster made up of one or more units of related information that has become a familiar pattern from earlier repeated encounters and thus can be recognized as a single item (Larkin et al, 1980)
- easy loss of information through distraction.

These constraints shape strategies involved in effective clinical reasoning (Elstein et al, 1978; Carnevali and Thomas, 1993). Such strategies include:

- assigning more specific descriptors and interpretation to mental information received from sensory memory
- rehearsal for maintaining or elaborating on information received
- clustering information into related chunks to permit more effective judgements and to save space in working memory
- transferring information to and from long term memory (Craik and Lockhart, 1972; Ashcraft, 1989; Baddeley, 1990).

Each of these strategies will be discussed below.

Assigning more specific meaning

The initial encoding of stimuli in sensory memory tends to be a general tag or label. For

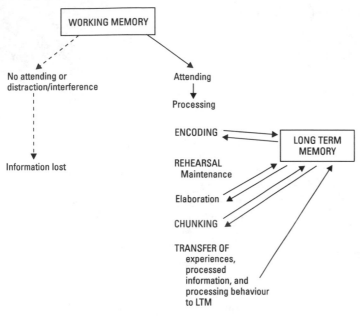

Figure 14.2   Working memory. From Carnevali and Thomas (1993) with permission

example, a pulse may be identified as to location (e.g. radial, pedal, carotid), strength (e.g. full, weak), rate (e.g. rapid, slow) and pattern (e.g. rhythmic, arrhythmic). However, it can be more precisely encoded in terms of an actual numerical rate, a 0 to 4+ volume and the specific rhythmic pattern (Wild et al, 1991). Richness and precision in encoding information in working memory has been found to be useful in subsequent cognitive tasks such as discrimination and differential diagnosis (Moscovitch and Craik, 1976; Baddeley, 1990). Professional growth requires clinicians to continually evolve qualitative and quantitative language or imagery to accurately and precisely describe and interpret clinical information being received in working memory.

WORKING MEMORY ENCODING EXERCISES

1. In reading and lectures about specific clinical phenomena or situations in your discipline or sub-speciality, identify the precise language or imagery for describing and assigning meaning to recognition features (e.g. risk factors, etiology, manifestations) associated with these phenomena or situations, including variations associated with closely-related phenomena or situations. Notice the manifestations that tend to be clear and obvious. Identify phenomena in which some manifes-

tations tend to be subtle in amplitude or occurrence, or to be disguised or ambiguous. Examples of such manifestations include: the physiological signs of risk for sudden infant death syndrome, manifestations of loneliness (Carnevali, 1986), elder abuse (Copstead, 1993), chronic cancer pain (Foley, 1987), some aspects of role dissatisfaction (Carnevali and Reiner, 1990), and confabulation used to cover memory loss in early Alzheimer's disease (Wills, 1993). Many of these are conditions to which society attaches stigma or blame. Seek to identify the subtle cues and also the kinds of disguising of manifestations that can occur.

2. As you read, listen to, and observe other clinicians, consciously critique their use of general versus precise, and qualitative versus quantitative language or imagery. Listen also to patients and families to detect the variety of language they use to describe their situations, experiences, and responses. Compare these to the language you currently use. Purposefully seek to broaden, modify, and refine the vocabulary, numerical gradations, and imagery you have available for encoding risk factors and manifestations associated with a given phenomenon or situation. Notice how you need knowledge of normal ranges or baselines as a basis for assigning meaning to variations. Consider

different norms based on age, gender, environmental, or cultural variations.

3. Engage in a patient or family encounter. Try to be aware of the precision you can currently achieve in describing and interpreting the data you are collecting and using. Describe the patient and situation to a colleague, mentor or teacher and ask that person to question you in ways that could increase your precision and accuracy in describing your findings on risk factors and manifestations of phenomena and assigning meaning. Repeat the previous activity with another clinician in your own field and with a clinician in another health care discipline. What did you learn?

4. Periodically repeat the above exercises with other patients, and other clinicians in your own field and other disciplines.

Maintenance rehearsal

Information is readily forgotten in working memory. Therefore, if one is collecting patient data and does not have access to paper and pen to record these data when they are obtained, one can mentally rehearse or repeat the information several times so as to fix it more firmly into memory until it can be recorded.

Elaborative rehearsal

Elaborative processing of information is both a more effective and more demanding means of retaining information needed for clinical reasoning in one's working memory and it is thought to result in greater long-term learning and more effective recall. It involves semantics, previously stored knowledge, and clinical experience as a basis for processing current data. Elaborative processing can occur with or without awareness and involves drawing relationships between what is already known and the information currently being processed.

The following case illustrates elaborative rehearsal. A nurse is caring for a dying patient who is managing the experience by use of hope and denial. Today, for the first time she hears the patient speak of his impending death. The nurse links this to her knowledge of movement through the stages of grief. Later in the day, the patient again reverts to speaking about feeling better and expecting medical treatment to effect a cure. Throughout the next day the patient vacillates between hope of cure and awareness of the reality of impending death. Prior to this clinical experience the nurse's concept of grieving had not included repeated vacillation between the elements. In future encounters with dying patients her knowledge would incorporate possibilities of vacillation and the need to follow a patient's lead in each encounter (Carnevali and Reiner, 1990; Carnevali and Thomas, 1993).

EXERCISES IN ELABORATION IN WORKING MEMORY

1. In a patient encounter, take in data from the situation. Notice your initial (sensory memory) identification Then process those cues by describing them more precisely and by assigning meaning.

2. Try to remember a situation in which you made a clinical judgement about a patient situation without really being aware of having done it. Ask yourself 'How did I know that?', then try to recall the patient information you processed in working memory to have arrived at your clinical judgement.

3. Select a patient situation where you feel familiar with one or more of the patient's diagnoses. Notice how soon you begin to assign meaning to information coming in from the patient situation, based on that you already 'know' from theory and clinical experiences.

Clustering/chunking information

An important cognitive skill involved in using working memory for clinical reasoning is clustering incoming information into meaningfully-related clusters or chunks (Larkin et al, 1980). Most clinical judgements are based upon conscious or unconscious recognition of cue patterns. This pattern recognition emerges from knowledge or clinical experience previously stored in long term memory.

Chunking conserves space in working memory by clustering units of related information into a chunk. Then the entire chunk is 'tagged' and used as one unit. Clinicians who are expert in working with particular phenomena tend to integrate more pieces of information into each chunk and to assign useful 'tags'. A clinician viewing a patient with apparently normal respirations might cluster all of the sights and sounds into a chunk and tag it 'respiration'.

On the other hand, a clinician seeing a patient as described below might group these ten cues into one chunk and tag them 'emphysema'.

> The patient is a thin person with normally pink skin colour. The breathing pattern is laboured particularly on exertion, and involves a prolonged expiratory phase, pursed lips during expiration and the use of scalene and sterno-cleidomastoid muscles. The patient has elevated shoulders, increased anteroposterior diameter of the chest and commonly sits with his elbows on his knees or on a table. His speech pattern involves sentences interrupted by laboured breathing.

A physician would use this cluster of information and the tag 'emphysema' to develop additional chunks containing more refined ventilatory test data. A nurse would move toward developing chunks related to how the person's functional capacities and daily living were affected by the breathing difficulties and infection risks (Carnevali and Reiner, 1990; Carnevali and Thomas, 1993). It can be seen that expertise in 'chunking' patient information is a complex process aimed at promoting pattern recognition and that it is essential for accuracy in clinical reasoning. The nature and labelling of the chunks would tend to be discipline-specific.

Chunking is learned from both theory and clinical experience. Lectures, books, and encounters with health care professionals provide knowledge about a discipline's or sub-specialty's usual and variant clustering of information relating to risk factors, the manifestations of clinical phenomena and the underlying dynamics that produce clinical findings. They also provide discipline-specific norms for precision in descriptors and the most useful 'tags' used by the discipline. However, clinicians need personal experiences with commonalities and variations in conditions, situations, and responses in order to store living, working knowledge of patterns and chunks of related findings (Schmidt et al, 1990).

Clinicians in varying health care fields and even sub-specialties will find different perspectives for their chunks. They will combine the same cues in different patterns and label them with different tags. This contributes to the richness but also the complexity and difficulties of inter-disciplinary practice.

Novices will tend to have fewer items in each chunk, not having had the clinical experiences needed to 'put things together' effectively (Tanner, 1984; Tanner et al, 1987). Clinicians who have sound, current theoretical foundations and multiple experiences with particular phenomena will unconsciously 'chunk' more items and integrate them at more sophisticated levels within their area of expertise (Corcoran, 1986a; 1986b).

EXERCISES IN CHUNKING

1. Think about a diagnosis, situation or response in your discipline that you know well; one where you believe you can 'chunk' clinical information easily and effectively. Identify and 'tag' the different chunks or patterns of information associated with that phenomenon. Under each chunk heading list the kinds of data you would incorporate. Then, repeat this exercise with a phenomenon with which you are less theoretically and clinically familiar. Compare the familiar with the unfamiliar exercise in terms of: (a) the speed with which you could make the lists, (b) the numbers of chunks and items in each chunk, (c) the sophistication and integration of items within the chunks, and (d) your feelings of satisfaction with your knowledge. Think about how your chunks in each instance would fit the 5–9 chunk limitation of working memory and how they could affect your clinical reasoning expertise.

2. Encounter a patient. Gather data and group them in chunks. 'Tag' the chunks. Ask a health care professional from a different field or sub-specialty (e.g. a medical–surgical nurse and a psychiatric nurse) to either look at the patient's record, see the patient or listen to your full, unchunked description of the patient. Ask that person how she or he would cluster the data. Compare it with your own. Would you chunk any differently the next time based on this experience? Why?

Transfer of information to and from long term memory

As can be seen from the discussion of the activities taking place in working memory, movement of information between working memory and long term memory is almost constant. New information and experiences taken into working memory move on to long term memory. These include:

- experiences, stored in episodic memory
- knowledge (new or revised) stored in semantic memory
- the activities of processing, retrieval and transfer thought to be stored both in episodic memory and an area identified sometimes as production memory (Anderson, 1985).

Repeated practice and building of efficient, often complicated organizational systems for storing information in long term memory eventually allows clinicians to move between working memory and long term memory so quickly that the boundaries between the two components of memory become blurred. At this stage the clinician is said to have developed *skilled memory* (Ericsson et al, 1980; Waldorp, 1987). Development of skilled memory can be enhanced by processing and systematically storing both knowledge and experience with the thought of its retrieval in mind. This will be discussed in the next section. In addition, repeated experiences of making clinical judgements and treatment decisions about specific phenomena tends to build the connections (Squire et al, 1992).

Long term memory in clinical reasoning

Long term memory acts like a 'library' of knowledge and experience that a clinician consults to identify and interpret information in working memory. Long term memory appears to have unlimited capacity and little forgetting. However, problems can occur in gaining access to and retrieving knowledge and experience when they are needed.

The two major divisions of long term memory are semantic memory, containing knowledge, and episodic memory, containing experiences. These are highly interactive in clinical reasoning. Schmidt et al (1990) hypothesize that novices in clinical reasoning primarily use theoretical knowledge from semantic memory, gradually adding clinical knowledge, called 'problem scripts'. Expert clinicians rely more on 'patient instance scripts' drawn from episodic memory for comparison with findings in the current situation as a basis for making clinical judgements.

Access is gained to both semantic and episodic memory by transmission of a unit or chunk of information from working memory to long term memory. This accessing information from

the current situation tends to communicate common, essential properties associated with the phenomenon to be recognized and understood. Gaining access to the needed diagnostic concepts in long term memory is thought to begin with one concept and then to spread along connecting pathways to other related concepts as shown in Figure 14.3. This suggests that clinicians need to store theoretical knowledge by 'cross filing' it in terms of other potential diagnostic explanations as well as clinical ramifications. The term 'diagnostic explanations' is used in this paper in a generic sense as a category of problem or as a label for such a category within any health care discipline. It is not limited to the fields of pathology, pathophysiology or psychopathology (US Department of Health and Human Services, 1980; North American Nursing Diagnosis Association, 1984; Williams et al, 1989).

Findings in the current patient situation that confirm previous knowledge can be processed to strengthen that part of the semantic diagnostic concept or linkages between concepts. Those which extend or are at variance with one's currently-held knowledge can be used to modify the stored concept, as should disconfirming findings. In this way clinical practice and new knowledge are used in an ongoing way to sharpen one's diagnostic concepts and linkages in long term memory.

Patient instance scripts can be processed before storing these in episodic long term memory. Here too, one can think about the possible ramifications. The following is an example of a patient instance script.

> A woman with advanced Parkinson's disease is having increasing difficulty with self-feeding. She is also experiencing associated problems with disturbed self-esteem, nutritional deficit, satisfaction with food, dependence on others for food preparation and feeding, and environmental distractions. In addition, her care giver is experiencing problems of being 'tied down', and feeling inadequate and unappreciated.

In the patient instance and care giver instance files, the problems could be filed under Parkinson's self-feeding difficulties and cross-filed with the related problems.

EXERCISES ON STORING KNOWLEDGE AND PATIENT INSTANCES

1. As you learn about phenomena or situations in your discipline, think about the conditions

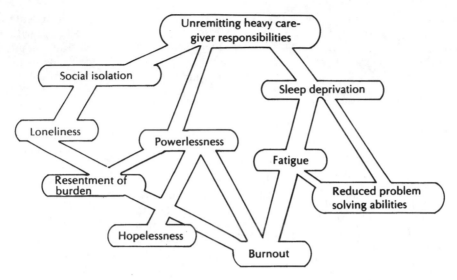

Figure 14.3 Example of linkages between diagnostic concepts in long term semantic memory. From Carnevali and Thomas (1993) with permission

under which you might need to retrieve this knowledge for use in clinical reasoning. Consider not only the main heading, but other possibilities. Identify the headings you would use if you were to file and cross-file this information in a filing cabinet or computer.

2. During your clinical experiences with patients, think about the patients' main problem and the ramifications or related difficulties they are experiencing. Identify the main heading and the cross-headings you might find useful if you were to seek to retrieve it.

3. When you are using either this knowledge or the related patient instance scripts at a later time, think about the earlier elements you stored and 'update your long term memory files' based on similarities or differences in the current patient instance.

Organization of knowledge for clinical reasoning

Diagnostic concepts (i.e. knowledge about any discipline-specific phenomenon or situation) which are stored with a consistent structure can offer greater ease of access for future clinical reasoning and ongoing storage of new knowledge. In the medical field, knowledge about pathology is usually organized to highlight the nature of the phenomenon, recognition features, prognostic variables, complications,

and treatment options. Other disciplines can use a comparable organizational structure to advantage (refer to Carnevali and Reiner (1990) for examples of organizational structures in nursing).

Since professional expertise in clinical reasoning is based upon access to correct, up-to-date knowledge and appropriate use of earlier clinical experiences, efficient storage and updating of one's clinical (knowledge) files is an ongoing professional responsibility. There is no question that new knowledge and experience regularly move from working memory to long term memory without awareness. On the other hand, thinking about future uses of new information and about patient instances in relation to clinical reasoning can provide a useful basis for the effective storage of such information in long term memory, and can make it more accessible for future clinical reasoning (Moscovitch and Craik, 1976; Baddeley,1990).

EXERCISES IN THE USE OF AN ORGANIZATIONAL SYSTEM FOR STORING KNOWLEDGE

1. Set up a structural outline for storing knowledge in your discipline, preferably one that highlights recognition features such as risk factors and manifestations, underlying mechanisms differential diagnoses or problem categories, prognostic variables, complications of untreated problems and

iatrogenic complications, treatment or management options and evaluation criteria. After each heading, identify relevant content in each category based on the knowledge and perspectives of your discipline.

2. Select a diagnostic concept or problem area commonly occurring in your discipline with which you are personally familiar. Using the theoretical and clinical knowledge and experience you already possess, organize your knowledge using the structural guidelines developed in Exercise 1. Refine your diagnostic concept by consulting the literature as needed, and by testing it in your encounters with patients who have problems within this diagnostic concept. Repeat this exercise with additional concepts until your concept library attains consistent structure.

Using patient instances

As clinicians develop professional practice expertise a transition is made in the clinical reasoning process they adopt. Initially their reasoning relies heavily on the use of theoretical knowledge. Increasingly, however, their reasoning relies more on the recall and use of patient instances scripts as the basis for recognizing and understanding the presenting situation (Schmidt et al, 1990). This suggests that patient instances, like new knowledge, need to be 'filed' in some systematic way. Each patient instance offers either confirmation of, or variation from, earlier patterns of risk factors, etiology and manifestations. It can also offer a strengthening of previously encountered linkages with related problem areas or new areas. Some degree of awareness of the need to update one's patient instance script file with new patient encounters is important for professional growth.

EXERCISES ON STORING PATIENT INSTANCES

1. Using a diagnostic concept and related problem areas developed in the exercise on structuring knowledge, recall patients who fall into this category. Assign a specific recognition tag to each patient instance, such as 'miscommunication, Parkinsonian facial immobility, Mary and her sister, Jim and wife' (Carnevali and Thomas, 1993; Linde, 1993). Consider the linkages to related problems being experienced by the patient or others and crossfile the patient instance also under these headings. Identify previously encountered patients, family members or care givers who might fit under the heading and tag them with the identification feature that highlights the differences. As you encounter new patients or family members who evidence variations within the major problem area, apply the same analytical tagging and linking processes.

Using the clinical reasoning process

Activities actually undertaken in the processing of information involved in clinical reasoning are certainly not linear, even though diagrammed steps and logic would make them seem to be so. However, it is possible to:

- identify components of the reasoning process (see Table 14.1)
- achieve a working understanding of them
- develop skill in the use of each of them.

For a full description of and additional exercises for each of the components, see Chapter 3 in Carnevali and Thomas (1993).

The clinical reasoning process can be used with or without awareness. Therefore it seems wise to initially and periodically check on one's current practices in the clinical reasoning process to determine whether unwanted or ineffective strategies are being used.

EXERCISES IN COMPONENTS OF CLINICAL REASONING

1. *Use of pre-encounter information*

   (a) Examine completed admission or intake forms for several patients. Notice items such as name, sex, age, marital status, address, religious preference, ethnicity, and other categories of information. Identify how each item of pre-encounter information directs your attention or otherwise affects your subsequent data gathering and clinical reasoning about the patient.

   (b) What pre-encounter information do you prefer to have before entering a patient situation for the first time? Why is this particular information important to

Table 14.1 Components of the diagnostic reasoning process

- Collection of pre-encounter data about patient situation*
- Entry into the patient situation

  Make a quick overview
  Do an urgency scaling for data collection or action
  Determine strategies for gathering patient data
  Structure role and nursing perspective for patient

- Collection of data using screening or problem-oriented approach
- Coalescing of data into related chunks in working memory
- Selection of cue or cue cluster of highest priority for initial diagnosing
- Retrieval of possible diagnostic explanations or patient instances from long term memory

  Move from general to specific
  Consider competing or alternative diagnostic explanations

- Utilization of recognition features associated with the retrieved diagnostic concepts as guides for observation of patient and situation
- Comparison of data in patient situation to recognition features in diagnostic concept, problem script or patient instances
- Assignment of a diagnosis if the data fit the recognition features of one of the retrieved diagnoses, problem scripts or patient instances

OR IF NONE FITS

* Pre-encounter data may or may not involve clinical judgement. If information is deliberately sought out by the nurse, judgement is involved. If the nurse is exposed to data without taking initiative, no clinical judgement is involved.
From Carnevali and Thomas (1993) with permission.

you? How does it make you feel more comfortable in the patient encounter? Ask others the same question and compare your findings. What are the advantages and disadvantages of obtaining pre-encounter information?

2. *Entry into the patient situation*

   (a) Initial scanning of the patient situation. What pattern or sequence of observation do you use to gain a quick grasp of clinical situations? Compare your patterns with those of others in your own field, in other specialties in your field, and in other health care disciplines.
   (b) Urgency scaling.
   After initially scanning a patient situation rank the identified data in terms of their relative urgency for data collection using a 5 point urgency scale with descriptors of your own devising for each urgency level. Engage in cross-specialty or cross-discipline comparisons of urgency scaling on patients.

   (c) Determining strategies for data gathering.
   Encounter several patients. Make initial scanning observations of each one and then make a conscious judgement about how you will purposefully adjust your data collection to take into account their psychophysiological status, age, ethnicity and language.
   (d) Structuring the patient/person's role and perspective.
   Role play a patient situation in which you as a professional in your own health care field help the 'patient' to become aware of your focus for data collection and the way in which you wish them to participate in the subsequent assessment.

3. *Determining whether to use a comprehensive or problem-oriented approach to the patient data base*
   Identify variables used in your discipline to determine the circumstances under which comprehensive versus focused approaches

are more appropriate and cost effective. Test these criteria with patients who have different pathology, medical treatment plans, length of stay, and care settings.

4. *Coalescing data into related chunks*
Gather data on a patient. During or after the data collection identify the data chunks you developed. Describe the patient to colleagues from another clinical specialty or discipline (without chunking the data) and ask them how they would cluster the data. Compare your results.

5. *Selecting the cue or chunk for initial assessment*
Using the patient on whom you gathered data in (4), determine which patient cue or cluster of cues you would select as a focus for initial follow-up in data collection. Which other cues or chunks would you later pursue in your assessment?

6. *Retrieving possible diagnostic explanations or patient instances from long term memory*
Using the cue or cue cluster from (5), retrieve from your long term memory possible diagnostic explanations for them. Move from general to specific. How many possibilities or related problems did you retrieve? Think of other closely linked (alternative) problem areas or diagnostic explanations that should also be considered in order to obtain the most precise identification of the problem

7. *Utilization of recognition features as observation guides*
Using the specific, alternative diagnostic explanations generated in Exercise 6, list the recognition features associated with each one. For instance such a list could be as follows: anger stage of grieving, event experienced as a loss of sufficient magnitude to generate an emotional response, versus anger as a response to frustration, a significant goal, a barrier, strong dissatisfaction (Carnevali and Thomas, 1993). Use these lists as observational guides in patient situations.

8. *Comparison of data in a patient situation to identified features*
Use the observational guides of recognition features to observe data in patient situations. Compare your findings with the patterns in the observational guides. Do the guides allow you to recognize problem areas or to differentiate between problem areas that have some of the same manifestations and risk factors? Modify and sharpen your observational guides from both ongoing theoretical and clinical encounters.

9. *Options if none of the original 'diagnoses' adequately fit and explain the situation*
It is not unusual, given the complexity of patients' problems that initial problem identifications do not fit. Then clinicians return to earlier components in the clinical reasoning process such as gathering additional data or considering other explanations for the current findings. Recall situations in which your earlier 'diagnoses' did not fit. Identify the strategies you used to proceed. What additional data did you seek? What other diagnostic avenues did you consider? How would you modify the diagnostic concepts and patient instances in your long term memory to incorporate this diagnostic experience?

Conclusion

The people who depend upon professionals for care in health and illness bring with them the complexities inherent in all human beings. Their presenting problems in health promotion, risk reduction, or in living with pathology and its treatment are rarely simple. Therefore, real challenges face health care professionals in any discipline who seek to provide care that is tailored to the individual's situation and is also rational, therapeutic, and cost effective.

Clinical reasoning is the critical foundation to problem identification and resultant treatment decisions. Individuals in some disciplines have thought that the process should be made simple. Unfortunately this is not possible, given the complexity of human beings and their health problems. The only solution is to accept the difficulty as given and then to strive to master the knowledge base, the data collection skills, and the cognitive processes needed to adequately address the requirements in the situation.

Achieving and maintaining excellence in clinical reasoning in any health care field is a lifelong pursuit. Only by acknowledging its difficulties and regularly engaging in critical practice is it possible to gain the consistent competence required to effectively and predictably meet patients' and their families' health care needs.

References

Anderson, J.F. (1985) *Cognitive Psychology and its Implications.*, 2nd edn. Freeman, New York

Ashcraft, M. (1989) *Human Memory and Cognition.* Scott Foresman and Co, Glenview, Illinois

Baddeley, A. (1990) *Human Memory.* Allyn and Bacon, Boston

Benner, P. (1984) *From Novice to Expert: Excellence and Power in Clinical Nursing Practice.* Addison-Wesley, Menlo Park, California

Carnevali, D. and Reiner, A. (1990) *The Cancer Experience: Nursing Diagnosis and Management.* J.B. Lippincott, Philadelphia

Carnevali, D. (1986) Loneliness. In *Nursing Management for the Elderly*, 2nd edn (eds D. Carnevali and M. Patrick). J.B. Lippincott, Philadelphia, pp. 287–298.

Carnevali, D. and Thomas, M. (1993) *Diagnostic Reasoning and Treatment Decision Making in Nursing.* J.B. Lippincott, Philadelphia

Coltheart, M. (1983) Iconic memory. *Philosophical Transactions of the Royal Society of London*, **B302**, 283–294

Copstead, L.E. (1993) Families and caretakers of the elderly. In *Nursing Management for the Elderly*, 3rd edn (eds D. Carnevali and M. Patrick). J.B. Lippincott, Philadelphia, pp. 239–249

Corcoran, S. (1986a) Task complexity and nursing expertise as factors in decision making. *Nursing Research*, **35**, 107–112

Corcoran, S. (1986b) Expert and novice nurses' use of knowledge to plan for pain control: How clinicians make their decisions. *The American Journal of Hospice Care*, **3**, 37–41

Craik, F. and Lockhart, R. (1972) Levels of processing: A framework for memory research. *Journal of Verbal Learning and Verbal Behavior*, **11**, 671–684

Dawson, N. and Arkes, H. (1987) Systematic errors in medical decision making. *Journal of General Internal Medicine*, **2**, 183–187

Elstein, A.S., Shulman, L.S. and Sprafka, S.A. (1978) *Medical Problem Solving: An Analysis of Clinical Reasoning.* Harvard University Press, Cambridge, Massachusetts

Ericsson, K., Chase, W. and Faloon, S. (1980) Acquisition of a memory skill. *Science*, **208**, 1181–1182

Foley, K. (1987) Pain syndromes in patients with cancer. In *Cancer Pain* (eds M. Swedolow and V. Ventafridda). Hastings Hilderly, London

Larkin, J., McDermott, J., Simon, D. and Simon, H. (1980) Expert and novice performance in solving physics problems. *Science*, **208**, 1135–1142

Linde, M. (1993) Parkinson's Disease. In *Nursing Management for the Elderly*, 3rd edn (eds D. Carnevali and M. Patrick). J.B. Lippincott, Philadelphia, pp. 334–347

Miller, G. (1956) The magical number seven, plus or minus two: Some limitations on our capacity for processing information. *Psychological Review*, **63**, 81–97

Moscovitch, M. and Craik, F. (1976) Depth of processing, retrieval cues and uniqueness of encoding as factors in recall. *Journal of Verbal Learning and Verbal Behavior*, **15**, 447–458

North American Nursing Diagnosis Association. (1984) Classification of nursing diagnoses. In *Proceedings of the Fifth Conference of the North American Nursing Diagnosis Association* (eds M.J. Kim, G.K. McFarland and A.M. McLane). Mosby, St Louis

Salame, P. and Baddeley, A. (1982) Disruption of short-term memory by unattended speech: Implications for the structure of working memory. *Journal of Verbal Learning and Verbal Behavior*, **21**, 150–164

Schmidt, H., Norman, G. and Boshuizen, H. (1990) A cognitive perspective on medical expertise: Theory and implications. *Academic Medicine*, **65**, 611–621

Squire, L., Ojemann, J., Mielin, F., Peterson, S. Videen, T. and Raichle, M. (1992) Activation of the hippocampus in normal humans: A functional anatomical study of memory. *Proceedings of the National Academy of Sciences*, **89**, 1837–1841

Tanner, C.A. (1984) Toward development of diagnostic reasoning skills. In *Diagnostic Reasoning in Nursing* (eds D. Carnevali, P. Mitchell, N. Woods and C. Tanner). J.B. Lippincott, Philadelphia, pp. 57–104

Tanner, C.A., Padrick, K.P., Westfall, U. and Putzier, D. (1987) Diagnostic reasoning strategies of nursing and nursing students. *Nursing Research*, **36**, 358–363

US Dept of Health and Human Services (1980) *International Classification of Diseases*, 9th revision. *Clinical Revision*, 2nd edn. Washington, DC

Waldrop, M. (1987) The workings of working memory. *Science*, **237**, 1564–1567

Wild, L., Craven, R. and Cunningham, S. (1991) Assessment of vascular function. In *Medical Surgical Nursing: Pathophysiological Concepts* (2nd edn) (eds M. Patrick, S. Woods, R. Craven, J. Rokosky and P. Bruno). J.B. Lippincott, Philadelphia, pp. 802–811

Williams, J.B., Karls, J.M. and Wandrei, K. (1989) The person-in-environment (PIE) system for describing problems of social functioning. *Hospital and Community Psychiatry*, **40**, 1125–1127

Wills, R. (1993) Delirium and dementia. In *Nursing Management for the Elderly*, 3rd edn (eds D. Carnevali and M. Patrick). J.B. Lippincott, Philadelphia, pp. 265–278

Section Four

Approaches to teaching clinical reasoning

15

The case study as an instructional method to teach clinical reasoning

Susan Prion and Robert P. Graby

Schools of nursing are becoming increasingly cognizant of the need to teach students the clinical reasoning skills that they will need to be successful as practising nurses. Studies of the clinical reasoning of experienced nurses have provided great insight into the processes that they use in day-to-day problem solving regarding patient care (Carnevali et al, 1984; Corcoran, 1986; Tanner et al, 1987; Radwin, 1990; Fonteyn, 1991). However, studies of the educational methods useful for teaching clinical reasoning are limited in number and scope.

The current work at the University of San Francisco described in this chapter is an attempt to meet the challenge of teaching clinical reasoning. Based on a model suggested by the survey of research on clinical reasoning by Radwin (1990), the authors have developed a system for teaching clinical reasoning using case studies to simulate the reality of patient care situations. This case study approach promotes a realistic analysis of patient condition, a holistic application of the clinical reasoning process and an opportunity to apply information from the entire nursing curriculum.

Case studies as an instructional method are particularly useful to provide a model of the clinical reasoning process for students. The opportunity for questions to the expert instructor about specific content, inferences that were made, cue groupings, decision making about relevant and irrelevant cues, and the types of additional information that would be needed are all very helpful for the beginning student

to start to approximate the clinical reasoning processes of competent nurses.

The chapter will briefly describe a clinical reasoning model used by the authors as the theoretical basis for a successful educational strategy using case studies. The chapter will explain and describe the case study method, outline the different types of case studies, discuss how to design an effective case study and describe the factors to consider when using a case study as an educational tool. Finally, we will provide an example of a case study that has been used to teach didactic content and also to demonstrate the clinical reasoning process to beginning student nurses.

The clinical reasoning model

The clinical reasoning process model (see Figure 15.1) used by the authors at the University of San Francisco is loosely based on the work of Radwin (1990) who surveyed research on diagnostic reasoning carried out in the 1970s and 1980s. These studies describe components and stages that are common to most models of the diagnostic reasoning process. From Radwin's delineation of diagnostic reasoning stages, the authors have formulated a model of clinical reasoning that is used as a basis for educational methods that elicit the desired clinical reasoning behaviours in students.

In any clinical situation, the nurse is initially confronted with a set of presenting cues that the

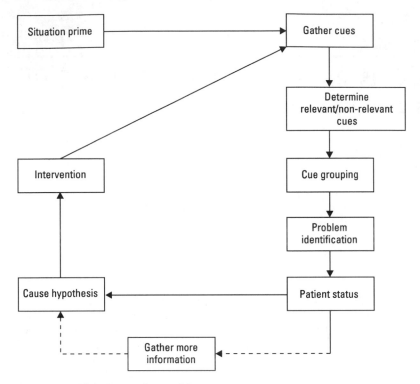

Figure 15.1   Clinical reasoning model

authors have designated as the 'situation prime'. Cues may consist of the patient's medical diagnosis, the topic of the practice case study or the patient's chief complaint. The situation prime acts as a crude sifting mechanism which immediately narrows the field of possible diagnostic hypotheses. If the situation prime predicts that this is a cardiac patient, an array of non-cardiac diagnoses are immediately eliminated, and those areas of potential cardiac problems and interventions are promptly activated in long-term memory. The nurse now has a framework or template against which to begin the process of specific cue gathering

Guided by the situation prime, the nurse begins to gather cues (pieces of information) that will help identify the specific patient problem. These may be laboratory or diagnostic test results, clinical signs and symptoms, physical assessment data and/or information from reports of other health care team members. Again, the situation prime has focused the nurse's investigation on a limited number of diagnoses. Cue gathering is the first step towards identification of the presenting problem from that limited list of possible diagnoses.

A critical feature of the cue gathering stage is the grouping and prioritizing of cues. This involves the examination of available patient information and a discrimination is made between relevant and non-relevant cues. For example, shortness of breath is a relevant cue for a cardiac patient. A slight rise in body temperature is usually an irrelevant cue for this type of patient. The outcome of this reasoning stage is a number of cues which the nurse has concluded are related to the situation prime or presenting problem.

Once these relevant cues are gathered, the nurse then begins to infer relationships among cues and groups cues together. These groupings may be by subjective features, physical signs and symptoms, organ systems and/or potential clinical disease patterns. All the groups combine to build an accurate picture of the patient situation.

This process of cue grouping is guided by two factors: the situation prime and existing patterns of knowledge (called schemata) in memory. The situation prime has already introduced our hypothetical cardiac patient situation. This contextual clue has limited the list of possible presenting problems but still leaves a large number of potential causes for the current situation. It is now that the nurse begins to compare these relevant groups of cues to patterns of knowledge of similar situations stored in memory. Simply put, the question is: 'What does this look like that I have seen before?'. In our education for clinical reasoning these patterns of knowledge are established through the repeated use of the case studies, which become reasonable adjuncts to clinical experience.

After cue grouping, the nurse considers possible hypotheses that might explain these groups. This step is labelled 'Problem Identification Hypothesis'. At this point, there may be more than one plausible hypothesis that may explain the patient's condition. A hypothesis is now retained or rejected depending on its alignment with the grouping of relevant cues.

The goal here is the identification of the problem. For example, the cues 'pallor' and 'diaphoresis' could indicate chest pain, a cardiac arrhythmia and/or hypotension. At this point, the patient's clinical status may demand that the nurse initiate emergency care for the patient, regardless of the cause of the presenting problem. For example, if our cardiac patient has extremely high blood pressure, the nurse may not have time to identify the cause of the rise in pressure. The critical issue is to deal with the immediate symptom and lower the blood pressure before it becomes life threatening. If the pressure is high but not life threatening, the nurse may have the time to gather additional information to determine the cause of the problem and then move to an intervention.

This stage in the clinical reasoning process is the identification of the Cause Hypothesis. The nurse asks 'Why is the patient experiencing this problem?' Determining the cause of the presenting problem is necessary to differentiate the appropriate interventions. The nurse continues to gather and group cues for ongoing evaluation of the correctness of the identified hypothesis and treatment. Once an intervention has been enacted, the clinical reasoning process revolves back upon itself, and the nurse again gathers and groups cues, hypotheses, checks the status of the patient and intervenes as required to stabilize the patient.

Of clear and obvious importance is how this theoretical model is translated into practice in the nursing school classroom. Research has shown that clinical reasoning skills are best acquired in settings that most closely approxi-mate the real patient situations that the nursing student will face in actual clinical practice (Resnick, 1987a; Tanner et al, 1987; Brown et al, 1989; Resnick, 1987b). However, it is not possible nor particularly desirable to duplicate the reality of the clinical situation in the classroom, especially for beginning nursing students. Despite the limitations of simulations as an educational methodology in health care settings, the rudimentary concepts of the clinical reasoning model can be instantiated through the use of case studies. This educational tool provides the nursing student with the closest approximation to real patient situations within the classroom.

There are many significant reasons for using a case study as an educational method to teach the clinical reasoning process to nursing students. When utilized with the appropriate guidance, questioning and feedback from experienced clinical nurse educators, case studies offer numerous opportunities for the student to exercise clinical reasoning in a simulation of a real situation, model exemplary decision-making behaviour, demonstrate accurate thought processes used to solve clinical problems, make and correct mistakes in a controlled and safe situation, identify assumptions, biases, and values that impact in a given situation, integrate information from the entire nursing curriculum, apply knowledge, acquire new knowledge, measure and evaluate knowledge acquisition and measure and evaluate the outcomes of the clinical reasoning process.

Case studies have been used very successfully as an educational method in the professions of medicine, law and business, engineering and education (Epstein, 1981; Oldham and Forrester, 1981; Bernheimer, 1982; Zarr, 1984; Kreps and Lederman, 1985; Christensen, 1987; McCarthy, 1987; Baxter, 1988; Carter and Unklesbay, 1989; Rasinski, 1989; Taylor, 1989; Boehrer and Linsky, 1990; Sansalone, 1990; Harrington, 1991; Merseth, 1991; Nagel, 1991; Boyce, 1992; Feinstein and Veenendall, 1992; Gist, 1992; Hartman, 1992; McWilliam, 1992; Gale, 1993). They are particularly useful in nursing education because the case study approach is one of the few educational methods that promotes the integration of the psychological, social, emotional, physical, and affective aspects of patient care in a controlled situation that prevents harm to the patient. In addition, varying the complexity of case studies allows the teacher to help students progress in their ability to deal with increasingly difficult and complex clinical problems.

Case study development

The process of writing a valid and reliable case study is labour-intensive but not complicated. The first and most important question the author needs to ask is 'What is the purpose of this case study?'. There are four major reasons for using a case study: (a) to teach students patient assessment and evaluation of patient data; (b) to promote integration and application of knowledge; (c) to teach specific content; and (d) to teach and evaluate reasoning skills.

The second step is to articulate clearly the specific objectives that the case study is designed to achieve. These objectives should be written according to the criteria for optimal behavioural objectives: measurable behaviour, conditions for accomplishment and criteria for successful performance (Mager, 1975). Next, the case study author needs to describe in detail the learners who will use the case study. Previous knowledge, age, level in school and timing during the semester all factor into the type and level of the case study.

The priorities and constraints of the educational situation require serious consideration. First, the size of the class must be taken into account. An educator may use a case study as a small group or individual student written task, or may discuss it with all the students participating during class. Student participation could be difficult in very large classes, but would work quite well in small ones. In addition, the classroom size and configuration should be examined. A large classroom with fixed chairs and desks does not lend itself to small group work.

Next, the case study author should determine the amount of time allotted for the class. The case study format may be determined by the time available to work on the case study. A more complex case study requires more time for effective use.

The purpose of the case study should be determined early in the development process. Does the instructor plan to use the case study instead of the content lecture, as a basis for the class discussion? Or, does the instructor plan to use the case study as an example to illustrate the points made in the class presentation? The complexity of the case study will be partially determined by its purpose.

The educational materials that are currently available to both instructors and students need to be catalogued. Some universities have a rich library of print, audiovisual and computer-assisted case studies that can be easily integrated into the classroom. If the appropriate materials are not easily available, then the instructor will need the time and resources to develop those materials. Complete and comprehensive case studies take time and careful thought to prepare.

The delivery logistic of the case study needs to be determined. Options include handing out the written case study in class, handing out the written case study before class, handing out the case study after class, using the case study as an audiovisual display, and presenting the case study verbally. If class time is limited, it would be better to give out the case study before class rather than allowing time in class for reading it. If a collaborative analysis of the case study by the entire class is planned, then using the case study as an audiovisual display or presenting the case study verbally would be most useful. Each option depends upon the purpose for the case study and the logistics of the individual class.

The author next needs to consider the specific content to be included in the case study. Categories of content can include the general information about the simulated patient such as name, age, gender, height, weight, social habits, profession/job and education, past medical/surgical history, patient's current status, the chief complaint, physical exam results, lab values, medications, and psychosocial information. Information about the patient's environment, or a specific patient situation can also be provided. This is information that the student would be expected to collect from the patient, the patient's chart or the patient's situation before providing care.

We find three major types of case studies to be most useful. The selection of case study format will depend upon the purpose of the case study and the other considerations discussed previously.

The first type of case study is the *stable case study*. This presents a body of static information and then asks the student about that information. Its purpose is to transmit information, identify assumptions and/or allow assessment of general or specific information contained in the case study. Stable case studies are relatively easy to write and are the easiest type for students to engage in. Stable case studies are very useful with beginning students. The most significant disadvantage to the use of stable case studies is their lack of approximation to a real, dynamic patient situation. That is, students are not required to judge what information is needed or extract the information themselves. Stable case studies can be helpful to demonstrate reasoning about a set of patient data, but cannot demonstrate the clinical reasoning process over time. Table 15.1 gives an example of this type of static case study.

The *dynamic case study* is a more sophisticated format in which the students are given a body of patient information, questioned about it, then given more information and more questions. Built into this case study format are changes in the patient's status. Dynamic case studies can be used to assess or predict changes in the patient's physical, emotional or psychological status over time, and are excellent tools to demonstrate and evaluate application and synthesis of complex information. They are more realistic and more sophisticated than the

stable case study. Care must be taken to manage dynamic case studies so that the student does not become lost or overwhelmed by the complexity of information provided. This is especially true if the case study is being used in a small group, and each student takes a different amount of time to answer the questions posed about the case. The amount of information provided and the level of probing questions used with the dynamic case study can vary with the level of student and the time available for case study analysis. Table 15.2 illustrates an example of a dynamic case study.

The third major case study format is the *dynamic case study with expert feedback*. This approach combines the advantages of the dynamic case study with the educational benefit of immediate feedback to student responses. It is a very effective method to illustrate one or more satisfactory reasoning pathways by comparing student responses and decisions with satisfactory or exemplary decisions made by identified experts. While all case study formats provide feedback upon completion of the case study analysis, the dynamic case study with expert feedback builds in written or verbal expert feedback after they answer each set of questions. The case study analysis involves

Table 15.1 Static case study example

Mrs. Smith is a 47 year old woman admitted with a pain in her left side. She has a 3 day history of nausea and vomiting. She complains of severe pain unrelieved by aspirin or Tylenol.

Vital signs: heart rate 112, blood pressure 145/72, respiratory rate 28, temperature 101.2 °F
Labs: Na 144, K 4.9, glucose 122

1. List 3 important assessment cues about Mrs. Smith
2. What would your most immediate nursing priority be for Mrs. Smith?

Table 15.2 Dynamic case study example

Mrs. Smith is a 47 year old woman admitted with a pain in her left side. She has a 3 day history of nausea and vomiting. She complains of severe pain unrelieved by aspirin or Tylenol.

Vital signs: heart rate 112, blood pressure 145/72, respiratory rate 28, temperature 101.2 °F
Labs: Na 144, K 4.9, glucose 122

1. List 3 important assessment cues about Mrs. Smith
2. What would your most immediate nursing priority be for Mrs. Smith?

Three hours after admission, she vomits 250 cc of bright red blood.

3. What other information do you need to assess Mrs. Smith's clinical status?
4. What is the first thing that you would do for her?

---

several sets of questions, after each new block of information is added to the case. By receiving feedback on their evolving thoughts and decisions, students are able to adjust their reasoning during the case and come to a solution along with the expert rather than simply be 'corrected' in hindsight. There may be more than one feasible reasoning pathway, of which the expert response is only one. Students are encouraged to examine both their own and the expert's responses and rationalize or explain their choice of response. We have found that the most important point here is to stress the role of the expert response. The expert's answers are not the only correct answer, but the expert's response also provides a framework for the students to study the method and outcome of the clinical reasoning process. Table 15.3 provides an example of a dynamic case study with expert feedback.

Case study question development

The final step in constructing an educational case study is to formulate a list of questions for the students that will help to promote the critical thinking and discussion which will thereby fulfil the purpose of the case study. The educational motive for the case study, whether to review important information, provide a knowledge application/integration

opportunity or test clinical reasoning ability, will be an invaluable guide for structuring questions. The level of the student in his/her program of study and timing of the case study use within the specific course (early or late), will affect the questioning strategy. Beginning nursing students have less clinical experience than more advanced students. Their facility with medical terminology is often primitive, and they are less knowledgeable than more experienced students about lab values and medications. For these reasons, the case study should be carefully written and reviewed by several educators to make sure that the overall structure of the example (wording, content, assumptions about supporting knowledge) is consistent with the level of the student group. Many students have not worked with case studies in previous classes, and take some time to become familiar with the process. Case studies used early in the course should be more straightforward and shorter in length than those examples used towards the end of the course.

The sequencing of questions about the case study can follow one of several formats. A hierarchical approach, such as Bloom's taxonomy (Bloom et al, 1956) or Belenky's structure (Belenky et al, 1986) can be useful to move from primitive, low cognitive level questioning, to more generalizable, sophisticated queries. Low cognitive level questions ask the

Table 15.3   Dynamic case study with expert feedback

Mrs. Smith is a 47 year old woman admitted with a pain in her left side. She has a 3 day history of nausea and vomiting. She complains of severe pain unrelieved by aspirin or Tylenol.

Vital signs: heart rate 112, blood pressure 145/72, respiratory rate 28, temperature 101.2 °F
Labs: Na 144, K 4.9, glucose 122

1.   List 4 important assessment cues about Mrs. Smith
2.   What would your most immediate nursing priority be for Mrs. Smith?

Expert response: You have a lot of info about this patient. She has severe pain in her abdomen, nausea and vomiting, ×3 days and her vital signs (VS) are all elevated. The VS could be up because of her pain or because she is having some other sort of stress, like a peptic ulcer bleed. After 3 days of nausea and vomiting, I'd really worry that she was dehydrated – in fact, her Na is 144, probably due to fluid loss. My first concern would be for pain relief, but I would also want some more information about her fluid status.

Three hours after admission, she vomits 250 cc of bright red blood.

3.   What other information do you need to assess Mrs. Smith's clinical status?

Expert response: Well, now we have a better idea of what's going on. I would immediately want a set of VS and to subjectively assess how Mrs. Smith is doing.

learner to recall a fact in a similar form to that in which it was presented ('What was the patients blood pressure? Is this higher or lower than a normal blood pressure?'). Higher cognitive level questions require some analysis, synthesis or evaluation of the information presented and the decisions made based on that information ('How do you know that your intervention was effective? What would you tell the patient's family at this time?'). A time-oriented questioning strategy ('What comes first? What would you do next') can help clarify and consolidate a dynamic case study. A priorities-oriented strategy ('What is your first concern? Next priority?') is useful to promote application, synthesis and problem formulation.

The questioning sequence we use flows directly from our conceptual model of clinical reasoning (see Figure 15.1.). The questions are structured as follows:

1. State the situation prime.
   i.e. What does your knowledge of the patient's history, chief complaint, diagnosis, and/or current situation lead you to suspect about the patient?
2. List all the available cues that are present in the case study.
3. In writing, categorize these cues into relevant and irrelevant cues categories based on the situation prime.
4. Organize the cues into meaningful groups based on your previous knowledge.
   i.e. Do these relevant cues suggest a disease or patient condition? Does this 'sound like' anything you already know?
5. List all plausible hypotheses that you can think of that would fit (explain) these cues.
6. Under each hypothesis, list all other infor-, mation you would need to gather to accept or reject each of the alternatives.
7. Based upon available and accessible information, select and state a problem/diagnosis hypothesis.
8. List the status of the diagnosis as emergency (immediate intervention), high risk or low risk, or potential risk.
9. Regroup available cues to develop a hypothesis about the possible cause(s) of the patient's condition.

Regardless of the case study format selected, the sequencing and alignment of questions with the conceptual model of reasoning presented in Figure 15.1 promotes modelling of orderly and effective reasoning, and provides frequent opportunities for the instructor to correct knowledge demonstrated errors in the student's reasoning process.

Application

What follows is an example of this case study process in an actual classroom situation. The authors expect that this case study method could be used effectively for any nursing content area, including traditionally 'difficult' subjects such as anatomy and physiology, pathophysiology and pharmacology.

This particular case study is used to teach clinical reasoning about congestive heart failure (CHF) to nursing students in an undergraduate pathophysiology course.

Purpose

The purpose of this case study is to provide a model of the clinical reasoning process concerning the patient with CHF and to reinforce content about CHF.

Learners

The students using this case study are all first or second year undergraduate nursing students who have as general prerequisites an anatomy and physiology class, basic normal physical assessment and basic lab value assessment skills including normal values for sodium (Na), potassium (K), glucose (gluc), blood urea nitrogen (BUN), creatinine, and creatinine phosphokinase–myocardial band (CPK–MB). Specific prerequisite knowledge for this case study includes: anatomy of the cardiovascular system; the normal route of blood flow through the body, traced from the left ventricle; definitions of preload and afterload; how to calculate cardiac output (CO), stroke volume (SV), ejection fraction (EF), left ventricular end diastolic pressure (LVEDP); normal pressures in the 4 chambers of heart and the pulmonary circulation; neural regulation of heart rate (HR), contractility and vascular diameter. Before the class in which this case study is to be used, the students have completed reading assignments in the assigned pathophysiology text about CHF.

Objectives:

The objectives of this case study are to:

1. Identify the relevant cues that indicate the clinical status of a given patient with CHF.
2. Identify all potential complications for the patient with CHF.
3. Describe nursing interventions to manage these complications.
4. Describe the expected medical interventions to treat these complications.
5. Explain the pathophysiological cause of each sign and symptom of CHF.
6. Relate the clinical signs and symptoms and treatments of CHF to the pathophysiology changes.

Priorities and constraints of situation

The priorities of the situation are the class size (40 students) and the timing of the class (halfway through a fifteen week semester). The class is scheduled for 80 minutes in the late afternoon in a classroom with movable desks. The case study was developed by the instructor, and is given to the students at the end of a lecture/discussion about the topic congestive heart failure. In class, the students form small groups of five to six students. The groups work on the case study for about 20 minutes, then share their answers with the entire class. Because the learners are beginning nursing students and the case study is used about halfway through the semester, the instructor has chosen to use a stable case study. The focus of this exercise for these beginning students is identification and interpretation of clinical cues and recognition of pattern in the information. In other activities where inquiry, planning and evolution of thought processes are stressed, a dynamic case study format would be preferred. Table 15.4 shows the case study information and the questions asked as they would appear on a single piece of paper for the student groups. Each student receives his/her own copy of the case study.

This case study aimed to exemplify the patient with congestive heart failure, a common clinical situation encountered by nursing students. Numerous cues are presented that allow the students to think about the physical, emotional and psychosocial implications of this disease for this patient. His physical status is that of a stereotypic congestive heart failure patient. In addition, his laboratory values and vital signs provide information very common for patients with this disorder. The psychosocial information gives the student some ideas for discharge planning for this patient.

The systematic progression of student and instructor through the case study questions at the end of the case study gives opportunities to assess the student's knowledge of CHF and his/her ability to apply this cognitive information to a simulated patient situation. The student can identify relevant and irrelevant cues and receive immediate feedback about those choices from the instructor. In addition, the student can make incorrect decisions without harm to the patient.

Conclusions

The case study approach has been used successfully as an instructional method for undergraduate nursing students at the University of San Francisco. We have not directly assessed their critical thinking skills through a test such as the Watson–Glaser (1964), but we have measured instructional effectiveness in several other ways.

First, we have tracked the final course grades for classes of students in pathophysiology, both before and after case studies were instituted as a primary teaching/learning technique. The overall course averages have increased approximately ten points (one letter grade for our school) since case studies were formally integrated into the lesson plans.

We have systematically investigated the students' perceptions of their learning achievements and also of the teaching method. Through the use of a validated survey, focus groups, open-ended written evaluations and specific classroom assessment techniques, we have gathered rich data about the case study method. The students consistently rate the case study activities 'thought aloud' with the instructor as the most valuable and useful part of the course. A typical student comment is: 'The case studies make it real for me. You retain the information much better than if you had to memorize a list of signs and symptoms. And when we talk about it, I can see how my

Table 15.4   Congestive heart failure case study

Mr. Jones is a 64 year old man with a history of two prior myocardial infarctions. He is admitted to your unit complaining of extreme shortness of breath, dispnoea on exertion, 2–3 pillow orthopnoea and ankle oedema, all increasing over the last 3 days. He was a postal worker forced to retire after his second heart attack 3 years ago.

Physical exam: Elderly-looking man in moderate respiratory distress, sitting upright at side of bed; lung sounds – bilateral crackles 1/2 way up, heart sounds – inaudible because of loud lung sounds; +3 oedema of lower extremities to knees, feet cool and unable to palpate pedal pulses, present with Doppler; Foley catheter to gravity draining scant amounts of dark yellow urine.

Psych/social: He lives in a third storey apartment with his wife of 42 years.

Meds: Digoxin 0.25 mg orally every day, Lasix 80 mg orally three times a day and as needed, KCL 40 mEq orally every day

Vital signs: heart rate 126, blood pressure 104/78, respiratory rate 28, temperature 99.6 °F

Labs: Na 145, K 3.7, gluc 148, BUN 18, creatinine 1.9, CPK–MB 5%

Intake and output: 24 hour intake = 800 cc 24 hour output = 240 cc

Urinalysis: Sp.G 1.022, dark yellow, pH 5

1. What do you expect to find?
2. List all the available cues.
3. Categorize the cues:

   Relevant
   Non-relevant

4. The most likely explanation/diagnosis is:
5. Other explanations/diagnoses could be:

   (a)
   (b)
   (c)

6. List the additional information you would need to confirm/reject these alternative explanations.
7. The correct diagnosis is:
8. The status of this diagnosis is:

   ☐ emergency
   ☐ high risk
   ☐ low risk
   ☐ potential

9. Describe the probable cause of this diagnosis, based on available information.

instructor is thinking about it. That really helps me to hear how an expert approaches the situation'.

Structured interviews have been conducted with several nursing instructors who teach clinical and theory class assignments during the junior and senior years. These instructors have been asked to rate the classroom and clinical performance of students both before and after the case study method was begun. One instructor sums it up well: 'I have much less need to review pathophysiology. They (the students)

seem to have learned and remembered much more than ever before'.

We have gathered some very preliminary narrative data from junior and senior students about their clinical performance. Questions such as 'How useful was the case study as a teaching/learning method?' and 'How much do you feel that you remember from pathophysiology?' are asked and the responses recorded. The students interviewed so far have been very positive about the usefulness of both the case study method and the opportunity to model an expert's clinical reasoning process. One student had a clinical experience in which she was the only person present initially at a patient emergency and she commented, 'I could hear your voice the whole time, helping me figure out what to do, talking through the case study we had in class about this very problem! I felt like I knew what to do because I had already gone over this situation in class and had a good idea of what was happening'.

Obviously, much more research needs to be done to investigate the educational possibilities of the case study method as a way to teach clinical reasoning. A study is currently underway at the University of San Francisco to compare the learning effects of two types of case studies. Until more is known about how and why case studies succeed instructionally, we can only suggest that a carefully developed and thoughtfully implemented case study seems to be the best way to model clinical reasoning in a classroom setting.

References

Baxter, V. (1988) A case-study method for teaching industrial sociology. *Teaching Sociology*, **16**, 21–24

Belenky, M.F., Clinchy, B.M., Goldberger, N. R. and Tarule, J.M. (1986) *Women's Ways of Knowing: The Development of Self, Voice and Mind*. Basic Books, New York

Bernheimer, E. (1982) Teaching community agency referrals to medical students: the case method approach. *Journal of Medical Education*, **57**, 718–719

Bloom, B.S., Engelhart, M. D., Furst, E.J., Hill, W.H. and Krathwohl, D.R. (1956) *Taxonomy of Educational Objectives*. McKay, New York

Boehrer, J. and Linsky, M. (1990) Teaching with cases: learning to question. *New Directions for Teaching and Learning*, **42**, 41–57

Boyce, B.A. (1992) Making the case for the case-based method approach in physical education pedagogy classes. *Journal of Physical Education, Recreation and Dance*, **63**, 17–20

Brown, J.S., Collins, A and Duguid, P. (1989). Situated cognition and the culture of learning. *Educational Researcher*, **33**, 32–42

Carnevali, D.L., Mitchell, P.H., Woods, N.F. and Tanner, C.F. (1984) *Diagnostic Reasoning in Nursing*. Lippincott, Philadelphia

Carter, K. and Unklesbay, R. (1989) Cases in teaching and law. *Journal of Curriculum Studies*, **21**, 527–536

Christensen, R. (1987) *Teaching and the Case Method*. Harvard Business School, Boston

Corcoran, S.A. (1986) Planning by expert and novice nurses in cases of varying complexity. *Research in Nursing and Health*, **9**, 115–162

Epstein, W. (1981) The classical tradition of dialectics and American legal education. *Journal of Legal Education*, **31**, 424–451

Feinstein, M.C. and Veenendall, T.L. (1992) Using the case study method to teach interpersonal communication. *Inquiry: Critical Thinking across the Disciplines*, **9**, 11–14

Fonteyn, M.E. (1991) A descriptive analysis of expert critical care nurses' clinical reasoning. Unpublished doctoral dissertation,University of Texas at Austin

Gale, F.G. (1993) Teaching professional writing rhetorically: the unified case method. *Journal of Business and Technical Communication*, **7**, 256–266

Gist, G.L. (1992) Problem-based learning: a new tool for environmental health education. *Journal of Environmental Health*, **54**, 8–13

Harrington, H. (1991) The case as method. *Action in Teacher Education*, **12**, 1–10

Hartman, L.D. (1992) Business communication and the case method: toward integration in accounting and MBA graduate programs. *Bulletin of the Association for Business Communication*, **5**, 41–45

Kreps, G.L. and Lederman, L.C. (1985) Using the case method in organizational communication education: developing students' insight, knowledge and creativity through experience-based learning and systematic debriefing. *Communication Education*, **34**, 358–364

Mager, R.F. (1975) *Preparing Instructional Objectives*. Pitman, Belmont, CA

McCarthy, M. (1987) A slice of life: training teachers through case studies. *Harvard Graduate School of Education Bulletin*, **22**, 7–11

McWilliam, P.J. (1992) The case method of instruction: teaching application and problem-solving skills to early interventionists. *Journal of Early Intervention*, **16**, 360–373

Merseth, K.K. (1991) The early history of case-based instruction: insights for teacher education today. *Journal of Teacher Education*, **42**, 243–249

Nagel, G.K. (1991) The case method: its potential for training administrators. *NASSP Bulletin*, **75**, 37–43

Oldham, M. and Forrester, J. (1981) The use of case studies in pre-experience business education. *Vocational Aspects of Education*, **33**, 27–29

Radwin, L.E. (1990) Research on diagnostic reasoning in nursing. *Nursing Diagnosis*, **1**, 70–77

Rasinski, T.V. (1989) The case method approach in reading education. *Reading Horizons*, **30**, 5–14

Resnick, L. (1982a) *Education and Learning to Think*. National Academic Press, Washington, D.C.

Resnick, L. (1982b) Learning in school and out. *Educational Researcher*, **16** (9), 13–20

Sansalone, M. (1990) Teaching structural concepts through

case studies and competitions. *Engineering Education*, **80**, 474–475

Tanner, C., Padwick, K., Putzier, D. and Westfall, U. (1987) Diagnostic reasoning strategies of nurses and nursing students. *Nursing Research*, **36**, 359–363

Taylor, W.C. (1989) A first-year problem-based curriculum in health promotion and disease prevention. *Academic Medicine*, **64**, 673–677

Watson, G. and Glaser, E.M. (1964) *Watson–Glaser Critical Thinking Appraisal Manual: Forms YM and ZM*. Harcourt, Brace and World, New York

Zarr, M. (1984) Learning criminal law through the whole case method. *Journal of Legal Education*, **34**, 697–701

16

Teaching the components of clinical decision analysis in the classroom and clinic

Nancy T. Watts

Logically, discussion of methods for teaching clinical decision analysis must begin with a few comments on the nature of clinical reasoning itself. It is a complex and variable process composed of a series of interdependent steps. Each step in the process calls for a somewhat different type of judgemental skill, and each is guided by a complex blend of experience-based intuition and theory-based logic. One way to appreciate the challenges of clinical decision making is to reflect on a few of the many ways it can go wrong.

Some of the most common and serious judgemental errors clinicians make are described in Table 16.1. They have been labelled 'sins' to emphasize that they may be committed not only by novice therapists whose judgemental skills are still being formed but also by highly experienced graduates who clearly 'know better'. Although they violate the rules of decision making most professionals are taught to follow, these flawed methods of judgement offer tempting short-term gains. The time pressures of clinical practice are intense, the scientific basis for many practical decisions skimpy, and the apparent logic of many old and new techniques compelling. These flawed methods of decision making offer time-saving and reassuring shortcuts to the laborious uncertainty of a fully rational approach. We think of them as 'sins' however, because of the serious risks and losses they frequently create for patients and because they dilute and waste the clinician's hard-earned professional knowledge and skills.

Clinical decision analysis provides a demanding but powerful antidote to such flawed short-cuts in judgement. Developed originally by business planners (Raiffa, 1968) and adapted in recent years for application to health care (Weinstein et al, 1980), decision analysis provides a systematic method for choosing a course of action when the goals of action are important, the costs significant, and logical choice difficult because many of the factors that may influence outcomes are unknown or cannot be assessed with certainty.

For a complete analysis six different steps are required: defining the decision problem, defining successful and unsuccessful outcomes, describing several alternative courses of action and their possible consequences, estimating the probability that each possible consequence actually will occur, estimating the costs of alternative approaches, and selecting the strategy that promises the best combination of high effectiveness and low costs. Detailed descriptions of these steps and practice exercises to help clinicians learn to perform them have been developed for physicians (Weinstein et al, 1980). Less detailed descriptions show how the method can be applied by physical therapists (Coogler, 1985; Watts, 1985; Francis 1988; Watts, 1989).

Complete decision analyses have much to offer fields such as physical therapy, particularly as tools for applying research to practice and for comparing alternative approaches to treatment in areas of controversy. However, for the individual clinician a complete analysis

Table 16.1   Seven deadly sins of clinical decision making

Vagueness	The purpose of evaluation or treatment is unclear. The wisdom of decisions cannot be judged because it is uncertain what they are intended to accomplish or how soon desired results should be achieved.
Narrowness	Alternative methods are seldom considered. If a familiar approach seems effective, little effort is made to identify others that might be even better.
Rigidity	Standardized regimens of evaluation and treatment are routinely used with little regard for important differences in individual patient needs and response. Reactions to treatment are not monitored to detect unexpected results.
Irrationality	Choices are based on habit, convenience, subjective impressions and the charisma of individuals who endorse specific techniques rather than on objective evidence and tested theory.
Wastefulness	Evaluations are extensive, but results have little influence on selection of treatment. Elaborate treatment techniques are used without considering whether less costly methods might be equally effective.
Insensitivity	Personal values and psychosocial concerns of patients and families are ignored. Improvement in physical performance is given higher priority than enhanced quality of life.
Mystery	The process used to arrive at decisions cannot be explained in terms patients and colleagues can understand. Others cannot question or contribute to this process.

is too laborious an undertaking to be practical as a means of making the host of different decisions a busy day of practice involves. Fortunately, the component steps of decision analysis still have great utility even if they are used separately or are incorporated into other decision making approaches. These steps represent practical and logical ways of thinking about patient care and they can be readily incorporated into both the academic and clinical education of students. This chapter provides an illustrative sample of teaching methods that can help students improve their judgemental skills in a few of the areas included in a full decision analysis. It is hoped this will tempt readers to invent methods of their own and to learn more about the decision analysis method itself.

Component skills and illustrative teaching methods

Specifying a basis for evaluating the results of treatment

Goal setting has long been recognized as an essential skill all clinicians must learn. However, today's clinical practice places new demands on therapists to learn, to state their goals in an unambiguous way. In particular,

quality assurance programs, reimbursement regulations, clinical research projects and the responsibilities of independent practice all require that the purpose of treatment be described in clear, specific and measurable terms. In early lectures and in students' initial attempts to set goals for individual patients, the main emphasis usually is on the *types* of improvements to be sought or kinds of problems to be prevented.

Such statements of purpose are a useful starting point, but they do not provide an adequate basis for testing diagnostic hypotheses, judging whether a patient's progress is acceptable, comparing alternative approaches to treatment, or deciding when treatment can be discontinued. Such decisions are possible only if a goal statement is available that says not only what type of change is intended but also when results should be evaluated and what measurable amount of change should be seen for those results to be judged acceptable. This is the difference between simply saying that the goal of treatment is to improve range of motion in the knee and specifying that if the patient's progress is acceptable s/he will have at least 80° of active, pain-free flexion in the knee by the end of the second week of treatment. Such standards for evaluating care have three important characteristics: they are *time-based*, describe an objectively *measurable* result, and focus not on the ideal result we might hope for, but on the *minimum level* that should be achieved to regard the results of a treatment as acceptable.

Students can be introduced to these decision making concepts early in their curricula by such means as:

- discussing the time characteristics of both the normal and pathophysiological mechanisms explained to them
- asking students to suggest how the changes they are discussing might be measured
- including practice laboratory activities that ask students to plan and perform simple assessment procedures that would be practical to use in monitoring short term progress as an integral part of ongoing treatment.

As their clinical work begins students can be asked to start attempting to formulate time-based standards. Initially this should be done under circumstances where a logical time for judging results is fairly obvious, where a widely-used method for objective measurement of the change sought is available, and where the minimum level of achievement needed can be tied to some practical function. For example, a beginning student might be asked to describe the specific functional goals a hip fracture patient should be expected to achieve by the time she is discharged to her home, or to specify the minimum number of degrees of flexion an elbow fracture patient should have before attempting to drive his car. More difficult tasks, such as deciding when and how to assess improvement in spasticity in the arm of a patient with chronic hemiplegia, or specifying how much low back pain should be reduced after a three day trial of a TENS device will need to be postponed until the student has enough clinical experience to attempt the level of predictions these standards involve.

To help students learn what types and amounts of improvements it is realistic to expect, and to emphasize the need to use time-based standards as a tool for reviewing and revising treatment, students in the clinic can be assigned to monitor and chart the progress of some of the patients they treat. Once a time-based standard has been drafted the student can be asked to mark the expected achievement on a simple graph that shows time units on the horizontal axis and increments of measured improvement on the vertical. As treatment pro-

gresses the student is asked to make periodic measurements of the patient's status and to plot these points on the chart. The rate and pattern of progress towards the point specified in the standard thus become obvious. In discussions with the clinical instructor the student can then be encouraged to compare progress patterns for several patients with a similar disorder, explore possible reasons for differences, and consider whether any changes in the initial plan of treatment seem needed.

At a still more advanced level students can be asked to try formulating goal statements that incorporate several different dimensions of success. For example, a time-based goal for acceptable progress in ambulation skills for a recent stroke patient may need to specify the minimum distance to be walked as well as the maximum support that should be needed and the degree to which this should be done without verbal coaching from the therapist.

Identifying alternatives

Clinical problem solving often is seen as a logical, linear process that leads step by step to the right answers for important clinical questions. Such thinking may be called *convergent* for it pulls together a wide range of information to arrive at a decision about the cause of the patient's problem or the best way to prevent or solve it. Important as it is, however, this type of clinical decision making must be linked with a second, very different, type of thinking in order to be really useful. Referred to by such names as *divergent* thinking, imagination, creativity, synthesis, and lateral thinking this complementary process emphasizes not the selection of the best answer to a question but the richness of the alternatives to be considered before a choice is made. Among the decision making tasks in which this type of thinking is most important are generating competing diagnostic hypotheses, redesigning treatment for the patient who fails to progress as expected, and finding ways to adapt and improvise treatment without sacrificing effectiveness when time, space, equipment, or support services are unusually limited.

Both classroom and clinical teachers can model this component of problem solving in their lectures and conversations with students by pointing out alternative explanations of the problems they discuss and by suggesting a variety of options for intervention. However, the most powerful tool for helping students learn to do this type of thinking for themselves is the question that has more than one 'right' answer. Such questions ask the student to originate ideas and design alternatives by:

• suggesting alternative explanations: 'What else might account for that?'
• predicting diverse possible outcomes: 'Can you think of anything different that might happen?'
• proposing varied options for action: 'Is there any other way you might be able to accomplish the same thing?'

A wealth of references are available for teachers interested in learning more about divergent thinking and its role in practical problem solving. Among the most readable and thought-provoking of these are the books by Edward de Bono (1971; 1976; 1978). Abundant ideas on how to formulate questions and manage discussions in order to stimulate student use of specific thinking skills also are provided by the education literature (Sanders, 1966; Hyman, 1979; Watts, 1990; Christensen et al, 1991).

However, success in teaching students to generate alternatives depends on more than an ability to formulate provocative questions. It also often requires patience and flexibility on the part of the teacher in evaluating and responding to student responses. Some of the alternatives they suggest may seem incompletely thought through, naive, or impractical. Others may propose explanations or courses of action with which the instructor is not familiar. Clearly, major errors in reasoning should not go uncorrected. Particularly in working with beginning students, however, minor flaws may need to be ignored, unfamiliar ideas treated with respect, and positive feedback be given to what is sound in their suggestions. Premature emphasis on finding the best answer can block student development of confidence and skill in the essential process of identifying alternatives. Helping students master both convergent and divergent thinking requires teachers to have a vision of the purpose of questioning which is broad enough to include both the logical search for right answers and the creative search for new ideas. This creative process was described by poet John Ciardi when he wrote:

A good question is never answered.
It is not a bolt to be tightened into place.
But a seed to be planted and to bear more seed.
Toward the hope of greening the landscape of ideas.

(Ciardi, 1972)

Contingency planning

Even the most carefully designed initial plans for evaluation and treatment often need revision once they are put into effect. As a case evolves new dimensions of the problem may surface, unexpected responses may occur, and the actions of other care givers may alter what we need to accomplish or are free to attempt. As students learn to identify possible alternatives they also can be encouraged to look ahead, to consider how they will respond if they encounter obstacles, problems . . . or surprising success. This sort of 'What if . . . ' thinking is far more complex than simply suggesting alternatives for a single specific decision or response. It involves visualizing a series of interrelated choices which are spread out over time and associated with multiple possible consequences.

The decision tree diagrams used in decision analysis are one device for keeping track of these alternatives and for comparing them with one another. The format for a decision tree follows several simple conventions. A branching tree is drawn lying on its side with key events shown from left to right across the page in the order in which they are expected to occur. A square indicates each point at which a choice must be made between two or more alternatives for action, and circles show the points at which at least two possible consequences of an action will become known. Lines branching out from these choice and chance points carry short labels describing the options to be considered and consequences that may be seen. Decision trees give us a common language for describing different approaches, and they encourage us to anticipate possible problems and prepare contingency plans for revising care if this proves necessary.

Guiding questions once again play an important part in helping students and recent graduates develop contingency planning skills. In discussions of either real or hypothetical cases the novices are first asked to describe the initial course of action they propose and the results they hope this will produce. Follow-up questions then explore alternative scenarios. As these are developed they can be added to the original plan using a decision tree diagram. For example, one segment of such a discussion with a student preparing to begin post-operative treatment of a patient who has just undergone a total knee replacement might go like this:

- Instructor – Let's talk about how you think you'll want to manage this patient between now and the time he goes home. From your examination and review of his chart you know he is a healthy, 58-year-old man whose knee problems were a result of repeated injuries while playing soccer when he was at university. You have identified his main problems as decreased range of motion, poor muscle control of knee extension and pain which limits his active movement. What do you think you'd like to do when you treat him today?
- Student – Well, it's just the first day after his surgery and since he doesn't have any discomfort at rest and there are only minimal signs of inflammation, I guess I'd start him off on the level 1 exercise program we were taught at school: quadriceps setting, active assisted motion through the painfree range, and assisted straight leg raising while he's wearing a knee splint. His upper extremities, hip and lung function are very good so he won't need any particular exercises there.
- Instructor – O.K. Let's record that this way:

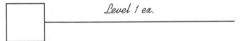

How long would you plan to continue with that? When do you think you might want to move on to something else?
- Student – Pretty soon I guess. As soon as he's doing O.K. with these easy exercises I'd advance him to the level 2 ones.
- Instructor – What do you mean by 'doing O.K.?' Can you be a little more specific about what you want to see him do before you advance to level 2, and tell me how soon you expect he'll reach that point?
- Student – Well, the paper on total knee patients we were assigned said that by the second day the patient should have at least

35° of motion with minimal discomfort and be able to do several straight leg lifts without help. If he could do that I'd go on to level 2 the second day.
- Instructor – All right, let's show that on the tree this way:

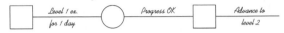

What next?

This is continued until the student's initial plan has been described and diagrammed up to the expected time of discharge from the hospital. Then:

- Instructor – That seems like a reasonable plan if your patient responds the way we hope he will. But let's go back and think about what you'll do if things don't turn out quite that way. For example, suppose when you see him the second day your patient complains of severe pain almost as soon as he begins to flex the knee. What would you do then?

Subsequent questions would be designed to help the student identify such contingencies and decide what changes in the original plan may be needed if they occur. As these are added to the decision tree the segment shown earlier might evolve into a branching pattern such as this:

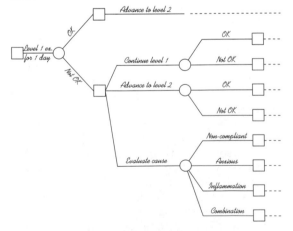

The example shown here is a rather simple one, representative of the way we might use decision trees to teach an inexperienced student. At a more advanced level more complex patients can be chosen for discussion, the student can be given less explicit guidance in identifying important contingencies, and more time can be spent in discussing the rationale for interpretation of different responses and in critiquing proposals for alternative action. A similar approach can be used to reflect on cases that have been treated already. This is particularly worthwhile when these cases have created particular problems or where patterns of progress have been different from what was expected.

The three areas of focus in all of these discussions and tree drawing exercises is on identifying key points at which progress should be assessed, on predicting some of the different ways in which individual patients may respond, and on deciding how such differences should influence the course of treatment. Such contingency planning clearly draws on the two decision making skills discussed earlier since at each step in drafting a tree the student must attempt to identify possible alternatives and describe these in time-based, objective terms. Some students will find this easier if they are reminded that the alternatives to be considered usually fall into one of a limited number of generic categories. For example, in considering alternatives for action early in a decision tree the options usually include two or more of the following:

- evaluation – gather further information about the patient or the treatment situation and evaluate it
- intervention – begin treatment on the basis of the information already available
- waiting – delay action for a specified period of time and then review the situation to decide whether to evaluate, intervene, wait longer or do nothing
- do nothing – in many cases this is combined with providing an explanation to the patient and referring colleague, or making a referral.

In deciding how to follow-up on the patient's initial response, if things go well we might:

- *continue* what we have been doing without change
- *do more* of the same thing to see if that works even better
- *do less* to see if we can get the same results more easily
- *do something different* to see if it is easier or more effective.

On the other hand, if the initial response is unsatisfactory we might:

- *keep trying* the same thing a little longer
- *try harder* – do more of the same thing
- *try something else* to see if it gets better results
- *evaluate* WHY the response is not as good as expected
- *ask for help* while we either stop doing anything further ourselves or continue with one of the other options.

These categories are too general to be adequate as a basis for detailed planning; however, reminding the student of them sometimes helps in identifying specific options that might otherwise be overlooked.

Predicting results and coping with uncertainty

Hypothesis testing is an important component of many logical systems of decision making because even the most attractive theories may prove false when they are subjected to reality testing. However, unless such testing is done with realistic caution it can easily be misleading. The source of this problem lies in the many differences that exist between the scientific laboratory and the clinical world. As Bursztajn and his colleagues point out (Bursztajn et al, 1981), 'For every observed effect the scientist seeks to isolate a specific cause or set of causes, as if it alone can account for the effect.' The causal explanations derived from this process are seen as *deterministic*, that is, 'A scientist using such an explanation claims that it is complete – i.e. that the list of causes is exhaustive and that the way they come together to produce the effect in question does not change.' They also are seen as *universal*. 'That is, "A causes B" means that we can completely specify the conditions under which A causes B. When we have such a complete list of conditions, then we can count on A causing B whenever those conditions occur.' To develop such causal theories, the scientist relies whenever possible on 'crucial experiments' in which the 'experimenter varies A while holding everything else constant, and observes how B in turn varies.' When students are introduced to new clinical theories, and when they start to test clinical hypotheses their thinking is often strongly influenced by this laboratory science model. Even when their lecturers are careful to qualify their predictions, what uncertain students often hear is that if they use a particular treatment method it *will* have a particular result. In planning how they will test their clinical hypotheses their assumption is often if the predicted result fails to appear the hypothesis *must* be rejected.

However, the clinical world is too chaotic for such simplistic assumptions to hold true on a consistent basis. The clinician has only limited ability to identify, isolate, control, and manipulate all the factors that may influence the effects of treatment. Many clinical phenomena have multiple causes and causal relationships may be influenced by a confusing array of individual differences among patients, therapists and treatment situations. As a result, observed results may fail to confirm hypotheses that are in fact true, or appear to support hypotheses that are actually false. We are used to guarding against such Type A and Type B errors in interpreting research data, but we often place less emphasis on them in our presentations of clinical theory and methods for testing of clinical hypotheses. Our students need to learn that such theories and hypotheses represent at best our educated guesses about what will happen when we use different therapeutic methods. We also can help them learn how to cope with this uncertainty and how to reduce it.

Decision analysis recognizes the uncertainty of clinical expectations by assigning quantitative probability estimates to all chance point branches on a decision tree. These estimates express the clinician's strength of belief that each of the consequences identified as possible at that point actually will occur. For example, in the segment of the decision tree shown earlier the probability of this patient responding badly to the level 1 exercises seems low. Yet this certainly is not impossible. We might then decide to assign a 90% probability to the 'OK' branch after the first circle, and only a 10% probability to the branch for 'NOT OK'. On the other hand, if the patient's initial response is unsatisfactory, the likelihood that simply continuing the same treatment will remedy the situation seems low. At that chance point we might then assign only a 30% probability of an 'OK'

response and say there is a 70% chance the response will remain problematic.

Assigning such definite quantitative values to our expectations is an unfamiliar and somewhat intimidating process for many clinicians despite the fact that all clinical choices are based on some type of assessment about the probability of success associated with the treatment alternatives we consider. These estimates usually are expressed by using qualifying terms rather than number: 'There's very little risk of a bad side effect here'; 'I think this patient is going to be a problem'; 'This approach usually gets results'. The advantages of quantitative estimates are that they reduce the ambiguity of terms such as 'usually', facilitate comparison of alternative approaches, and confront us forcefully with the need to examine the sources of our beliefs about what to expect. Probability estimates, both quantitative and verbal, draw on three quite different sources of guidance: the clinician's own experience with similar cases, objective data from directly related clinical research or quality assurance outcome studies, and the logical application of less directly related, but still relevant, basic and applied science theory. Students can be helped to make intelligent use of all three sources by using teaching methods such as these:

- Making frequent reference to the research evidence that both supports and casts doubt on the purported effects of the therapeutic methods students are taught.
- Encouraging analysis of opposing points of view and discussion of the strengths, weaknesses, contradictions, and unanswered questions that exist in research currently available on these methods.
- Emphasizing major factors that may alter, interfere with or enhance the usual pattern of response to each intervention we teach.
- Including a major emphasis in courses on scientific method on topics such as external validity, the use of meta-analysis (Norton and Strube, 1989) and the questions to be answered in research utilization (Stetler and Marram, 1976).
- Arranging for students to take part in quality assurance programs that involve the establishment of outcome standards and their use in auditing the actual results of care.
- Setting aside time during the student's clinical experience for repeated contact with a

number of patients who share a similar disorder or complaint, and arranging for the student to stay in contact with at least a few patients long enough to see first hand how they progress and how treatment evolves.

Such experiences as these will not teach the student to carry out the interesting statistical analyses of combined probabilities that have attracted such attention in the medical literature on clinical decision analysis. They will, however, foster students' recognition of the uncertainty that surrounds many clinical decisions and help them deal with that uncertainty in a way that can make their future practice more realistic.

Conclusion

The teaching methods outlined in this chapter represent only a tiny sample of the many ways students can be taught to use components of decision analysis methodology in their day-to-day work with patients. The list of decision analysis components discussed is equally incomplete. Among the other steps that deserve equal attention are:

- analysis of the costs of care
- assignment of values or utility ratings to the possible outcomes of a clinical decision
- determination of the best strategies for evaluation of patients and critical analysis of how clinical data are used as a basis for practical decisions
- comparison of the overall cost-effectiveness of different approaches
- collaboration with patients to incorporate their preferences and concerns in the decision making process.

None of these component skills can be fully mastered in the time available for entry level education. Graduate clinicians, including those of us responsible for teaching students, will need to continue work on clinical decision making methods throughout our careers. This will be easiest if we find ways to support and teach one another. A few of the ways in which this can be done include:

- Regularly scheduled case conferences in which staff compare ideas for management based on different models for decision making and in which they share ideas on treatment alternatives, probability estimates, and methods of gathering objective data on the outcomes of care.
- Development of multicentre data banks and projects such as that undertaken recently by Partridge and her colleagues in Britain to document milestones in recovery among patients with a common disorder such as stroke (Partridge, 1992).
- Staff journal clubs that focus on issues related to the application of research findings to practice.
- Expanded publication of books and papers that present, compare, criticize and synthesize different methods for making clinical decision processes more effective.

Effective clinical decision making is a difficult job. Fortunately engagement in the process also is contagious. As you do your best to help students learn such component skills as the ones discussed here, you may be pleasantly surprised to find how much you are learning yourself.

References

Bursztajn, H., Feinbloom, R.I., Hamm, R.M. and Brodsky, A. (1981) *Medical Choices, Medical Chances: How Patients, Families, and Physicians Can Cope With Uncertainty*. Delacorte Press/Seymour Lawrence, New York, pp. 24–25

Ciardi, J. (1972) *Manner of Speaking*. Rutgers University Press, New Brunswick, NJ

Christensen, C.R., Garvin, D.A. and Sweet, A. (eds) (1991) *Education for Judgment: The Artistry of Discussion Leadership*. Harvard Business School Press, Boston

Coogler, C.E. (1985) Clinical decision making among neurologic patients: spinal cord injury. In *Clinical Decision Making in Physical Therapy* (ed. S.L. Wolf). F.A. Davis, Philadelphia, pp. 149–170

de Bono, E. (1971) *The Use of Lateral Thinking*. Penguin Books, Harmondsworth, Middlesex

de Bono, E. (1976) *Practical Thinking*. Penguin Books, Harmondsworth, Middlesex

de Bono, E. (1978) *Teaching Thinking*. Penguin Books, Harmondsworth, Middlesex

Francis, K. (1988) Computer communication: decision analysis using a spread sheet. *Physical Therapy*, **68**, 1409–1410

Hyman, R.T. (1979) *Strategic Questioning*. Prentice-Hall, Englewood Cliffs, NJ

Norton, B.J. and Strube, M.J. (1989) Making decisions based on group designs and meta-analysis. *Physical Therapy*, **69**, 594–600

Partridge, C.J. (1992) Describing patterns of recovery as a basis for evaluating progress. *International Journal of Technology Assessment in Health Care*, **8**, 55–61

Raiffa, H. (1968) *Decision Analysis: Introductory Lectures on Choices Under Uncertainty*. Addison-Wesley, Reading, MA

Sanders, N. (1966) *Classroom Questions, What Kinds?* Harper and Row, New York

Stetler, C. and Marram, G. (1976) Evaluating research find-ings for applicability in practice. *Nursing Outlook*, **24**, 559–563

Watts, N.T. (1985) Decision analysis: a tool for improving physical therapy practice and education. In *Clinical Decision Making in Physical Therapy* (ed. S.L. Wolf). F.A. Davis, Philadelphia, pp. 7–23

Watts, N.T. (1989) Clinical decision analysis. *Physical Therapy*, **69**, 569–579

Watts, N.T. (1990) *Handbook of Clinical Teaching*. Churchill Livingstone, Edinburgh

Weinstein, M.C., Fineberg, H.V., Elstein, A. S., Frazier, H.S., Neuhauser, D., Neutra, R.R. and McNeil, B.J. (1980) *Clinical Decision Analysis*. W. B. Saunders, Philadelphia

17

Teaching clinical reasoning to occupational therapy students

Judy Ranka and Christine Chapparo

Occupational therapists are viewed as successful clinical reasoners if they can identify the problem, understand the client's view of the problem, decide on which is the best, just and non-harmful course of action and predict the outcome of therapy for the client. This involves multiple processes that result in ongoing decision making that is characterized by dimensions of knowledge, reflection and intuition. As Rogers (1983, p. 615) has stated, these dimensions 'are inextricably entwined' in a clinician who is simultaneously a scientist, ethicist and artist: a clinical reasoner.

If clinical reasoning is the core of occupational therapy practice, the responsibility of the occupational therapy curriculum must be to facilitate its students to become effective clinical reasoners. This means that the curriculum must provide opportunities for students to develop the knowledge, skills and attitudes associated with being a clinical reasoner. We believe there are five core dimensions to this process. One, students need to develop and learn to use knowledge stores that contain information about occupational therapy theory, health and disability, and the tools of occupational therapy practice, as well as experiential knowledge of outcomes. Two, students need to develop the specific interpersonal skills required to glean information about another person's perspective of illness and the skill to affect change. Three, students need to develop insight and the use of intuition to create images of future potential for clients with disability. Four, students need to become cognizant of

their own moral positions and ways of dealing with ethical dilemmas that arise during the course of therapy. Finally, students need to be able to reason a best course of action within the context of restrictions imposed by current health care systems.

The purpose of this chapter is to outline major aspects of the undergraduate occupational therapy curriculum at The University of Sydney that develop clinical reasoners. Two perspectives will be presented. First, aspects of curriculum structure, philosophy and assumptions which support and extend outcomes of clinical reasoning units that exist within our curriculum will be examined. These aspects are based on the results of three major curriculum evaluations. The purpose of these evaluations was to review our undergraduate course content and teaching strategies in light of the current and future needs of the profession. One outcome of these evaluations is the evolution of a curriculum framework which integrates occupational therapy philosophy and content with educational strategies based on adult learning principles and problem solving modes of instruction. The assumptions, values and principles that were developed as part of the revised curriculum framework provide the foundation for teaching clinical reasoning throughout our curriculum.

Second, this chapter will give examples of the specific clinical reasoning learning units presented in our bachelor's program to illustrate how students develop the major processes involved in clinical reasoning in occupational therapy. This curriculum graduates approximately 150 students each year. Classes are presented to large groups of students in lecture format and in tutorials consisting of approximately 18 students per group.

Curriculum framework for development of an occupational therapy clinical reasoner

In our view the curriculum within which occupational therapy education occurs is formed by a number of overlapping and integrated contexts which include physical, personal, social, historical and political dimensions. Clinical reasoning units that we teach are embedded in this context. The meaning and value students place on various clinical reasoning learning experiences are largely derived from the total curriculum context. If students are to internalize and value the specific clinical reasoning processes taught, the total curriculum context must be viewed by the student as supporting those behaviours. If this does not happen, students are likely to perceive reasoning processes as dichotomous with occupational therapy practice and devalue them. For example, if a clinical reasoning unit that teaches the value of client participation in the problem solving process is embedded in a curriculum context where problem solving leading to prescriptive types of intervention are paramount, then students will perceive the two approaches as in conflict and are likely to adopt a clinical reasoning style that

conforms to the dominant mode. Congruence across the whole curriculum in terms of philosophies, assumptions and values is therefore preferred.

Curriculum values and assumptions that support clinical reasoning

In structuring our curriculum to support the development of students as clinical reasoners, five basic educational values and assumptions that most closely align with the practice and philosophy of clinical reasoning were considered. These curriculum values and assumptions about learning are congruent with the values and assumptions about occupational therapy clinical reasoning. Table 17.1 demonstrates this congruence.

Curriculum principles that support clinical reasoning learning units

The values and assumptions outlined in Table 17.1 form the basis for the curriculum principles we employ. These principles provide the educational rationale driving our clinical reasoning learning units. We believe that the development of students as clinical reasoners is predicated on a curriculum which considers:

1. Facilitation of the gradual development of higher order problem solving skills through the application of theoretical knowledge and therapeutic skills (Skager, 1978; Starratt,

Table 17.1 Values and assumptions that support clinical reasoning learning experiences

Values and assumptions about learning	*Values and assumptions about clinical reasoning*
People learn differently	Therapists use highly individual and different modes of reasoning
Learning is a cognitive process that is coloured by individual beliefs and values of the teacher and learner	Clinical reasoning in occupational therapy is a process of cognition that is coloured by the therapist's own beliefs and values about the outcome of therapy
Effective learning is prompted by problem solving and by presentation of incomplete information that motivates the learner to complete the picture	The process of clinical reasoning is triggered by clinical problems and by incomplete information about a client situation
Learning is developmentally acquired and is affected by maturation, experience and situation	There are stages in the development of clinical reasoning ability that differentiate novice and expert clinicians
Continued engagement in learning is a valued process	Clinical reasoning has been identified as the core of occupational therapy practice, and as such is valued by the occupational therapy profession

1974). This can be accomplished by incorporating experiential learning methods into the curriculum, and by the appropriate use of modelling of the educator's own clinical reasoning processes (Mezirow, 1981).

2. Facilitation of the development of clinical reasoning through a progression involving instrumental learning (use of facts and knowledge), dialogic learning (questioning and critical analysis), and self-reflective learning (self-appraisal) (Jelinek, 1978; Mezirow, 1985; Schon, 1987).

3. Supporting students in developing their ability to make intelligent choices about the direction, focus and priority in treatment (Brookfield, 1985; Mezirow, 1981; Skager, 1978). This can be accomplished through learning units that require the students to make choices, expand their range of options, and participate in discussion on the perspectives of others who have alternative ways of understanding (Mezirow, 1981).

4. Incorporation of opportunities for students to both solve problems that are presented, and identify problems that require solutions (Burns and Brooks, 1974; Grundy, 1987; Skager, 1978). This can be accomplished by the presentation of client cases that have incomplete information, and by helping students to understand how to use their own knowledge as well as the experience of others to create an image of the problem (Mezirow, 1981).

5. Progression from external feedback to internal self-assessment of the clinical reasoning process (Knowles, 1984; Mezirow, 1985; Schon, 1987; Skager, 1978). This can be accomplished by creating experiences which promote progressive mastery in clinical reasoning ability. We believe this requires a supportive climate with feedback that encourages a change in thinking style as well as risk taking.

6. Providing direction and opportunities for students to transfer reasoning strategies from the classroom to the clinical environment (Skager, 1978). This can be accomplished by encouraging students to reflect on the decisions they make in both simulated and real fieldwork contexts and to develop criteria for judging these decisions (Mezirow, 1981).

7. Providing opportunities for students and educators to engage in dialogue and reflection on their individual clinical reasoning processes without fear of judgement (Cunningham, 1982; Skager, 1978). This involves setting a climate for the development of clinical reasoning skills that avoids competitive judgement of performance.

We argue that a curriculum based on these principles has potential to produce an occupational therapist whose clinical reasoning style is characterized not just by intelligent problem solving but by a mode of problem solving that is based on understanding, insight, adaptability and personal responsibility for the sincerity of beliefs and the appropriateness of actions. However, the overall curriculum goal in developing such a clinical reasoner is not to dominate individual reasoning. Rather, the curriculum aims to develop the student's mastery of his or her own reasoning style in a way which makes possible the ability to choose therapeutic action freely from a large range of alternatives.

Clinical reasoning learning units

The ability to operationalize these principles in specific clinical reasoning units requires occupational therapy educators who are capable of functioning simultaneously as directors of the reasoning process, facilitators of the reasoning process and models of reasoning processes as determined by their perceptions of the maturity of the student (Brundage and MacKeracher, 1980). This section of the chapter describes examples of learning units which facilitate four specific types of clinical reasoning in our undergraduate curriculum: procedural reasoning, interactive reasoning, ethical reasoning and the use of multiple reasoning modes. An outline of the aims, structure and content is presented for each unit.

Facilitating procedural reasoning: learning to use knowledge to develop a picture of the problem

Various conceptualizations of what Fleming (1991) refers to as procedural reasoning have been described in occupational therapy literature (Gale and Marsden, 1982; Hopkins and Tiffany, 1988; Neuhaus, 1988; Pelland, 1987; Rogers and Masagatani, 1982), and are familiar to occupational therapists. Generally, these perspectives involve facilitating the use of procedural reasoning strategies which are synonymous with 'treatment planning', a process of problem solving, hypothesis generation and testing, and more recently, constructing an occupational therapy diagnosis (Rogers and Holm, 1991).

Reported approaches to facilitating the development of aspects of procedural reasoning ability in occupational therapy students are limited. The units described in this section have largely been constructed through a synthesis of information from occupational therapy literature presented in Chapter 7, literature from the field of education specifically concerned with adult, self-directed and lifelong learning, and our own ideas and experiences (Ranka, 1986, 1990). We suggest that learning experiences designed to facilitate procedural reasoning in occupational therapy students involve providing them with mechanisms to construct an occupational therapy diagnosis and structure a plan of intervention. This requires that students gain knowledge of the processes involved in procedural reasoning including the dimensions of cue acquisition, hypothesis generation, cue interpretation and hypothesis evaluation (Rogers and Holm, 1991). We also assert that students should have opportunities to practise the application of these processes in a non-judgemental environment in order to develop skill and confidence in their ability to function in this role (see Bittel, 1989; Brookfield, 1981, 1983, 1985; Pratt, 1987).

Aim

We address this aspect of clinical reasoning through learning units which provide students with a model for procedural reasoning. This model includes a problem solving structure, and a strategy for using the direction provided by theory and personal views of practice. We evaluate these learning units by assessing how well students can construct a comprehensive occupational therapy program to manage clinical problems which is framed by theory and reflects a critical appraisal of the literature.

The structure of learning experiences and the role of facilitator

Our experience suggests that students require opportunities to develop these procedural reasoning abilities throughout the course. Three sequential phases may assist in organizing this progression: (a) learning to use knowledge to develop a general picture of the problem and possible course of action; (b) using theory to complete the picture when portions of knowledge are missing; and (c) integrating experience with knowledge to construct a personal theory capable of structuring the process when problems are complex and many factors remain unknown.

A. Using knowledge to construct a picture of the problem. This learning unit is organized around incomplete and 'ill-structured' case studies which mirror usual clinical conditions. The content of the case studies gradually evolves as the unit progresses. Students have an opportunity to practise and discuss all the stages involved in procedural reasoning from initial assessment through to termination of therapy. The initial focus of the case studies varies and is determined by the level of maturation of the learning group and the skills of the tutor/facilitator. For example, some cases focus on the major occupational areas affected (self-maintenance, productivity, leisure, rest), while others focus on the causes of dysfunction (psychosocial, biomechanical, sensory–motor, cognitive, environmental).

Cases are presented initially in the form of written referrals to occupational therapy. The teachers and learners in each group form into small collaborative groups: 'occupational therapists'. Each 'therapist' compiles a list of cues from the referral by formulating responses to the questions:

'What do I know?'
i.e.: What knowledge do I have that may be relevant to this case? What cues have I noticed?

'What do I need to know?'
i.e.: What is missing from my knowledge store? What seems irrelevant?

'How can I find out?'
i.e.: What human resources (experts, the client) may expand my current knowledge? How do I consult with them? What material resources

may expand my current knowledge or confirm my impressions? How do I access them?

In this problem sensing stage, each group formulates initial hypotheses about the nature of dysfunction in occupational performance, the nature of disease, tentative theoretical frameworks for practice and ideas about a suitable occupational therapy program. These questions form the substrates of each successive phase of the process.

As the unit progresses through stages of the reasoning process, additional cues are introduced through combinations of written case notes, videotaped excerpts of client performance, and/or through experiential role plays involving the use of actors or former occupational therapy clients employed as tutor assistants for this purpose. The content of this supplemental information is partially determined by the types of hypotheses generated by the various collaborative groups. In this way each case becomes unpredictable: several courses of action may be appropriate, and decisions made at one stage will influence the outcome at subsequent stages. For example, one collaborative group may decide to assess the home environment of their 'client' while another may focus on upper limb function. Based on these decisions each group receives different information and continues to pursue different lines of reasoning.

The role of the facilitator in this learning unit is complex. Of prime importance is the ability to sense when to become an intrinsic member of each collaborative group and when to encourage independent reasoning. Because the outcome of procedural reasoning for each case is shaped by the 'occupational therapists', the facilitators need to be comfortable with uncertainty. It has been suggested that such abilities are predicated on the facilitators having a level of expertise in the content area (Bittel, 1989; Brundage and MacKeracher, 1980), as well as confidence and maturity.

B. Using theory to complete the picture. This phase requires that students apply conceptual models of occupational therapy practice to the process of procedural reasoning. Students examine the philosophical base of a variety of conceptual models of practice, identify and define the dominant concepts and constructs of each model, outline major principles and describe underlying assumptions of selected models. Cases are used to explore how each model frames the process of procedural reasoning. Students have an opportunity to select and apply an appropriate occupational therapy conceptual model to an ill-structured case study similar to those described in the previous phase. Comparing and contrasting various models and their application provides students with an opportunity to examine how various theories can shape the process of procedural reasoning.

The facilitators in this group act as resources to help students to clarify their perceptions and further the students' understanding of theory. The classroom atmosphere is one of permission giving: students are encouraged to provide personal comment on their views of the usefulness of various conceptual models without concerns about expressing opposing views.

C. Using experience to construct a personal theory. Phase three of developing procedural reasoning is necessarily the most mature phase. Again, a case-based approach is used. In this unit collaborative groups of students examine complex cases which contain many conflicting cues. Students then attempt to link their acquired knowledge of health and disease, knowledge of occupational therapy conceptual models for practice and knowledge gained from experience, to construct individual 'pictures' of the problem and a proposed course of action. We refer to these individual pictures as 'personal theories'. Students are assisted to develop a supporting rationale for their personal views and present this to the other learners in the group. Through this process students learn to articulate their own views and respect the views of others.

We have found that this unit is most effective when the facilitators create an environment which supports the presentation of incomplete ideas and encourages discussion of conflicting viewpoints. This usually occurs when facilitators become members of the collaborative groups and are willing to articulate their own personal theories concerning the cases presented.

Facilitating interactive reasoning: learning to understand the client's perspective

As discussed in Chapter 7, creating an image of the meaning of disability and illness from the client's perspective is a primary goal of clinical reasoning in occupational therapy. Critical self-reflection is central to this outcome. Communication and dialogue become salient factors in the process of critical reflection because this type of reasoning involves testing the justification or validity of presuppositions or assumptions about the client (Mezirow, 1991). It is through the interactive system of skilled communication that occupational therapists attempt to understand what is valid in the assertions made by others and attempt to achieve consensual validation for their own assertions about clients' problems and potential. Fleming (1991) referred to this process as interactive reasoning.

This section describes how skill in interactive reasoning is facilitated within the academic context of our undergraduate occupational therapy curriculum. Information presented is drawn from research on reflective judgement from the field of education, from knowledge of the process of interactive reasoning as it occurs in occupational therapy practice and from our experiences of teaching student occupational therapists about clinical reasoning.

Research about the process of reflective judgement from the field of adult education indicates that students at different ages and educational levels enter courses with markedly different assumptions about what and how something can be known or understood (Mezirow, 1991). Our experiences in teaching undergraduates suggest that many first year students in occupational therapy enter the course believing that they can 'know' absolutely through concrete observation and knowledge about what is the 'right' thing to do in therapy. Some students at this level view clinical reasoning as discovering 'the truth'. Others rely on occupational therapy educators to explicate it. However, many of the problems faced by occupational therapists involve uncertainty, are incomplete, or cannot be articulated by clients (Chapparo, 1993; Rogers, 1983). If students are to develop clinical reasoning strategies that are based on understanding of the client's perspective of the problem, they must learn to construct a therapeutic solution to the existing problem that is justifiable after consideration of all perspectives of the problem and all interpretations of the problem. This can only occur if students begin to accept that for some problems, there are no absolutely 'true' answers.

Based on the work of adult educators (e.g. Mezirow, 1991) we have found that specific educational experiences in both the academic and clinical portions of the curriculum are ideally designed to focus on ways that students can discover the meaning other people have of illness and disability.

Aim

The aim of these learning experiences is not only for students to understand the perspectives of others but to be challenged to examine their own perspectives about illness, therapy and disability. These challenges, along with appropriate environmental support, promote an interactive clinical reasoning style that is based on reflective thinking.

We have come to realize in facilitating these learning experiences, that there are developmental limits to how far or how fast students at a given age can advance in their ability to construct a mental picture of another person's perspective. Development of this type of reasoning appears to occur slowly, and, in our opinion, it is unlikely that young adults, even given the best educational environment, will easily use the kind of reflective judgement that experienced therapists employ. Therefore, expected outcomes of learning experiences designed to promote interactive reasoning need to be adjusted by occupational therapy educators to suit the experience and maturity of the students in the group.

We have evaluated the effectiveness of these learning experiences by assessing how well students are able to communicate effectively with a variety of people. From the perspective of clinical reasoning, critical communication skills include identifying and interpreting another person's beliefs and values about disability; phrasing interpretations of another person's views of disability in non-judgemental terms and comparing and contrasting client problems from the perspectives of the medical diagnosis, the occupational diagnosis and the client who is ill.

The structure of learning experiences and the role of facilitator

In our program we pay attention to the development of student abilities through three increasingly complex stages of interactive reasoning as presented by Chapparo (1993). First, students work on developing the antecedent skills required for client-focused communication. These antecedent skills are largely interpersonal and include observation, listening, questioning, and feeling at ease with entering purposive social interactions within the context of an interview. Second, students work on developing an ability to accurately record and interpret information they obtain from others during discourse. This phase could be conceptualized as testing out the interpretations of other people's stories and metaphors of illness and disability. Third, students engage in the process of exploring another person's personal causality. This involves students engaging in purposive discourse in which the structure, duration, context and conditions are set by the client's situation. The primary function of this aspect of interactive reasoning is to let the student explore issues of maintaining and relinquishing control and authority, thereby facilitating clients and others to become participants in the reasoning process.

Facilitation mechanisms that can be used by educators to develop abilities at each of the three developmental phases of narrative reasoning include, but are not limited to, the following.

A. Antecedent phase. Practice of communication skills within the context of interactive reasoning consists of intensive practice of interacting with others, with the goal being to understand other people's perspectives about disability. Students are required to encourage others to voice their views about disability and illness. These practice interview sessions are videotaped and then discussed by the whole tutorial group. Ultimately, students obtain a range of different perspectives of disability that are held by different people. In such situations the risks and pressures of voicing personal opinions are minimized by the educator who models the kind of listening, observing, and interviewing that is essential to the student's role as an interactive reasoner; encouraging the student to examine information gathered and identify gaps that pose problems in creating a picture of another person's perspective.

B. Interpretation phase. During this interactive phase of learning, facilitators question students about the dimensions of the information obtained through interviews and observations of clients and others. This includes prompting when information has been missed or when assumptions have been made in the absence of direct information from the client. Students are encouraged to interpret the narratives of others and rephrase them in a form that they understand. They are encouraged to identify aspects of client narratives that are puzzling and to create an explanation that could account for the puzzling phenomena.

C. Personal causality phase. In this aspect of developing interactive reasoning skills, students engage in exploration of the perspectives of others in situations that are characterized by risk taking, pressure and accountability. Students participate in a series of 'hypotheticals' that require them to role-play various dichotomous scenarios (as described by Donelly, 1992).

The technique of dichotomous scenarios employs a forced-choice format, where the student is assigned one of a number of alternative perspectives concerning some aspect of a clinical situation. One such example involves a case history of an occupational therapist who is engaged in helping parents place their child with developmental disability into a regular school. Students are required to take the part of the child, the parents, the classroom teacher, the school principal and the occupational therapist. They develop arguments for and against such a placement from the perspective of one particular person in the scenario. Underpinning the development of positions for placement (therapist, child and parents) and against the placement (teacher and principal) is information regarding ideology, educational policy, hegemony, general views of people about children with developmental disability, the students' own views about developmental disability and their interpretations of videotapes of interviews with parents of children with developmental disability. The purpose of these exercises is to help students learn to develop a client-centred reasoning process. Facilitation consists of helping students identify and confront the issue of their degree of commitment to the clients' perspectives, goals and needs, versus the students' perspectives, goals and needs; helping students confront and understand hostile judgements and reactions; and helping students expand the extent to which they are conscious of client-centred issues in their reasoning processes.

Facilitating ethical reasoning in occupational therapy

Although occupational therapy interventions are not often directly concerned with ethical issues of life and death, they are concerned with issues of quality of life, the consequences of many modern life saving techniques. The most common ethical question to be answered by occupational therapy practitioners today is concerned with 'who will be treated when not all can be treated' (Neuhaus, 1988, p. 288). Having the knowledge, the clinical judgement and the clinical skill but not the funding, the time or resources to enhance a client's quality of life is a constant dilemma for today's practising therapist.

The realism of these ethical dilemmas is often far removed from the idealism that is a feature of many curricula. Students often report back from clinical sites about difficulties they had with clinical reasoning that led to decisions about the amount, type and intensity of actual treatment versus the treatment that should have been given. Students in these situations speak of feelings of helplessness, ineffectiveness and in many cases anger towards therapists, patients, educators and the health system in general. They have difficulty using their reasoning processes to imagine how they, as future therapists, will work in environments where such decisions must be made. Students often lack three ingredients that offer a sense of direction to experienced therapists: facts, experience (Neuhaus, 1988) and wisdom.

It is clear that students need useful and timely learning experiences that bring ethical questions closer to reality. These learning experiences can illustrate how clinical decision making must always be tempered with open acknowledgment that it may not always be possible to decide the 'right' thing to do in a clinical situation. In many instances, it is a matter of deciding that one decision is better than other less desirable options.

Aim

The general aim of learning experiences that facilitate a process of ethical reasoning is to help students consider alternative solutions to clinical problems involving ethical dilemmas in a systematic way, and to increase students' understanding of the psychological dimensions of ethical decision making. We evaluate these learning experiences by identifying how well students are able to: identify ethical issues in clinical situations; articulate ethical reasons for treatment choices they make; appropriately tolerate and/or resist ethical disagreement and ambiguity in clinical situations; and ultimately, articulate a personal ethical framework that can guide decision making.

The structure of learning experiences and the role of facilitator

There are two primary processes involved in ethical reasoning. One involves a cognitive process whereby students identify and understand ethical principles and issues that relate to health care and disability. The other involves interpersonal and intrapersonal processes that incorporate individual values, perceptions, opinions and feelings. As with the development of interactive reasoning, learning experiences that facilitate ethical reasoning are structured in consideration of students' levels of maturity and their increasing ability for self-reflection. Harnessing the interpersonal communication skills acquired in other parts of the curriculum, together with knowledge about disability, students can begin to engage in the process of ethical reasoning.

First, students' ethical imagination is stimulated by increasing their knowledge of key ethical principles (autonomy, beneficence, truthfulness, and justice) and by exposing them to many ethical issues in occupational therapy practice. One of the most effective teaching tools to stimulate ethical imagination is the use of case studies. Through case studies, students can be guided to identify ethical issues, apply ethical principles to real life clinical situations and determine their own ethical position. Supervision in these learning experiences requires an educator who can create a 'safe' learning environment where students are free to express their own opinions and feelings. The educator gives explicit permission for the variety of ethical positions that will exist within the student group. The most helpful facilitators are those who can act as role models for students, not in asserting the 'correct' ethical position, but in demonstrating how ethical questions can be openly discussed.

Second, students are required to start making decisions that involve ethical reasoning and build a strong case for the decision that is made. Structures for facilitating this level of reasoning, again, involve case studies. One example of how this could be done is an exercise where students are asked to determine who will be treated in an occupational therapy program that is limited by staff shortages. Out of five clients of varying age, sex and disability, students are to choose which two will receive immediate therapy. Each student is required to outline the line of reasoning that led to this choice and articulate how the choice reflects his or her personal, ethical and moral values.

Using case studies, the following exercise also contributes to helping the student become aware of the ethical issues implicit in reasoning a course of action. After presentation of a case, students are required to analyse the implied contract between the occupational therapist and client(s) in the case. This analysis incorporates such aspects of ethical action as rights, obligations of the therapist and client, the nature of the relationship, determining who makes the decisions about the course of action and the handling of conflicting ethics (Haddad, 1988). Students are then required to articulate how the implicit ethics of the situation impact on the clinical reasoning process which culminates in treatment.

Third, students are helped to appreciate the emotional and affective reactions that accompany ethical dilemmas and to channel these responses into a feeling, but logically reasoned response. As with interactive reasoning, role-playing dichotomous scenarios allows students to simulate clinical experiences initially within a 'safe' environment. As Haddad (1988) reports, role-playing demonstrates the difference between doing and thinking. It permits students to practise developing reasoned affective responses that are often required for maintaining good interpersonal relationships between health care workers who have disparate ethical positions. It illustrates how a therapist's behaviour is a function not only of personality, but also of role expectation. Last, students become

aware of the feelings of others and learn that it is usual for others to hold different points of view.

In using this method, students are encouraged to display genuine responses and ask questions as the scenario progresses. Volunteers for each scenario are sought and others act as participant observers of the decision making process. The primary focus of the technique at this level is that it is focused on process, rather than solution (as described by Donelly, 1992) .

Putting it all together using multiple reasoning modes

Ultimately students require opportunities to orchestrate multiple reasoning modes and learn about the 'art' of clinical reasoning. Functional performance requires motivation, physical action and understanding social meaning within social and cultural contexts. It is necessary, therefore, that students engage in learning experiences that challenge them to consider all aspects of the client and the presenting problem.

Aim

Of the clinical reasoning modes described, this is perhaps the most difficult for undergraduate students as it requires professional and life experience to construct images of client potential. We expect that students will be able to change from one reasoning mode to another in describing a course of action in therapy.

The structure of learning experiences and the role of facilitator

The stimulus we use to promote the development of multiple reasoning modes is a detailed case history that incorporates complex and conflicting information about diagnosis, client perceptions, social, physical and cultural environments and organizational variables. Students are encouraged to use multiple reasoning modes by answering stimulus questions such as the following:

'What is the problem?'
Answers to this question are identified from several perspectives: the client, care giver, doctor and the therapist, thereby challenging the

student to use both procedural and interactive modes of reasoning.

'What should be done?' and 'What can be done?'
Answers to these contrasting questions challenge students to shift from procedural modes of reasoning to making ethical decisions about what can be done within the social and economic constraints imposed by the variables in the case.

'What will I do?' and 'Why?'
Answers to these questions challenge students to make decisions based on the information at hand about their own actions and give reasons for their choice based on personal theoretical and ethical notions of the case.

'What will be the outcome?'
The ability to answer this question comes later in the curriculum when students have had considerable fieldwork experience. At earlier stages of learning it is important that educators fill out this part of the story of cases presented. Through experiential narratives from educators and from clinicians, students develop images of therapy outcomes. Story-telling within the context of case scenarios becomes a useful technique in developing skill at this stage of developing a clinical reasoner.

Conclusion

Facilitation of students' clinical reasoning incorporates scientific and artistic elements that are directed to a specific conclusion: the most appropriate action for a particular client. Since this process calls for judgement and decision making as well as science, the ethical and intuitive elements of the reasoning process must be equally recognized as significant facets of the educational process. We have suggested in this chapter that effective clinical reasoning can be facilitated through the use of two related structures. The first is a curriculum context that supports the values and assumptions of clinical reasoning in occupational therapy, and ultimately provides a vehicle for translating clinical reasoning into the total occupational therapy process. The second is through specifically structured learning units that facilitate both specific modes and integrative modes of clinical reasoning.

References

Bittel, B. (1989) *Make Your Own Tomorrow: Adult Learning and You.* Hyde Park Press, Adelaide

Brookfield, S. (1981) Independent adult learning. *Studies in Adult Education,* **13**, 15–27

Brookfield, S. (1983) *Adult Learners, Adult Education and the Community.* Teachers College Press, New York

Brookfield, S. (1985) Self-directed learning: A critical review of research. In *New Directions for Continuing Education* – Number 25: *Self-Directed Learning: From Theory to Practice* (ed. S. Brookfield). Jossey Bass, San Francisco

Brundage, D. and MacKeracher, D. (1980) *Adult Learning Principles and Their Application to Program Planning.* The Minister for Education, Toronto

Burns, R. and Brooks, G. (1974) Processes, problem solving and curriculum reform. In *Conflicting Conceptions of Curriculum* (eds E. Eisner and E. Vallance). McCutchan Publishing Corp, Berkeley

Chapparo, C. (1993) Clinical reasoning: A model for occupational therapy in the practice area of neurology. Unpublished PhD Thesis. Macquarie University, Sydney

Cunningham, P. (1982) Contradictions in the practice of nontraditional continuing education. In *New Directions for Continuing Education,* No. 25: *Linking Philosophy and Practice* (ed. S. Merriam). Jossey-Bass, San Francisco

Donelly, M. (1992) *Integration Issues in Occupational Therapy. Fourth Year Curriculum Hypotheticals.* School of Occupational Therapy, The University of Sydney, Sydney

Fleming, M.H. (1991) Clinical reasoning in medicine compared with clinical reasoning in occupational therapy. *American Journal of Occupational Therapy,* **45**, 988–996

Gale, J. and Marsden, P. (1982) Clinical problem solving: the beginning of the process. *Medical Education,* **16**, 22–26

Grundy, S. (1987) *Curriculum: Product or Praxis.* The Falmer Press, London

Haddad, A.M. (1988) Teaching ethical analysis in occupational therapy. *American Journal of Occupational Therapy,* **42**, 300–304

Hopkins, H.L., and Tiffany, E.G. (1988) Occupational therapy – A problem-solving process. In *Willard and Spackman's Occupational Therapy,* 7th edn. (eds H.L. Hopkins and H.D. Smith). J.B. Lippincott, Philadelphia, pp. 102–111

Jelinek, J. (1978) The learning of values. In *Improving the Human Condition: A Curricular Response to Critical Realities* (ed. J. Jelinek). Association for Supervision and Curriculum Development, Washington DC

Knowles, M. (1984) *Andragogy in Action: Applying Modern Principles of Adult Education.* Jossey-Bass, San Francisco

Mezirow, J. (1981) A critical theory of adult learning and education. In *Education For Adults,* Vol. 1: *Adult*

Learning and Education (ed. M. Tight). The Open University, London

Mezirow, J. (1985) A critical theory of self-directed learning. In *New Directions for Continuing Education – Number 25: Self-Directed Learning: From Theory to Practice* (ed. S. Brookfield). Jossey-Bass, San Francisco

Mezirow, J. (1991) How critical reflection triggers transformative learning. In *Fostering Critical Reflection in Adulthood* (ed. J. Mezirow). Jossey-Bass, San Francisco

Neuhaus, B.E. (1988) Ethical considerations in clinical reasoning: The impact of technology and cost containment. *American Journal of Occupational Therapy*, **42**, 288–292

Pelland, M.J. (1987) A conceptual model for the instruction and supervision of treatment planning. *American Journal of Occupational Therapy*, **41**, 351–359

Pratt, D. (1987) Curriculum design and humanistic technology. *Journal of Curriculum Studies*, **19**, 149–162

Ranka, J. (1986) Occupational therapy theory and Process 1 subject description. In *Stage 4 Review: Bachelor of Applied Science (Occupational Therapy)*. School of Occupational Therapy, University of Sydney

Ranka, J. (1990) *Occupational Therapy Theory and Process 1 Subject Workbook*. School of Occupational Therapy, University of Sydney

Rogers, J.C. (1983) Eleanor Clarke Slagle lectureship – 1983: Clinical reasoning: The ethics, science and art. *American Journal of Occupational Therapy*, **37**, 601–616

Rogers, J.C. and Masagatani, G. (1982) Clinical reasoning of occupational therapists during the initial assessment of physically disabled patients. *Occupational Therapy Journal of Research*, **2**, 195–219

Rogers, J.C. and Holm, M. (1991) Occupational therapy diagnostic reasoning: A component of clinical reasoning. *American Journal of Occupational Therapy*, **45**, 1045–1053

Schon, D.A. (1987) *Educating the Reflective Practitioner: Toward a New Design for Teaching and Learning in the Professions.* Jossey-Bass, San Francisco

Skager, R. (1978) *Lifelong Education and Evaluation Practice.* Pergamon Press, New York

Starratt, R. (1974) Curriculum theory: Controversy, challenge and future concerns. In *Heightened Consciousness, Cultural Revolution and Curriculum* (ed. W. Pinar). McCutchan, Berkeley

18

Issues in teaching clinical reasoning to students of speech and hearing science

Janet Doyle

In this chapter I hope to convince the reader of the need for closer examination of the links and distinctions between the teaching and learning of clinical reasoning on the one hand, and clinical reasoning as practised by clinicians on the other. In particular I will be arguing for a better data base on which to draw when assisting students to develop clinical reasoning skills consistent with good clinical practice. I also make a related plea for a greater degree of connection between academic activity and clinical practice. The views expressed here have developed from my experience in the field of speech and hearing sciences, as a practising audiologist and as an educator of student speech pathologists. My colleagues Susan Block, Louise Brown, Georgia Dacakis, Jacinta Douglas, Jenni Oates and Shane Thomas have each assisted significantly with the development of some of the thoughts presented.

For the purposes of this chapter, clinical reasoning is defined as the application of relevant knowledge and skills to the evaluation, diagnosis and rehabilitation of client problems (Jones and Butler, 1991). Hence clinical reasoning is an essential aspect of clinician activity. However, in my view clinical reasoning is only part of what may be termed the clinical decision-making system, in which the major and interrelated components are clinician, client, task and environment (Doyle and Thomas, 1988). This concept of a dynamic system acknowledges the natural complexity of the clinical situation, reminding us of the

interactive character of these four components and of their influence on system output.

Each component is also complex in itself. Clinicians have attributes which include: knowledge base, length, type and variety of clinical experience, style of interpersonal interaction, role perception, perceptions of the problem or task, professional ethos, clinical policy and habit, need for and response to decision feedback, response to environmental constraints and expectations, and clinical reasoning ability. The clients have a similar range of attributes, including their own perceptions of the problem or task. The task will have attributes which include: explicitness, complexity, familiarity, and relationship to other tasks. The environment component has attributes which include: the prevailing style of clinician–client interaction, the relative emphasis on individual versus group decision-making among clinicians, physical and financial resources, treatment philosophy and protocols, stated aims and responsibilities of the facility and its funding sources, and decision making balance between clinicians and administrators. This environment overlaps with the personal environment of the individual client and his or her family.

Given this framework, clinical reasoning may be seen as an aspect of the clinician component of the complex natural system which is clinical activity. Clinical reasoning involves formulating and then choosing among various options which are identified and described in terms of data variables (Hammond et al, 1980). This is done by the exercise of judgement which is the cognitive process of evaluating those data (Schwartz and Griffin, 1986). Clinical reasoning results in a decision to behave in a certain way. Although not usually the case, this behaviour may include taking no action (Schwartz and Griffin, 1986).

Clinical reasoning may be further conceptualized in terms of broad cognitive strategy and in terms of how informational cues are used. General cognitive approaches to judgement, such as the 'exhaustive', 'hypothetico-deductive', and 'pattern recognition' strategies have been proposed. The hypothetico-deductive approach for example, described by Elstein et al (1978) is thought by many decision researchers and clinical educators to be a highly effective general cognitive strategy. Such strategies are not necessarily used consistently by individuals who employ them, the decision strategy possibly varying with the nature of the problem (Politser, 1981). At a more detailed level, clinical reasoning involves the use of clinical data in the form of a range of informational cues. Decision makers use these cues in various ways, generally placing more importance on some cues or combinations of cues, than on others. Hence, even given the same general cognitive approach to a clinical problem, individuals may weight informational cues differently. This latter aspect of clinical reasoning will be addressed in the present chapter.

In the context of this paper the client base of interest comprises persons with communication disorders. Such disorders include problems with articulation, language, fluency, voice, hearing, cognition, social interaction, and certain motor functions such as swallowing. Speech pathologists diagnose and treat a broad range of such communication problems, although many develop a speciality practice with particular client groups. Audiologists diagnose and treat those persons whose communication difficulties primarily lie with hearing loss.

Speech pathologists from the La Trobe University program in Victoria qualify after completing a four year, full-time Bachelor of Speech Pathology degree, during which they experience a minimum of 300 directly supervised contact hours with clients, and a similar number of hours in related clinical activity such as case discussions, report writing and administration. In Australia audiologists qualify for clinical practice after completing a graduate diploma or degree in Audiology, following a first degree in Psychology, Science, Speech Pathology, or Medicine. Audiology programs usually involve at least 200 contact hours of directly supervised clinical practicum.

Clinical practice in speech and hearing sciences

It is useful to review some of the characteristics of clinical practice in the field of communication disorders which impinge on the clinical reasoning process and on our attempts to develop the clinical reasoning skills of students. Firstly, the presenting symptoms of persons with communication problems can be diffuse and can involve complex relationships between component communication skills. The fact that an individual's communication is intimately linked to their particular life setting further complicates the picture. As a result of these factors a sequential process of diagnosis and treatment may not be possible in many cases. Rather, diagnosis and treatment may be concurrent processes, each process contributing to the refinement of the other. Additionally, there may be a need to assess and continually evaluate priorities and goals where multiple aspects of communication are involved. These implications for reasoning and clinical practice need to be considered during the teaching or fostering of students' hypothesis generating skills and the development of judgement necessary for treatment selection decisions.

Secondly, although the use of technology in speech pathology practice is increasing and has always been a feature of audiology practice, the prime vehicle of assessment in communication disorders remains communication itself. Whilst speech pathologists and audiologists may observe client interaction with others, they are typically involved in the processes they are attempting to evaluate. This means that they must not only concurrently observe and interact with the client, but that they must also observe the interaction to which they contribute. During communication assessments speech pathologists and audiologists may need to make a range of judgements to interpret client responses as either diagnostic signs, or as features of the interpersonal process between clinician and client. A corollary of this is the influence of the clinician's interpersonal skills on assessment and treatment processes and outcomes. Conventional wisdom among speech pathologists and audiologists is that the individual clinician's personality and clinical approach can be a highly significant influence on the interaction process.

Thirdly, as in other health science areas, there is a range of potentially suitable approaches to the treatment of many communication problems. For example, fluency problems can be treated with an intensive program, or with longer term, intermittent, individual speech therapy, and may be addressed with relaxation, prolongation, delayed auditory feedback and other techniques (Ham, 1986). Choices in voice therapy for laryngectomees include oesophageal speech, electronic devices, and surgically implanted prostheses (Edels, 1983). Hearing problems may be addressed with hearing aid amplification, development of speech reading skills, use of assistive listening devices, environmental manipulation, assertiveness training, or some combination of these approaches (Alpiner and McCarthy, 1987). The potential benefits and risks of these various options for individual clients are not always easy to predict. In my view this is partly due to insufficient data from comparative studies of the therapeutic outcomes associated with various treatments for particular communication problems. In fact we know relatively little about the prevalence of different treatment approaches. The clinician is generally faced with several treatment choices and with some difficulty in assessing the relative merit of these.

Further, the culture of particular clinical environments may influence treatment choice. In a given clinic, there may have developed over time a clinic preference for a particular approach to diagnosis and treatment for various problems. For example, the rationale underlying the management of common vocal disorders may be a traditional symptom-based orientation (e.g. Colton and Casper, 1990) in one clinic, and a more global philosophy (e.g. Aronson, 1990), in another. Similarly, assessment and management of persons with acquired brain damage may be characterized in one clinic by a psycholinguistic approach (e.g. Lesser, 1989), whereas other clinics may have a pragmatic (e.g. Davis and Wilcox, 1985) or localizationist orientation (e.g. Goodglass and Kaplan, 1983). In some areas of communication therapy, treatment given

may be overtly connected to the personal beliefs and cultural values of clinicians and clients. The area of hearing impairment in children, for example, is known for the vigour with which oral versus manual approaches to communication development and rehabilitation are discussed, and for the sometimes zealous commitment of clinicians to one or the other approach (Schlesinger, 1986).

Implications for teaching clinical reasoning

Given these and other natural complexities associated with clinical practice in speech and hearing sciences, how is clinical reasoning best taught? Our general approach in the Department of Communication Disorders at La Trobe University has been one of encouraging the development of reasoning skills by providing opportunities to observe, discuss, exercise and evaluate clinical reasoning. This fostering approach is consistent with that proposed by Gale (1982) and by Higgs (1990).

We do not have a compulsory unit or subject in our degree program for speech pathologists titled 'Clinical Reasoning' or similar. Rather we attempt to develop clinical reasoning skills through experiential learning. There are three reasons for this. Firstly, we are not convinced that a theoretical coverage of clinical reasoning will result in generalization to clinical practice. Research has shown that studying the process of decision analysis for instance does not necessarily result in more efficient decision behaviour, and the knowledge gained in formal study of clinical reasoning may not be applied to practice (Grant and Marsden, 1986; Schwartz and Griffin, 1986; Doubilet and McNeil, 1988). Secondly, we acknowledge that for many communication disorders there are a range of approaches to diagnosis and treatment, each of which may be equally valid. We wish to develop some acknowledgement of this among students, and to promote flexibility in student responses to clinical problems. Thirdly, the majority of our teaching staff are themselves practising clinicians, and this has led to an educational environment which favours an integrated approach to the development of student skills.

One of our key teaching strategies is the use of simulated patients in classroom learning contexts. The goal of these sessions is to enable students to experience their reasoning role and develop their skill in reasoning in a protected, simulated environment which provides them with feedback on their performance and opportunities for discussion and reflection on their reasoning. The chapter by Edwards, Franke and McGuiness in this volume discusses the use of this strategy in the speech pathology course and in other courses at La Trobe University. Such conscious experience of clinical reasoning in a safe environment is complemented by 300 hours of client contact experienced in a range of clinics during the speech pathology course, and the corresponding opportunity to observe and benefit from the clinical reasoning of experienced clinicians, who in some cases are acknowledged experts.

The need for real world data

In this paper my concern is to discuss a fundamental problem which I believe applies not only to speech and hearing sciences, but across much of health science education. This problem is the lack of a comprehensive data base concerning how clinicians reason in practice, drawn from the everyday practice of qualified clinicians, on which we can draw when discussing the notion of good practice in clinical reasoning, and to which we can refer for educational purposes.

Data from the real world practice of speech pathologists and audiologists have the potential to form an invaluable feedback loop, connecting academic activity and student learning to clinical practice. At this point in time we do not know (empirically) whether the majority of persons who graduate from our program continue to develop their clinical reasoning skills, perhaps later becoming 'experts'; we do not know to what degree the clinical reasoning abilities of our graduates interact with the clinical environment of their workplace; we do not know if and how individual speech pathologists and audiologists differ in their approach to particular problems; and we know very little about how the clinical reasoning and the resultant decisions of clinicians relate to outcome measures in health care. These are all important issues for practising clinicians and educators alike, and need to be addressed if we are to link student learning to the demands of clinical practice in an optimal manner. In particular we need the courage to evaluate our clinical behaviour in relation to the optimality of client out-

comes. So how best to gather data to provide the necessary description of clinical reasoning as it occurs in practice?

There is good reason to believe that research aimed at addressing these and other issues is best conducted in the real world of clinical practice, rather than in the laboratory, or in the university teaching clinic. Although the latter settings offer opportunities to refine the knowledge gained by studies of real world practice, and are excellent for studying aspects of student learning, they cannot be assumed to yield data which generalize to everyday practice of qualified speech pathologists and audiologists. The settings are often simply too different. In general, the external validity of research findings conducted in laboratory settings, and those derived purely from the study of hypothetical cases, is questionable (Ebbeson and Konecni, 1980; Thomas et al, 1990). In 1980 Ebbeson and Konecni published a paper in which they reviewed comparisons of decision making behaviour in natural and laboratory settings. In a series of studies with judges and car drivers, Ebbeson and Konecni were able to demonstrate that the use of particular items of information (cues) by the same decision makers varied significantly in the two settings. They concluded that 'the external validity of research that relies on laboratory simulations of real-world decision problems is low. Seemingly insignificant features of the decision task and measures cause people to alter their decision strategies' (Ebbeson and Konecni, 1980, p. 42).

This comment might also apply to the use of simulated patients to study clinical reasoning. Colleagues and I have provided a more recent review of this problem as it pertains to the clinical situation (Thomas et al, 1990). Two main points were made in this review. The first was that the methodology frequently used to study as well as to teach clinical reasoning and decision making in controlled settings may yield data that do not relate well to clinical behaviour in natural settings. Judgement behaviour in simulated Paper Patient Management Problems for example, may differ from that in the real clinic (Goran et al, 1973; Page and Fielding, 1980). Additionally, with the notable exception of Elstein et al (1978), the issue of realism in other pen and paper clinical tasks is rarely discussed. Therefore, as with the judges in Ebbeson and Konecni's (1980) studies, we would assert that it is possible that both student and practising speech pathologists and audiologists might behave differently in laboratory and natural settings.

The second major point made by Thomas et al (1990) was that clinical reasoning in natural settings may be influenced by a range of factors simply not encountered in controlled settings. These factors include sociological influences (Eisenberg, 1979), stress (Cleland, 1967; Lippincott, 1979; Bourbonnais and Baumann, 1985), time pressures, and circadian rhythms (Watkins, 1984). Time pressures and other aspects of the clinical environment are known to be problems for many audiologists and speech pathologists (Doyle, 1989; Meggs and Doyle, 1992). This is not to say that situations in which, for instance, time pressure is absent or deliberately controlled are not very useful for aspects of teaching clinical reasoning, but simply that any research data derived from such situations may have limited applicability to the real world clinic.

An additional problem with trying to study clinical reasoning processes solely in the laboratory or teaching clinic is that the task is usually designed to assist with particular research or educational objectives, and therefore may not be fully representative of the tasks which test the clinical reasoning of practitioners. Further, the manner in which a task is presented may influence judgement (Tversky and Kahneman, 1981; Payne, 1982). The effects on decision behaviour of redundant information, the temporal order of information acquisition, and the amount and manner of information presentation, have been reviewed by Einhorn and Hogarth (1981), Larichev and Moshkovich (1988), and Levin and Reicks (1990).

Framing (i.e. the manner in which information is presented to judges) and other task effects in clinical decision-making have been clearly demonstrated (Eraker and Sox, 1981; Tversky and Kahneman, 1981; McNeil et al, 1986). For example, McNeil et al (1986) found that choice between alternative therapies for lung cancer was influenced by whether the likely result was framed in terms of mortality (probability of dying) or in terms of survival (probability of living). Additionally, as already indicated, judgement may be affected by the context in which the judgement is made, the decision maker being influenced by aspects of the environment not directly presented as part of the decision task (Einhorn and Hogarth, 1982).

The cognitive processes involved in solving tasks in some laboratory settings have been demonstrated to be volatile, and may easily change in response to minor changes in task presentation (Dawes, 1975; Hayes and Simon, 1977). Hayes and Simon (1977), in a series of experiments involving problem isomorphs, demonstrated that changing instructions can affect the time required to solve problems. This was because subjects adopted different representations of the problem in response to different instructions. Dawes (1975) argued that if there is a single model of appropriate task performance, then that model is primarily related to the task, rather than the subject undertaking the task. In other words, however we present the task when studying clinical reasoning in a controlled way, we may influence the processes we are seeking to document.

As is evident from the preceding discussion, it is important that more research is carried out in natural field settings if we are to develop a good description of the clinical reasoning behaviour of practitioners. Natural field settings contain the complexity of problems as encountered by decision makers (Wigton, 1988). Such field studies are appropriate to the discovery and prediction of decision behaviour (Carroll and Johnson, 1990), allow researchers to select those tasks which are representative of the clinical practice under study, and have the potential to establish the prevalence of heuristics and treatment decisions (Hershey and Baron, 1987).

Not only should we study clinical reasoning in the real clinic, but we should study practising clinicians. To date, many studies of clinical reasoning and decision making have used students instead of, or in addition to, practising clinicians. For example, Norman et al (1990) reported a study designed 'to explore the nature of diagnostic errors in dermatologic diagnosis' (p. 19). Subjects were 16 first year family medicine residents, and the study provided subjects with educative examples of the clinical cases they were later asked to judge. Thus not only was the research situation controlled, but the study concurrently addressed learning and decision behaviour. The use of student or novice practitioners in many studies of clinical reasoning and decision making remains common. This is perfectly appropriate if the aim is to develop effective methods of teaching decision making and evaluating student learning (Balla, 1982; Balla and Edwards, 1986; Eisenstaedt et al, 1990; Papa et al, 1990). However, it is not valid if we wish to study what clinicians do when they are no longer students. It is important to avoid confusing the study of student learning with the study of practitioners' clinical reasoning.

Brehmer and Brehmer (1988) argued that student subjects will not usually have a developed approach or judgement policy for the clinical reasoning task in question, but will develop their policies during the course of the experiment. Brehmer and Brehmer (1988) also made the point that because student subjects have little or no experience of the characteristics of real cases relevant to the judgement task, their judgements are unlikely to be affected by deviations from representativeness in the task. Thus results of policy-capturing studies (i.e. studies that analyse judges' behaviour to derive a profile of how judges weight the relative importance of informational cues) which employ students cannot generalize well to the judgements of experienced subjects. The evidence firmly suggests that the use of subjects who are experienced and typical practitioners is necessary if research findings are to be valid representations of the clinical reasoning and decision behaviour of speech pathologists and audiologists.

A study of practising audiologists' decisions

I will now briefly describe a study of practising audiologists' reasoning and decisions conducted by myself and a colleague Shane Thomas. The study addressed a very common, and presumably relatively simple, clinical task: whether or not to recommend hearing aid amplification. Subjects were sixteen Australian audiologists (eight females and eight males). Assessing client suitability for hearing aid amplification was known to be a normal part of the client practice of each audiologist.

Each of the sixteen audiologists was asked to study the same set of 80 cases (70 different cases, and 10 of the 70 which were repeated for purposes of assessing reliability), and in each case to note whether they would, or would not, recommend hearing aid amplification. They were not asked to make any deci-

sions about hearing aid style or electroacoustic characteristics, but simply whether they would recommend aiding to the client. Each audiologist made his or her recommendations independently, over two sessions.

The cases were designed to be representative of naturally-occurring cases. This was achieved by using audiograms from real clients, and including information which audiologists were known to seek in consultations with clients (Doyle, 1990). The task was designed only after extensive observation of practice in real clinics. The presentation of each case was in a format typical of audiological data, and each case had passed a prior realism assessment. In these and other ways, the task was constructed to be typical of cases encountered by the audiologists in clinical practice.

There were six informational cues embedded in each case. These were: the average pure tone loss (Cue #1), the hearing threshold at 2000 Hz (Cue #2), the slope of the hearing loss (Cue #3), speech discrimination ability (Cue #4), the degree of hearing difficulty reported by the client (Cue #5), and the client's attitude towards aiding (Cue #6). Thus four of the six cues represented information derived from test procedures, and two of the cues represented information gained from interaction with the client. I was interested to discover how practising audiologists utilized these cues to reach the aiding/not aiding decision. What degree of agreement would there be among audiologists? If they differed in their opinions, could those differences be explained by different clinical reasoning, even though they were given exactly the same data? The methodological difficulty remained that audiologist behaviour might be different if faced with real clients, rather than representations of real clients (no matter how good those representations were). However, the study had potential to compare the clinical reasoning of individual practising audiologists for the same, very typical, problem.

The results were quite startling. As shown in the left hand column of Table 18.1, the number of cases for which aiding was recommended ranged from 15 to 61. That is, one audiologist recommended hearing aid amplification for 15 of the 70 cases, whereas another audiologist recommended aiding in 61 of the same cases. In general there was only a moderate level of agreement ($r = .49$) among the 16 audiologists.

Table 18.1 Hearing aid decisions, and standardized discriminant function coefficients for judgement cues, by audiologist

	Aiding recomendation		Cues					
	No	Yes	Average pure tone loss	2 KHz threshold	Slope	Speech discrimination	Client report	Client attitude
1	34	36	0.40573	0.39373	0.08212	−0.03289	0.38748	−0.53281
2	17	53	−0.42598	−0.57532	0.02330	0.48327	0.11636	0.41898
3	27	43	0.44732	0.45263	0.09631	0.07485	−0.01130	−0.64250
4	12	58	−0.11984	1.03781	0.06710	−0.05794	0.02834	−0.22561
5	22	48	0.04020	0.83323	0.01949	−0.18647	0.57289	−0.08584
6	21	49	0.19160	0.87474	0.10924	−0.16406	−0.08907	−0.12914
7	11	59	0.05142	0.48066	−0.08496	0.12464	0.88089	−0.34551
8	23	47	0.07032	0.91362	0.05259	−0.33148	−0.08500	−0.22129
9	9	61	−0.09846	0.93606	0.01689	0.03107	0.59053	0.16070
10	24	46	0.21373	−0.58749	−0.01680	0.02001	−0.16698	0.87141
11	15	55	−0.04677	0.97282	0.05971	−0.06532	0.16111	−0.22139
12	55	15	1.48515	−0.84557	−0.28671	−0.10670	0.18838	−0.34628
13	14	56	−0.12367	0.95520	−0.01013	−0.14080	0.35265	−0.35495
14	24	46	−0.32679	0.89558	0.01931	−0.01569	0.37650	−0.69859
15	11	59	0.47770	0.02033	−0.14068	−0.30489	0.55652	−0.60312
16	33	37	0.59132	0.45346	0.17251	0.10975	0.35282	0.06977

In order to determine how informational cues were used by individual audiologists to reach these obviously different decisions, estimates were calculated, for each audiologist, of the standardized discriminant coefficients (Klecka, 1975) with the six cues as the discriminating variables and the yes/no hearing aid recommendation as the criterion variable. Table 18.1 also shows these standardized canonical discriminant function coefficients for each of the six cues, by audiologist. The relative importance of each type of information is indicated by the size of the coefficient.

For example, the data for audiologist #4 show that Cue #2 (the client's hearing threshold at 2000 Hz) had a coefficient of 1.03781, much greater than any other cue. Thus, as the value of the 2000 Hz threshold changed, so was the audiologist's opinion about aiding likely to change. Cases in which there was a severe loss of hearing at the 2000 Hz frequency would very probably be recommended for aiding, whereas cases in which hearing at 2000 Hz was relatively good, would not. In contrast, changes in the values of other cues, such as Cue #5 (the degree of hearing difficulty reported by the client) were not likely to influence audiologist #4's recommendation. Whether the client reported little or great difficulty hearing mattered hardly at all in the clinical reasoning of this particular audiologist.

Study of Table 18.1 shows that other audiologists had very different approaches to the use of the clinical data. Audiologist #10 for example was influenced primarily by the client's attitude to hearing aids. It is clear that among audiologists there was a range of judgement policies reflecting differences in weights given to test data versus client reports.

A classification analysis (Norusis, 1988) showed that the discriminant functions describing audiologists' policies were very robust, with a mean correct classification rate of 89.9%. Thus audiologists' different recommendations for the same cases were not the result of any random behaviour, but of highly predictable, yet individualistic, patterns of clinical reasoning.

This demonstration of individualistic decision-making approaches is consistent with audiologists' own general observations of clinical practice. For example, Yeend and Dillon (1992) state 'It is also clear that, at least within NAL Hearing Centres, different audiologists make very different recommendations regarding fitting milder losses'. The study I have described here provides some empirical evidence of what many clinicians suspect to be the case: that the individual practitioner can be a potent factor in the delivery of speech and hearing services.

Implications of different clinical approaches for practice and teaching

The fact that individual clinicians may apply clinical reasoning in very different ways to particular decision tasks is not surprising, given that outcomes of our intervention frequently are not easy to predict. If decision outcome is likely to be variable and related to a number of interacting factors, it is unlikely that clinicians can readily develop their reasoning based on a knowledge of typical outcomes. In the absence of this knowledge, a range of potentially adequate approaches to the problem develop. Lack of data linking the outcomes of our decisions with the clinical reasoning which resulted in those decisions, means that we do not have the ready means of deciding whether one clinical reasoning approach is any better than another. This is a significant problem for clinicians, such as speech pathologists and audiologists, who deal routinely with questions for which there is no single, clear cut, obviously correct solution.

What constitutes a good outcome for a particular client? This is by no means an easy question to answer. To continue with the example of hearing aid amplification, the question of what constitutes an adequate or optimal hearing aid fitting has not been systematically addressed by audiologists. Demorest (1986) is of the view that this is because the benefit of hearing aid fitting has not been clearly defined, and hence there can be disagreement about criteria for an adequate solution to the task of providing amplification. In the absence of generally agreed outcome criteria, the task remains ill-defined because it is not clear whether or not a solution has been reached (Miller et al, 1960).

Current audiological approaches to outcome evaluation in hearing aid fitting fall into two broad categories. These are: surveys of client aid use and/or satisfaction, and audiological test measures such as real ear gain, aided thresholds or aided speech perception. The survey approach involves client centred criteria and therefore assumes that a successful fitting is one which is associated with user competence, high user satisfaction and hours of regular daily aid use in a range of situations (Brooks, 1981, 1985; Hawes et al, 1985; Hickson et al, 1986; Cox et al, 1991; Dawson et al, 1991). The test approach involves audiologist-centred criteria and therefore assumes that a successful fitting is one which is associated with a significant degree of test-demonstrated improvement in auditory perception of speech and/or its component frequencies (Mueller and Grimes, 1987; Byrne and Cotton, 1988).

Consistency between performance on these two broad criteria is not always evident (Brooks and Chetty, 1985) and this reflects in part some tension between client and audiologist perspectives to outcome evaluation. Moreover, within each approach, the methods employed may influence results. For example, in the client-centred survey approach the design of the survey instrument may significantly affect apparent outcome (Cox et al, 1991).

Regardless of the criteria used to judge the adequacy of hearing aid fitting, there is some evidence suggesting that optimal results may not be the norm (Upfold and Wilson, 1980; Upfold and Smither, 1981; Goldstein, 1984; Gray-Thompson and Richards, 1987). Can this situation be linked to variation in clinical reasoning approaches? We cannot know this if we have not yet agreed on what is the benefit to be expected, if we do not do more outcome studies, and if we do not study the clinical reasoning of the practitioners involved.

What does this all mean for educators? Which of the sixteen audiologists shown in Table 18.1 has the correct approach to the problem of assessing a client's need and suitability for hearing aid amplification? Is there a single correct approach, or a set of equally correct approaches? Which approach(es) serve(s) as a good model for student audiologists and speech pathologists? How should we use this information to inform our teaching?

I again state that a major limitation to answering these questions is the lack of information about the outcome of decisions resulting from different judgement processes such as those indicated here. There is much to be done if we are to first adequately describe what we do, then study the optimality of the decisions resulting from our clinical reasoning, and finally feed that information back into our teaching programs. The study of the development of clinical reasoning in students is an equally important matter, but I suggest that it is vital not to confuse this with the study of the reasoning of practising clinicians.

In summary, we need to describe the clinical reasoning and decisions of practising clinicians (in this case, speech pathologists and audiologists), to examine reasoning and the resultant decisions in terms of optimal client outcomes. Then we can consider what aspects of clinician behaviour are important to foster among student clinicians. In the meantime it is important to provide opportunities, in the clinic and in the classroom, for students to develop cognitive strategies, such as effective hypothesis generation and testing, that are known to be associated, at least in the case of experts, with accurate and efficient decision making.

References

Alpiner, J.G., McCarthy, P.A. (1987) *Rehabilitative Audiology: Children and Adults*. Williams and Wilkins, Baltimore

Aronson, A.E. (1990) *Clinical Voice Disorders*, 3rd edn. Thieme, New. York

Balla, J.I. (1982) Critical cues and prior probability in decision-making. *Methods of Information in Medicine*, **21**, 9–14

Balla, J.I. and Edwards, H. (1986) Some problems in teaching clinical decision-making. *Medical Education*, **20**, 487–491

Bourbonnais, F.F. and Baumann, A. (1985) Stress and rapid decision-making in nursing: An administrative challenge. *Nursing Administration Quarterly*, **9**, 85–91

Brehmer, A. and Brehmer, B. (1988) What have we learned about human judgment from thirty years of policy capturing? In *Human Judgment: The SJT View* (eds B. Brehmer and C.R.B. Joyce). Elsevier Science Publishers, Amsterdam, pp. 75–114

Brooks, D.N. (1981) Use of post aural hearing aids by NHS patients. *British Journal of Audiology*, **15**, 79–86

Brooks, D.N. (1985) Factors relating to the under-use of post aural hearing aids. *British Journal of Audiology*, **19**, 211–217

Brooks, D.N. and Chetty, M.V. (1985) A comparison of two hearing aid selection methods. *British Journal of Audiology*, **19**, 43–47

Byrne, D. and Cotton, S. (1988) Evaluation of the National Acoustic Laboratories new hearing aid selection procedure. *Journal of Speech and Hearing Research*, **31**, 178–186

Carroll, J.S. and Johnson, E.J. (1990) *Decision Research: A Field Guide*. (Applied Social Research Methods Series, Vol. 22). Sage Publications, Newbury Park, CA

Cleland, V.S. (1967) Effects of stress on thinking. *American Journal of Nursing*, **1**, 108–111

Colton, R.H. and Casper, J.K. (1990) *Understanding Voice Problems: A Physiological Perspective for Diagnosis and Treatment*. Williams and Wilkins, Baltimore

Cox, R.M., Gilmore, C. and Alexander, G.C. (1991)

Comparison of two questionnaires for patient-assessed hearing aid benefit. *Journal of the American Academy of Audiology*, **2**, 134–145

Davis, G.A. and Wilcox, M.J. (1985) *Adult Aphasia Rehabilitation: Applied Pragmatics*. College Hill Press, San Diego

Dawes, R.M. (1975) The mind, the model, and the task. In *Cognitive Theory: Volume I* (eds. F. Restle, R.M. Shiffrin, N.J. Castellan, H.R. Lindman and D.B. Pisoni). Lawrence Erlbaum Associates, Hillsdale, New Jersey

Dawson, P., Dillon, H. and Batlaglia, J. (1991) Output limiting compression for the severe–profoundly deaf. *Australian Journal of Audiology*, **13**, 1–12

Demorest, M.E. (1986) Problem solving: Stages, strategies and stumbling blocks. *Journal of the Academy of Rehabilitative Audiology*, **19**, 13–26

Doubilet, P. and McNeil, B.J. (1988) Clinical decision analysis. In *Professional Judgement: A Reader in Clinical Decision Making* (eds J. Dowie and A. Elstein). Cambridge University Press, Cambridge, M.A., pp. 255–276

Doyle, J. (1989) A survey of Australian audiologists' clinical decision-making. *Australian Journal of Audiology*, **11**, 75–88

Doyle, J. (1990) *Talk, Test and Tempt: What Happens in Audiological Consultations*. Paper presented to the 9th National Conference of the Audiological Society of Australia. The Audiological Society of Australia, Thredbo, N.S.W.

Doyle, J. and Thomas, S.A. (1988) Clinical decision-making in audiology: The case for investigating what we do. *Australian Journal of Audiology*, **10**, 45–56

Ebbeson, E.B. and Konecni, V.J. (1980) On the external validity of decision-making research: What do we know about decisions in the real world? In *Cognitive Processes in Choice and Decision Behaviour* (ed. T.S. Wallsten). Lawrence Erlbaum Associates, Hillsdale, New Jersey, pp. 21–45

Edels, Y. (ed.) (1983) *Laryngectomy: Diagnosis to Rehabilitation*. Croom Helm, Beckenham, Kent

Einhorn, H.J. and Hogarth, R.M. (1981) Behavioural decision theory: Processes of judgment and choice. *Annual Review of Psychology*, **32**, 53–88

Einhorn, H.J. and Hogarth, R.M. (1982) *A Theory of Diagnostic Inference: II. Judging Causality*. Centre for Decision Research, Graduate School of Business, University of Chicago

Eisenberg, J.M. (1979) Sociologic influences on decision-making by clinicians. *Annals of Internal Medicine*, **90**, 957–964

Eisenstaedt, R.S., Barry, W.E. and Glanz, K. (1990) Problem-based learning: Cognitive retention and cohort traits of randomly selected participants and decliners. *Academic Medicine*, **65**, S11–S12

Elstein, A.S., Shulman, L.S. and Sprafka, S.A. (1978) *Medical Problem Solving: An Analysis of Clinical*

Reasoning. Harvard University Press, Cambridge, Massachusetts

Eraker, S.A. and Sox, H.C. Jnr. (1981) Assessment of patients' preferences for therapeutic outcome. *Medical Decision Making*, **1**, 29–39

Gale, J. (1982) Some cognitive components of the diagnostic thinking process. *British Journal of Educational Psychology*, **52**, 64–76

Goldstein, D.P. (1984) Hearing impairment, hearing aids and audiology. *American Speech–Language–Hearing Association*, **26**, 24–38

Goodglass, H. and Kaplan, E. (1983) *The Assessment of Aphasia and Related Disorders*, 2nd edn. Lea and Feibiger, Philadelphia

Goran, M.J., Williamson, J.W. and Gonnella, J.S. (1973) The validity of patient management problems. *Journal of Medical Education*, **48**, 171–177

Grant, J. and Marsden, P. (1986) Medical students as adult learners: Implications for an innovative short course in the clinical curriculum. *Medical Teacher*, **8**, 243–251

Gray-Thompson, M. and Richards, S. (1987) A computer program for hearing aid selection: Its trial and development. *Australian Journal of Audiology*, **9**, 19–23

Ham, R. (1986) *Techniques of Stuttering Therapy*. Prentice Hall, Englewood Cliffs, New Jersey

Hammond, K.R., McClelland, G.H. and Mumpower, J. (1980) *Human Judgment and Decision-Making: Theories, Methods, and Procedures*. Praeger, New York

Hawes, N.A., Durand, R.M. and Clark, S.R. (1985) Understanding desired benefits of a hearing aid: A consumer behaviour perspective. *Journal of the Academy of Rehabilitative Audiology*, **18**, 112–122

Hayes, J.R. and Simon, H.A. (1977) Psychological differences among problem isomorphs. In *Cognitive Theory, Volume 2* (eds N.J. Castellan, D.B. Pisoni, and G.R. Potts). Lawrence Erlbaum Associates, Hillsdale, New Jersey, pp. 21–41

Hershey, J.C. and Baron, J. (1987) Clinical reasoning and cognitive processes. *Medical Decision Making*, **7**, 203–211

Hickson, L., Hamilton, L. and Orange, S.P. (1986) Factors associated with hearing aid use. *Australian Journal of Audiology*, **8**, 37–41

Higgs, J. (1990) Fostering the acquisition of clinical reasoning skills. *New Zealand Journal of Physiotherapy*, **18**, 13–17

Jones, M.A. amd Butler, D.S. (1991) Clinical reasoning. In *Mobilisation of the Nervous System* (ed. D.S. Butler). Churchill Livingstone, Melbourne, pp. 91–106

Klecka, W.R. (1975) Discriminant analysis. In *Statistical Package for the Social Sciences*, 2nd edn (eds N.H. Nie, C.H. Hull, J.G. Jenkins, K. Steinbrenner and D.H. Bent). McGraw-Hill, New York, pp. 434–467

Larichev, O.I. and Moshkovich, H.M. (1988) Limits to decision-making ability in direct multiattribute alternative evaluation. *Organizational Behaviour and Human Decision Processes*, **42**, 217–233

Lesser, R. (1989) *Linguistic Investigations of Aphasia*, 2nd edn. Studies in Disorders of Communication. Cole and Whurr, London

Levin, I.P. and Reicks, C.J. (1990) Contemporary application of research on judgement and decision making (Commentary). *Journal of the National University of Singapore Society*, **8**, 3–8

Lippincott, R.C. (1979) Psychological stress factors in decision-making. *Heart and Lung*, **8**, 1093–1097

McNeil, B.J., Pauker, S.G., Sox, H.C. Jnr., and Tversky, A. (1986) On the elicitation of preferences for alternative therapies. In *Judgment And Decision Making: An Interdisciplinary Reader* (eds H.R. Arkes and K.R. Hammond). Cambridge University Press, New York. pp. 386–393

Meggs, C. and Doyle, J. (1992) Job satisfaction. *Australian Communication Quarterly*, **Spring**, 12–15

Miller, G.A., Galanter, E. and Pribram, K.H. (1960) *Plans and the Structure of Behaviour*. Rinehart and Winston, New York

Mueller, H. and Grimes, M.A. (1987) Amplification systems for the hearing-impaired. In *Rehabilitative Audiology: Children and Adults* (eds J.G. Alpiner and P.A. McCarthy). Williams and Wilkins, Baltimore. pp. 115–160

Norman, G.R., Brooks, L.R., Allen, S.W. and Rosenthal, D. (1990) Sources of observer variation in dermatologic diagnosis. *Academic Medicine*, **65**, SI9–S20

Norusis, M.J. (1988) *SPSS-X Advanced Statistics Guide*. SPSS Inc., Chicago

Page, G.G. and Fielding, D.W. (1980) Performance on PMPs and performance in practice: are they related? *Journal of Medical Education*, **55**, 529–537

Papa, F.J., Shores, J.H. and Meyer, S. (1990) Effects of pattern matching, pattern discrimination, and experience in the development of diagnostic expertise. *Academic Medicine*, **65**, S21–S22

Payne, J.W. (1982) Contingent decision behaviour. *Psychological Bulletin*, **92**, 382–402

Politser, P. (1981) Decision strategies and clinical judgment. *Medical Decision Making*, **1**, 361–389

Schlesinger, H. (1986) Total communication in perspective. In *Deafness in Perspective* (ed. D . M. Lutterman). Taylor and Francis, London

Schwartz, S. and Griffin, T. (1986) *Medical Thinking: The Psychology of Medical Judgment and Decision-Making*. Springer-Verlag, New York

Thomas, S.A., Doyle, J. and Browning, C. (1990) Clinical decision making: What do we know about real world performance? In *Judgment and Decision Making* (ed. W.H. Loke). Scarecrow Press, Chicago

Tversky, A. and Kahneman, D. (1981) The framing of decisions and the psychology of choice. *Science*, **211**, 453–458

Upfold, L.J. and Smither, M.F. (1981) Hearing aid fitting protocol. *British Journal of Audiology*, **115**, 181–188

Upfold, L.J. and Wilson, D.A. (1980) Hearing aid distribution and use in Australia: The Australian Bureau of Statistics 1978 survey. *Australian Journal of Audiology*, **2**, 31–36

Watkins, S. (1984) How to live with rotating shifts. *Registered Nurse*, **March,** 57–58

Wigton, R.S. (1988) Use of linear models to analyze physicians' decisions. *Medical Decision Making*, **8**, 241–252

Yeend, I. and Dillon, H. (1992) Minimum aidable loss in infants and primary school aged children. Paper presented to the 10th National Conference of the Audiological Society of Australia. The Audiological Society of Australia, Barossa Valley, South Australia

19

Teaching towards clinical reasoning expertise in physiotherapy practice

Judi Carr, Mark Jones and Joy Higgs

Effective clinical practice in physiotherapy requires more than concern for others' welfare and competence in a range of treatment skills. It also requires an intellectual problem solving approach to the clinical encounter. This problem solving, or clinical reasoning, provides the framework within which the physiotherapist's concern and technical competence is applied so that the client can achieve the desired outcome.

However, there is more to being a professional physiotherapy practitioner than being a competent clinical care giver. Our undergraduate courses move ever further away from the model which successfully produced practitioners who worked essentially under medical referral, and even medical supervision, to models which strive to educate autonomous professionals. Undergraduate and postgraduate physiotherapy courses emphasize learning and research which extend and validate our unique knowledge base and our methods of assessment and treatment. Our courses must produce graduates who are capable of sound problem analysis and client management within their area of expertise, and who are able to recognize and refer on to others problems which are outside that area. Physiotherapists are part of the wider health and welfare industry. They need to be able to set their practice within recognized social, ethical and legal mores, and work co-operatively and communicate effectively with others. Such knowledge and skills are required for the physiotherapy profession and its members to be accountable to the community which they serve. The authors of this chapter regard the intellectual development which is encouraged in the learning of clinical reasoning as vital not only for clinical competence, but also for the conduct of other aspects of the physiotherapist's professional role.

Clinical reasoning can be defined as the cognitive processing, or thinking, used in the evaluation and management of clients. This thinking guides the direction and content of the client interview and the physical examination. It enables analysis of data collected during assessment and the synthesis of this information into diagnosis. And, it enables the clinician to make decisions about whether or not to intervene, which type of intervention is more likely to be successful, and when physiotherapy intervention should cease. As such, the reasoning process is not the only factor leading to clinical efficiency and effectiveness, but we believe acquiring proficiency in clinical reasoning is a vital step in developing expertise in physiotherapy practice.

Chapter 6 by Jones, Jensen and Rothstein discusses clinical reasoning in physiotherapy in detail, and the reader is referred to that chapter for further information. The main focus here is the way we help students in our programs to develop their clinical reasoning competence. The chapter briefly outlines a clinical encounter in physiotherapy and a theoretical basis for clinical expertise. The major areas of learning common to our programs are then presented, and the chapter concludes with a description of three clinical reasoning learning programs conducted by the authors.

The clinical process and clinical expertise in physiotherapy

Effective physiotherapy practice involves a series of investigation loops, commencing with an initial client assessment and proceeding through the initial problem formulation, intervention, reassessment, reformulation of the problem, if necessary, and further intervention, until a final outcome is reached. 'Diagnosis' is part of problem formulation, but a conception of the client and presenting problem which is much broader than merely diagnosis is required to allow appropriate treatment to be initiated. This clinical reasoning process can be characterized, then, as an action learning spiral, with successive loops built on the base of the previous ones (see Figure 19.1). At a simplistic level, each loop can be interpreted as one encounter, or 'treatment session', with a client. At a more sophisticated level, each client encounter in itself can be regarded as a series of investigation loops.

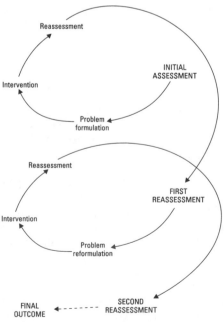

Figure 19.1   The clinical reasoning spiral

Clinical expertise, or 'efficient effectiveness', is what we want our students to achieve in the long term through this action learning. Two major schools of thought regarding the basis for professional expertise are the knowledge-based theory and the information processing theory. The existence of superior information processing skills in experts, although the early favoured theory, proved insufficient by itself to account for expert–novice differences. For example, novices confronted with clinical problems generally engage in a similar type and level of problem solving process as do experts (Barrows et al, 1978; Neufeld et al, 1981). And experienced clinicians, when confronted by common presentations of common conditions, do not appear to regard these even as problems needing solution; in these cases, diagnosis is made rapidly, apparently on the basis of a pattern recognition system (Groen and Patel, 1985). Although some type of information processing framework is therefore required for decision making by both experts and novices, the theory currently favoured in the literature proposes that what most characterizes the expert is 'specialist' knowledge. This is regarded as an extensive, context-specific and domain-specific knowledge base which enables the problem solving process to produce a better result because the expert can readily recognize patterns within data generated by client assessment (Patel et al, 1986; Schmidt and Boshuizen, 1993).

Educational content and process – what do we want our students to learn?

Cognitive psychologists studying the learning process see all learning resulting from information processing. That is, learning results from each person constructing an 'own reality', not just by adding additional bits of information to an existing knowledge bank, but by assimilating and integrating new information into existing organized knowledge structures (referred to as 'schemas'), or by creating new schemas which take account of the newly acquired information (Anderson, 1990). Hence, for the clinician who is intent on developing expertise, it is important to recognize that knowledge base and cognitive processing skills are interdependent, not independent, factors. It can be argued that ongoing participation in action learning (or experiential learning) during clinical practice is one means by which physiotherapists can acquire the knowledge base typical of the expert. Therefore, a major aim of educational programs for clinical physiotherapists should be to foster effective, independent, active learning in our students.

The authors of this chapter are involved in physiotherapy education programs at undergraduate, postgraduate and continuing professional education levels. These programs emphasize that the clinical reasoning process is synonymous with clinical learning and they aim to produce graduates who deliberately evaluate their own knowledge, reasoning and other clinical skills with the intention of improving their performance. Five major areas of learning are addressed in these programs.

Cognitive skills

These allow the intellectual processing to occur and include the following:

Cue perception refers to the ability to recognize a piece of information as relevant to the problem under consideration. This term is used to indicate an intellectual skill (involving information processing) rather than a physical ability such as touch or visual perception. The recognition that a visible swelling or a client's age are highly relevant components of the presenting problem is an example of cue perception. The importance of this skill is obvious if it is realized that these cues provide essential ongoing input to the clinical problem solving process.

Data evaluation is the examination and prioritizing of data recognized as cues, and it is inextricably tied up with cue perception itself. Items of information need to be considered with reference to the clinician's knowledge base in order to identify their accuracy and real relevance, and need to be weighted against each other to determine their relative importance. In most clinical cases conflicting evidence will exist, and the physiotherapist must be able to critically consider the place of each piece of data in the overall picture that is building. This means some data will be ignored, discarded or devalued in the eventual problem formulation. Having reasons for assigning differing weightings to data is vital in the clinical reasoning

process because, if the client fails to progress as anticipated, cues that were originally perceived, but initially were judged to be unimportant, will need to be re-evaluated. Reasons for assigning varied weightings include rules of interpretation (if/then propositions) based on currently accepted biomedical or clinical knowledge.

Problem formulation is the ability to construct an abstract concept from a collection of factual information. The initial conceptualization of the person and the problem confronting the physiotherapist will determine the line of inquiry to be followed in further assessment, and hence will greatly affect the type of information that is fed into the clinical reasoning process during both assessment and treatment phases. The conceptualization of a forty year old man following a severe cerebrovascular accident as 'a young person concerned with his physical appearance' or as 'a practical person concerned with resuming his regular life as quickly as possible' should suggest the quite different approaches that could be taken with the same client.

Generalizing from instances is the process by which concepts or schema for certain objects or events are compiled. It is the ability to recognize or construct a class of things on the basis of a pattern of characteristics rather than on the basis of detail. Common schema which even young children construct include concepts of furniture (a chair versus a table), concepts of letters and numbers (a vs b, i vs 1, 1 vs 7) and concepts of family members and their roles (mother vs father, mother vs aunt, sister vs brother). The possession of such schema greatly facilitates thinking and language in everyday life, and the possession by physiotherapists of concepts specific to their field of practice similarly advantages their thinking, their problem solving, and therefore, their learning. The ability to build concepts such as stiffness, structural weakness, muscle 'weakness', and spasticity from a combination of factual knowledge learned in the classroom and clinical knowledge learned from ongoing experience is vital to the physiotherapists' ability to function efficiently and effectively.

'Instancing' from generalizations is the ability to recognize a particular object as an example

of a class of objects, without being deterred by details which are atypical. Being able to characterize a knee problem as primarily one of poor muscle power, even where there is a component of joint stiffness, is an example of this.

Hypothesis generation and testing   is the operation of collecting and examining data during a clinical encounter in an attempt to actively confirm or negate the various hypotheses that have been proposed. These hypotheses may be concerned with explanations for the client's problem, or they may relate to propositions about the most appropriate management of that condition. Hypotheses are determined on the basis of cognitive processes such as those outlined in the preceding paragraphs, and are tested using logical inference in combination with the additional cue perception, data evaluation, problem formulation, etc., which result from further client assessment. The two way relationship between knowledge and reasoning is highlighted here: the reasoning process is the mechanism by which knowledge (be it of facts or principles or if/then 'rules') is continually generated and tested, yet this generation and testing process cannot proceed unless some information, some 'knowledge', can be used in the first place as a benchmark for decision making.

Knowledge base

Because our educational programs require students to justify their reasoning through assessments and treatments involving either real clients or clinical case studies, students need to revisit, or perhaps to encounter for the first time, information from the basic physical and biomedical sciences such as anatomy, physiology, pathology and kinesiology. The facts and principles used in this way are likely to remain more accessible to memory because of the relevance of the context in which they are used (Tulving and Thompson, 1973, Cervero, 1988) in contrast to the limited clinical relevance of the classroom in which these subjects are normally 'taught'.

Through experience with real clients or case studies, students are also exposed to clinical facts, principles, concepts and procedures of importance to the physiotherapist. These may be quite specific to physiotherapy practice, such as the concept of irritability, or they may

be more general, such as the relationship between psychosocial profile and health status. Similarly, the outcomes of different interventions can be learned. All this clinical knowledge is then available to be utilized in the reasoning process in future clinical encounters.

Even though the input would appear to be similar for different students engaged in a particular learning activity, the learning that actually occurs in each student is likely to be different because of the differing backgrounds that our students bring to their physiotherapy studies and the variety of clinical experiences encountered by different individuals. Both the prior knowledge, with which any new information will be integrated, and the particular ways in which students process information best will be different. Hence the learning that is derived from a given experience will be unique to each individual.

Metacognition and self-evaluation

As with all independent practitioners, physiotherapists must rely on themselves to monitor and judge their own performance. There is no external assessor to assist with this process in real life clinical practice. A major skill required by physiotherapists, then, is the ability to engage in reflective practice. In the simplest sense, this means acting as the 'fly on the wall' during their clinical contacts, observing their own actions and reviewing their own thinking processes in an objective and dispassionate way. The awareness and monitoring of one's own thinking is called metacognition, and it requires the clinician to be able to process two types of information simultaneously. On one level, the clinician is gathering, analysing and synthesizing data related to the client being assessed, but on another level, the clinician is evaluating the quality of this information processing itself. If practitioners are to evaluate their own performance at the same time as they are evaluating their clients, they must be able to recognize the basis for their clinical reasoning and the potential for errors. Incorrect or inadequate reasoning can occur at any stage of the clinical process. There may be errors of perception, interpretation, synthesis, planning, or even errors in the reflection process itself.

By reflecting on their performance, then, clinicians gather evidence to help in judging the merit of that performance and in identifying aspects of it which are either good or poor. These evaluations may result in immediate adjustments to decisions or actions, may increase the physiotherapist's knowledge of how to perform more efficiently or effectively in future, or may act as the stimulus for further academic learning.

Interpersonal and verbal communication skills

Interview skills are vital because it is by questioning clients that much of the information required for feeding into the clinical problem solving process is obtained. If the physiotherapist asks questions that are poorly understood by the client, or initially fails to establish a climate in which the client feels comfortable to truthfully answer questions, the quality of data used by the physiotherapist in the clinical reasoning process will be poor, and the outcome of the clinical encounter will therefore also be poor.

In clinical practice physiotherapists may work mostly as independent sole practitioners, interacting little with people other than their own clients. However, more commonly they function as members of health care teams, and have a broader community education role in addition to their therapeutic role. The ability to communicate articulately and in a professional manner with one's peers and associates is therefore an essential skill. This requires the physiotherapist to be able to construct a valid argument and then to phrase it in terms appropriate to the audience, whether that audience be other health care workers, politicians, legal practitioners, manual workers in a back care program, or children at the local primary school.

Other skills which support clinical reasoning effectiveness

The level of skill with which the physiotherapist is able to apply physical examination techniques and detect the tactile or visual responses to these techniques is, again, a major determinant of the quality of data fed into the clinical reasoning process. So also is the physiotherapist's ability to, for example, critically read and extract relevant information from laboratory reports and X-rays. Because of the cyclical nature of clinical practice in physiotherapy, knowl-edge of the results of any intervention (physical or otherwise) contributes to the ongoing clinical reasoning process. The physiotherapist's counselling and teaching skills, as well as manual or other technical treatment skills, affect the outcome of treatment and, hence, it is also essential for these skills to be performed effectively.

Educational programs – how do our students learn these things?

If knowledge, including knowledge of procedures, and the skills of clinical reasoning are to be used eventually in clinical practice, then their recall will be enhanced if the original learning occurs in a similar context (Tulving and Thomson, 1973; Cervero, 1988). Our learning programs use a variety of activities which encourage students to practise and recognize the elements which we believe will lead to 'expert' performance. These activities occur in simulated clinical contexts, with case studies having a high profile, and also in real time clinical practice. Three examples from our programs are described in the following pages.

First year undergraduate preclinical learning

The first learning program to be discussed is a subject titled *Introductory Physiotherapy*, taught in the first year of the Bachelor of Applied Science (Physiotherapy) course at the University of South Australia. This subject exists within a quite traditional course, where the majority of the first year curriculum is dedicated to the teaching of basic physical, social and biomedical sciences by lectures and practical classes. The aims of this subject are multiple, but they all fall within four broad goals: to introduce students to the complex role of the physiotherapist, to give students a clinical focus for their other first year learning, to help students develop a positive attitude to and skills in independent learning, and to introduce students to a basic clinical problem solving model.

The central feature of the subject design is the small group problem-based tutorial, modelled on the format used at the University of Newcastle Medical School in Australia (Clarke, 1979). A wide variety of physiotherapy cases are introduced to students in this subject, including ones involving orthopaedic, cardiorespiratory, neurological, paediatric and psychosocial problems. Each problem is addressed over two tutorial sessions, separated by several days.

At the beginning of each problem, the student group is given the task and a trigger containing some information about the client and the presenting problem. Students list any cues that they can identify in the trigger, make reasonable inferences based on the cues (e.g. looks fit, looks like it's just her shoulder) and then develop an initial summary of the client and the problem which attempts to encapsulate and categorize all the important information so far (e.g. an elderly woman with a problem of general stiffness and discomfort). The group then generates a set of hypotheses which they think may explain the client's problem, and sets about trying to clarify which of the possibilities is correct through 'interviewing' the client (role played by the tutor). In discussing how the information gained seems to support or negate these hypotheses, the list of possibilities may be added to, refined or reduced, and cues that were not perceived as relevant initially may be recognized. At the end of the first session, students identify what information they need to go away and research in order to further clarify the problem, and allocate these learning goals to individual group members. The research required usually includes anatomy, physiology, kinesiology and pathology, and sometimes includes aspects of physiotherapy assessment and treatment.

In the second group tutorial session, students report back their research findings, commenting on how the information they found contributes to clarifying the problem, and suggesting further questions that need to be asked of the client or additional aspects of the physical examination that should be performed. Again, cues that were originally missed may be identified in the light of new information, or discussion from the previous session may be revisited in more detail, sometimes resulting in quite different conclusions. The examination of the client is continued (albeit in an abbreviated and superficial way because of the students' inexperience) and this additional information is also added to the group's clinical reasoning process. At the end of this second tutorial session, a final client/problem summary is constructed and the argument which led to that conclusion is recorded.

The emphasis in tutorials is on the students identifying what is known (individually or collectively), what they need to know to be able to progress towards the problem solution, the use of evidence and sound reasoning to support or negate hypotheses, and student responsibility for their own learning. The tutor acts as a resource person, giving client information through role play, keeping students reasonably 'on track', modelling how to present, for example, an argument or a clinical summary, suggesting alternative learning resources, providing feedback on group performance, and especially early in the year, helping the group to establish a productive working pattern.

The group tutorial program is complemented by written assignments designed to lead students individually through other clinical problems. These mirror the group problem solving format as closely as possible while allowing students to complete the tasks alone and obtain feedback about their individual achievement and progress.

The earliest problems that are dealt with are ones which all students will have some knowledge of at a lay level, such as the sprained ankle, stress-induced illness in the 'middle-aged executive', and the reciprocal effects of the aging process and lifestyle on each other. These topics are treated fairly simply with the aims of familiarizing students with the problem solving format to be used, and starting the move away from the use of lay knowledge to more scientific knowledge such as the structure of muscles, the mediation of pain, the biochemical nature of the inflammatory process, and how physical assessment, for example, movement and palpation, can be used to analyse the cause of the presenting problem. All the early problems use visual triggers in the form of brief video clips. These are deliberately rich in cues and a relatively large proportion of time is spent on the perception–evaluation–analysis of these cues. As the year progresses, the problems themselves become more complex and there is a shift in emphasis from the consideration of initial cues and derivation of reasonable inferences to the planning and carrying out of interviews and physical examinations, progressive reasoning through these assessments, and planning approaches to intervention based on decisions made.

At various stages of the year, students are asked to reflect on questions such as: What did I learn from working on this problem? What learning resources that I used were most helpful? What is it that contributes to this learning group working well or working poorly? and, How has our learning been helped or hindered by the tutor? In addition to promoting self-appraisal in a hopefully non-threatening manner, reporting on these activities contributes to the evaluation of the subject.

Subject evaluation has been multi-faceted, incorporating formal methods such as anonymous questionnaires and informal methods such as unsolicited reports. It has involved students, tutors, other members of the Physiotherapy School staff and outside observers. Resulting data have been used both formatively, to develop and improve the subject, and also summatively, to judge its worth as an ongoing component of the undergraduate curriculum. Some students initially seem to struggle with the concept of the subject, but by the end of the year the majority of feedback is very positive and students feel all subject goals are being achieved. Tutors and observers of the subject have been impressed by students' ability to use the basic sciences to explain clinical features and to construct arguments using clinical data, and by their ability to plan logical assessment procedures. Other Physiotherapy School staff have incorporated aspects of the subject's design into their own subjects in later years of the undergraduate course. On the basis of these results, *Introductory Physiotherapy* has been deemed to be a successful innovation and maintains its place in the curriculum.

Postgraduate clinical reasoning program in manipulative physiotherapy

A subject titled *Clinical Reasoning* has been taught for several years within the Graduate' Diploma and Master of Applied Science (Manipulative Physiotherapy) courses at the University of Sydney. These courses are designed for qualified physiotherapists and the curricula therefore build on the students' considerable base of professional knowledge and skill. The applied sciences, physiotherapy theory and practice subjects, and clinical education are closely integrated to enhance the transfer of knowledge and skills from the classroom into clinical practice. The specific aims of the clinical reasoning subject are to enable students to become aware of how they reason in

relation to clinical problems, to understand the theoretical processes of clinical reasoning, to critically evaluate clinical reasoning literature in the light of their own clinical experience, and to develop their skills in the areas of clinical reasoning, self-evaluation of their reasoning abilities and communication of their reasoning to others.

These aims highlight the need for students to become aware of their thinking, and to practise, describe, examine and receive feedback on their reasoning. If clinical decisions are to be explored in depth and students are to be free to attempt and evaluate different reasoning strategies and decision alternatives, the real life clinical setting with time pressures and possible negative consequences for clients is not ideal. A classroom setting allows for taking 'time out' to discuss students' thinking and the potential consequences of their decisions. It also allows students to hear the different reasoning and decisions of others so they can consider the relative merits of alternative positions. In the classroom students can discuss their reasoning in groups and receive feedback from their peers and teachers. Classroom activity, followed by subsequent integration of reasoning skills into clinical education, is therefore used as the format for this subject.

An experiential learning strategy is used. The class is set up with a 'fish bowl' or discussion group in a semi-circle facing the audience. The discussion group comprises two groups of students, an expert panel and a chairperson. One group of three or four students is rostered each session to act as the physiotherapist whose task it is to work through and discuss a hypothetical client case. This group is known as 'the student panel'. The second group of three students represents the client in the activity. These students have previously prepared a case study in consultation with an experienced physiotherapist.

The expert panel consists of physiotherapy and applied science teachers and clinicians. Their role is to challenge students' knowledge, their use of knowledge and their clinical inquiry strategies, and provide feedback to the students on these areas. They engage students in exploration of the relative advantages of different inquiry methods, investigation techniques and intervention strategies. Their particular concern is to help students evaluate the validity of their own knowledge and critically review their clinical strategies. Students' reasoning and investigations are examined via questions such as 'What information would you like to obtain next and why?' and 'What use can you make of the data you have just received in relation to your working hypotheses?' Questions such as these require students to become more conscious of what and how they are thinking, and to express and critique their thoughts. The questioning itself and the subsequent feedback to the students encourages them to use and develop their ability in reflective self-awareness and self-evaluation.

The chairperson is the overall manager of the learning activity, guiding the general direction of the discussion and allocating time to various segments such as history taking, data collection relating to physical examination, management decisions, or management evaluation. This person may facilitate discussion of the case by inviting questions or comments from the expert panel, or may 'short cut' the process, for instance if time becomes a problem, by requesting particular information from the student group which represents the client. The chairperson may call 'time out" to discuss with the whole class more general aspects of clinical reasoning. Other issues of importance to clinical practice are also critically explored in these discussions including the need for effective reasoning and decision making skills as first contact practitioners, the value of an extensive and sound knowledge base as a foundation for that reasoning, the role of the client in clinical decision making, and the use of assessment and treatment protocols as opposed to reasoning through each individual client case.

During the panel session students acting as the physiotherapist are assessed by teachers on their reasoning, knowledge and ability to communicate their reasoning. The students acting as the client are assessed on the adequacy of preparation and the accuracy/consistency of the case they present. The student panel also receives feedback from peers in the audience in the general discussion at the end of the session. The teachers record their results on rating scales and discuss these with students after the class, giving feedback on their performance.

In preparation for these panel sessions, some classes early in the program examine theories and research associated with clinical reasoning. Student activities include writing an assignment in which they compare their own reasoning strategies to models identified in the literature, and drawing cognitive maps. Drawing these maps, which represent their knowledge of a particular topic in diagrammatic form, helps students to assess and revise their knowledge base in terms of its accuracy, comprehensiveness and its organization. The process of map drawing can also help students to learn how to organize their knowledge so it can be accessed more readily. Students learn a great deal about their own knowledge from the activity itself and from the feedback given by their peers and teachers on knowledge content demonstrated and the links being made between knowledge components in the maps.

Evaluation of the subject has included student evaluation questionnaires, an open discussion session at the end of the course, and review of student results by the teachers involved. Results indicate that participants have learned a great deal about the nature of clinical reasoning, about how they reason and about the soundness, relevance and breadth of their knowledge. They have developed skills in metacognition and in communicating their reasoning, a very necessary part of being a collaborative and credible member of the health care team. Further, they have had opportunities to explore their attitudes and values regarding clinical practice and clinical decision making, to experience the client's role and to examine how the client influences the physiotherapist's reasoning and decision making.

Postgraduate supervised clinical practice in manipulative physiotherapy

The clear intent of the preceding examples of experiential learning activities is to help students recognize and develop skills in the process of clinical reasoning. The various formats of simulated patients have distinct advantages over real life clinical practice as a medium for teaching, such as better control over problem type and complexity and avoidance of the safety risks associated with incorrect clinical decisions. However, the clinical setting is where students will eventually be required to function, and no degree of simulation can replicate the unpredictability and variability which exists in real life client presentations. This example illustrates learning during supervised clinical education in the Graduate Diploma and Master of Applied Science (Manipulative

Physiotherapy) courses at the University of South Australia.

Clinical placements are an integral component of physiotherapy curricula at both undergraduate and postgraduate levels. They always involve teaching students safe and effective client care based on accepted modes of practice, but they do not necessarily identify the development of clinical reasoning as an educational objective. Because students will have varying levels of skill in problem solving or critical, logical thinking which they can apply to the physiotherapy domain, to simply require them to examine and treat real clients is probably not sufficient to optimize their clinical learning.

A stated major aim of the supervised clinical practice component in the postgraduate programs in manipulative physiotherapy at the University of South Australia is to encourage students to develop skills in clinical reasoning. In particular, students learn to use a hypothetico-deductive process of reasoning throughout their clinical encounters. In a manual therapy course, much attention must also be directed towards achieving competence in client interviewing and manual assessment and treatment procedures. However, these skills need to be integrated within a coherent clinical reasoning framework.

Students are introduced to the concept and a process of clinical reasoning in physiotherapy during preclinical learning activities, and are encouraged to use this process in their clinical work on course. For discussion of this physiotherapy reasoning process, the reader is referred to Chapter 6 and Jones (1992). In order to teach clinical reasoning, supervisors must have means of accessing the student's thoughts. One way of doing this is via a clinical reasoning 'worksheet'. Students are required to pause at key points, for example, after taking a history, and complete relevant sections of the worksheet. These enforced periods of 'time out' encourage the student to review information that has just been found and to plan the next section of assessment or management. Too many interruptions can be time consuming and disturbing to the student's flow of thought, but in manual therapy such planning can be critical, not only for the student's reasoning, but also for the client's well-being, as excessive examination or treatment can result in worsening of some clients' symptoms.

Ideally, the supervisor will review all worksheets within days of their completion and provide students with feedback about them. However, even when time does not allow this, experience has shown the process of reflecting on the client examination or management in order to answer the worksheet questions is in itself an excellent independent learning activity. Students may recognize, through their own difficulty in answering certain questions, that they have insufficient information or understanding about the case. While this clinical reasoning form is designed for postgraduate manual therapy students, the concept of such a worksheet which encourages retrospective reflection together with planning for future action is applicable to all areas of physiotherapy practice and all levels of professional education.

Another way of accessing student thinking is by discussion during the actual clinical encounter. Clearly it is neither practical nor desirable to interrupt the student after every inquiry to question interpretation of information, but, again, strategically placed 'time out' periods at key stages of the examination and treatment can be very effective. At these stages, students are encouraged to make interpretations of their observations, formulate hypotheses, identify interview or physical examination measures that could be used to test these hypotheses, consider the examination and management implications associated with different hypotheses, and specify supporting or negating evidence to substantiate their judgements. In addition to these planned 'time-outs', students are interrupted if it appears they are following incorrect or unexplained lines of inquiry. There needs to be advance agreement between student, client and supervisor about these 'time out' discussions. Client co-operation is usually easily obtained if they are aware of the purpose of the interruptions, and informal contracts between individual students and supervisors are used to delineate the extent and method of such discussions. When the discussions are an agreed part of the learning process, and when they are conducted in a non-threatening manner, students enjoy the opportunity for ongoing reflection during the clinical encounter.

The extent and nature of the interaction, guidance and feedback provided during clinical sessions varies considerably. For example, working interpretations or hypotheses are based on the students' conceptualization of the client data. Students' ability to perceive and evaluate relevant cues is influenced by their existing knowledge schemas. Schemas are partly developed by common classroom activities conducted during the present course, but they also depend on each individual's unique base of knowledge and experience gained from previous academic education, clinical experience and life in general. Different students' conceptualizations of the same client presentation may therefore be quite different. If there is to be growth in a student's clinical proficiency, supervisors must deal with each student according to level of knowledge and reasoning ability. To assist their learning, students need also to be able to test for themselves the implications of their own conceptualizations or working hypotheses. This can be difficult in the clinical setting where there is always some degree of ethical constraint for the correct solution to the client's problem to be obtained as quickly as possible. Thus, supervisors must balance their own involvement in the clinical decision making process to ensure safe and reasonable judgements are reached and acted upon, while at the same time enabling students to experience for themselves the results of their own reasoning.

Because reasoning proficiency and knowledge base are viewed as interdependent factors, another major aim of clinical practice in the postgraduate manual therapy programs at the University of South Australia is trying to promote students' acquisition of declarative knowledge such as clinical patterns of presentation (for example, syndromes) and procedural knowledge such as if/then guides to action.

To encourage students to expand their knowledge in relation to patterns of client presentation, they are required to maintain a 'Diary of Clinical Patterns'. They are provided with forms on which to record the typical features of the most common clinical patterns encountered in manual therapy practice. Students keep the diary for the duration of their course, adding information to it as the year progresses. These patterns are not taught directly to students, rather students are expected to extract the relevant information from their involvement in classroom activities, private reading, and their clinical practice with real clients.

The diaries serve several purposes. Firstly, they provide a form of advanced organizer for learning, priming students to look for information to add to their evolving diary during clinical practice and other learning activities. The exploration of clinical patterns through a hypothetico-deductive reasoning process encourages students to test the consistency of the patterns and their response to alternative treatment approaches. The diaries also provide a stimulus for independent study, with students seeking out additional information from other sources (textbooks, journals, peers, experienced therapists) to support their clinical observations. Lastly, the inevitable overlap in clinical patterns that emerges assists students to learn not only the classical features of a pattern, but also the range of features which may be shared by several patterns, the variation of features within one pattern that are encountered in real clients, and treatment principles and techniques associated with effective management of the different patterns.

Evaluation of the supervised clinical practice component of the course is undertaken as a round table student–staff discussion at the end of the course. It is almost always cited as the most valuable component of the course because of the way it encourages students to think logically and because of the attention it allows to individual needs. Course review sessions are also conducted between staff members, usually with an independent facilitator. Developments in the program, such as modifications to the clinical reasoning worksheet, have been outcomes of these review sessions.

Conclusion

Clinical reasoning proficiency is central to the physiotherapist's ability to manage clients efficiently and effectively because this thinking process guides the entire clinical encounter. Each treatment session and each case are powerful sources of learning for the physiotherapist if a clinical reasoning process is followed and the therapist engages in reflection and self-evaluation during and after the process. Such experiential learning facilitates the building of an extensive body of clinically relevant declarative and procedural knowledge and the ability to readily access this knowledge during clinical practice. If these are hallmarks of expertise, then the educational programs described above aim to move students closer to this position by encouraging learning within the appropriate clinical context and by promoting reflective and independent learning skills which will ensure students' knowledge acquisition does not stop on completion of their university courses.

References

Anderson, J.R. (1990) *Cognitive Psychology and its Implications* (3rd edn). WH Freeman and Company, New York

Barrows, H.S., Feightner, J.W., Neufeld, V.R. and Norman G.R. (1978) *Analysis of the Clinical Methods of Medical Students and Physicians.* McMaster University, Hamilton, Ontario

Cervero, R.M. (1988) *Effective Continuing Education for Professionals.* Jossey-Bass, San Francisco

Clarke, R.M. (1979) Design and implementation of the curriculum in a new medical school. *Programmed Learning and Educational Technology*, **16**, 288–295

Groen, G.J. and Patel, V.L. (1985) Medical problem solving: some questionable assumptions. *Medical Education*, **19**, 95–100

Jones, M.A. (1992) Clinical reasoning in manual therapy. *Physical Therapy*, **72**, 875–884

Neufeld, V.R., Norman, G.R., Feightner, J.W. and Barrows, H. S. (1981) Clinical problem-solving by medical students: a cross-sectional and longitudinal analysis. *Medical Education*, **15**, 315–322

Patel, V.L., Groen, G.J. and Frederiksen, C.H. (1986) Differences between medical students and doctors in memory for clinical cases. *Medical Education*, **20**, 3–9

Schmidt, H.G. and Boshuizen, H.P.A. (1993) On acquiring expertise in medicine. *Educational Psychology Review*, **5**, 205–221

Tulving, E. and Thompson, D.M. (1973) Encoding specificity and retrieval processes in episodic memory. *Psychology Review*, **80**, 352–373

20

Teaching clinical reasoning to occupational therapists during fieldwork education

Susan Ryan

The fieldwork education setting provides the ideal forum for teaching and developing the clinical reasoning abilities of students. In this setting there are many experiential learning opportunities which the educator can use, create and facilitate meaningfully. To make best use of these opportunities fieldwork educators need to be knowledgeable about different approaches to reasoning and how it develops. They also have to understand educational principles that can be used to elicit and develop these abilities.

The first section of this chapter will examine issues in the profession of occupational therapy and in the nature of fieldwork that have a direct bearing on the facilitation or restriction of reasoning abilities. The second section will examine the development of the reasoning process during the fieldwork experience. Boud and Walker (1991) propose a three stage model for reflective learning. They are: preparing the experience, experiencing the experience, and reflecting on the experience. In this chapter ideas and exercises for developing and teaching reasoning skills in students will follow this framework.

Professional issues

Traditionally, occupational therapists have worked in hospitals under the aegis of the medical system. Their practice, however, and therefore the types and patterns of reasoning they use, is inherently different from that of medi-cine, physiotherapy and certain aspects of nursing. The essential difference between occupational therapy and more medically-oriented professions is that occupational therapists who work within the hospital system, especially those using treatments, do not follow a diagnostic pattern of reasoning which is similar to medicine and involves problem sensing, diagnosis, and problem resolution (Rogers and Holm, 1989). Clinical reasoning patterns appear to be contextual and to vary with the practice setting.

The over-riding philosophy of occupational therapy is holistic and humanistic and is mainly concerned with the person's functional performance in all aspects of daily living. This sits at odds with the scientific medical models. Presently, the focus of occupational therapy practice is shifting away from the hospital towards various settings in the community such as people's homes, doctors' surgeries, community centres, schools, correction centres and industrial settings. If clinical reasoning patterns are contextual then certain types of reasoning will predominate over others in these different settings. Future research may clarify this.

As discussed in Chapter 7 of this book (and by Fleming, 1991 and Mattingly, 1989b), occupational therapists use at least four forms of reasoning in practice: procedural, interactive, conditional and narrative. Because practice is so diverse, different forms of reasoning may predominate or be given variable weightings in different practice areas. This has implications in fieldwork education. Because certain ways of reasoning can be generalized while others are specific, educators cannot assume that students will be able to transfer their reasoning abilities from one setting to another. A number of recent studies (Patel and Cranton, 1983; Maxim and Dielman, 1987; Tanner et al, 1987), suggest that interpersonal skills, technical skills, attitude to health care, selection of data acquisition, history and interview, and professional responsibility are in the category of generalized skills. By comparison, they have found that problem solving, factual knowledge, number and earliness of hypothesis activation, diagnostic accuracy, and physical examination are task specific. Therefore, each time students start a placement in a different setting the educator needs to identify what existing knowledge the students have in relation to this setting, and help the students develop both their knowledge and reasoning skills within that context.

Fieldwork issues

The duration and position of fieldwork placements within courses is a critical factor in promoting the development of specific reasoning abilities. Fieldwork education may constitute up to one third of the total basic education syllabus. The World Federation of Occupational Therapists (WFOT) requires a minimum 1000 hours of fieldwork in entry-level occupational therapy courses and many schools exceed this amount.

The usual model for occupational therapy fieldwork placements involves one student working with one therapist, usually in one setting. The premise underlying this model is that students receive individual attention and have a consistent role model to follow. There are several disadvantages to this system and many formative learning opportunities for developing reasoning abilities are lost. Some of the factors to be considered are:

- The fieldwork educator's primary responsibility is with the client not the student. Therefore the amount of time spent with the student is limited and is primarily concerned with planning procedures and doing formative and summative assessments with the student.
- The crucial relationship between teacher and student must be one of trust and if this factor

is missing the student has little chance to change educators without causing some degree of disruption in the placement.
- The student's development is strongly influenced by the knowledge of one educator and by the content and nature of the program that is offered. Both of these factors could limit the learning experience.
- There is little or no peer support or exchange of ideas with peers at the actual time of the experience.
- The same educator is both educating and assessing the student. Most of the methods used to promote reasoning require the student to share feelings. They may feel inhibited to voice their feelings or concerns to their teacher if that person is also the assessor.

Another model which I experienced in Australia gave one senior clinician responsibility for a group of students. Daily group meetings each having a different theme were organized and these were often facilitated by other professionals. During the placement students sometimes worked alone but more often worked in pairs. They worked with one therapist for a two week period and then changed and worked with another in the same setting and so received different points of view. Group visits were arranged and were discussed jointly afterwards. Assessments were made by all the people involved. Collective professional assessment, individual self-assessment and peer assessment provided considerable support for both teacher and students. In this model the educational input received and the opportunities for developing reasoning were much greater for the student.

Group interpretation of practice is an ideal forum for examining and developing reasoning abilities or exposing faulty reasoning processes, because it provides different perspectives. Sessions following problem-based learning methodologies can be facilitated by a professional who withdraws as students' competence and confidence develops. Structured carefully, this approach could increase the students' depth of understanding in a particular area of clinical practice.

The clinical reasoning process – implications for fieldwork education

The occupational therapy (reasoning) process

Many schools in the United Kingdom put a great deal of emphasis on the study of the occupational therapy process which includes seven phases: data gathering, assessment, problem identification, therapeutic intervention, problem resolution, closure, and evaluation. Fieldwork placement assessment forms echo this logically-ordered process.

However, Higgs (1990) and Schon (1987) and many other authors express concern that professional education is being presented in too simplified a manner that is not reflective of clinical practice. Schon states that professional education should prepare students to deal with the complex and unpredictable problems of actual practice with confidence, skill and care. The complexity of clinical practice is apparent in the findings of the joint American Occupational Therapy Association/American Occupational Therapy Foundation study described by Mattingly and Gillette (1991). This study suggests that experienced therapists constantly revisit and re-evaluate situations even within a single practice session. That is, these therapists are constantly revising their reasoning during their actions, or reflecting-in-action. This highly sophisticated ability runs contrary to logically-ordered models of reasoning, recipe formulas, checklists and memorized data.

Developmental stages of clinical reasoning

The study of reasoning development also suggests ways to educate students during fieldwork placements, particularly ways that build up the clinical picture from the simple to the complex. Methods that encourage construction of knowledge and the development of understanding, where an individual's conceptual framework serves as the foundation upon which further learning is built, can be particularly powerful and are likely to be more congruent with the actual complexities of practice. For instance, the educator could use videotapes with concepts maps to promote students' reflection on their knowledge base, their use of knowledge and their clinical reasoning.

Mattingly (1989a) discusses the phenomenon of the occupational therapist 'being in a different story' from that of the client, or not seeing the situation from the client's perspective. This can also occur in fieldwork education between teacher and student, for instance when the educator is not aware of, or does not consider the student's stage of development. The educator's expectations of the student's abilities and understandings can be mismatched.

A similar finding was made by Ryan (1990) who identified that inexperienced therapists extracted only 27% of key data from the same amount of information on medical charts as did experienced therapists. The inexperienced therapists needed to be in the actual situation with the client before they could form images or make decisions. These findings suggest that students need help with interpreting written material and with forming images of the disability or the person prior to meeting them. The educator could give this area of practice more time and attention. Self-directed learning or group exercises with incomplete handouts could facilitate the extraction and formation of prospective procedural reasoning. Images of the client may be heightened by viewing videos of the client prior to the actual meeting and many varied experiences can be structured around the client even in early fieldwork placements. For example, investigating the life story of the patient with their friends and family will enhance an interactive image and will contribute to the narrative history of that particular person. This will assist the formation of a more accurate conditional image.

The development of expertise

Another way of understanding reasoning development is from models which describe the development of expertise in practice. Presently theories from a number of disciplines provide this framework. These include theories stemming from cognitive development models (Perry, 1979), skill acquisition models such as Dreyfus and Dreyfus' model (1986), and the development of occupational therapy competence (Frum and Opacich, 1987). Understanding these models will enable the fieldwork educators to facilitate the clinical reasoning development in their students. In addition, our understanding of the development of occupational therapists' reasoning will continue to be enhanced by current research activities in this area (Mattingly 1989a,b; Munroe, 1992; Salz, 1991).

Development, although a continual process, is not linear. That is, reasoning needs to fold back on to previous levels of understanding so that each individual encounter with a client builds up a bank of knowledge and experience which enhances understanding. Table 20.1 illustrates a staged progression of activities which enhances reasoning skills. It has been developed from my experience of working with students in the fieldwork setting. The stages along the horizontal axis show the development of insights into specific understandings. Each step augments the previous one. Looking at the sections of each stage in the vertical columns the activities not only build on to each other but they use an overlapping technique that folds back onto previous knowledge.

The diagram depicts the development of contextual learning of specific reasoning which needs to occur each time a student starts in a different practice setting or when working with a different client population. The first stage starts with the student examining his or her knowledge base which will be different for each person. The educator should not assume the starting point. This is why mutual learning contracts between the teacher and the student are so important. As awareness increases so does the ability to recognize cues, to sense and to begin to solve problems. Reflecting on action from the videotapes leads gradually to the ability to begin the process of reflecting-in-action during practice. The educator can facilitate the formation of multiple hypotheses quite quickly by providing comparisons and comparable stories. Reasoning is developed in a dynamic, complex and cumulative way which is unique for each person. Educators who use videotapes throughout the placement as their means of educating can show the first and the last recorded tapes to the student to illustrate how his or her expertise has developed. These can also be used as a means of assessment.

Strategies for developing clinical reasoning ability in fieldwork education

Case studies and case stories

Case studies are another mechanism for enhancing clinical reasoning. They normally focus on the medical and procedural aspects of client care and this reinforces the objective, professional line of inquiry and enhances procedural reasoning. However, one of the most crucial aspects for the therapist during a session is to enter part of the client's world and to empathically experience his or her unique situation. Case stories which are of a narrative nature enter the client's world and promote the development of narrative reasoning abilities and personal image formation. Both these methods can be used at different times and they can also be compared and contrasted to show different facets of practice.

Experiential learning

Experiential learning is not merely the act of experiencing. It is much more dynamic and complex. It should also incorporate the values of critical and objective reflection on subjective experiences according to Rowan (1981) (cited in Weil and McGill, 1989). Experiential learning encourages openness to new experiences, and lateral and critical thinking which challenge established ways of looking at the professional experience. This subjective reflection can result in reconceptualization and reframing of ideas which leads to new integrations and applications.

It has been my experience that most fieldwork educators provide for the student (or negotiate with the student) a desirable and varied fieldwork program. Also many educators are aware of different learning approaches used by adults. Unfortunately, it appears that less thought is commonly put into the structure of the learning experience itself or ways of facilitating reasoning within those structures. Even negotiated programs need to be individualized according to the student's level of reasoning. With a knowledge of the educational principles and strategies which are outlined below, some creative ideas, and a bank of projects at hand, the task for the educator becomes easier to organize and personalize.

Table 20.1 The development of clinical reasoning in a specific practice setting

First stage	Second stage	Third stage	Fourth stage	Fifth stage
	Cue acquisition begins	Comparative practice starts		Decision making begins and practice develops
		Hypotheses are generated	Cue acquisition becomes more accurate	Strategies for individual intervention develop
	Student senses problems	Problem solving develops	Pattern recognition strengthens	Hypotheses become more refined
	Student begins initial awareness	Cue acquisition strengthens	Student forms multiple hypotheses	Pattern recognition differentiates and strengthens
	Joint reflection on action–educator facilities	Pattern recognition begins	Joint reflection on action and interpretation of differences and similarities	Cue acquisition becomes more acute
	Student participates in selected area of practice (videotaped)	Student leads reflection on action from videotape	Student observes actively	Student leads reflection on action and examination of individual practice begins
	Student observes activity	Student begins reflecting in action	Compare knowledge	Reflecting in action continues
Student builds bank of knowledge from different perspectives	Student develops initial understanding	Student leads part/whole session	Compare stories of two clients	Student works with both clients
Student examines knowledge base	Educator and student share knowledge and stories of one client	Student's awareness and understanding increases		
First stage	*Second stage*	*Third stage*	*Fourth stage*	*Fifth stage*

Ongoing generalization and interpretation of practice →

Clinical reasoning develops in a specific setting →

← Knowledge and understanding increase

A variety of experiences can enrich students' learning. Students need to have many experiences with clients to enrich their own personal library of stories and to compare and contrast the therapist's way of interacting. This should include working with clients with a range of diagnoses and working with a number of clients with the same diagnosis who require different approaches to management. These experiences can be structured in increasing levels of contrast and complexity. For example students working with a 50-year-old businessman suffering from clinical depression and a 17-year-old school girl with the same medical diagnosis will learn that these two clients will need a completely different form of management. For a student on an early fieldwork experience such a marked contrast in clinical practice strategies could be difficult to comprehend and the reasoning behind the actions would need to be carefully explained.

Viewing clinical problems from different perspectives can broaden students' learning and reasoning approaches. Examining the same problems or clients from different perspectives will provide more opportunities to develop the procedural, interactive, narrative, and conditional forms of reasoning. Even during early placements this activity will enrich a student's understanding. The perspectives of the occupational therapist, the client, the carer or family, as well as the student, can all be incorporated into the learning experience and into the clinical reasoning process. If the placement is short and time is a limiting factor a group of students could each examine one perspective and then bring this back to the group for discussion.

Different learning approaches can be incorporated during educational program planning activities. Students have often developed their own favoured way of learning. Instead of matching learning styles, designing sessions using different learning approaches can enrich each student's experience. When structuring the learning program the fieldwork educator may ask if it fosters self-directed learning, problem-based learning, experiential learning, trial-and-error learning, or problem solving. Sessions may have a combination of approaches but if they are designed for a specific situation, one approach usually predominates. However, the approach chosen should take into account the student's stage of professional development.

Reasoning can be enhanced by providing learning experiences with varying degrees of complexity. The fieldwork educator can structure the experience to provide similar tasks in varying degrees of complexity, and thereby help students learn to reason in simple and complex clinical problem situations. Sometimes in the work environment it is not always possible to have clients that have the same diagnosis and yet present differently. A bank of videotapes of different clients can help to overcome this difficulty.

A variety of methods of questioning can be used to enhance learning. Questioning is one of the most essential skills that a fieldwork educator can develop because there are many ways of using questions to explore and develop students' clinical reasoning, especially in early or difficult placements. Gradually, however, teacher questioning should be supplemented or largely replaced by student questioning. That is, students should be encouraged to question themselves and other people, and to find their own answers from within their experiences. Questioning each other in groups is another way to stimulate reasoning and to form connections. This is often referred to as 'inter-connected knowing'. Questions may be:

- Procedural, factual and precise, e.g. 'What would you do next?'
- Open-ended and broad, e.g. 'What are the motivational strategies you could try with this client?'
- Provocative and challenging, e.g. 'If you had said it this way instead of saying it that way, how might the session have finished?'
- Projective and conditional, e.g. 'How do you think Mrs Cuthbert will manage her cooking in three months time?'
- Retrospective and reflective, e.g. 'Why did you plan this session the way you did?' 'How would you plan a session differently for this client if you could do it again?'

Each of these approaches to questioning can stimulate students' thinking, help them to challenge their knowledge base, values and assumptions, and critique their reasoning strategies.

Reflection is a valuable catalyst for developing clinical reasoning. It plays an important part in fieldwork education, particularly in helping students to make sense of their experiences, and provides a useful mechanism for helping students to become aware of and develop their clinical reasoning. Different authors propose various approaches to this important aspect of reasoning development. A central theme in all the methods is the personal impact that experience has on the people involved in the action.

Fish et al (1991) propose a framework using four 'strands of reflection' to promote reasoning abilities. These strands are:

- the factual reflection strand which describes the actual procedures that were followed in a therapy session and the feelings which they aroused. It sets the scene, tells the story, pinpoints critical incidents and identifies views about future practice.
- the retrospective reflection strand which views the entire therapy session. It is in this mode of reflection where patterns and new meanings emerge.
- the substratum reflection strand which uncovers and critically explores personal theory and then relates it to formal theory.
- the connective reflection strand which links present theory to future theory and practice.

This framework can be used effectively after particularly difficult clinical encounters. It is also useful in group work when each person's reflections provide other perspectives.

Schon (1987) provides three models for educating reflective practitioners: 'joint experimentation', 'follow me', and 'hall of mirrors'. These methods of reflecting are particularly useful in educational practicums where the student can rehearse practice in safe surroundings with a senior practitioner. 'Joint experimentation' involves the experimenter and student working together exploring and testing possible actions. In 'follow me' the educator presents a whole performance then breaks it down into parts and analyses each in turn before putting the whole performance back together again. In 'hall of mirrors' the student and the educator continually shift perspectives, one moment enacting practice, another moment, discussing it.

A third model of reflection is that proposed by Boud and Walker (1991) who have revised their original thinking concerning reflection. In Boud et al's first model (1985) the student was encouraged to return to the experience, attend to his or her feelings, and then re-evaluate the experience. As stated in the introductory paragraph of this chapter, these authors now believe that reflection after the event is not enough and that more emphasis must be put on preparing for the experience, reflecting-in-action during the experience through noticing and intervening, and that this should then be followed by reflection after the experience.

Implementing reflective learning during fieldwork

Preparing the educator

As discussed above, the quality of the fieldwork experience for the student depends heavily on the knowledge and ability of the educator. Therefore the nature and content of fieldwork education programs can play an important role in the success of fieldwork education. In the United Kingdom the present fieldwork education programs for occupational therapists were designed in the 1980s. These courses do not embrace reasoning development or reflective practice. They are now being revised. In addition, post-graduate courses have been developed and multi-disciplinary courses for occupational therapists, teachers, social workers, and nurses are being designed. In the United States a self-study series (Crepeau and LaGarde, 1991) with video vignettes of scenarios from practice has been introduced as an alternate educational route.

Reassuringly, the educator does not have to be an expert. Cohn (1988), for instance, argues that the fieldwork educator does not necessarily have to have a full understanding of each clinical problem or client because the clinical reasoning process is also a learning experience for themselves. Educators need to expand the students' reasoning abilities from the students' current level. In doing so the educator's own understanding will deepen.

Preparing learning activities and resources in the fieldwork setting

Apart from their personal preparation, fieldwork educators have to prepare their setting. They need to ensure that up-to-date factual material is available as a resource and that reference books, articles and research projects are available to the students to provide a wide spectrum of knowledge. Some references should support the content of the educational establishment where the student studies, while others should provide contrasts. Similarly, induction and departmental policy documents designed for accreditation procedures should describe the philosophy of the service, the setting, and the procedural routines currently being used. Possible learning opportunities, as opposed to learning objectives need to be specified and should include the entire service area. With this material at their disposal students can influence meaningful ways of developing their own reasoning.

There are many other specific things that the educator can prepare that will nurture the development of one type of reasoning or another. Narrative reasoning can be facilitated by having a library of video stories, photographs, and case stories written by previous students. These can be accompanied by guided observation sheets with questions which require varying degrees of complexity in clinical reasoning, for the student to complete. These sheets may involve the students in examining observed behaviours, interpreting interactions, and describing procedures and then putting them into the client's life context. The student could also be asked to view a section of a videotape and to pose questions about the action.

Conditional and prospective narrative reasoning can be developed by getting the student, or a group of students, to create the next chapter in the patient's story. At a later time this chapter can be compared with the real situation. Cognitive reasoning can be facilitated by the educator who designs the frameworks of practice and concept maps which gradually become less prescriptive. More competent students may be asked to develop their own maps by first brainstorming the many factors that need to be considered and then grouping these into different concepts.

Procedural reasoning can also be developed through the use of training videos, manuals, and leaflets that demand active participation from the learner. Incomplete handouts, quizzes, and videotapes with pauses and questions can encourage this. The students' personal views of the situation always need to be included and elicited in some way in order to help them relate new knowledge to their existing knowledge base.

Preparing the student

Students can also prepare themselves for the experiences of fieldwork before the placement. It is important to encourage students to take an active and responsible role in this preparation since they are not only learning to be self-directed learners but also they are developing their identity and skills as independent clinicians and clinical decision makers. Students bring with them to the fieldwork placement a personal frame of reference based on their knowledge and prior experiences. According to Boud and Walker (1991) individuals bring their own 'personal knowing' and 'intent' to any situation and these factors create a unique situation and experience for each individual. Therefore it is advisable to encourage students to examine and then remedy their own preparedness (e.g. their present base of knowledge) in relation to the impending fieldwork placement. For instance, students could prepare a self-evaluative diary which could serve as the foundation for the placement.

Such a diary would include a number of different sections. For instance, one section could relate to the source of existing knowledge. Looking at their present store of knowledge students can ask themselves where it came from. Was it from formal lessons at school, anecdotal stories, personal experiences, or from background reading from books, the popular press or television? What can they do to augment this foundation? Can they write to organizations, view videos, read, ask questions, or interview other people such as professionals, clients or others who work in similar services? This section of the diary will facilitate students' cognitive and procedural reasoning.

Another section of the diary could look at the anticipated ages and backgrounds of the clientele they would be working with. How near or far is this group from their own age, their own experience? What do they know about that group's culture, history, ways of living and talking? Who can they ask and how can they find out? This section will facilitate their narrative reasoning abilities and will also help interactive reasoning when they are in the actual situation with the client.

Another section of the diary could be prospective. What are the sorts of questions the students will need to find answers for? What are they expecting? What would they like to know or experience? How do they plan to design their own learning opportunities? These questions challenge the students to think about and mentally prepare for the experiences they will encounter and can also identify learning weaknesses which they need to address prior to the placement. Finally, a section should be included in which the student explicitly examines feelings and expectations prior to the placement. This can be exceptionally revealing if it is linked into the reflective experience at the end of the placement.

Each section of the diary is initially written on the left page of the book leaving the right page empty. During the end-of-placement reflective exercise, notes could be made with a different coloured ink on that opposite page. Compiling the diary in this manner will reinforce meanings and deepen understandings, and pinpoint critical incidents. Developing this foundation diary not only makes this knowledge explicit for the student but it will provide a valuable source of information to the educator.

Reading phenomenological books such as *The Man who Mistook his Wife for a Hat* (Sacks, 1986), illustrates professional thinking styles, reactions and reasoning and provides a model for reflection and self-review. Other books on clients' personal experiences can also be illuminating. Students could be asked to read such books and write about how they think they would cope under similar circumstances. This will develop an understanding of the client's thoughts and needs which should play a role in collaborative decision making.

Preparing to be an explicit reasoner or reflective learner is not easy. Students need to practise thinking aloud to themselves and with other people. The distinction between 'thinking aloud' and 'talking aloud' needs to be made clear. Students need to be able to voice their thinking rather than simply describing incidents or experiences. Many occupational therapists find this aspect of reasoning difficult. Vocalizing their thoughts on an audiocassette, either alone or with a peer, will enable students to practise voicing, justifying and examining their reasoning while on placement.

Reflecting-in-action – experiencing the experience

At the beginning of fieldwork placements individual agreements (mutual learning contracts) with students should be clearly established. These agreements can deal with mutual expectations, learning goals and strategies, and assessment goals and methods. In each of these areas clinical reasoning abilities can be targeted.

Traditionally, students follow a procedural route with their educator looking at processes and skills from the professional viewpoint. However, in my experience it is preferable to create a foundation on which to build reasoning rather than rushing in to the procedural aspects of work. This can be facilitated by concentrating on the exercises which encourage interactive and narrative reasoning through story telling, observation and interactive encounters early in the placement.

Students need to understand why they are doing these activities and to actively participate in their choice and design so that they actively 'own' their experiences. Otherwise they may well become confused or disillusioned. A sense of expectation needs to be created. The following learning strategies can be used to embellish procedural tasks and create richer meanings.

Observations and noticing

As illustrated in Table 20.1 it is from detailed noticing that cues are picked up and patterns are formed. The student and the educator can work through prepared exercises to discuss cues that can be obtained from clinical cases and to consider how these cues influence clinical reasoning. Direct contact with clients will provide another means for developing observational skills and awareness of cues, and can be started at the beginning of the fieldwork placement. Guided observation sheets can facilitate this. Students can join an interview conducted by the educator and be asked to follow a parallel framework by writing down their own interpretations of what they hear and see and then comparing these with the educator's notes.

This 'noticing' framework, which is different from the professional procedural one, can be deepened through discussion. For instance, the student could be asked: What similar personal encounters have you experienced? What are your views about this person? What feelings did you experience? And, in order to expand the students' thinking the teacher could also ask questions such as: How do you think the client's family felt? How might members of the public react? What other agencies or disciplines work with these problems? What other things would you have asked? What further knowledge would you need to gather?

Simulations provide another powerful experience and they may be appropriate in some settings. Apart from the usual physical simulation tasks in occupational therapy like being in a wheelchair, other experiences could be explored such as sensory deprivation, sitting or lying and waiting for hours. This may strengthen the student's understanding of various patterns of behaviour often seen with clients like anger, depression, and passivity. Comparing this experience with the experiences of a peer or even with a client will add other perspectives. Each of these activities serve to expand and strengthen the students' knowledge base and act as a foundation for effective clinical reasoning.

Interactions and revelations

According to Fleming (1991) interactive reasoning is often a neglected area of practice. Even interactive sessions such as interviewing are usually learned in a procedural manner. 'Talking to' the client can be a valuable precursor to the formal interview and this will combine both narrative and interactive reasoning. One of the essential requirements in this type of encounter is active listening and trying to understand the client's story. Audiotaping a session with a client (with permission) and then writing down everything that can be remembered afterwards and comparing it to the taped version will develop this skill.

Empathic sharing and self disclosure is another aspect of interactional reasoning that was studied in clinical reasoning studies of experienced and effective therapists conducted at Boston (Schwartzberg, 1992). The therapists seemed to change and adjust their way of talking and behaving in order to fit in and enter the client's world. Spending time informally with clients and then viewing videotapes of themselves in this dialogue will heighten the student's sense of empathy. Vocalizing and

exploring feelings will also aid interactive reasoning.

Students working in pairs can prepare and conduct unstructured interviews When one student gets 'stuck' the other can continue. This helps to develop their interactive abilities and confidence. It will also accommodate the unexpected twists and turns which are usually lost in a structured interview and these can be dealt with in group sessions. Students can then progress to developing their own framework for an interview, constructing the questions to ask and providing the reasoning for these. Peer projects where one student challenges another's reasoning will encourage students' confidence to practise in uncertain situations. This can be made more challenging by having therapists join this session as they can not only question the student's thinking but they can also expand it through questioning and sharing their own practice perspective. These informal methods can then be contrasted with formal, structured interviews to illustrate which method gathered more useful information and what information was most relevant to the client's actual situation.

Procedures and interventions – reasoning patterns

This is the area of practice widely acknowledged and viewed as being 'professional' (Fleming, 1991). Ryan (1990) found that experienced therapists used different patterns of procedural reasoning from that of inexperienced therapists. They were able to think in 'wholes' rather than in isolated events. This implies that educators need to be aware of the patterns of reasoning students use. Experienced therapists consider multiple strategies whereas novice therapists seem to consider one hypothesis and then another. An educator, by questioning the student carefully, could encourage the use of more advanced multiple reasoning strategies. Students also need much more time to generate their thoughts, ideas and decisions than do experienced clinicians. In the same study Ryan (1990) found that students took three times longer to make decisions.

As mentioned earlier, the student's reasoning during medical chart inspection or other forms of data-gathering in the period before meeting a client has been found to be very sparse (Ryan, 1990). Group exercises which seek out factual knowledge, and which voice, share and question personal opinions, will augment procedural reasoning at this point. Prior to meeting a client the group could brainstorm possibilities for procedural actions and develop between them a range of strategies and rationales. Images would form more quickly by pooling and linking their collective knowledge and experiences. This reasoning then needs to be challenged by the educator who can point out apparent assumptions students are making, expand reasoning and correct erroneous ideas. In this way ideas are tested, problems shared, and solutions generated and this gradually unfolds an anticipated image of the client which enhances conditional reasoning. Sharing with peers is a powerful medium that enhances reasoning.

This 'connected knowing' can be further facilitated by the educator linking knowledge and experiences from other sessions or from formal theory learned at school. Other ways of facilitating procedural reasoning and therapeutic interventions can be developed by directly watching the educator in action. Like Schon's (1987) reflection methods, this can be facilitated by active 'listening and telling' during the experience which expands the usual demonstrating, questioning and reflecting. It is necessary to choose clients carefully and to include them in the planning so that they are active participants and can contribute to the session themselves. It is important to remember also, that safe practice and ethical considerations have priority when planning these sessions especially when pairs of students or a single student tries a procedure alone.

The students can also develop a form of questioning where they actively talk to themselves during a situation, either aloud or silently. Such questions could include: 'Do I understand what is happening?' 'Does it make sense to me?' 'Could I be doing this another way?' 'Is this better than the last time?' Writing all these questions and feelings in the reflective section of a diary during the placement will add breadth to the present experience and will form a base for later reflection on action.

Reflecting on the experience

Debriefing stages such as those strands suggested by Fish et al (1991) can illuminate the fieldwork experience. Interpreting the experi-

ence, searching for critical incidents, and patterns, thinking laterally of other ways of doing, critically analysing, comparing and contrasting other sessions and other experiences, becomes an essential form of reflective practice. Attending to feelings, particularly obtrusive ones, is a part of occupational therapy practice often left unexpressed. Reviewing feelings captured at a particular moment and then comparing them to present feelings about the situation may help the student to re-evaluate the experience and form other interpretations. Finally, thinking about one's thinking which is known as metacognition or metareasoning will enrich the individual's store and foundation of experience and will promote critical reflection on one's reasoning ability.

Conclusion

Because practice is so uncertain the processes through which the student has to pass must accommodate this. In this chapter many practical suggestions have been given in a staged manner which reflects the development of clinical reasoning as well as the complex whole. To simplify the process defies the reality of clinical situations. By combining knowledge of the students' stages of development, the process of professional development, learning strategies, and reflective methods and continuing to explore ways of enhancing clinical reasoning, the educator will be able to present students with valuable clinical learning experiences which will facilitate the development of the students' reasoning abilities.

References

Boud, D., Keogh, R. and Walker, D. (1985). Promoting reflection in learning: a model. In *Reflection: Turning Experience Into Learning* (eds D.J. Boud, R. Keogh, and D. Walker). Kogan Page, London. pp. 18–40

Boud, D. and Walker, D. (1991) *Experience and Learning: Reflection at Work*. Deakin University Press, Geelong, Victoria

Cohn, E.S. (1988). Fieldwork education: Shaping a foundation for clinical reasoning. *American Journal of Occupational Therapy*, **43**, 240–244

Crepeau, E.B. and LaGarde, T. (eds) (1991) *Self-Paced Instruction for Clinical Education and Supervision*. The

American Occupational Therapy Association. Inc., Baltimore

Dreyfus, H. and Dreyfus, S. (1986) *Mind Over Machine: The Power of Human Intuition and Expertise in the Era of the Computer.* Free Press, New York

Fish, D., Twinn, S. and Purr, B. (1991) *Promoting Reflection: Improving the Supervision of Practice in Health Visiting and Initial Teaching Training. Report Number Two.* West London Institute of Higher Education, Twickenham, U.K

Fleming, M.H. (1991) The therapist with the three-track mind. *American Journal of Occupational Therapy*, **45**, 1007–1014

Frum, D.C. and Opacich, K.J. (1987) *Supervision: Development of Therapeutic Competence.* The American Occupational Therapy Association, Inc., Baltimore

Higgs, J. (1990) Fostering the acquisition of clinical reasoning skills. *New Zealand Journal of Physiotherapy*, **18**, 13–17

Mattingly, C. (1989a) The narrative nature of clinical reasoning. American Association of Occupational Therapists, Baltimore

Mattingly, C. (1989b) *Doing with patient: Occupational therapy as a collaborative practice.* American Association of Occupational Therapists, Baltimore

Mattingly, C. and Gillette, N. (1991) Anthropology, occupational therapy and action research. *American Journal of Occupational Therapy*, **45**, 972–978

Maxim, B.R. and Dielman, T.E. (1987) Dimensionality, internal consistency and interrater reliability of clinical performance ratings. *Medical Education*, **21**, 130–137

Munroe, H. (1992) Clinical reasoning in community occupational therapists: Patterns and processes. Unpublished doctoral thesis, Heriod-Watt University, Edinburgh.

Patel, V.L. and Cranton, P.A. (1983) Transfer of student learning in medical education. *Journal of Medical Education*, **58**, 126–135

Perry, W. (1979) *Forms of intellectual and ethical development in the college years.* Holt, Rinehart and Winston, New York

Rogers, J.C. and Holm, M.B. (1989) The therapist's thinking behind functional assessment I. In *American Occupational Therapy Association Self Study Series: Assessing Function* (ed. C.B. Royeen). American Occupational Therapy Association, Rockville, MD

Rowan, J. (1981) A dialectical paradigm for research. In *Human Inquiry: A Sourcebook for New Paradigm Research* (eds P. Reason and J. Rowan). John Wiley, Chichester, U.K. pp. 93–112

Ryan, S. (1990) Clinical reasoning: A descriptive study comparing novice and experienced occupational therapists. Master's thesis, Columbia University, New York

Sacks, O. (1986) *The man who mistook his wife for a hat and other clinical tales.* Perennial Library, New York

Salz, K.L. (1991) Study participants anticipate benefits for students. *OT Week*, **5**, 7, American Occupational Therapy Association, Rockville

Schon, D.A. (1987) *Educating the Reflective Practitioner.* Jossey-Bass, San Francisco

Schwartzberg, S.L. (1992) Self-disclosure and empathy in occupational therapy. Paper presented at the Occupational Therapy Conference, Trinity College, Dublin, Ireland, July 1992.

Tanner, C.A., Padrick, K.P., Westfall, U.E. and Putzier, D. J. (1987) Diagnostic reasoning strategies of nurses and nursing students. *Nursing Research*, **36**, 358–363

Weil, S.W. and McGill, I. (1989) *Making Sense of Experiential Learning: Diversity in Theory and Practice.* St Edmundsbury Press, Suffolk, U.K.

21

Teaching clinical reasoning to nurses in clinical education

Sheila A. Corcoran-Perry and Suzanne M. Narayan

Clinical reasoning has been integral to nursing education for decades in both academic and staff development programs. Beginning in the early 1960s, clinical reasoning was taught as 'the nursing process'. This general process involved linear steps of assessing patient needs, planning and implementing nursing care to meet the identified needs, and evaluating outcomes. While 'nursing process' outlined the steps, it did not describe the underlying thinking involved when nurses assessed, planned, implemented, or evaluated patient care.

Research on nurses' clinical reasoning conducted since the late 1970s has revealed the inadequacy of 'nursing process' as a representation of how nurses actually reason and make clinical judgements (Corcoran, 1986; Tanner, 1987; Tanner et al, 1987). The findings have demonstrated that, similar to other health professionals, nurses use a wide range of analytical processes as they encounter patient situations that are characterized by complexity, uncertainty, ambiguity, and instability. Therefore, the teaching of clinical reasoning has changed from focusing on a single, linear process to that of developing a variety of clinical reasoning skills.

Nurses use clinical reasoning to make both autonomous and collaborative, interdisciplinary judgements about patient care. The scope of nursing practice includes diagnosing and treating human responses to actual or potential health problems (American Nurses' Association, 1980). Nursing practice encompasses helping people to cope with their illness experiences. This occurs within a perspective that focuses on persons as holistic beings and on a broad concept of health that includes illness. As participants in the health care team, nurses also engage in collaborative judgements regarding the diagnosis and treatment of patients' disease conditions. Given the complexity of clinical reasoning in nursing and the range of health care issues involved, nurse educators use many instructional methods to help learners develop the necessary reasoning skills and knowledge base.

In this chapter, we describe five instructional strategies that are used in nursing education to teach aspects of clinical reasoning. The strategies are: analogy, iterative hypothesis testing, interactive model, 'thinking aloud', and reflection-about-action. Some of these strategies emphasize cognitive processes, while others emphasize knowledge organization. Still others stress both process and knowledge. Each strategy is briefly described including a summary of the phases or components of the strategy. Then, an example is provided to illustrate how the strategy has been used to teach clinical reasoning to nurses in the classroom or clinical setting. Finally, the discussion concludes with consideration of the particular aspects of clinical reasoning that are enhanced by the strategy.

Analogy

An analogy is defined as 'a resemblance in some particulars between things otherwise unlike, i.e.

a similarity' (Jorgensen, 1980, p. 2). It is a simple, but powerful linguistic tool for developing both creative and critical thinking abilities. Often analogies are used to make the unfamiliar familiar, or to make the familiar unfamiliar (Alexander et al, 1987). The latter is useful for prompting review of fixed perspectives.

Nursing educators often use analogies to simplify the mental image of a task, or to view a situation from another perspective (Elsberry and Sorensen, 1986). For example, when students are struggling to understand the circulatory system, an instructor might have students imagine that it is a closed system of tubing (blood vessels) with a pump (the heart) to circulate fluid (blood). Then the students can speculate about what would happen if the tubing were constricted, if there was a hole in the tubing, or if the pump failed.

The 'synectic' model of teaching is a formal instructional approach that incorporates analogies. It has five phases: (1) describe the present situation or problem; (2) present and describe an analogy for the situation; (3) describe the similarities between the analogy and the situation; (4) describe the differences between the analogy and the situation; and (5) re-explore the original situation on its own terms (Joyce et al, 1992).

The following example illustrates how one nursing faculty member used this model to help nursing students develop a simple but powerful mental representation (Corcoran and Tanner, 1988). In a medical–surgical setting, the teacher often heard students describe patients only in terms of their diseases. In their written assignments, students referred to patients as persons, but usually in terms of a combination of biological, psychological, social, and spiritual parts. To counter these reductionistic perspectives and to develop a sense of patients as whole indivisible persons, the teacher came to the next class with an analogy to represent holism. The teacher began with Phase 1 in which she acknowledged the difficulty many people have grasping the concept of holism. She shared statements that she had heard and read which reflected this quandary.

In Phase 2, the teacher presented an analogy. She began by setting on the table jars of flour, water, sugar, butter, eggs, and baking powder. The teacher asked, 'What do I have here?' The students listed the ingredients. Then the teacher took all the ingredients out of the jars, put them into a bowl, mixed them together and asked, 'What do I have now?' The students indicated a mixture of ingredients. The next question was, 'Can I retrieve any of the individual ingredients?' to which the answer was 'No.' Next the teacher said, 'Imagine that I have put these mixed ingredients into a pan and placed them in an oven at 350 degrees for one hour. Here is what I have,' as she revealed a cake. Then the teacher asked the students to describe the analogy. The students stated: 'We ended up with something very different from the ingredients with which we began, a cake'; 'The separate ingredients to make the cake are not visible'; 'The ingredients cannot be pulled out'; and 'A transformation occurred in the ingredients as they were mixed and heated'. This phase helped students gain insight into the meaning of the term 'whole'. They came to view the 'whole' of a cake as something greater than and different from the sum of its ingredients. Their creative abilities were promoted as they visualized the ingredients being combined and taking on a new identity.

In Phase 3, the teacher asked the students to describe the similarities between the cake and a whole person. The students repeated the statements about the inability to distinguish or extract the parts, whether of a cake or a person. They talked about both the cake and a person being greater than and different from the sum of the parts. They concluded that persons are more than their physical, psychological, social, and spiritual parts. The students also indicated that one could examine the parts, for example the quality of the flour or the quality of a person's heart; the quality of the parts could influence the quality of the whole, but did not describe the whole.

In Phase 4, the teacher asked the students to focus on the differences between a cake and a person. They identified the primary differences between the nature of a cake as an inanimate object and of a person as a living, dynamic being. Then they explored these differences in greater detail. Phases 3 and 4 involved the students' critical thinking abilities as they analysed the similarities and differences between the cake analogy and the concept of a person. The students were required to compare and contrast these two seemingly different entities.

In Phase 5, the teacher and students re-examined the concept of holism. For example, they explored the language that would represent a view of persons as holistic beings. After completing this activity, the teacher and students reflected on the thinking processes they had used in working with the analogy.

Analogies promote both creative and critical thinking, two processes central to clinical reasoning. Creative thinking abilities are relevant to hypothesis generation during the diagnostic reasoning process, as well as to the generation of possible interventions. For example, analogies can help one visualize multiple interpretations of cues or causes of presenting symptoms. Similarly, analogies can promote both multiple and innovative ways for treating a given condition or situation. The critical thinking abilities promoted by the use of analogies are relevant to hypothesis and treatment evaluation. For example, the generated alternatives and/or treatments must be compared and contrasted for potential effectiveness and efficiency. Therefore, an analogy can be exploited more consciously as a conceptual tool for teaching aspects of clinical reasonmg.

Iterative hypothesis testing

Recent research in nursing and in medicine provides evidence that clinicians use an iterative (repetitive) hypothesis testing approach in their diagnostic reasoning (Elstein et al, 1978; 1990; Tanner et al, 1987). The findings show that clinicians form diagnostic hypotheses based on minimal clinical data, activate hypotheses very early in the process, and use the activated hypotheses as a context for gathering additional relevant data to confirm or eliminate hypotheses.

This repetitive approach enables the decision maker to cope with the limits of short-term memory because only a few diagnostic hypotheses are kept in working memory at one time. Each hypothesis represents a cluster of cues, a single 'chunk'. Such 'chunks' place less demands on one's working memory than do many pieces of unrelated data. One can then rule-in or rule-out single hypotheses. For example, several cues from a patient may suggest a particular diagnosis. Then the clinician can use the hypothesized diagnosis to collect additional data to either support or reject the hypothesized diagnosis. Or one can compare two or three hypotheses at a time. Also, the diagnostic hypotheses help the decision maker

distinguish relevant from irrelevant data. This is possible because the classifications of most medical and nursing diagnoses include defining characteristics or critical symptoms. These characteristics or symptoms become the relevant data to collect.

Kassirer (1983) proposed a comparable strategy called iterative hypothesis testing for enhancing clinical reasoning. It is composed of three phases: asking questions to gather data about a patient, justifying the data sought, and interpreting the data to describe the influence of new information on clinical reasoning.

Iterative hypothesis testing is illustrated as follows: A nursing staff development instructor worked with a group of telephone triage nurses in a seniors' clinic. The nurses wanted to improve their diagnostic reasoning skills. They acknowledged that the goal of triage is proper disposition of patients who call the clinic; that is, referral of the patient to an appropriate health care provider at an appropriate time and place (Corcoran-Perry and Bungert, 1992). However, they did not feel confident about their approach to triage.

One of the nurses, Jim, indicated that he recently encountered a situation that he would like to re-examine. He agreed to serve as a source of information about the patient for the other nurses as they used an iterative hypothesis testing approach to collect data and decide about the appropriate disposition of the patient. The process of questioning, justifying, and interpreting occurred as follows.

Jim began the session by saying that the patient, Samuel Morris, called the clinic indicating that he wasn't feeling well and was having pain. A member of the group began data collection by asking: 'What history information is on Mr. Morris' written care plan?' When asked to justify the question, the nurse indicated that she did not know Mr. Morris and wanted some background that might allow her to help Mr. Morris more efficiently and effectively. The group concurred with this justification. Jim provided the following information in response to the question: 'Mr. Morris' care plan indicates a history of degenerative joint disease, hypertension, and obesity'. Then the nurse who requested the data interpreted the new information. She stated that it made her think of several possible sources of pain, including joint pain associated with his degenerative disease.

Next, another member of the group indicated that she would greet Mr. Morris and ask him, 'Where is your pain?' Her justification was that she associated pain with four classic categories of description: location, duration, intensity, and distress. The group concurred with this justification. Jim provided the information that Mr. Morris' response was, 'It feels like it is right under my breastbone.' The nurse who asked for the data interpreted this response by indicating that it made her think immediately of a myocardial infarction (MI). Substernal pain did not seem connected to his degenerative joint condition.

This approach was continued as the next nurse asked for duration of pain with the justification that she was pursuing the primary descriptors of pain, as well as classic symptoms of an MI. Jim provided the information that Mr. Morris' pain had occurred on and off for the past two days. It hurt when he took a deep breath. The nurse interpreted that this new information did not fit the classic symptoms of MI and made her think that perhaps he had a recent mechanical injury to his chest.

The questioning, justifying, and interpreting continued as the nurses pursued the pain descriptors and tested the competing hypotheses. They gathered data about the intensity of pain, prior activity that might indicate either injury or stress, radiating pain, and other associated symptoms. Upon learning that Mr. Morris could not recall a recent activity that might cause injury, but that his chest felt 'tight' and that he experienced sweating and feelings of indigestion, the group concluded that he probably had not suffered a mechanical injury, but that he might be experiencing a life-threatening condition. They chose to have Mr. Morris brought to the emergency room (ER) by ambulance for immediate medical attention. Jim, the nurse who brought this incident to the group, indicated Mr. Morris was brought into the ER and had, in fact, suffered an MI.

As the group re-examined their reasoning processes, they became more aware of their previously unconscious use of hypothesis generation and testing. They requested more staff-development sessions directed at developing this approach. Also, the nurses indicated that Mr. Morris' situation helped them refine their knowledge of MI symptoms in elderly persons. For example, they described being distracted by the information that Mr. Morris' pain occurred on and off for two days. Now they realized that elderly persons might not experience the sudden, sharp, and intense pain often described by younger persons with myocardial infarctions. In addition, they explored how a nursing perspective influenced their approach to this type of collaborative, interdisciplinary decision. In doing so, they focused on Mr. Morris and his family as well as on his possible life-threatening condition. They expressed concern about: (1) how Mr. Morris and his family might respond to the information that paramedics would be sent to bring him to the ER, and (2) ways in which they might support Mr. Morris and his family and help them cope with this frightening experience until the paramedics arrived.

As just illustrated, iterative hypothesis testing can be used to enhance diagnostic reasoning. It is helpful for discriminating among specific competing hypotheses and for clarifying the defining characteristics which differentiate them.

Interactive model

The interactive model is a strategy that is designed to teach new knowledge by building on and refining previous learning (Eggen and Kauchak, 1988). The model stresses the interaction between and among the learner and new content, what is already known and what is to be learned, and abstract, text-book knowledge and knowledge gained through practical experience.

The conceptual foundation of the interactive model is schema theory (Rumelhart, 1977; Rumelhart and Norman, 1981). Schemata are mental structures that organize knowledge and guide the way we perceive and categorize information from the world around us. Rumelhart and others suggest that people try to make sense of what they encounter based on prior knowledge and experience. Schemata serve as a way to store this information as elaborated networks of interconnected ideas. Schemata are not static. They are active processes that are constantly being re-evaluated for fit and usefulness. When learning occurs schemata are tuned and refined to accommodate new knowledge.

The interactive model includes three components: advance organizers, progressive differentiation, and integrative reconciliation (Ausubel,

1963). The following example illustrates the use of the interactive model to teach the concept of peripheral oedema.

The faculty member began by presenting an advance organizer. An advance organizer is a blue print or framework that previews the material to be learned and connects it to information already familiar to the student. Advance organizers present content at a more abstract level than the information they organize. Advance organizers subsume the content to be learned. An effective organizer links new information to an existing schema and provides a way for the student to refine the old schema or create a new one. The advance organizer presented by the faculty member was a brief statement about the concept of oedema.

> Oedema is the abnormal accumulation of fluid in the interstitial spaces of the body. Oedema originates due to several aetiological processes. Its presentation may be generalized or local. It may be subtle or grossly evident. While many forms of oedema are of concern in patient care, our focus will be on peripheral oedema, especially oedema affecting the lower extremities.

Then, the faculty member used the process of progressive differentiation to help the students examine the relationships within the new content on peripheral oedema and to link the new content to their previous knowledge about the general concept of oedema. In progressive differentiation, the more general concept is presented first and is then broken down into subordinate concepts or ideas. For example, the instructor put on the board the diagram shown in Figure 21.1. The instructor pointed out that there are several kinds of oedema, but that this class discussion would focus on peripheral oedema. She further differentiated peripheral oedema into several types. Then she distinguished each type according to usual cause, nature, pigmentation, ulceration, foot involvement, and other relevant characteristics.

Notice that the example shows how the ideas in the refined schema of peripheral oedema are related to previous ideas in an organized way that can be diagrammed. This linking of concepts provides a basis for the nursing students to encode the information and to store it in long-term memory. Students' refinement of a schema is not just passive learning of the instructor's schema. Instead, students are actively engaged in forming new relationships among ideas, connecting this new content to previous knowledge, and building upon their own existing schema.

Finally, the faculty member applied integrative reconciliation, the third component of the interactive model. Integrative reconciliation is a method that enables the instructor to actively engage the student in: recognizing similarities and differences, exploring the relationships between concepts, and making inferences about underlying causes or other critical features.

All three components of the interactive model can be used in the classroom or clinical setting. The nursing instructor decided to employ integrative reconciliation as a teaching method in the clinical setting. The following example illustrates her use of three types of integrative reconciliation.

After the content on peripheral oedema had been formally presented in class, the instructor gave the students an opportunity to assess several patients, each experiencing a different type of peripheral oedema. She asked students several questions: 'Now that you have observed Mr. Young and Mrs. Stone, how do orthostatic oedema and oedema due to chronic venous insufficiency compare? What are the similarities in appearance? What are the differences?' These questions required the nursing students to make simple comparisons of similarity and difference between the two types of oedema they had observed. This type of integrative reconciliation is referred to as horizontal reconciliation because the comparisons are made between concepts at the same level of generality.

Next, the instructor said, 'Let's consider the statement: "the most frequent vascular cause of peripheral oedema is an increase in capillary pressure which can result whenever the venous pressure is increased". How do these two types of oedema relate to this statement?'

This statement and question illustrate the second type of integrative reconciliation, vertical reconciliation. In vertical reconciliation, the student relates subordinate ideas back to the broad concept presented in the advance organizer. This activity reinforces the relationship between the advance organizer and the new content and helps the student refine old schemata.

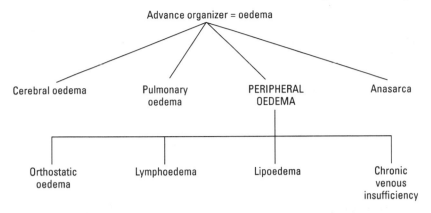

Figure 21.1 Progressive differentiation of the concept of oedema

Finally, the instructor asked the students, 'Would you expect to see bilaterality more often in orthostatic oedema or in chronic venous insufficiency? Why or why not?' These last two questions required the students to make an inference about the underlying processes that lead to the two kinds of peripheral oedema. This third type of reconciliation enables the student to relate these concepts not only in terms of general features or characteristics, but also the physiological processes that cause them.

Through the activities involved in integrative reconciliation, students link the knowledge gained in using advance organizers and progressive differentiation to the process of clinical reasoning. Learning to identify similarities and differences among signs and symptoms and exploring relationships among concepts enhance cue and pattern recognition. Practice in making inferences about patient data reinforces students' skills in accessing their own knowledge base and thinking deductively.

Learning through the interactive model promotes what Higgs (1992) calls deep learning, i.e. learning for understanding and meaning rather than rote learning of facts and principles. Use of this teaching strategy strengthens the content and organization of the knowledge that the nurse uses during clinical reasoning. The nurse who reflects on the learning that has occurred using the interactive model gains an appreciation for the enriched knowledge structures developed through the use of advance organizers, progressive differentiation, and integrative reconciliation; and the vividness and salience of concepts that are not just abstractions, but are associated with actual observations of patients

in the clinical setting. Furthermore, the interactive model also fosters essential skills that underlie clinical reasoning, including cue and pattern recognition and hypothetico-deductive reasoning.

'Thinking aloud'

'Thinking aloud' is a teaching strategy that is helpful in developing nurses' knowledge and clinical reasoning processes. Originally, 'thinking aloud' was used as a data collection method in research on the cognitive processes people use to solve problems or make decisions. Corcoran and colleagues (1988) suggested that since this method had proved effective in revealing the requisite factual knowledge and its structural organization, and the cognitive processes used by research subjects during clinical reasoning, the strategy would also be beneficial in teaching clinical reasoning skills.

In this strategy, the nurse is given a particular clinical situation (either real or simulated) and asked to think aloud while making a decision. The 'thinking aloud' verbalizations may be tape-recorded and later transcribed. Analysis of the recorded transcriptions reveals the cues to which the nurse attends, the hypotheses or inferences generated, and the nursing actions proposed.

This strategy is illustrated with an excerpt of a transcript of a cardiovascular clinical specialist 'thinking aloud' about a simulated patient case (see Tables 21.1 and 21.2). The clinical specialist shared this transcript with new nurses being oriented to a cardiovascular step-down unit. The situation involved a man who had

Table 21.1   Clinical situation

Four days after admission to CCU for an inferior MI, Mr. Seitz is transferred to the coronary step-down unit. He talks very little with the nursing staff, turns away when people come into the room, and is reluctant to ambulate in his room although his order is up ad lib.

In a high-pitched voice, Mrs. Seitz says that she must stay at her husband's bedside 24 hours a day because 'He's too sick to be left alone and you nurses don't seem to realize this.'

Mr. and Mrs. Seitz have two sons ages 10 and 15 who have been staying with neighbours while their father has been hospitalized. Mrs. Seitz says that the older boy, Mark, is quite upset and got into a fight with another boy at school today.

Table 21.2   Transcript excerpt and analysis of 'thinking aloud' session

Verbalization	Coding
Reluctant to ambulate in his room	Cue 1
That suggests to me that he may be depressed	Hypothesis 1
It doesn't really say that he's anxious but there is probably some underlying anxiety as well	Hypothesis 2
It says here that the older boy Mark is quite upset and got into a fight at school	Cue 2
Mrs. Seitz may feel guilty that she's staying here and neglecting her children	Hypothesis 3
I don't know the situation when he first noticed chest pain	[Unavailable information not coded]
It could have been something between the two of them So she may be going into a rescue mode She is going to save him from the awful nurses	Interpretation of cue
Because she inherently feels guilty	Restate hypothesis 3
It may be simply a matter of she just never heard or was not told enough times that he would not stay in the CCU for ever and ever and so she's not ready to have him transferred at all	Hypothesis 4
So I guess she's saying this to me: 'He's too sick to be left alone and you nurses don't seem to realize that.'	Cue 3
I guess she's probably telling me that	
And so my reaction would be to acknowledge that she is going through a really hard time	Action 1
And I think I would say, 'You seem very anxious about him being here in this unit and transferring out of the coronary care unit' and I would let her reflect on that	Action 2
And then I would try to find some positive meaning for the transfer But I would also identify that the transfer is a very important step in the progress toward getting back to a normal life and that he is ready for it physically	Action 3
And it is quite safe and I would outline whatever safety features I think would be helpful to her so that he is cardiac monitored	Action 4

been transferred from a coronary care unit (CCU) to a step-down unit four days after experiencing a myocardial infarction. His wife was quite concerned about the transfer. Table 21.1 presents the clinical situation and Table 21.2 provides a transcript excerpt and an analysis of the excerpt.

Together the clinical specialist and the new nurses analysed the transcript for the cues to which the specialist attended, her interpreta-

tions of cues, the hypotheses generated, and the nursing actions proposed. With a more advanced level of nurses, the clinical specialist might examine the transcript for the ways in which cues are combined, evidence of ruling hypotheses in or out, and the rationale for nursing actions.

As she reviewed the transcript, the clinical specialist asked: 'Now as you look at my comments, what are the cues that I focused on?' The nurses agreed that the cues to which the clinical specialist attended were: Mr. Seitz's reluctance to ambulate, the information that the older boy, Mark, is quite upset and got into a fight with another boy at school, and Mrs. Seitz's statement, 'He's too sick and you nurses don't seem to realize this'.

The nurses commented that they found the clinical specialist's hypotheses about Mrs. Seitz's motivations and behaviour helpful. Several nurses admitted that they would have identified Mrs. Seitz's anxiety, but not the possibility that she might be feeling guilty.

As the clinical specialist and the nurses reflected on the situation, they identified four nursing actions that the clinician had proposed: acknowledging that Mrs. Seitz is going through a hard time, recognizing Mrs. Seitz's anxiety, finding positive meaning in the transfer from the CCU to the step-down unit as an indication of progress toward normality, and outlining ways in which the step-down unit nurses provide for the patient's safety such as cardiac monitoring.

In addition, the nurses summarized what they had learned from the session. They commented that it was useful to think about the positive meaning in the transfer of a patient from CCU to a step-down unit. This led to a discussion of other ways in which a patient and family could 'draw a positive meaning' from the experience of having a myocardial infarction. For example, they might gain greater appreciation for the value of each and every day of life, or the experience could motivate them to develop healthier life styles.

The 'thinking aloud' method can be adapted and used to enhance clinical reasoning skills in many situations. Instructors may find it a useful strategy in teaching students in clinical settings. For example, an instructor might ask a student to 'think aloud' as nursing care is planned. The instructor supports and reinforces the student's appropriate use of knowledge and clinical reasoning processes and helps the student become aware of lack of knowledge or errors in reasoning.

Experienced nurses may use the 'thinking aloud' method to enhance their own clinical reasoning skills. They could share 'thinking aloud' verbalizations with each other as they make diagnostic or treatment decisions for patients who are particularly challenging or difficult. These verbalizations would enable

them to acquire a better understanding of their reasoning processes and to appreciate the richness of their clinical knowledge. In addition, nurses can improve their clinical reasoning by linking the knowledge and processes used to specific patient outcomes. Finally, 'thinking aloud' may reveal underlying causes of errors in clinical reasoning. Such errors may be revealed through feedback from peers or experts during 'thinking aloud' sessions or by the nurse's enhanced ability to justify clinical inferences and correct his/her own errors in reasoning.

Refection-about-action

'Reflection-about-action' is a strategy for promoting deliberation about one's practice within the context of particular clinical situations (Harris, 1993; Schon, 1987). Reflection-about-action occurs when one contemplates prior clinical situations, especially situations that were puzzling, troublesome, or particularly interesting (Harris, 1993). Since the reflections occur after a particular event, the knowledge gained usually cannot make a difference to the event at hand. However, the new knowledge can influence future clinical reasoning in similar situations.

The theoretical underpinnings for this strategy come from the work of Benner (1984), Schon (1983; 1987), and Harris (1993). All effectively argue for a new epistemology of professional practice. This epistemology conceptualizes professional knowledge as being gained from actual experience in clinical situations. One does not simply apply theoretical knowledge to a clinical situation. Instead, one gains this type of knowledge through the experience of making decisions about clinical situations, particularly situations characterized by complexity, uniqueness, uncertainty, instability, and/or conflicting values (Harris, 1993). Clinical reasoning in such situations cannot rely simply on acontextual facts, rules, and/or procedures that were learned in a classroom or from the literature. Instead, much of the required knowledge and the clinical reasoning processes are developed in the experience of practice. However, experience in the usual sense is not adequate. One does not develop this type of knowledge and skill from simply 'doing' something, but from reflecting on clinical judgements made, feelings generated, and actions taken within the context of particular situations.

While the clinical setting traditionally has been used as a learning laboratory in nursing education, this site has been considered the place where students develop skill in applying what they already know. It has been assumed that the theoretical knowledge gained in the classroom provides the foundation on which clinical practice is based. Gaining new knowledge, or transforming old knowledge during clinical experiences often has not been explicitly recognized or intended. Benner's (1984) work and that of Schon (1983; 1987) has caused many nursing educators to rethink the purposes for using the clinical setting as a site for learning. Instead of conceptualizing clinical activities as opportunities for students to simply 'apply' theoretical knowledge, these educators view such activities as a means for students to develop new and different types of knowledge. This knowledge is integrated with the theoretical knowledge that students bring to their clinical activities and incorporated into their clinical reasoning about particular patient situations.

Reflection-about-action is a strategy that promotes pondering about a particular situation in relation to the environment in which it occurs, as well as the feelings experienced, the judgements made, and the actions taken. Consequently, the theoretical and professional knowledge and the reasoning processes implicit in clinical practice can be delineated, elaborated, criticized, and transformed for future practice (Harris, 1993). Schon (1987) suggested that clinicians (whether students or professionals) reflect together on practice, using specific examples in the form of cases or demonstrations.

The following example illustrates how reflection-about-action was used in a senior nursing student's elective clinical experience. The student observed and worked with an expert hospice nurse mentor as she cared for several patients who were experiencing severe pain. At the end of each clinical session, the student and mentor reflected together on how they made clinical decisions about the recurrent, troublesome problem of pain control for the particular patients.

During these reflections-about-action, the mentor referred to aspects of each patient's condition that she thought contributed to the experience of pain. For example, she commented that the woman with ovarian cancer not only had physiological sources of pain, but her sense of guilt about having several abortions and her lack of a social support system seemed to intensify her pain. The mentor attended to multiple, diverse cues and related them to her diagnostic conclusion about the patient's level of pain. In contrast, the student had noted the same patient concerns, but interpreted them as being separate issues. She recognized the cues and generated separate diagnostic hypotheses about each. However, upon hearing the mentor's reflections, the student realized that she had not considered these aspects of the patient's situation as being interdependent and pain related. As a result of this dialogue, the student gained a greater appreciation for the complex nature of pain as a human experience.

As the mentor went on to describe her selection of particular drugs and their dosages to control the woman's pain, the student asked about the 'rules' that the mentor used. When the mentor indicated that she had few rules because each case was unique, the student commented, 'But you made statements that sounded like rules or guidelines. And they were statements that I hadn't read in my textbooks or in the studies that I reviewed about pain control'. When the mentor asked the student what rules she heard, the student said: 'Well, you said things like "Keep it chemically simple"; "It is better to increase the dosage than to increase the frequency of an analgesic"; and "This woman is likely to have constipation as a side effect of the analgesic; I should start a laxative to prevent or at least control that" '. The mentor was surprised to hear these statements, not realizing that she had made them. Then she shared with the student particular clinical situations earlier in her practice that had made these informal rules (heuristics) meaningful to her.

As the mentor reflected on other treatments she used for the woman's pain control, the student was amazed by the multiple and diverse interventions considered and used. While the student tended to think of analgesic medications as the major treatment for pain, the expert often combined analgesics with comfort measures, diversion, relaxation, and encouragement to verbalize feelings and concerns.

Together, the mentor and student recalled the woman's comment that their presence and 'being with her' for a quiet time of meditation was very helpful. This reinforced for both of them the importance of being physically and emotionally 'present' with patients.

This illustration exemplifies how reflection-about-action can be an important strategy for enhancing the clinical reasoning of both nursing experts and nursing students. Taking time to ponder particular clinical experiences enables one to: gain new insights; integrate theoretical and professional knowledge with feelings, actions, and outcomes; and use the experience as a basis for clinical decision making in future practice. In this sense, experience is not simply the passage of time, but rather a source of new knowledge, a challenge to clinical reasoning skill, and an opportunity to transform one's practice. The theoretical knowledge that one brings to clinical reasoning can be refined and transformed as it is combined with professional knowledge and used in the process of making judgements. As Schon (1987) pointed out, reflection is critical for both experienced practitioners' and novices' development, renewal, and self-correction.

Conclusion

Clinical reasoning has been a part of nursing education for decades. Initially it was taught as 'nursing process', a variation of the scientific method. Its introduction in the early 1960s was important in emphasizing that nurses use a systematic process and that they are thinkers as well as doers. However, recent research has shown that 'nursing process' is an inadequate representation of how nurses actually make clinical judgements. The research findings indicate that nurses, like other health professionals, use both domain-specific knowledge and a wide range of analytical processes during clinical reasoning (Corcoran, 1986; Tanner, 1987; Tanner et al, 1987). Therefore, the teaching of clinical reasoning has changed from focusing on a single, linear process to developing a variety of clinical reasoning skills and a broad, well-organized knowledge base.

Since no educational method addresses all aspects of clinical reasoning, we selected five strategies that nursing educators use to teach diverse clinical reasoning skills. The strategies are: analogy, interactive model, iterative hypothesis testing, 'thinking aloud' and reflection-about-action. Examples from classroom and clinical teaching in both academic and staff development programs were included. There are many other strategies that have been used to enhance nurses' clinical reasoning skills, including computer assisted instruction, use of decision analysis, and simulated laboratories for teaching and testing clinical reasoning.

Two excellent resources for other educational strategies to promote development of general reasoning skills are *Models of Teaching* by Joyce et al (1992) and *Strategies for Teachers: Teaching Content and Thinking Skills* by Eggen and Kauchak (1988). It is important for educators to develop a repertoire of strategies, beginning with one or two and adding others over time.

References

Alexander, P., White, C., Haensly, P. and Crimmins-Jeanes, M. (1987) Training in analogical reasoning. *American Educational Research Journal*, **24**, 387–404

American Nurses' Association. (1980) *Nursing: A Social Policy Statement*. ANA, Kansas City, MO

Ausubel, D. (1963) *The Psychology of Meaningful Verbal Learning*. Grune and Stratton, New York

Benner, P. (1984) *From Novice to Expert: Excellence in Clinical Nursing Practice*. Addison-Wesley, Menlo Park, CA

Corcoran, S. (1986) Task complexity and nursing expertise as factors in decision making. *Nursing Research*, **35**, 107–112

Corcoran, S., Narayan, S. and Moreland, H. (1988) 'Thinking aloud' as a strategy to improve clinical decision making. *Heart and Lung*, **17**, 463–468

Corcoran, S. and Tanner, C. (1988) Implications of clinical judgment research for teaching. In *Curriculum Revolution: Mandate for Change* (ed. National League for Nursing). National League for Nursing, New York, pp. 159–176

Corcoran-Perry, S. and Bungert, B. (1992) Enhancing orthopaedic nurses' clinical decision making. *Orthopaedic Nursing*, **11**, 64–70

Eggen, P. and Kauchak, D. (1988) *Strategies for Teachers: Teaching Content and Thinking Skills*, 2nd edn. Prentice Hall, Englewood Cliffs, NJ

Elsberry, N. and Sorensen, M. (1986) Using analogies in patient teaching. *American Journal of Nursing*, **86**, 1171–1172

Elstein, A., Shulman, L. and Sprafka, S. (1978) *Medical Problem Solving*. Harvard University Press, Cambridge, MA

Elstein, A., Shulman, L. and Sprafka, S. (1990) Medical problem solving: A ten-year retrospective. *Evaluation and the Health Professions*, **13**, 5–36

Harris, I. (1993) New expectations for professional competence. In *Educating Professionals: Responding to New Expectations for Competence and Accountability* (eds L. Curry, J. Wergin et al). Jossey-Bass, San Francisco

Higgs, J. (1992) Developing clinical reasoning competencies. *Physiotherapy*, **78**, 575–581

Jorgensen, S. (1980) *Using Analogies to Develop Conceptual Abilities*. ERIC Reports, #ED 192 820, U.S. Department of Health, Education and Welfare, National Institute of Education, Washington, DC

Joyce, B., Weil, M. and Showers, B. (1992) *Models of Teaching*, 4th edn. Allyn and Bacon, Boston

Kassirer, J. (1983) Sounding board: Teaching clinical medicine by iterative hypothesis testing. *New England Journal of Medicine*, **309**, 921–924

Rumelhart, D. (1977) *Introduction to Human Information Processing*. Wiley and Sons, New York

Rumelhart, D. and Norman, D. (1981) Analogical processes in learning. In *Cognitive Skills and Their Acquisition* (ed. J.R. Anderson). Erlbaum, Hillsdale, NJ, pp. 335-359

Schon, D. (1983) *The Reflective Practitioner*. Basic Books, New York

Schon, D. (1987) *Educating the Reflective Practitioner*. Jossey-Bass, San Francisco

Tanner, C. (1987) Teaching clinical judgment. *Annual Review of Nursing Research*, **5**, 153–173

Tanner, C., Padrick, K., Westfall, U. and Putzier, D. (1987) Diagnostic reasoning strategies of nurses and nursing students. *Nursing Research*, **36**, 358–363

22

Using simulated patients to teach clinical reasoning

Helen Edwards, Miranda Franke and Bill McGuiness

This chapter discusses how and why we have used simulated patients in clinical education particularly in teaching clinical reasoning at Lincoln School of Health Sciences, La Trobe University. The account focuses on considering the reality for teachers and students of using simulated patients and the processes required to make a simulated patients program work.

Simulated patients are not intended to replace the experience gained in working with real patients. They are seen as an optimal pre-clinical experience, where students have the chance to develop clinical reasoning skills at a deep level before having to deal with the complexity and unpredictability of the real world.

Simulated patients were introduced into the medical education literature by Barrows and Abrahamson as far back as 1964, and in a more detailed format by Barrows (1971) in his textbook *The Simulated Patient*. Barrows defined a simulated patient as 'a healthy person who has been trained to portray the historical, physical and emotional features of an actual patient'. This definition incorporates the essential characteristics of simulated patients. They are based on actual case histories, not an amalgam or 'ideal' case developed for teaching or assessment purposes. Lay people are trained to portray all aspects of a real case: historical, physical, social and emotional. After training, the simulated patients are checked for accuracy by an experienced clinician before being used with students. Once trained, simulated patients are used in a structured way in student education most commonly as a bridge into working in clinics or in assessment.

Simulated patients have been used to teach and assess a wide variety of clinical skills including interviewing and counselling, data gathering, performing a physical examination, conducting psychosocial assessment, and developing skills in clinical reasoning and decision making. Simulated patients are commonly used in assessment, both of individuals and groups.

Our rationale for developing simulated patients in the 1980s was to attempt to improve aspects of students' clinical education, in particular to prepare students for clinical settings and to reduce the variability and lack of control which often happens in clinical teaching. We adhere closely to the Barrows' model. Other users modify the original concept, often altering the case, training or presentation to suit their philosophy or circumstances.

The use of simulated patients is supported in the literature. Evidence points to the reliability, value and efficacy of using simulated patients. Gordon et al (1988) reported that experienced clinicians cannot differentiate between real and simulated patients during history taking or physical examination. In addition, evaluations of the use of simulated patients report that students relate well to simulated patients (Sanson-Fisher and Poole, 1980). Elstein et al (1978) were sufficiently confident of the reliability and validity of simulated patients to use them in research on cognitive processes in diagnosis. The nomenclature 'simulated patient' has been gradually replaced, in the USA in particular, by the term 'standardized patient' to emphasize the scientific basis and application of this teaching approach.

In a well documented paper, Vu et al (1992) described the development and application of simulated (or standardized) patients as they have been used over six years in a comprehensive assessment program at Southern Illinois School of Medicine. From their experience these authors identified an 'increasing feasibility, validity, reliability, and utility of performance based examinations' using simulated patients. They found cost to be a drawback.

Another study by Ainsworth et al (1991) reported on using simulated patients in all years of the medical course at The University of Texas. In this program simulated patients were employed for both teaching and assessment, in a range of areas including introduction to patient evaluation, history taking and physical examination skills, introduction to clinical medicine, integrating clinical skills, clinical clerkship, demonstration of competence, the senior assessment exercise and finally during the postgraduate medicine residency.

While papers such as these convince us of the reliability, validity and usefulness of simulated patients, it must be emphasized that simulated patients are not seen as a replacement for real patients. Rather they are an educational tool used to develop and refine students' learning and clinical skills, such as clinical reasoning, as students progress to becoming practising clinicians.

Reasons for using simulated patients

The most important reason for using simulated patients is that teachers can manage and manipulate the use of such patients for student learning in a wide range of areas such as programming, level of content, environment, ethics and safety, economy and reproducibility. Other advantages include using the process of 'time out' and feedback from patients to improve the educational experience for students.

Manipulating programs

Using simulated patients enables the clinical teacher to program student/patient interactions to suit the curriculum. That is, teachers can select a particular type of case, nominate the time to study that case and be reasonably assured that the interaction will actually occur at that time and with the designated case. Similarly the teacher can pre-determine the level of clinical reasoning involved in the learning activity. In real clinics plans are frequently disrupted by reality, for instance if the patient has gone to the X-ray department. This capacity to program with confidence results in efficient use of the clinical teachers' and the students' time.

Manipulating the level of content

One of the great assets of working with simulated patients is that teachers can be very specific about the type of encounter that we offer to students. This is achieved by manipulating the variables of type and complexity of the disorder to be studied, the level of interpersonal skill required for a successful interaction, the complexity of the therapeutic/assessment task that is required, the duration of the encounter and whether the student deals with a part or the whole of a treatment or assessment session.

For instance, we can give novice students a theoretically less complex disorder to manage in their early encounters with clinical reasoning, in order to build confidence. We can match current levels of acquisition of theory to practice, or organize to practise specific skills such as interviewing while not allowing students to be overwhelmed by the complexity of the patients' disorder. We may wish to specifically challenge our students' interpersonal skills and for example, offer them an encounter that will really test their ability to keep a patient motivated.

Using simulated patients allows us to be extremely prescriptive and to use educational theory to select the particular encounter which best matches the students' learning needs and best suits teacher planning. By manipulating variables associated with the use of simulated patients we can teach clinical reasoning in appropriately small chunks and at a pace that matches the students' learning and level of experience. We still expect students to cope with and adapt to the unexpected and to be flexible in the clinical setting but with simulated patients we control when and how our students have to be flexible.

Manipulating the environment

Simulated encounters allow control over the type of environment in which encounters take place. Thus at certain times we may wish the student to have to deal with noisy, distracting or threatening environments and at other times we may wish to have the environment as conducive as possible to a successful encounter. We can create hospital-like environments, outpatient clinics, home-based situations, etc. to best meet the learning goal. By comparison, in the real clinical setting, the teacher will need to deal with whatever situation happens to be present.

Other advantages – ethics and safety, economy and reproducibility

Using simulated patients makes some aspects associated with ethics and safety in clinical practice easier to deal with. Since simulated patients do not really have the conditions for which they are being assessed or treated, they can for example, be used for long sessions or be exposed to many repetitions of the same procedure, neither of which would be ethical or practical with a real patient. There is also a reduced risk that the simulated patient can actually be harmed by the students.

It is possible to have many students working with the one simulated patient which results in economic use of students' and teachers' time and thus reduced time and budget expenditure. Teachers can have greater confidence that every student working with a particular simulated patient is receiving the same kind of clinical experience. Simulated patients are trained to accurately reproduce their symptoms, case histories and psychosocial backgrounds across different encounters. They are therefore predictable and consistent over time. Real patients are far from this!

Time out

Using 'time out' in working with simulated patients is of great benefit when teaching clinical reasoning. The student (or teacher) can call 'time out' at any point during an encounter with a simulated patient to break from the interaction and seek assistance/feedback/reassurance from peers or the facilitator. During 'time out' the simulated patient freezes, staying in role but not interacting with the student until 'time in' is called. At that point the encounter resumes as though there had been no break in the interaction. 'Time out' is used for discussion, group input, problem solving and reviewing performance. With no time pressure, students are often able to reason creatively about the current situation, resume with new strategies and then complete a more successful encounter, thereby furthering their confidence.

There is also the possibility of trialing various interventions, calling 'time out', getting some feedback or having time to reflect and then retrialing with a different approach. These 'time outs' are a rich source of opportunities for development of clinical reasoning. This is because the details are fresh in the student's mind, there is space to reflect and there is the chance to immediately resume and try again rather than having to wait until the next real patient encounter (and perhaps develop some performance or anticipation anxiety in the meantime).

Feedback from patients

At the completion of the encounter, simulated patients de-role and return as themselves to give feedback to the students. The simulated patient can be requested to provide feedback about any aspect of the encounter. Students are encouraged to seek specific feedback about their own particular performance providing a rich opportunity for further development of clinical reasoning. As issues about the encounter arise the facilitator or other students may bring in examples from clinical work or theory to attempt to assist the student in devising a maximally effective encounter.

Educational focus

The sole aim in using simulated patients is educational. This contrasts with the mix of education and service delivery which occurs with real patients. In an encounter with a simulated patient the student can be encouraged and permitted to experiment. This is an acknowledged process where students can make mistakes and learn from them without endangering the patient. There are few opportunities for students in the real clinical health sciences for experimentation and yet this is an important experience for students to have. It helps them develop deep approaches to learning and to discover their own individual style of working rather than simply adopting that of their clinical teachers.

Example one – simulated patients in use

The following section provides an example of using simulated patients with students. This example reflects the planning, reality and dynamic nature of teaching using this method. The descriptions are deliberately presented in the teachers' own words to highlight the experience of teachers in using simulated patients.

Background

One of the difficulties faced by many third year speech pathology students when first attempting to diagnose a communication disorder of neurological origin can be the enormous amount of information about their clients that they have to observe and process. Benner (1984) suggests that skilled practitioners have a filtering and 'clinical chunking' process operating, where they see patterns and parts of wholes rather than thousands of individual symptoms/behaviours. Novice practitioners are less able to see clinical patterns and thus observe and mentally record many individual pieces of information before attempting to make sense of this and see some patterns. Therefore in a teaching/learning session it is an advantage to be able to present just a part of the overall neurological problem so that students can begin to see some patterns.

The simulated patient

In this exercise the simulated patient portrayed a 36 year old mother of two, who was unemployed and on a single parent pension. The patient sustained a cerebrovascular accident some three months ago and a diagnostic CT scan revealed a large area of decreased attenuation in her left fronto-parietal region. She presents with a dense right upper limb hemiparesis and resolving Broca's type aphasia and is currently an inpatient in a fast stream rehabilitation centre.

The students

The group comprised twenty speech pathology students in the third year of their four year undergraduate program. They were completing their theoretical studies of neurological disorders and were about to enter an off-campus clinical placement in this area.

The learning task

The task assigned to the students was to accurately diagnose the communication disorder of the simulated patient while maintaining rapport and attending to any patient queries. The students were given the case history the previous week and asked to gather and practise relevant testing materials and bring these along to the session. The tests were divided amongst the four groups of five students and dealt with the areas of: general interview and conversational sample, auditory comprehension testing, verbal expression testing and reading, writing and computational testing. Each group had fifteen to twenty minutes to complete its section.

The exercise

The session, from the teacher's viewpoint occurred as follows. The teacher is designated as 'I', the patient as 'Joan' and the students as 'Jill' and 'Sarah' (Group 1).

Time in: Joan presents with a flat affect and gives short telegrammatic responses to the students' questions. They find it difficult to get a sample of her speech and call 'time out' and come behind the one way screen.

Time out: Jill (student) reports 'She seems so depressed, I can't get her to talk. What should I do?' I ask for suggestions from the group. There is much talk about the need to motivate her (Joan), to explain why we need the speech sample, to find out if there is something bothering her, to ask if she needs to talk to someone, and to ask if we can help her in some other way. Jill and Sarah take heart and return.

Time in: 'Joan we need to get an example of you talking so we can see what things we could help you with in therapy, but you seem a bit down today. Is there something troubling you?' Sarah enquires. 'Well . . . my son, bad, in trouble . . . not stop him . . . speech no good . . . not listen', Joan painfully and slowly replies. The students are off now and although Joan struggles, she wants to communicate. The interview finishes after twenty minutes and we all regroup behind the one way mirror.

Time out: 'So what have we observed about Joan and does that knowledge suggest we should alter our testing plans?', I ask the group. There is much discussion about what we already know about Joan and redundancy in testing.

Time in: Group 2 begin the auditory comprehension testing and all goes well until they reach some higher level items, where Joan begins to look flustered and confused. The students push on and Joan becomes more agitated until she breaks down and pushes the testing items off the table. The students did not seem to see it coming and are shocked at her response.

Time out: 'What's the matter with her? What's she crying about?' implore the pair. More discussion about Joan's responses over the past few minutes, about failure, about the nature of these test items and her probable lack of pre-morbid exposure to such vocabulary/concepts. The group suggest ways to keep her motivated and her need for reassurance. They decide that it is not worth upsetting her just to complete this section of the test which is not giving us much information anyway. We talk about what we have found out about her auditory comprehension thus far and make plans for what specific areas we need more information about and how to go about getting this for next week. The pair plan to go back in and suggest finishing after giving her a task which we are confident that she will succeed on and tell her about the need for some more small, specific tasks for next time. They also plan to give her a brief summary of what they have observed to date and to ask her whether she has noticed these things affecting her everyday conversation.

Time in: The last two groups follow on.

Time out: These groups have several trips behind the mirror for time out discussions during which clinical reasoning is very active. Students have the benefit of time, lack of pressure without the client present, and peers to add ideas. My role is to steer their thinking/logic and to avoid faulty reasoning or incorrect facts. I am also a resource person who can confirm students' observations and interpretations or direct them to reading/materials to further their knowledge.

Feedback: After the sessions, Joan de-roles and comes to give the group feedback on how it was to be assessed, to fail, to not understand the purpose of the testing, and to have deficits so plainly demonstrated. She also gives reinforcement to the students about their interaction styles, their obvious concern for her well being, and their empathy. The students talk about optimal ways of indicating errors in client responses without making the client feel poorly, their difficulty in continuing testing when clients are failing. They ask lots of questions about how they could have worded things so that Joan really understood what they were doing.

Reflection/review

This is the opportunity to summarize the facts we have gathered, to check for comprehension of these, to discuss interpretation of the behaviours and patterns observed, and to plan for the next encounter with this patient.

Discussion of this example and how it facilitated clinical reasoning

This example illustrates the richness in learning to be derived from using simulated patients in teaching clinical reasoning. Here the students were able to observe client behaviour and then with the benefit of 'time out', verbalize these observations and check them against their teacher's and peers' observations. They had time to reason out the current situation, generate strategies for change and receive feedback about their reasoning before trialing new approaches. This is a very powerful means of helping students to become aware of their own reasoning and to learn to critique their reasoning. Students were also able to try out different approaches or ideas with the simulated patient, to receive feedback from their peers and the teacher, and then correct or retrial their approach if their hypotheses did not work well. In addition, students were able to match their observations to a theoretical management model and discuss how the model accounted for some of the behaviours and what the model failed to account for.

The use of real patients in this example would not have allowed the students to have the freedom to make mistakes, to change their management approach or to learn from their mistakes in such an effective manner. Neither could we have comfortably had the 'time out' from a real patient situation, to allow for the much needed mental space for such processing, or for students' self-evaluation and development of their reasoning abilities. Most importantly, the feedback from the simulated patient adds a true verification of the level of success of the strategies employed. We have found that students appear to place considerably more value on the direct feedback from the simulated patient, as compared to the teacher's perception of how it was for the simulated patient.

Example two – simulated patients in use

The following section provides a second example of the use of simulated patients with students. In this case, the learning experience is conducted with a large group of students. It is presented as the reflections of the teacher who designed and conducted the activity.

Background preparation

Interactions with clients are central to successful clinical management of the clients and to the effectiveness of clinical reasoning which drives this management. The process of history taking, in particular, is not only a means of providing data for reasoning which leads to decisions regarding diagnosis and management, but it also involves clinical reasoning. That is, the clinician relies on effective reasoning and decision making during the history taking phase to help guide this process, to test the reliability of the data collected and to pay attention to the needs of the client, e.g. for a break in the process if it becomes distressing. Students, therefore, need to learn how to reason during client interactions and how to make use of the data they obtain for diagnostic and management decisions. This example focuses on reasoning during history taking.

We have found that students often experience anxiety when confronted with the task of planning and implementing client interactions in the clinical setting, for the purpose of history taking. This exercise aimed to prepare year one nursing students for this task through practice with simulated clients. It occurred one week prior to students' first clinical fieldwork experience.

The exercise was designed to allow students, in the simulated environment, to practise their history taking and reasoning without the client suffering any consequences from student mistakes. Also, it was intended that feedback from the simulated patient, teacher and peers would help develop students' data collection and reasoning abilities. The specific task was for students in small groups to take the client's history, and in particular to explore the reasons behind timing and technique decisions associated with collecting client information of a more intimate nature.

Organizing the learning activity

To enable two hundred and fifty students to participate, four simulated patients were used over a two day period. The case studies were chosen to provide a mix of common scenarios. They included depression, cerebrovascular accident, head injury and arthritis, each combined with a variety of social problems. One teacher was assigned to two simulated patients for the purposes of introducing the students, monitoring the interaction, and calling time out where appropriate. Students were divided into groups of four and were allocated twenty minutes to conduct the interview.

In an attempt to help students develop a real appreciation of the variety of emotional responses they might experience and the variety of decisions they would need to make during initial interactions with clients, the students were not told that the patients were simulated. They believed that a group of patients with a variety of chronic illnesses had agreed to an interview with the students. During the interview students were asked to assess the patient's reactions to the level of information (general and intimate) obtained, and to document their reasons for the time and techniques they selected to elicit intimate information. These findings as well as the students' feelings, were documented in a journal.

The majority of students were obviously very nervous when entering the interaction. Some repeated in intricate detail the verbal patient description which was provided by the teacher immediately prior to the interaction. Others sought verbal reassurance that the teacher would be close by if required. The students were then introduced to the patients and the interaction began.

The power of the simulated patients to generate the emotions commonly experienced during nurse–client interactions was continually evident. Helen, a patient rehabilitating from a closed head injury with an adynamic affect, proved to be the most difficult for the students. Helen's lack of non-verbal feedback increased the students' unease. There were often long periods of silence accompanied by nervous glances between students and teachers. The prolonged periods of silence not only caused unease for the students, but I too found myself considering interjections to help the conversation from time to time. It required a constant effort to remind myself that the focus for this was experiential learning and that the confusion and unease the students experienced was a necessary motivator to encourage them to explore their reasoning, feelings and behaviour. Many of the students assigned to Helen were unable to elicit more than basic information.

Other simulated patients who exhibited more 'normal' responses helped the students to feel more at ease. Conversations with these patients helped students elicit more useful data and also a greater amount of intimate information. In fact, so personal was the information given by Sheila, a woman caring for her sick husband at home, as well as running the family business, that it brought a tear to some students' eyes. Another group of students were convinced that they could actually see the knee swelling described by Patsy (another simulator), even though the knee was normal.

Once it was obvious that a lull had developed in the conversation, usually approximately twenty minutes into the exercise, time out was called and the patient was asked to de-role. This event, was for me, the most dramatic. Some students began to laugh stating that they felt like they were 'on candid camera'. Others became very angry saying that they felt 'cheated'. One student said to me that she felt that she could no longer trust me and that she would not be able to be sure that patients she encountered in her clinical rotation were real. Fortunately the angry students were in the minority with most students experiencing relief that the patients were simulated.

The sense of relief following the disclosure provided a comfortable platform for the students to discuss their performance and reasoning. Students who had gathered little intimate information were able to describe how they had had difficulty deciding when to seek this information because of the absence of appropriate cues. The simulator and teacher were able to help the students explore other possible indicators and techniques for gathering this information. Students who had been more successful were able to describe the reasons for their timing and use of techniques for data collection. Client cues, student comfort level, age and sex of the client and the severity of the presenting symptoms were commonly identified by this group as factors contributing to their successful reasoning and performance.

The students' written feedback restated and expanded upon the feedback discussions. The majority of students were able to identify key elements to be considered when deciding when and how to explore client information of a more personal nature. Students also discussed how they had performed in relation to these elements and how they would make improvements. Some students stated that they had not recognized the complexity of this type of clinical decision until completing and analysing this simulated patient session. This observation provides an insight into an important advantage of the use of simulated patients over actual clinical practice, in that simulated learning experiences more frequently and readily promote reflection by students on their learning experiences. Such reflection actively encourages students to turn their experiences into learning.

In our exercise students' feelings also became the focus for reflection. Students identified a sense of empathy with their clients and compassion for them, even after they had learned that the clients were simulators. The anxiety witnessed by the monitoring teachers was also mentioned in the students' journals. Many questioned their abilities to carry out the interaction prior to the exercise, but later reported that they felt more comfortable about performing this task in the future. All students stated that they found the exercise to be of benefit, including students who had felt angered by the deception.

Evaluation

I believe that the aim of enabling students to develop their reasoning and interaction skills with patients, buffered by the security of simulation, was met in this exercise. The interaction provided the necessary vehicle and motivation for students to analyse their own reasoning and interactions and it provided some positive feedback about their existing skills. Subsequent journal entries from students' clinical rotations demonstrated an increased awareness of their own and their colleagues' reasoning and interpersonal behaviour. The client histories collected by the students also demonstrated that desirable learning had occurred, including an enhanced ability by the students to decide when and how to elicit relevant information.

With the benefits of hindsight I would have informed the students that the patients were simulated. The literature recommends this, asserting that once the interaction begins the student forgets that the patients are simulated. This was an assertion that I chose to ignore, believing that the experience would be more meaningful and effective if the students thought the patients were real. The anger expressed by some students indicated that this course of action could be detrimental. In fact, the assertion that simulation is forgotten was supported during this exercise. That is, even though some students had been told by their peers that the patients were simulators, this made little difference to the outcome. One student, for instance, stated in her journal 'I felt silly at first because she wasn't a real patient, but after a while I forgot as she was very believable' .

Apart from being effective educationally the use of simulated patients in this exercise demonstrates how simulated patients can be used in a cost-effective manner with large groups of students. Students were able to explore their reasoning and behaviour in a secure environment and were better prepared for the demands the real-world clinical rotation would place upon them.

Making simulated patients work for you

Deciding to incorporate simulated patients in a teaching program requires commitment at a number of levels in order to 'make it work'. Our experience of ten years of using simulated patients suggests that four areas are particularly crucial to successful use of simulated patients. These are the teacher's approach, quality control, financial arrangements and organizational commitment.

The first factor in making a simulated patients program work is the attitudes of teachers and students. Teachers are the key to this. They must be committed to using simulated patients properly. Simulated patients are not like a book which can be borrowed from the library shelf just when needed. They need to be 'looked after' and treated respectfully and humanely and with consideration for the arduousness of their role. Teachers must be very clear about how they wish to use the simulated patients in their teaching and what is appropriate training and debriefing for such a teaching session. Students also need to be adequately prepared, to act in an appropriate manner and to take the teaching session seriously. Our experience has been that students very quickly forget the 'artificial' nature of the encounter and participate in a real way with the simulated patients.

Simulated patients are used with students at different year levels in a number of courses and settings. A system of quality control is necessary to ensure that simulated patients are being trained and used properly and in particular that they perform consistently across time and across different situations. Our quality control strategies include very careful selection of people to become simulators, careful consideration of possible cases for simulation, systematic training involving a clinician, 'checking out' sessions with 'outsiders' as part of training, a user's manual for teachers, feedback sheets from teachers after each session, debriefing between teachers in meetings and an annual meeting between teaching staff and simulators.

As our simulated patients scheme has become devolved from school to department level to meet financial pressures and to comply with the 'user pays' philosophy which is increasingly common in higher education, we have found the task of ensuring quality becoming increasingly difficult. At the same time, this difficulty has made us more acutely aware of the need to have quality control measures built into the system.

Using simulated patients is a labour intensive and expensive operation. Therefore teachers planning to adopt this teaching strategy need to be clearly aware of the financial implications and necessary organizational arrangements. To fit into the traditional university financial system and thus avoid financial problems that we have had in the past, we use the Tutors pay scale for our simulators and pay for training at the same rate as actual simulation. By comparison, other organizations use different rates depending on type of use of simulated patients such as prolonged sessions, giving extensive feedback, particularly taxing roles or undergoing invasive procedures. Whatever rate is agreed it is necessary to budget for this, and while it may be cheaper than operating in the 'real' clinic there can be resistance to adding another expense to teaching the curriculum.

The final prerequisite for successful implementation is organizational commitment. This is essential because the infrastructure required to run a successful simulated patients program is more than an individual or even a small group of staff can expect to provide successfully. A successful simulated patients program depends on having a bank of appropriately trained simulators. Planning for this involves deciding on cases to be simulated, recruiting and training patients and organizing and monitoring their use. We have found it best to have one person who can be the main focus of the scheme and can interact with simulators throughout their recruitment training and use. Devolving responsibility to several people in smaller units loses this focus.

Conclusion

Using simulated patients to teach clinical decision making is a particularly rich and flexible teaching approach which allows students to develop skills in a safe structured environment. With appropriate activities in place at the organizational level, teachers will be able to use simulated patients to help students become aware of how they behave in interacting with clients and how and why they make clinical decisions. These skills can be directly transferred into the 'real' clinical setting.

References

Ainsworth, M.A., Rogers, L.P., Markus, J.F., Dorsey, N.K., Blackwell, T.A. and Petrusa, E.R. (1991) Standardized patient encounters. A method for teaching and evaluation. *Journal of the American Medical Association*, **266**, 1390–1396

Barrows, H.S. (1971) *The Simulated Patient*. Charles Thomas, Springfield, Illinois

Barrows, H.S. and Abrahamson, S. (1964) The programmed patient: a technique for appraising student performance in clinical neurology. *Journal of Medical Education*, **39**, 802–805

Benner, P. (1984) *From Novice to Expert: Excellence and Power in Clinical Nursing Practice*. Addison-Wesley, Menlo Park, California

Elstein, A.S., Shulman, L.S. and Sprafka, S.A. (1978) *Medical Problem Solving: An Analysis of Clinical Reasoning*. Harvard University Press, Cambridge, Massachusetts

Gordon, J., Sanson-Fisher, R. and Saunders, N.A. (1988) Identification of simulated patients by interns in a casualty setting. *Medical Education*, **22**, 533–538

Sanson-Fisher, R.W. and Poole, A.D. (1980) Simulated patients and the assessment of medical students' interpersonal skills. *Medical Education*, **14**, 249–253

Vu N.V., Barrows, H., Marcy, M.L., Verhulst, S.J., Colliver, J.A. and Travis, T. (1992) Six years of comprehensive, clinical, performance-based assessment using standardized patients at the Southern Illinois University School of Medicine. *Academic Medicine*, **67**, 42–50

23

Teaching clinical reasoning to orthoptics students using problem-based learning

Linda McKenzie

Orthoptists are allied health personnel who work in the area of applied ocular physiology as part of eye health care and rehabilitation teams. Orthoptists are trained in the assessment and treatment of patients who have defects of eye movement or binocular vision and the loss or reduction of visual function that accompanies such disorders. The overall aim of the orthoptics course is to produce competent clinicians, i.e. health professionals who are able to manage effectively the clinical problems presented to them in practice. Therefore, the development of competence in clinical reasoning is a necessary part of the orthoptist's education. This chapter presents a problem-based learning program which addresses this issue.

The educational program for orthoptists at La Trobe University is a three year Bachelor of Applied Science degree. In addition to core theoretical and clinical subjects, areas of study include: optics; ocular and neuroanatomy; general, ocular and neurophysiology; medical sciences, ophthalmology and pharmacology; behavioural sciences and health education. Problem-based learning was introduced into the orthoptics course in 1981 to promote the integration of the theoretical and clinical aspects of the course and to facilitate the development of the students' clinical reasoning skills. Due to the multidisciplinary nature of the Lincoln School of Health Sciences, many of the subjects are taken in conjunction with students of other disciplines. Consequently, it was decided that the problem-based program in the orthoptics course include only the core subjects Orthoptics I, II and III, in years one to three of the course, respectively. Throughout all years of the course the students attend clinical placements, in which they gain clinical experience concurrently with their theoretical concepts, and learn to transfer their knowledge and skills to clinical practice.

Clinical reasoning and problem-based learning

Clinical reasoning has been defined as 'the skills necessary to evaluate and manage patient problems effectively, efficiently and humanely' (Barrows and Tamblyn, 1979). The process of clinical reasoning has been described as one of hypothesis generation and testing (Barrows and Tamblyn, 1979; Barrows and Feltovich, 1987). This process includes: formulation of an initial concept of the problem from the patient's presentation and from other cues, initial data collection and problem distillation, generation of diagnostic and management hypotheses, implementation of an inquiry strategy and clinical investigation, problem synthesis and formulation of diagnostic and management decisions. This is followed by patient management and evaluation of management.

It is well established that problem-based learning offers one of the best methods for developing clinical reasoning skills (Barrows and Tamblyn, 1979; Barrows, 1985; Norman, 1988). In problem-based learning the student is presented with a clinical problem to solve in a simulated situation. This problem acts as a stimulus to the development of reasoning skills and to the acquisition of clinical knowledge and experience by the student. Using a simulated clinical experience has the advantage that students gain knowledge and skills in a setting where common clinical pressures such as time restrictions, patient welfare priorities and taking responsibility for clinical decisions, are lessened.

Cox (1987) states that 'teaching . . . should be designed to provide the usable knowledge and skills that the students can apply to health problems . . . and that . . . in an applied science, students must learn how to apply that science, in addition to knowing the concepts and principles of the science'. The use of clinical problems as the framework of a curriculum allows students to apply their existing knowledge and clinical experience to the management of clinical problems. Their simulated experience in solving the clinical problem replicates the process which occurs during clinical practice.

Problem-based learning encourages the achievement of various educational objectives (Barrows, 1985). These include:

- development of clinical reasoning skills
- integration of information into a cohesive learning unit
- consolidation, application and integration of theoretical and clinical knowledge
- development of self-directed learning skills, and the motivation to become self-initiating and self-evaluating learners
- development of critical thinking
- ability to function as an individual within a group setting, and development of independence, collaboration and co-operation in a functioning team
- development of communication skills
- development of appropriate attitudes and values through discussion of social, ethical and medico-legal issues.

Problem-based learning promotes 'deep' learning. In a 'deep' approach to learning students aim to gain an understanding of the subject and are motivated by an interest in the subject. This is a desirable approach for students in the health sciences to adopt because it promotes effective learning and parallels the behaviour

expected of competent clinicians. That is, competent clinicians are expected to seek meaning and demonstrate internal motivation both in their everyday clinical reasoning and patient management activities and in their lifelong professional development.

It appears that although individual students may have a preferred learning style, their approaches to learning are also influenced by the teaching they receive and the learning environment (Newble and Clarke, 1986). Problem-based, self-directed learning programs strongly encourage a deep approach to learning by allowing students to gain a deeper understanding than is possible through programs which encourage rote learning. Deep learning is promoted by stimulating the students' interest and motivation to learn and by providing a framework for students to learn to apply their learning to a clinical problem.

Problem-based learning in the orthoptics program

In the Orthoptics program at La Trobe University the method of problem-based learning used varies over the three years of the course. The program changes from being more teacher-directed to more student-directed as the students progress. Using a taxonomy of problem-based learning methods developed by Barrows (1986), which describes a range of methods from lecture-based cases through to closed-loop problem-based learning, the method used in both the first and second years of the course would be labelled as the 'case method'.

The 'case method' involves the presentation of a case vignette, or a summary of the patient problem for discussion. This method strongly encourages student-directed learning, and is supported by teacher-direction in the amount and sequencing of information to be learned. Students are challenged to develop their knowledge and collect patient data in order to decide the cause of the problem. Using this knowledge and data students then practise hypothesis generation, information analysis and decision making.

However, the case method has some potential limitations. In particular, the amount of clinical reasoning that occurs can be limited to some extent if the patient information is presented as a complete case, in comparison to the real clinical setting where the student or clinician would have to deal with incomplete presenting information. Because inquiry skills are not highly challenged if the information is presented as an organized unit, the method used in our course involves presenting the case vignette on a step-by-step basis. This promotes the use and development of inquiry skills without expecting students early in the course to employ the full extent of free inquiry that an experienced clinician would use in actual clinical practice with a real case.

As the students progress in the course the problem-based learning format moves towards the method designated in Barrows' taxonomy (Barrows, 1986) as 'problem-based' and 'closed-loop problem-based' learning. These use sequential management problems or patient management problems. In this situation the students develop their knowledge, apply this to patient diagnosis and management, and evaluate previous decisions. Using this method, students are challenged in all steps of clinical reasoning and the learning process is very strongly student-directed, with the role of the teacher being that of facilitator.

This progression in the extent of student direction in learning and in the clinical reasoning demands placed on the students is supported by both Barrows (1986) and Norman (1988). The latter suggests that the presentation of prototypical problems in the early years assists the students to understand basic mechanisms and concepts, and that the use of more complex problems subsequently aids the development of clinical diagnosis skills and the discovery of discriminating features.

Throughout the course the time allocated to problem-based learning classes varies from two one hour sessions per week in first year to one three-hour session per week in third year. These sessions are run with the entire student groups, which means up to thirty in first year and between sixteen and twenty four in second and third years.

The first and second year programs

Session 1

In first year the students study the sensory systems of vision and binocular function. This includes the diagnosis, investigation and princ-

iples of management of concomitant strabismus and its sensory complications. Second year focuses on the ocular motor control systems and ocular motility disorders, particularly paretic strabismus and disorders of the eye movement control systems.

As previously stated the first and second year programs mostly use a 'case method', where the patient details are presented by case notes, photograph or video (refer to Tables 23.1 and 23.2). Group discussion then evolves around such general questions as 'What do I know about this?', 'What appears to be the problem?' and 'What do I need to learn about this?'. Such questions relate primarily to the hypothesis generation stage and the recall and application of previous knowledge. They also enable students to refine their knowledge needs into learning goals under direction from the tutor who helps them to sequence their learning tasks and identify the amount of content to be learned.

Table 23.1 First year problem 1, session 4

Trevor presents to your clinic for an orthoptic assessment. He is six years old and his general medical history is uneventful. His father wears glasses, but there is no other ocular family history and he has no visual complaints.

Clinical findings
Visual acuity without glasses R 6/6 N5 L 6/18 N6

Table 23.2 Second year problem 3, case vignette

Referral from rehabilitation centre
Thank you for seeing Mrs Laws, aet 56 yrs, who has had multiple sclerosis diagnosed 20 years ago. At present she is having problems with her reading, having to close one eye to read easily. Could you please assess and manage appropriately.

On assessment
Cover test (N and F)
  Straight in primary position

Ocular movements
  Dextro-version   Full
  Laevo-version   Limitation of R adduction
                          Nystagmus of L abducting eye
                          Diplopia on left gaze
  Vertical movements intact
  Convergence intact

The cases presented are simple, with the aim of stimulating the learning and application of particular basic concepts such as anatomy, physiological mechanisms, optical principles, disorders of the systems and the clinical consequences of diagnosis and management. Consequently the learning needs are largely predictable, and on completion of the discussion period during which the students define their learning needs, they are provided with a set of learning goals for the problem.

These learning goals are given to assist the students and to act as a study guide as described by Laidlaw and Harden (1990). Each learning goal provides an introduction to an area of content and a framework for the learning task, emphasizing the important concepts, directing the student to the most appropriate reading and adding further information or explanations as necessary. The study guide assists in defining knowledge that is necessary for the problem and distinguishing this from the extra knowledge that is available, but not necessary. This is very valuable for the beginning clinician since it assists in setting limits on the expected level of knowledge to be acquired (Cox, 1987; Laidlaw and Harden, 1990). Such limits are of concern to the student, especially at the beginning of the course when they feel unable to differentiate between necessary and unnecessary information, and are faced with the rather daunting task of gaining an entirely new body of knowledge. One of the major aims at this stage is to help students understand key concepts and their application and avoid an over-emphasis on particular details.

Subsequent sessions

After the students have individually collected the information set out in their learning guides they return to the group with the knowledge gained. At this stage discussion involves the clarification of this new knowledge, further discussion of the problem and elaboration or rejection of diagnostic hypotheses.

The content is aimed at outlining the major physiological process under discussion and the effects of disorders of this process. This is related to the particular case being studied. In terms of the clinical reasoning process, the class is now at the stage of formulating the problem. At this level an actual diagnosis may not be made, but some statement concerning the nature of the problem, based on a synthesis of the information collected, and a statement of the underlying cause or process, is encouraged. In addition the class would generate some management hypotheses. During the discussion the tutor directs questions to allow the students to identify and demonstrate their areas of confidence and ascertain areas which may require assistance in relation to the problem objectives.

The whole class discussion sessions are supported by further small group learning sessions such as tutorials and seminars. At the completion of some problem units the students are given a self-assessment problem which allows them to test the application of their knowledge on another clinical problem, and to question their knowledge of the underlying concepts and their ability to generate hypotheses, to formulate a diagnosis and to propose a management plan.

The third year program

Objectives and format

At the completion of the third year orthoptics subject the students are expected to be able to:

- demonstrate appropriate application and interpretation of investigative procedures and competence in diagnosis of problems of both the sensory and ocular motor mechanisms
- demonstrate an understanding of the management of clinical problems by the selection and planning of appropriate treatment regimes for these patients, with regard to the likely prognosis
- demonstrate the ability to evaluate and appropriately modify methods of treatment
- demonstrate an awareness of relevant general medical areas, the implications of systemic disorders and a basic knowledge of the roles of other health professionals and the role of the orthoptist in the multidisciplinary team
- demonstrate an awareness of relevant ophthalmic conditions and procedures which will have an effect on orthoptic management
- demonstrate an awareness of the need to modify orthoptic management in different clinical situations in sympathy with the patient's age and general condition

- demonstrate the development of communication skills and an appreciation of appropriate ethical conduct
- appreciate the need for a positive attitude to self-evaluation and continuing education both through individual effort and formal learning situations.

In the third year, the program is presented in the free-inquiry format of patient management-problems. This method has been outlined previously (McKenzie, 1987). The student group proceeds through a patient problem. At any stage this is both an individual and group process where students have their own ideas, but may be challenged by other students. Where a diagnostic or management decision must be made, this is a group decision.

Problem discussion sessions

The problems in third year commence with the initial or presenting information of the patient as this would occur in a clinical setting. This information is provided by the tutor according to a guide for tutors developed for the program. The information may be in the form of a referral letter, a tape (audio or video) of a patient interview, a hospital record summary, a photo, or simply the appointment booking by the patient (refer to Table 23.3). Presenting information is analysed to decide on the important data and to formulate the students' initial concept of the patient's problem. This process leads to the generation of working hypotheses, and to a decision concerning further information required about the patient i.e. the inquiry strategy.

At this stage students may seek details of the patient's history or relevant medical, ophthalmic and orthoptic assessment results from the

tutor. The information may be given either verbally, as handout charts or overhead projections as relevant. During the inquiry stage the discussion involves such areas as the optical and physiological basis of testing procedures, anatomical and physiological development and function, aetiology and pathogenesis of the ocular and systemic problems, the patient's signs and symptoms, diagnostic hypotheses, and investigative procedures and their efficiency.

If results to a requested test are not on the information sheet then this is stated by the tutor, promoting a critical evaluation of the investigative procedure. After the group has decided that sufficient investigation of the patient has taken place, the group discusses diagnostic hypotheses. These may be confirmed or negated by the group and a preliminary diagnostic decision made. Through participation in this process students develop an important skill, i.e. the ability to be able to make an initial diagnostic decision for an unfamiliar problem based on what may seem to be incomplete data, or despite what might appear to be conflicting data.

The problem also requires management decisions which involves discussion of treatment options and a group decision for the preferred management option. The management plan should include a plan for treatment at this first visit, long-term management including prognosis and a general outline of the proposed treatment procedures. The group discussion at this stage includes areas such as relief of the patient's symptoms, urgency of the condition, further tests or procedures needed to confirm the diagnosis, and specific treatment procedures. Discussion of treatment procedures involves the optical, physiological or pharmacological basis of the procedure, expected outcome, time period and review period for any procedure and patient or parent instructions.

Having made an initial diagnostic and management decision the group then decides on when it will 'review' the patient. At the next visit the students are told the procedures that were actually performed which may or may not coincide with their management decisions. This leads to a critical evaluation of the treatment hypothetically performed in comparison to the treatment the group had chosen. If the patient has a general medical condition the discussion will include consideration of the management

Table 23.3 Third year problem 1 presentation

Referral of baby George
Re: Simpson, baby George
To: Eye Clinic, for ophthalmic assessment. Aet 6/52
From: Paediatric Registrar

This babe was born of normal delivery at 35/52 gestation. Birth weight 2510 g. Apgar score at birth 6/10, later 10/10. Ophthalmic assessment on day 3 showed normal fundi. I am now referring him to you for further assessment and would be grateful for your advice.

procedures performed by other health personnel, and the reciprocal relationship of the ocular status to other aspects of the patient's management. Awareness is also raised of the behavioural, social, economic, ethical and medico-legal aspects of patient management. As discussion of the problem continues, critical evaluation of the management becomes a major area for discussion.

The process is ongoing and circuitous, involving continual data and information collection, analysis, synthesis and decision making. The students experience the need to learn, the process of applying knowledge to clinical cases and situations, and the process of critically analysing and synthesizing theoretical and clinical information in order to make clinical decisions.

This procedure continues throughout the patient management problem. The problems are set over a typical clinical time span which may be anything from a few months to several years. Discussion of each problem normally takes place over two weeks. During the problem discussion any topics the students consider they do not understand are written on a learning needs list. At the completion of the first session the students allocate these topics to be researched either individually or as a group before the next session. At the beginning of the next session the students report back to the group, discussing these topics in relation to the patient problem, and evaluating the decisions that they had previously made in the light of their new knowledge. This skill of evaluating the effectiveness of their learning and re-applying the knowledge to the problem is an important extension of the problem-based learning process (Barrows, 1986).

For each problem the group elects one student to be a scribe. This student records the group discussion on a portable whiteboard, so that the data are available to them from one week to the next. This avoids all students trying to record details instead of participating fully in the group discussion. The responsibility of the scribe is to record accurately all the patient information and to give a representative account of the group discussion. The report is then compiled and a photocopy given to each student.

Seminar

A seminar is conducted at the completion of each problem. It aims to provide feedback on the students' management decisions, to present and discuss alternative methods of investigation and treatment and allow further discussion and clarification of areas of difficulty in the problem. This seminar serves to highlight the areas of differential diagnosis and alternative management strategies in a discussion setting which allows presentation of the tutor's personal views and the opinions of others. This is in contrast to the problem discussion sessions when the students should not be given feedback during their reasoning process to avoid disruption of the students' decision making process and to facilitate discovering learning.

The seminar is conducted by a different staff member from the group tutor and is held approximately two weeks after completion of the current problem. During this time another problem is commenced. The two weeks', delay allows the lecturer time to read the group reports and the students to further study the topic. The seminars encourage students to organize their learning and apply the knowledge to other examples, thereby enhancing retention and recall (Barrows, 1985). There is also discussion of the problem objectives, to ensure that the group feels they have adequately covered the subject areas concerned.

Problem design and choice of problems

As previously discussed the problems selected for the earlier years of the course represent cases and situations commonly found in the clinic and tend to be of the case vignette format. In third year problems are of the patient management problem type. They are chosen as examples of diagnostic problems, common disorders that require on-going or long-term management, or less-frequently-occurring disorders which require particular treatment procedures that are applicable to a wide variety of patients.

The patient management problems have been chosen after consideration of essential subject areas to be covered and problems that will be encountered in practice, as advocated by Cox (1987). To ensure adequate coverage of all the areas necessary for clinical and theoretical competence, the problems used during the year are plotted on a matrix with particular disorders, signs or symptoms cross-referenced against investigative or treatment procedures, administrative and ethical procedures, general medical conditions, different age groups and other factors such as rehabilitation or hospitalization. The choice of problems then allows study of examples of the most common conditions and some examples of the less frequently occurring problems. This facilitates the development of the skills required to investigate and treat most conditions which present in the clinical situation.

The problems are taken from actual case histories of patients, and are chosen for various reasons. Generally cases are selected because of a complicating feature or treatment procedure that sets them apart from what students regard as 'classical text book patients', thus stimulating wide discussion. Because the patient management problems are actual patient histories, they include information concerning the choice and results of particular treatment procedures. The alternative of providing a scenario for various choices of treatment procedures was discussed in our school, but it was felt that this would be too complex, and would detract from the reality of the patient's case history. Apart from changing the patient's name and the name of the hospital to preserve confidentiality, the case details are not altered, and therefore totally free inquiry is not possible as some results are not available. However, these absent results serve as the basis for discussion of all the options available, and the students are asked to decide what they consider is the best option at any particular stage of the patient's progress.

The majority of the problems are in written format, many accompanied by photographs, results charts or other illustrative material. Time and resource pressures due to the small numbers of staff involved in the development of these materials means that only a few of the problems have an audio-visual presentation or supporting material. The paper format is the simplest to produce, but we have found it to be a very effective method of presentation.

The problem file consists of a summary page, a tutor guide, an information sheet, objectives, a resource file and a seminar outline. The tutor guide is presented in two sections, one half of the page giving instructions on the problem presentation, the other half on the student discussion. There is also a time scale of the patient's visits. The student discussion section lists the major points to be covered by the students during the course of the problem. The tutor may need to direct appropriate questions to the students if they have not discussed some aspect of the problem. This section also includes a list of assignment topics suitable for the problem. The information pages contain all the details of each step of the patient's progress and the method of presentation of each, and include any photographs, attachments or overhead projections. There are objectives for each problem which are available to the students at the completion of the problem in order for them to review their understanding of the topic.

A resource file is compiled for each problem and consists of articles or information relevant to the problem. It is available to the students after the completion of the problem. This encourages the students to research their own material, rather than following teacher-prepared objectives. It is primarily used as a guide for further reading.

The role of the tutor

'The skill of the tutor is to make learning student-centred instead of teaching-centred; facilitating learning instead of dispensing knowledge' (Barrows, 1985). The role of the tutor in a group discussion session is to facilitate and guide student learning. The tutor provides the patient information on request from the group and is there to aid students in determining what they need to know. The tutor initially must establish a good working climate and assess and facilitate group dynamics. The students are encouraged to both give and receive constructive criticism of their viewpoints.

The tutor's role is continually active. Non-directive comments and questions may be required to challenge the students to elaborate and justify their views, to encourage all students to give their opinion and to encourage the group to reach consensus. The tutor ensures that the entire clinical problem-solving process is followed. In addition, the tutor encourages individuals and the group to recognize their own learning needs, and to take appropriate actions and use relevant resources to fulfil these needs.

In the early discussion sessions during the course the tutor needs to actively encourage all of these processes, but with time the students should become more self-sufficient as a learning group. It is the students' responsibility to facilitate the group process and thereby take responsibility for their own learning.

Tutors face the difficult task of not giving in to the temptation of providing the 'answers' during the group discussion. Instead, they need to accept the challenging role of guiding the students to their own achievements. It is important that the students not be given feedback during the process as to the right or wrong decisions, actions or thoughts but that they be allowed to reason through each step (Barrows and Feltovich, 1987). School staff and clinicians may be used by the students as resource persons to discuss the patient problems, giving of their knowledge and experience to the students. However, this advice is restricted to outside the problem discussion sessions which should be student-centred.

Assessment

The type of assessment used throughout the orthoptics subjects is of the type described as modified essay questions (MEQs) (Feletti and Engel, 1980). This method of assessment allows students to demonstrate their competence by applying their knowledge to a series of patient problems. It allows assessment of the students' ability to formulate diagnostic hypotheses, plan investigative procedures, diagnose, make appropriate management and treatment decisions and evaluate clinical results. The questions can be used to assess various levels of knowledge and aspects of the clinical reasoning process. The student may be requested to complete such tasks as generating hypotheses based on a patient presentation, listing further information that they would require in order to diagnose a problem, interpreting clinical data, suggesting a diagnosis, formulating a management plan or writing a report. For each of these tasks the students may be requested to give reasons for their answers, explain the physiological and pathological mechanisms and justify their decisions.

In first and second years, the MEQs are in a standard examination format where the entire paper can be viewed. Each question consists of the presentation of some case details followed by a series of questions. The first and second year papers consist entirely of short cases (see

Table 23.4   Second year assessment problem

Referral from Neurology Registrar
Thank you for assessing Mr. H. S. who is complaining of intermittent diplopia when he blinks. On examination it appears that instead of updrift occurring during eye closure, convergence occurs. This convergence is maintained for a few seconds, hence the diplopia.

Can you please examine Mr. S. and advise us as to the aetiology of this condition.

1.   What are your ideas at this stage as to the types of ocular movement disorders you may be expecting?
2.   How would you assess Mr. S?

Table 23.4), whereas the third year papers contain a combination of long and short cases.

In third year the assessment is by booklet-type MEQs consisting of ongoing patient management problems, as described by Feletti and Engel (1980). This format simulates the chronological nature of clinical decision making, where the students must complete each question independently, and are unable to preview the coming questions or return to change previously answered questions. In using this type of assessment it is necessary to provide the student with some guidelines as to the suggested time to be spent on each section because they are unable to gain an overview of the paper as is common during reading time at the commencement of the examination. The timing guidelines are printed on each page as part of the questions and are also on a summary sheet separate to the paper.

The cases chosen for examination are selected to achieve several goals. These are to cover a wide range of the typical cases seen in practice, to assess students' performance in relation to cases where significant consequences may arise from diagnosis or management decisions, or to test different aspects of the clinical reasoning process. Standard answers are compiled by consultation between examiners and other orthoptists. The assessment results in these subjects are norm-referenced, the students receiving a grade level.

As part of the overall assessment, a number of assignments are completed during the year. The assignments vary for each problem and include such tasks as a literature review, a critical evaluation of the management performed, a report to a referring health professional or teacher, or a patient management problem similar or contrasting to the one completed.

Evaluation

The orthoptics program is evaluated annually via course evaluation questionnaires completed by students. Prior to 1987 when the problem-based learning program was introduced into the second year of the course, evaluation by students who had experienced the lecture-based program included such comments as:

'Too much, too fast'
'Boring, difficult, involved memorizing rather than understanding'
'A very difficult area'
'Complicated at first, but with revision became easier'.

By comparison, after the new program had been introduced, students who experienced the problem-based program commented:

'One of the high points is . . . not being lectured to'
'Interesting, made you think, history to diagnosis and lesion site, did not involve rote learning but actually applied it to the clinical situation'
(The course involved) 'working at my own pace, active seeking of information rather than passive reception'
'I learned quite a lot from this because I actually had to find out the information for myself and then summarize it. It forced me to study more than I would have with lectures.'
'Too much information, not enough guidelines'
'Initially (I was) unsure about how to go about preparing work and detail needed'
(I needed to) 'work with a partner' . . . 'keep up' . . . 'do lots of reading'
'Get as much feedback as you can'
'If you don't understand, see someone'
'Quite successful; you only get out what you put in, rather than being spoon fed'.

It was apparent, after a major portion of the second year had been converted to a problem-based learning mode, that the students found the content difficult regardless of the teaching method. However, it was evident that the problem-based learning students appeared to be more positive in their comments concerning this method of learning and the perceived relevance of the knowledge to clinical practice. The major concern initially expressed by the students of the problem-based learning unit was their uncertainty of the requirements and expectations of the program. However, this anxiety decreased as the students became more familiar with the problem-based learning approach and its assessment. It was also apparent that the students become aware of their difficulties with the content much sooner with the problem format than they may do with the lectures, as they are made to clarify and apply their knowledge at every step.

Comments made by third year students indicate the particular advantages of the problem-based learning program were its promotion of integration between the theoretical and clinical subjects and the opportunity it provides to apply the clinical reasoning process to typical clinical problems. Typical students' comments were:

'The discussion allows the expression of various points of view and necessitates the clarification of different interpretations'
'The group discussion consolidates the knowledge gained in previous years, improving my ability to design and implement management plans'
'The group discussion allows the sharing of the different clinical experiences gained by each student'
'The discussion of problems with new and unexpected conditions allows me to feel able to cope better in clinical situations'.

Evaluation by the students also highlighted the importance of assessment and its effect on the style of learning. The advantage of adopting a clinical problem format for assessment was evident. The following are typical examples of third year students' comments:

'The assessment format allows me to assess my ability to treat a patient on an ongoing basis, and the booklet style (with the new information provided on each page) means I can start (thinking) again if I make a mistake rather than continue on the wrong track'
'The assessment format correlated with the subject style'.

Conclusion

As a staff member involved in both the lecture and problem-based programs I would add some comments to the student evaluation. I would suggest that more staff time is required initially in the preparation of the problems, compared to the preparation of a lecture. This time is spent in designing problems, ensuring that all necessary content areas are covered by the selected problems, searching for appropriate references, setting learning goals, preparing handouts and organizing all supporting resources. In subsequent years the time spent is probably similar to that spent in repeat lecture preparation, by up-dating references, revising problems, familiarizing yourself with the reference material, and administering learning goal and reference handouts. Time spent with individual students will probably vary from year to year.

I would emphasize the constant need to encourage the students through the first stages, as they may take time to adjust to this method. Their greatest concern is related to their confidence, being unsure of the amount of detail and knowledge that is required of them. In the first year we conducted the problem-based learning program many hours of staff time were spent with individual students discussing their difficulties and reading and confirming their notes. However, this workload decreased in subsequent years as both the teachers' and students' confidence in the method developed.

This is a very powerful teaching/learning method. The teacher's role as a 'facilitator of learning' is very different from that involved in presenting a lecture of summarized information. It involves facilitating a discussion, initially to raise an awareness of the students' learning needs and subsequently to discuss material previously studied by the students, and aiding the students in the final steps of understanding and applying that knowledge to the clinical problem. This is both an effective and enjoyable method of learning and great satisfaction can be achieved through the deeper and more informed student discussion which occurs as the students' knowledge base increases. As they progress through the course students are more readily able to see the relevance of their learning and become highly motivated to learn. In summary, the use of problem-based learning allows the students to learn within the context of a clinical problem, to gain an organized body of knowledge and to practise consciously their clinical reasoning skills.

References

Barrows, H.S. (1985) *How to Design a Problem-Based Curriculum for the Pre-Clinical Years.* Springer Publishing Company, New York

Barrows, H.S. (1986) A taxonomy of problem-based learning methods. *Medical Education*, **20**, 481–486

Barrows, H.S. and Feltovich, P.J. (1987) The clinical reasoning process. *Medical Education*, **21**, 86–91

Barrows, H.S. and Tamblyn, R.M. (1979) *Problem-Based Learning in Health Sciences Education.* National Medical Audiovisual Centre, National Library of Medicine, Atlanta, GA

Cox, K. (1987) Knowledge which cannot be used is useless. *Medical Teacher*, **9**, 145–154

Feletti, G.I. and Engel, C.E. (1980) The modified essay question for testing problem-solving skills. *Medical Journal of Australia*, **1**, 79–80

Laidlaw, J.M. and Harden, R.M. (1990) What is . . . a study guide? *Medical Teacher*, **12**, 7–12

McKenzie, L. (1987) Problem-based learning in the final year of orthoptics. *HERDSA News*, **9**, 3–4

Newble, D.I., and Clarke, R.M. (1986) The approaches to learning of students in a traditional and in an innovative problem-based medical school. *Medical Education*, **20**, 267–273

Norman, G.R. (1988) Problem-solving skills, solving problems and problem-based learning. *Medical Education*, **22**, 279–286

24

Teaching clinical reasoning in nursing: an environmental perspective

Gail Hart

Nurses have a critical role within the health care sector. In acute care institutions they provide a 24 hour service to individuals with life-threatening illnesses. In long-term health care institutions and in the community they provide ongoing care and continuity for a wide range of clients. While many other health care professionals contribute to health care services in all settings, the clinical decision making skills of nurses provide baseline data that inform all members of the team (Field, 1987).

In order to ensure that nurses are well prepared for their central role in the delivery of health care services they must develop effective clinical reasoning skills. Such skills are best tried and tested in the real world experience of clinical practice. The clinical setting, however, is a complex learning environment that lacks the order and control of a classroom. Students are bombarded with unfamiliar stimuli, their role is unclear, their level of autonomy is uncertain and sometimes their very presence is unwelcome. Not surprisingly they experience anxiety and their confidence falls. They have difficulty identifying learning opportunities and applying problem solving skills they have developed in other areas of study.

The principles of adult learning offer direction to assist in the development of clinical reasoning skills. Nursing students and experienced nurses need assistance to appreciate the importance of clinical reasoning within practice. They need encouragement to be self suffi-cient and self directed within the clinical setting in order to identify learning opportunities and access resources. The key for educators is to create a supportive and collegial learning environment which fosters adult learning. This involves acknowledging and building upon the learners' clinical experiences and their strengths as adult learners. It also involves creating opportunities for learners to reflect on their learning, to share their experience with peers and to engage in critical discussions and debate on clinical reasoning in practice. The experience of clinical practice is rich with clinical problems and tasks which illustrate the need for, and provide opportunities to develop and evaluate skills in clinical reasoning. When opportunities for peer consultation are structured and well facilitated they provide a forum for helping students learn to articulate their clinical reasoning and integrate their knowledge with practice.

Despite the significance of clinical decision making skills in nursing, preparation for practice has only recently demonstrated an equal emphasis on theoretical and practical knowledge. Only since 1993 have registered nurses in Australia, for instance, required baccalaureate preparation for entry to the profession. Hospital training programs of the past concentrated on the 'knowing how' rather than the 'knowing why'. A stereotype of the nurse as efficient and busy, a doer rather than a thinker, has dominated both the popular and professional culture.

Learning by doing

Learning by doing is an important concept in a practical profession such as nursing. It suggests that the development of knowledge, understanding and skills is linked in a significant way with experience. Learning through experience is particularly important in the development of clinical reasoning expertise since such expertise requires not only the development of a sound knowledge base, but also the acquisition of cognitive skills.

The phrase 'learning by doing' has sometimes been used to suggest that the only way of learning the practice of nursing is by rehearsing skills within a clinical setting. When used to express this perspective, the phrase is more accurately described as 'learning by doing (knowing how)'. Here the practitioner has observed and repeated a skill or procedure until it can be performed efficiently and demonstrated to others. Hospital-based nurse education programs provided the opportunity for such practice but did not ensure an understanding of the underlying principles. The application of theory and the transfer of principles to practice require a further step and a new phrase 'learning by doing (understanding why)'. At this level the practitioner is also able to explain 'why', to suggest further general applications, and to outline how this specific skill or procedure relates to a wider body of knowledge. Such understanding necessitates a strong theoretical base for nursing practice.

Beyond understanding is an additional step in clinical reasoning: 'learning by doing (adapting)'. Some practitioners move beyond the practical application of theory to practice by reflecting on their own practice and by adapting their approach. In effect, their practice becomes reflection-in-action and theoretical knowledge is generated from the practical situation (Jarvis, 1987).

Benner (1984) has outlined the development from novice to expert nurse and has differentiated five levels in terms of the approach of nurses to clinical decision making. According to Benner both the novice and the competent nurse make judgements on the basis of a set of rules acquired in a context-free situation. Students, recent graduates and even experienced nurses entering a new area will painstakingly follow a skills-oriented procedure step-by-step without being sensitive to patient cues or

data that suggest the need for a modified or alternative intervention. In contrast, expert nurses working in a familiar environment intuitively assess the situation in a holistic way and only later reflect on the process to identify the principles underlying their decision. Field (1987) has observed, however, that many expert practitioners are unable to explain the basis for their action. They 'know how' but they lack the ability to provide a theoretical rationale for their decisions. They are unable to share the basis of their expertise with less experienced nurses and they are unable to contribute to the knowledge base underlying nursing practice.

This paradoxical situation creates a problem for the development of nursing knowledge and theory in order to support clinical practice and provide the foundation (knowledge base) for clinical reasoning. Most, if not all nursing theories are incomplete and lack adequate testing and refining (Hoon, 1986; Field, 1987). It is important that nurses working in the field are able to utilize, test and refine nursing theory in order to reason effectively, since reasoning involves the ability to translate theoretical knowledge into the 'know how' of clinical practice. If many of the most expert practitioners are unable to justify clinical decisions and interventions according to a conceptual model or theory it is unlikely that the chasm separating theory and practice will be easily bridged. It is equally unlikely that the clinical reasoning skills of students and recent graduates will be able to be effectively fostered and developed by experienced practitioners within the clinical setting.

Clinicians as preceptors

The concerns identified above have important implications for the effectiveness of preceptor programs. The term preceptor is used to describe 'a unit-based nurse who carries out one-to-one teaching of new employees or nursing students, in addition to his/her regular unit duties' (Shamian and Inhaber, 1985). Preceptors have been widely used to assist recent graduates to make the transition from university to the workplace and in the supervision of nursing students during clinical placements. Both of these situations are critical periods in the development of graduate and student nurses' confidence in applying their skills in critical thinking to the clinical problems they encounter in practice. They are unlikely to meet this challenge successfully without the support, encouragement and example from more experienced colleagues.

The role of preceptors is a challenging one, particularly since the widespread introduction of tertiary-educated nurses into the workforce which has created role ambiguity and role confusion, not only for recent graduates but also for those experienced nurses with the responsibility of guiding recent graduates' beginning practice. Preceptors have a critical role in modelling clinical reasoning within the workplace environment. Yet many nurses identified as preceptors are either unable or unwilling to demonstrate and encourage clinical reasoning. According to Greipp (1989) staff shortages have limited the number of people available to act as preceptors and some nurses become preceptors 'by default'. They are often not adequately prepared or rewarded for their role (Young et al, 1989). The questioning and reflective approach to practice encouraged at university is threatening to nurses who feel unable or unwilling to provide the rationale for their practice. Del Beuno (1987) cautions that power may be misused in a preceptorship relationship to conceal vital information. 'Some nurses assigned to orientate novices may not share their own experiences, rationalizing that "I had to do it the hard way, so why don't they?" ' (Del Beuno, 1987).

In a recent study Ives and Rowley (1990) surveyed 750 registered nurses about their attitudes to tertiary education and teaching. Respondents were positively inclined towards teaching university-based students and the majority felt adequately prepared for the role. However, many were unclear of what was expected of them. The researchers concluded that general information about curricula, details of students' level and experience, and clear objectives should be provided to staff before the students arrived on the ward. This briefing information should be followed up with regular informal discussions during the clinical placement and should be supplemented by relevant documentation. Staff need encouragement to share their clinical expertise with students. This is most effectively achieved when staff feel confident enough to articulate their clinical reasoning and question students in a way that indicates support, but also challenges the students to think critically about their experiences in the clinical setting.

If clinical nurses are to participate in helping nurse students learn and develop their clinical reasoning skills, then the preparation of facilitators and preceptors needs to be conducted effectively. The calibre of research on the use of mentors needs to be improved to identify the type of phenomenon that is helpful in promoting individual and professional growth (Hagerty, 1986). One answer to this question is provided by Hsieh and Knowles (1990) who reported that one of the important conditions for a successful preceptorship relationship in nursing was the availability of peer support groups for both preceptors and learners. Another solution is to improve preceptor's preparation in such areas as understanding how to maximize the use of the clinical learning environment and how to utilize adult learning theory. The sections below discuss these areas.

The clinical learning environment

The experiences nursing students gain in the clinical setting offer the best opportunity to integrate skills learned in practice and in the university laboratory with theory learned in the classroom. This is particularly the case with clinical reasoning which cannot be fully appreciated or experienced in the absence of the complexity, consequences and reality of the clinical setting. It is the responsibility of the clinical educator to enable such integration to occur.

Unlike teaching in the laboratory or classroom, however, clinical education takes place in a complex setting much of which is beyond the control of the teacher. An important factor in this situation is that clinical educators are responsible for the safety of clients. Educators also need to be flexible enough to identify learning opportunities within a rapidly changing environment and then match those opportunities to students with varying learning needs and abilities. They need good public relations skills to convince busy nursing staff to co-operate with teaching and to support students. This process has been described as 'facilitating the entry of aliens within a hostile environment' (Townsend, 1989, personal communication).

In recognition of the complexity, labour-intensiveness and importance of clinical education it is desirable for each clinical facilitator to supervise a limited number of students (e.g. up to eight). Clinical facilitators are usually selected for their excellent clinical skills. However, it is probable that few will have adequate teaching experience and that even fewer will be familiar with the course curriculum and philosophy when they commence. It is within this context of risk and uncertainty, and with clinicians who are learning through experience how to be teachers, that students are faced with the demanding task of expanding their knowledge base, of integrating their theoretical knowledge with clinical practice, and of developing their reasoning and decision making abilities.

Most research related to clinical education has focused on teacher behaviours from the perspective of students (O'Shea and Parsons, 1979; Knox and Morgan, 1985; Ripley, 1986; Windsor, 1987). Despite the research interest in identifying effective clinical teaching behaviours, Karuhije (1986) found that few clinical teachers were adequately prepared for their role. Wong and Wong (1987) drew attention to the lack of preparation available for most clinical instructors and the low prestige associated with clinical teaching in nursing. Thus, while the clinical setting offers an ideal opportunity to test and revise clinical reasoning skills, the clinical educators' role in fostering the development of clinical reasoning may well be limited by several factors. These include inadequate preparation and teaching ability of the educator, limited access of students to the clinical expertise of unit staff, and an organizational climate which limits opportunities for peer consultation and critical debate about reasoning and decisions in relation to patient care. Without such opportunities there is little challenge to unit staff or clinical educators to develop, articulate and revise their clinical reasoning skills. Students have little opportunity to observe and share reflection-in-action or the application of clinical reasoning skills to specific patient care situations.

This problem was investigated by Fretwell (1983) who conducted an action research project to help ward sisters and charge nurses develop their teaching role and create an effective ward learning environment. Peer groups were established to provide support for experienced staff who wished to develop their teaching skills and abilities. The participants identified behaviours which improved the environment. These included an integration of theory and clinical teaching, a wider involvement of personnel in the teaching role, an ability to support and advise learners, opportunities for bedside teaching and the assignment of an experienced nurse to act as a personal tutor or 'preceptor' to the student. The peer groups provided nursing staff with the opportunity to share experiences and make explicit the process of clinical reasoning.

A further study on factors which enhance the ward as a learning environment was conducted by Smith (1987) who examined the importance of ward management styles to the ward learning and caring environment. She concluded that 'a central feature of the creation of a positive learning and caring environment is the accessibility and approachability of trained staff to students and patients' (Smith, 1987, p. 413).

In her action research work on clinical education Shailer (1990) has described the process of developing a clinical learning environment audit. Her work is based on a review of the literature related to performance indicators and ward learning environments, an evaluation of previous learning audits and discussions with clinicians and educators. Although Shailer's work is inconclusive, it represents an important step in the identification of the features of a clinical environment which support learning for nursing students. Included in her broad criteria for effective learning environments are the following:

- clear policies and a system of accountability for patient care
- peer support
- planned ward orientation
- availability of resources relevant to the clinical area
- educational opportunities that encourage active participation
- organizational commitment to on-going professional development
- a performance appraisal system
- regular communication forums
- a system of formally evaluating the quality of nursing care.

Another study on learning environments was conducted by Hart (1992) who surveyed 516 registered nurses to determine what attributes characterized a positive clinical learning

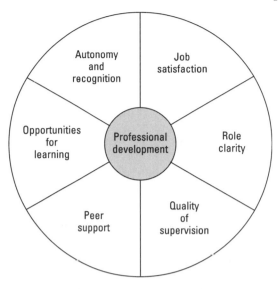

Figure 24.1 The clinical learning environment

environment. This research supported the significance of the social context of learning for nurses working in the clinical setting. Nurses perceived that they were developing professionally when the following six factors were evidenced within the workplace: autonomy and recognition, job satisfaction, role clarity, quality of supervision, peer support, opportunities for learning (Figure 24.1). Hart (1992) emphasized the value of a collaborative approach between administration and education for the development of effective strategies to:

- support professional autonomy by encouraging nurses to be responsible and accountable for their own practice and by valuing and acknowledging nursing expertise
- ensure that staff have the opportunity to negotiate and clarify their role and responsibilities at ward level
- improve the quality of supervision and foster a co-operative approach to performance appraisal which is directly linked to improving the quality of nursing practice
- support formal and informal opportunities for staff to develop a collegial work environment
- enhance learning opportunities within the workplace by utilizing experienced nurses more effectively as role models and preceptors and encouraging active participation within in-service sessions.

Another important aspect of the learning environment in relation to the promotion of clinical reasoning skills is the attitudes of nurses themselves and their colleagues to the nurses' clinical decision making role. The significance of clinical reasoning skills for good practice is only recognized if nursing expertise in clinical decision making is acknowledged and valued. Clinical reasoning skills are irrelevant in a workplace where nurses lack the autonomy to change practice. Similarly, reasoning skills are not challenged and further developed unless nurses are actively encouraged to share work experiences with peers and articulate the process of clinical reasoning. There must be an active commitment by practitioners and administrators to foster the development of nursing expertise. This is evidenced where nurses are expected to be accountable and responsible to their peers and clients for their practice. It is evidenced where scarce resources are allocated to support the development of clinical reasoning skills and the implementation of improved practices.

Adult learning theory

Educators need to be able to assess the clinical learning environment in order to identify appropriate opportunities for developing and evaluating students' clinical reasoning skills. As discussed above, a significant constraint to the facilitation of student learning is the lack of preparation for the clinical teaching role. This section examines key educational theory issues and practices which can be adapted to assist clinical nurse educators perform their teaching role effectively. The focus of this discussion is on adult learning theory since there is a fundamental link between the expectations of autonomous decision making and responsibility for one's actions which both adult learning and clinical reasoning place on the individual. In order to facilitate the development of clinical reasoning skills, educators are well advised to acknowledge and enhance students' strengths as adult learners and capitalize on the immediacy of practice as a powerful motivator for student learning and a trigger for clinical reasoning.

Until the late 1960s there was little systematic research in the field of adult learning. While research has expanded rapidly since the 1970s much of it has been practice-orientated rather than discipline-orientated and consequently the practice-orientated research has tended to be almost atheoretical (Rubensen, 1985). Jensen (1964) suggested that adult learning could develop a unique body of knowledge using two methods. Knowledge could either be generated from practice (grounded theory) or borrowed from relevant fields of study and synthesized to suit the special purposes of adult learning. This second approach has been adopted by Knowles (1990) to develop his andragogical model for adult learning. This model borrows from clinical psychology, developmental psychology, sociology, social psychology and philosophy.

Andragogy is in contrast to pedagogy which 'assigns to the teacher full responsibility for making all decisions about what will be learned, how it will be learned, when it will be learned and if it has been learned' (Knowles, 1990). The andragogical model makes the following assumptions.

Adults have a need to know

Adults are concerned about the benefits that will accrue from applying new knowledge. Friere (1970) developed an elaborate approach for the 'consciousness raising' of peasants in developing countries which he described in his *Pedagogy of the Oppressed*. He stressed the importance of helping learners to realize the 'need to know' in terms of improving their effectiveness and the quality of their lives.

The learner's self concept influences his or her approach to learning

Adults have a self concept as responsible decision makers and are capable of self-directed activity. Unfortunately many adults have been conditioned by earlier educational experiences to behave as passive recipients. There is a need to create learning opportunities that facilitate the students' transition from dependent learners to self-directed learners.

The learner's past experience plays a role in his or her learning

Adults bring a rich resource of life experience to any learning situation. Experiential techniques that tap this experience through group discus-

sion, simulation, problem solving, case methods and peer support techniques are most beneficial.

Adults have a readiness to learn

Adults demonstrate readiness to learn in response to developmental tasks. For example, new employees will usually demonstrate a readiness to learn those things that they need to know in order to cope effectively with their new responsibilities.

Adult learning is task-oriented or problem-centred

Adults are motivated to learn to the extent that they perceive it will help them deal with and resolve real life problems. Learning is most effective when new knowledge, skills and attitudes are presented in a context which closely approximates reality.

Internal motivation is a major factor in adult learning

The most powerful motivators for adults are internal pressures such as the desire for increased job satisfaction, self esteem and quality of life. Tough (1979) found that a motivation to grow and develop was intrinsic to adults but could be blocked by barriers such as a negative self-concept as a learner, inaccessibility of opportunities or resources, time constraints and programs that violate principles of adult learning. In other words, the motivation inherent in adult learners can be suppressed and thwarted by a working and learning environment which doesn't encourage individuals to be self-directed and autonomous practitioners.

Knowles (1990) outlines the contribution that the behaviourist, cognitive, personality and humanistic theorists have made in acknowledging the significance of the human and interpersonal climate of the learning environment. The behavioural psychologists stress the importance of recognizing and rewarding motivation to learn and apply new knowledge, skills and attitudes. Cognitive theorists emphasize clarity of roles, open communication and constructive feedback about performance. An environment that tolerates and even welcomes mistakes as evidence of risk taking and learning is also encouraged. Personality theorists stress the significance of a 'mentally healthful' climate that respects individual and cultural differences and moderates stress levels (Weatjen and Leeper, 1966). The humanistic psychologists suggest that collaboration rather than competition should be fostered in order to promote group loyalty, supportive peer interaction and a democratic approach to decision making. Management theory also lends support to an environmental perspective on learning and human resource development. The concept of organizational climate is central to Knowles' model of andragogy.

Adult learning theory has far-reaching implications for the working and learning environment of nurses. The design of learning programs and environments based on the above assumptions can facilitate learning. By promoting learner autonomy and self-reliance, a supportive environment can be created which can enable graduate and student nurses to develop their own knowledge and contribute to the development of the knowledge base of the nursing profession. In addition a supportive climate is desirable to allow learners to take the type of risks involved in practising their clinical reasoning using such activities as 'thinking aloud' about reasoning, exploring clinical reasoning with peers and testing their reasoning in new clinical situations.

Implementing a listening–dialogue–action sequence in clinical education

Paulo Friere (1970) argues that the social context of education is never neutral. Individuals carry with them a lifetime of experience which shapes their perspective and influences their interactions with others. Friere (1983) proposes a listening–dialogue–action sequence to encompass the principles of active learner participation and to acknowledge the social context of education. The first step is 'listening' to people's life experiences in order to assess needs. The second step is the development of a 'dialogue' to ensure a common interpretation of the issues raised and to promote critical thinking and problem posing. The third stage of 'action' emerges directly from the sequence of listening and dialogue. As individuals and groups test out their analyses within practice they set in place a recurring spiral of action–reflection–action. This framework of listening, dialogue and action will be used below to illustrate opportunities for developing clinical reasoning skills within the clinical setting.

Listening (reflection)

Clinical reasoning begins with the identification of a problem or issue encountered in practice. It requires a sensitivity evidenced by a willingness to listen or attend to one's own thoughts and feelings as well as those of others. Attending or listening provides a means of exploring experience in order to lead to new understanding and appreciation. This strong link between the learning experience and the reflective activity which follows is inherent in the concept of the reflective practitioner (Schon, 1983; Kemmis, 1985). The concept acknowledges the interdependence of theory and practice and highlights the potential contribution of practice to ongoing professional development, increased knowledge and skills and the development of theory.

In order to facilitate this link from practice to theory practitioners need opportunities to reflect on practice and develop an approach to practice that is actually reflection-in-action (Jarvis, 1987). One is often prompted to attend, listen or reflect when one experiences an uneasiness or inner discomfort about a situation or practice. Jarvis (1987) suggests that practitioners need assistance to crystallize ideas they generate in practice. Boud et al (1985) also support the value of creating time for reflection as a means of enhancing learning from experience. They advocate scheduling a debriefing period for a group or allocating specific time for maintaining a personal journal outlining experiences and reactions to them. Hart and Baume (1991) also describe the use of journal writing and peer consultation as reflective techniques to promote professional development within clinical settings. Powell (1989) notes that the development of reflective techniques does not replace formal programs of study but suggests that they could be used as a strategy to promote learning from experience throughout one's nursing career.

Reflective journal writing involves practitioners making a written account of critical incidents from their clinical experience. It allows the practitioner to reframe problems encountered in day-to-day practice and develop manageable solutions. In addition, they can learn to critique their reasoning strategies and knowledge base and, as a result, enhance their clinical reasoning ability. By documenting practice on a regular basis the complex and individualized nature of many health care situations is highlighted and nurses are less likely to develop the selective inattention that Schon (1983) describes as a response to engaging in repetitive and routine practice. They are more likely to be flexible and creative in their approach to problem solving. The unexpected changes that occur as a result of a more innovative approach to practice are welcomed by reflective practitioners as part of continuing inquiry or 'reflective conversation' (Schon, 1983). By sharing the 'reflective conversation' facilitated by journal writing, practitioners can engage in peer consultation and thus develop their expertise in clinical reasoning.

Dialogue (peer consultation)

Peer consultation is a process whereby a practitioner confers with a colleague or group of colleagues to seek resolution of a clinical or organizational issue. Within this process group members are valued as equals and peers, expertise and power is shared, active participation is encouraged and there is an atmosphere of openness and respect for differing values; group trust and co-operation is high. Numerous writers have advocated peer consultation and have highlighted the potential benefits as follows:

- establishment of a non-threatening learning community (Erickson, 1987)
- decreased work-related anxiety (Pasacreta and Jacobsen, 1989)
- self-discovery, insight and personal growth on the part of the participants (Fontes, 1987; Bilderback, 1989)
- increased acceptance, validation and support between group members (Fontes, 1987; Bilderback, 1989)
- recognition for, and promotion of professional expertise (Bilderback, 1989; Hart, 1990)
- enhanced self-esteem and increased confidence (Fontes, 1987; Hart, 1990)
- prompt evaluation of competency (Bilderback, 1989)
- improved communication and information sharing (Pasacreta and Jacobsen, 1989; Hart, 1990)

- a more professional and client-centred approach to care (Hart, 1990)
- improved staff morale (Pasacreta and Jacobsen, 1989)
- improved quality of care (Pasacreta and Jacobsen, 1989).

Peer consultation offers the opportunity for nurses to share their expertise in clinical reasoning. The group context is important because it provides the opportunity for nurses to pool their knowledge and skills to resolve a clinical problem. Shields et al (1985) advocate the use of peer consultation in a group context as a source of 'validation, counsel, and affiliation to clinicians during periods of risk-taking, conflict and role transition'. They suggest that as a model for professional development it exceeds traditional methods of education and clinical supervision. The main advantages are the active participation of the learner and the contribution of multiple viewpoints to a particular issue. The teacher acts as a facilitator or 'co-learner' rather than an instructor or supervisor.

Critical thinking and clinical reasoning within a group context can be encouraged by a facilitator using a five-step questioning strategy to shift the discussion from a personal description to critical analysis and action planning (Wallerstein and Bernstein, 1988). Group participants are invited to describe an incident from their clinical experience (step 1). Then all group members are involved in exploring the complexities of the problem (step 2) and sharing similar experiences (step 3). The group identifies psychosocial, biophysical, cultural, economic and political factors which contribute to the problem (step 4) and collectively develops a nursing care plan to address the problem (step 5). The goal of this process is to facilitate a shift in perception from powerlessness to empowerment. Through the group experience clinical reasoning skills are affirmed and necessary changes to the individual's knowledge base or reasoning process are identified and encouraged.

Action (collaboration)

The process of clinical reasoning is effective if it informs and improves clinical practice. To achieve this outcome it is essential to have administrative support of the decision making role of nurses and of the implementation of teaching/learning strategies to promote clinical reasoning. Support is particularly required in terms of staffing and the use of staff time. That is, both the development of clinical reasoning skills and implementation of clinical reasoning in nursing practice is resource-intensive in terms of staff time.

Teaching/learning strategies to promote clinical reasoning are many and varied. In this chapter the principal strategies advocated are reflection, peer consultation and thinking aloud. Urden (1989) asserts that professional knowledge is embedded in practice and recommends a range of strategies to support clinical knowledge development including joint rounds, clinical forums/discussions, peer review and specialty consultation. Each of these strategies incorporates the concepts of collaboration and peer consultation within a group context. Titchen (1987) outlines a problem-based approach to continuing education for physiotherapists which focuses on problems encountered in their daily work. This innovative approach is based on small group work, self-evaluation, self-initiated and self-directed learning, group learning and peer group teaching. It has been adopted and used successfully with registered nurses in New South Wales (Hart, 1990).

Hamilton (1984) used a similar approach with charge nurses in Melbourne, based on two assumptions adopted from Revans (1980) and Knowles (1980) respectively. These were that the people closest to problems are best suited to solving them and that adults learn best when their experience is utilized. The project involved a group of 11 charge nurses meeting regularly to identify problems encountered in their work and use the collective wisdom, experience and expertise of the group to resolve issues. This process of peer consultation and collaboration is one that the medical profession has used effectively to build and maintain an effective power base within the health care sector (Quinn and Smith, 1987).

Corcoran et al (1988) describe 'thinking aloud' as a strategy to encourage nurses to acknowledge and share their use of knowledge to make clinical decisions. They claim the potential benefits include:

- opportunities to extend, refine and verify knowledge and processes according to feedback from peers

- opportunities to share practical and rule-of-thumb knowledge and make explicit expert nurses' tricks of the trade
- increased self esteem by revealing a broad knowledge base, diverse cognitive processes and the complexity of decision making.

These authors suggest that peer dialogue is particularly useful for the continuing professional development of experienced nurses. They outline three aspects of implementing a thinking aloud strategy: (1) the selection of appropriate cases; (2) the use of coaching techniques to encourage nurses to articulate thought processes; and (3) the analysis of process to tease out the knowledge informing the clinical reasoning process. They suggest a model of diagnostic reasoning proposed by Elstein et al (1978) to structure the thinking aloud process and help analyse the data generated.

Harman et al (1989) describe a continuing education program to develop clinical decision making skills for experienced nursing staff. A one-day workshop plus a follow-up teaching session for small groups and individuals was introduced for 900 nurses representing 34 units at Toronto General Hospital. Nurses were encouraged to identify and use peer support to select appropriate nursing diagnoses and develop care plans. The authors suggested that the creation of an atmosphere which promoted the open discussion of common concerns and frustrations about nursing practice and clinical reasoning was important. Such forums encouraged nurses to question their longstanding beliefs and values about nursing. It was only then that they were able to proceed with learning and developing skills in clinical reasoning. The support, commitment and involvement of the work unit managers was considered critical to the success of the program. Regular meetings between the managers were organized to provide opportunities to discuss concerns regarding program implementation and receive peer support. In order to overcome initial resistance to the program a minimum of two months was needed to introduce clinical decision making and encourage behavioural change.

In a collaborative venture between a university school of nursing and a teaching hospital, Farrell and Bramadat (1990) developed two strategies to promote clinical reasoning skills.

The first, paradigm case analysis, allows students to 'share in the discussion of real life cases of experienced clinicians' (p. 154). This strategy provides an opportunity for dialogue, fosters openness to criticism and allows participants to trace the decision making process. Their second strategy, stimulated recall during action, was introduced in recognition of the limitation of retrospective case analysis and in an effort to stimulate reflection-in-action as opposed to reflection-on-action (as per Schon, 1987). Nurses were concurrently observed in practice and questioned about their process of clinical reasoning. Both strategies encouraged clinicians and students to verbalize and document their reasoning. They also provided support and recognition for nursing expertise and increased awareness of the complexity of nursing practice.

Maltby and Andrusyszyn (1990) discussed the value of a case-study approach to teaching decision making for post basic students. These students were divided into small groups to share their collective experience in order to address a broad range of case studies. Students commented favourably that the learning experience increased their awareness of their decision making and encouraged lateral thinking.

An educational game to enhance nurses' emergency decision making knowledge and skills was developed by Schmitz et al (1991) with attention to the principles of adult learning. It offered the advantage of acquiring and testing knowledge in a safe context rather than in the high risk environment of an accident and emergency unit. The game involved a team approach to encourage an exchange of ideas and insights and minimize errors by pooling expertise. The authors concluded that this learning experience helped 'foster co-operation, communication, cohesiveness and peer learning and support' and that 'the game in a novel, fun and challenging way helps build an underlying collegial frame work for nursing practice' (p. 156).

Ponte and Barrett (1992) introduced professional issues forums in order to support theory based practice amongst primary care nurses. The experience of discussing patient care within a theoretical framework helped practising nurses to reframe the unique aspects of each client, view the case within a social context and plan individualized interventions.

Conclusion

Any strategy to develop and enhance the clinical reasoning skills of students and recent graduates must be sensitive to the workplace culture and encompass both an educational and administrative focus. Many experienced and expert nurses need assistance to move from 'knowing how' to 'understanding why' and then developing the confidence to adapt their practice on the basis of reflection and peer consultation. Providing such opportunities within the workplace and ensuring a responsiveness to suggestions for improved practice demands both an administrative and educational commitment. Only when the workplace culture supports a commitment to professional development and quality will students be confident to use a process of continuous improvement that ensures that theoretical understanding is linked to and underpins clinical 'know how'. It is also such an environment that will encourage experienced nurses to contribute to the development of both the theory which underpins nursing practice and the process of clinical reasoning in nursing, by utilizing, testing and refining models and conceptual frameworks within their practice.

References

Benner, P. (1984) *From Novice to Expert: Excellence and Power in Clinical Nursing Practice.* Addison-Wesley, Menlo Park, California

Bilderback, B. (1989) Surviving the stages of peer consultation. *American Journal of Nursing*, **89**, 113–116

Boud, D., Keogh, R. and Walker, D. (1985) *Reflection: Turning Experience Into Learning.* Kogan Page, London

Corcoran, S., Narayan, S. and Moreland, H. (1988) 'Thinking aloud' as a strategy to improve clinical decision making. *Heart and Lung The Journal of Critical Care*, **17**, 463–468

del Bueno, D. (1987) How well do you use power? *American Journal of Nursing*, **87**, 1495–1498

Elstein, A.S., Shulman, L.S. and Sprafka, S.A. (1978) *Medical Problem Solving: An Analysis of Clinical Reasoning.* Harvard University Press, Cambridge, Massachusetts

Erickson, G.P. (1987) Peer evaluation as a teaching–learning strategy in baccalaureate education for community health nursing. *Journal of Nursing Education*, **26**, 204–206

Farrell, P. and Bramadat, I.J. (1990) Paradigm case analysis and stimulated recall: Strategies for developing clinical reasoning skills. *Clinical Nurse Specialist*, **4**, 153–157

Field, P.A. (1987) The impact of nursing theory on the clinical decision making process. *Journal of Advanced Nursing*, **12**, 563–571

Fontes, H.C. (1987) Small group work: A strategy to promote active learning. *Journal of Nursing Education*, **26**, 212–214

Fretwell, J.E. (1983) Creating a ward learning environment: the sister' s role. *Occasional Papers Nursing Times*, **79**, 37–39

Friere, P. (1970) *Pedagogy of the Oppressed.* Herder and Herder, New York

Friere, P. (1983) *Education for Critical Consciousness.* Continuum Press, New York

Greipp, M.E. (1989) Nursing preceptors – looking back looking ahead. *Journal of Nursing Staff Development*, **5**, 183–186

Hagerty, B. (1986) A second look at mentors. *Nursing Outlook*, **34**, 16–24

Hamilton, H. (1984) A resource unrecognized – creative management taps full potential of charge nurses. *Australian Journal of Advanced Nursing*, **1**, 6–10

Harman, L., Wabin, D., MacInnis, L., Baird, D., Mattiuzzi, D. and Savage, P. (1989) Developing clinical decision-making skills in staff nurses: An education program. *Journal of Continuing Education in Nursing*, **20**, 102–106

Hart, G. (1990) Peer consultation and review. *Australian Journal of Advanced Nursing*, **7**, 43

Hart, G. (1992) The clinical learning evironment: Nurses' perceptions of professional development in clinical settings. Unpublished PhD Thesis, University of New South Wales, Sydney

Hart, G. and Baume, P. (1991) Proletarianization of nursing research. In *Proceedings of International Nursing Research Conference*, Centre for Nursing Research, Adelaide

Hoon, E. (1986) Game playing: a way to look at nursing models. *Journal of Advanced Nursing*, **11**, 421–428

Hsieh, N.L. and Knowles, D.W. (1990) Instructor facilitation of the preceptorship relationship in nursing education. *Journal of Nursing Education*, **29**, 262–268

Ives, G. and Rowley, G. (1990) A clinical learning milieu: Nurse clinicians' attitudes to tertiary education and teaching. *Australian Journal of Advanced Nursing*, **7**, 29–35

Jarvis, P. (1987) Lifelong education and its relevance to nursing. *Nurse Education Today*, **7**, 49–55

Jensen, G.E (1964) How adult education borrows and reformulates knowledge of other disciplines. In *Adult Education: Outlines of an Emerging Field of University Study* (eds G.E. Jensen, A.A. Liveright and W. Hallenbeck). Adult Education Association of the United States, Washington, DC

Karuhije, H.E. (1986) Educational preparation for clinical teaching: perceptions of the nurse educator. *Journal of Nursing Education*, **25**, 137–144

Kemmis, S. (1985) Action research and the politics of reflection. In *Reflection: Turning Experience Into Learning* (eds D. Boud, R. Keogh and D. Walker). Kogan Page, London

Knowles, M.C. (1980) *The Modern Practice Of Adult Education: Andragogy Versus Pedagogy.* Cambridge Books, New York

Knowles, M.C. (1990) *The Adult Learner: A Neglected Species*, 4th edn. Gulf Publishing Co., London

Knox, J.E. and Morgan, J. (1985) Important clinical teacher behaviors as perceived by university nursing faculty, students and graduates. *Journal of Advanced Nursing*, **10**, 25–30

Maltby, H.J. and Andrusyszyn, M.A. (1990) The case study approach of teaching decision-making to post-diploma nurses. *Nurse Education Today*, **10**, 415–419

O'Shea, H.S. and Parsons, M.K. (1979) Clinical instruction: Effective and ineffective teacher behaviors. *Nursing Outlook*, **27**, 411–415

Pasacreta, J.V. and Jacobsen, P.B. (1989) Addressing the needs for staff support among nurses caring for the AIDS population. *Oncology Nursing Forum*, **16**, 659–663

Ponte, P.R. and Barrett, C. (1992) The professional issues forum for primary nurses: A method for professional development. *The Journal of Continuing Education in Nursing*, **23**, 34–37

Powell, J. (1989) The reflective practitioner in nursing. *Journal of Advanced Nursing*, **14**, 824–832

Quinn, C.A. and Smith, M.D. (1987) *The Professional Commitment: Issues and Ethics in Nursing.* W.B. Saunders Co., New York

Revans, R.E. (1980) *Action Learning: New Techniques for Management.* Blond & Briggs, London

Ripley, D.M. (1986) Invitational teaching behaviors in the associate degree clinical setting. *Journal of Nursing Education*, **25**, 240–246

Rubensen, K. (1985) Adult education research. In *The International Encyclopaedia of Education* (eds T. Heuson and N. Postlethwaite). Pergamon Press, New York, p. 170

Schmitz, B.D., MacLean, S.L., and Schidler, H.M. (1991) An emergency pursuit game: A method for teaching emergency decision making skills. *The Journal of Continuing Education in Nursing*, **22**, 152–158

Schon, D. (1987) *Educating The Reflective Practitioner: Toward a New Design for Teaching and Learning in the Professions.* Jossey-Bass, San Francisco

Schon, D. (1983) *The Reflective Practitioner.* Temple Smith, London

Shailer, B. (1990) Clinical learning environment audit. *Nurse Education Today*, **10**, 220–227

Shamian, J. and Inhaber, R. (1985) The concept and practice of preceptorship in contemporary nursing: a review of pertinent literature. *International Journal of Nursing Studies*, **22**, 79

Shields, J.D., Zagata, K.F. and Zander, K. (1985) *Peer Consultation in a Group Context*. Springer Publishing Co., New York

Smith, P. (1987) The relationship between quality of nursing care and the ward as a learning environment: developing a methodology. *Journal of Advanced Nursing*, **12**, 413–420

Titchen, A. (1987) Design and implementation of a problem based continuing education programme: a guide for clinical physiotherapists. *Physiotherapy*, **73**, 318–323

Tough, A. (1979) *The Adult's Learning Project*. Ontario Institute for Studies in Education, Toronto, Ontario

Townsend, S. (1989) Comment by a seconded clinical educator during clinical conference at Charles Sturt University, Mitchell, Bathurst, N.S.W.

Urden, L.D. (1989) Knowledge development in clinical practice. *The Journal of Continuing Education in Nursing*, **20**, 18–22

Wallerstein, N. and Berstein, E. (1988) Empowerment education: Friere's ideas adapted to health education. *Health Education Quarterly*, **15**, 379–394

Weatjen, W.B. and Leeper, R.R. (eds) (1966) *Learning and Mental Health in the School Association for Supervision and Curriculum Development*. National Education Association, Washington, DC

Windsor, A. (1987) Nursing students' perceptions of clinical experience. *Journal of Nursing Education*, **26**, 150–154

Wong, J. and Wong, S. (1987) Towards effective clinical teaching nursing. *Journal of Advanced Nursing*, **12**, 505–513

Young, S., Theriault, M.S. and Collins, D. (1989) The nurse preceptor: Preparation and needs. *Journal of Nursing Staff Development*, **5**, 127–131

25

Teaching clinical decision making

Bella J. May and Jancis K. Dennis

One of the major goals of the physical therapy educator is to help the learner develop the necessary skills to become an effective clinical decision maker. Considerable research in decision making is available to the educator. Much of the research and our own experiences have led to the development of a model of clinical decision making which has provided the background for the development of learning materials (May and Dennis, 1993). We have also used the case study approach quite extensively for classroom, clinical and continuing education learning experiences (May, 1992; Dennis, 1992). In this chapter, we share our experiences with a decision making approach to education.

Assumptions

There are a number of general assumptions which underlie our approach to education. The assumptions serve to focus our educational activities.

1. Students are assumed to be internally motivated, curious, and open to exploring clinical problems as a learning experience. Our focus is therefore on the development of higher order constructs, such as application of principles and multiple interpretations of information, instead of memorization and recollection of correct answers. Educational experiences should provide the opportunity for students to develop their awareness of the need to modify general management approaches for individual clients.

2. A model of decision making is not synonymous with a description of decision making in the real world. The model is useful in driving teacher behaviours when selecting learning experiences for students, in particular in the generation of case studies.

3. Decisions in physical therapy are seldom supported by outcome research and more than one management approach to a particular situation is often acceptable. When outcome data are not available, clinical decision making lends itself to exploration of the relationships between pathological processes and the problems as experienced by the client.

4. Decisions are constructed in the context of specific problems. Observation of clinicians supports the argument that specific schemata are constructed during the clinical evaluation process (Jensen et al, 1990, 1992, in physical therapy; Patel et al, 1986, in medicine). Experience allows the clinician to respond to salient information and change the course of inquiry as the clinical 'picture' evolves. Students often have more difficulty recognizing and interpreting the data to construct a cohesive view of the problem.

5. Decision rules are developed through experience and students do not have decision rules in place. Students may look to others for decision rules to manage large amounts of assessment data and to avoid the risk of making an incorrect decision.

6. Generation of multiple hypotheses is appropriate when exploring a case study. Although there is evidence that the generation of multiple hypotheses is not consistent with expert behaviour, students will develop multiple associations between pieces of information if they explore many possibilities as opposed to focusing on the single most appropriate problem definition or management approach.

7. Students will learn to be self-evaluative if they are given the opportunity to reflect on their clinical decision making behaviours.

A model of decision making

Decisions made by physical therapists can be characterized as falling along two continuums; from familiar to unfamiliar and from standardized to open. As Figure 25.1 indicates, decisions can fall in different areas of each continuum. A client who characterizes an easily recognizable clinical picture will prompt familiar decisions. The therapist has treated many individuals with similar problems and knows the most effective therapeutic approach. There are usually no questions about diagnoses or major problems. The decision is 'familiar' because it has been experienced many times before. By comparison, individuals who present with multiple problems or with conditions where the most desirable treatment may be contraindicated, exemplify unfamiliar decisions. Numerous factors may affect the decision making situation such as an unstable physiological state, limited economic resources and unavailability of equipment or personnel. For whatever reason, there is no readily available method of management and the situation requires adaptation of ideas and some creativity.

Similarly, the decision regarding treatment options may be fairly well defined either by established protocol or by the diagnosis. Such a decision can be considered as standardized. There is solid documentation regarding the effectiveness of the treatment options and the decision rules that accompany them are usually well documented and supported by research data. Alternatively, some decisions have little or no structure and can be considered as open

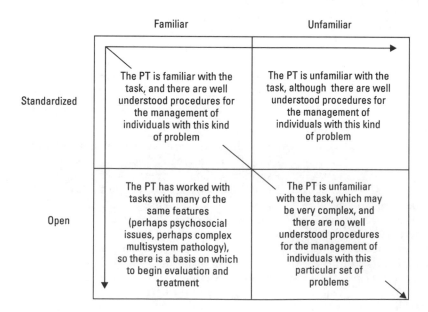

Figure 25.1 A continuum of decisions. Arrows denote increasing task complexity. From May and Dennis (1993) with permission

decisions. The therapist may not know the diagnosis, or one may not be established or there may be little or no supporting medical information. In such cases there are few guidelines for treatment either in practice or research.

With experience many decisions in physical therapy become closer to the familiar and standardized ends of the continua. Familiar and standardized decisions are made rather quickly and the experienced therapist may not be aware of the elements which go into the making of such decisions. Unfamiliar and open decisions, on the other hand, are made more slowly as all elements are carefully considered. Most therapists experience a variety of decisions in a usual work day or week. For students, most decisions are unfamiliar and open. Categorizing decisions is a useful means of communicating about a process which is generally internal and relatively subconscious. It is particularly helpful for the educator seeking to sequence learning experiences from simple to complex or from the familiar to the unfamiliar.

Definition of terms

The model presented in this chapter is designed as a tool for teachers rather than practitioners. It includes a task, something to be done, a decision maker and, eventually, a decision which, if implemented and evaluated, provides feedback to continue the process. There are three major sections called, for descriptive purposes, the task universe, the decision maker, and the task environment (see Figure 25.2). The terminology used in the model is designed to provide a frame of reference for the teacher and student in the design and use of learning experiences.

The task universe is all the potentially available information about the task and its context. It includes information about the client such as expectations, goals, physiological status, psycho-social orientation and lifestyle. The task universe also includes the environment in which the decision is to take place such as the hospital room or the rehabilitation setting, the time available for the treatment and so forth. Within the task universe are the expectations of others such as the supervisor or administrator. Factors in the task universe exist independently of the decision maker. All potential data, whether known to the decision maker or not, are part of the task universe. The concept of the task universe as discussed above clearly has implications in the structuring of learning experiences.

The decision maker brings a knowledge base, feelings about her or himself as a decision maker, a well established set of personal and professional values, a cultural background, a preferred style of thinking, and a variety of past experiences to the decision process. Students may be uncomfortable making

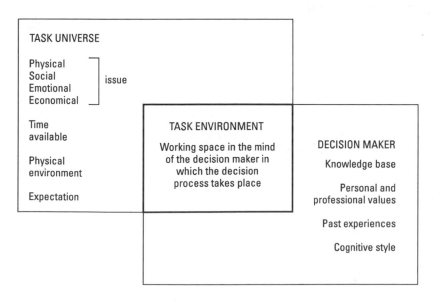

Figure 25.2 Definition of terms. From May and Dennis (1993) with permission

decisions even about paper and pencil case studies. Students may also have some beliefs about their role in making decisions. All of these feelings may affect their decision process.

The task environment exists in the mind of the decision maker. The focus of the decision process is this interaction between the task universe and the decision maker which we call the task environment. The decision maker places boundaries on situations, or frames the problem and the decision process takes place within the frame. The task environment, then, is the working space in the mind of the decision maker in which the decision process takes place. In the few minutes it takes to read a referral or look at a client waiting in the room, the experienced therapist begins the process of decision making. Almost automatically, the therapist looks for the critical cues. Something in the referral or in the way the client is standing or sitting evokes memories and patterns from the knowledge base and past experiences. Simultaneously, the therapist begins to create a mental image of the decision task and make some hypotheses about the major problems and possible interventions. Without the experience base, the student does not form this mental picture.

Critical cues can be defined as the keys in a set of data which serve to access the clinician's memory for specific diagnoses or problems. The critical cues are linked with data in memory and are used to frame the task environment. The decision process is affected by the way we frame a particular problem, the cues we attend to in the task universe, the particular relationships triggered in our memories. Critical cues vary with different task universes. For instance, the client in the outpatient centre presents somewhat differently than the client in the home. Helping students differentiate critical from non-critical cues and making the links between cues and data is an important aspect of teaching decision making.

The decision process

The decision making process is divided into five major activities which may appear to be linear and logical but which are actually ongoing and spiralling. Briefly, the therapist must first identify and clarify the client's major problems, decide what to do and do it, then determine if it worked. Figure 25.3 illustrates the activities described below.

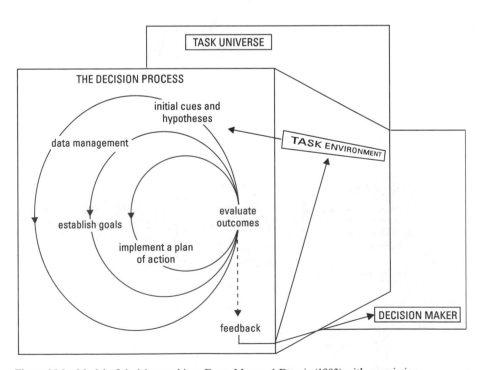

Figure 25.3   Model of decision making. From May and Dennis (1993) with permission

Initial cues, usually critical cues are key items which serve to access the clinician's memory for specific diagnoses, problems or actions. Pattern recognition is the phenomenon of making a judgement on the basis of a few critical pieces of information. The patterns have been laid down in memory through our past experiences and have been modified by increasing knowledge and experiences. In many instances the recognized patterns form hypotheses which help focus and guide further actions. Hypotheses are suppositions or assumptions about the client's diagnosis, major problems and possible management.

The data management process actually begins when the referral is read or the self-referred client begins to speak. Data management is a complex cognitive process in which data are perceived, attended to, structured and matched against other data stored in memory. Data management functions as a bridge between hypotheses and decisions regarding action. A wide variety of information gathering processes are used including routine history taking, formal assessment procedures, interviewing and observation. Data management is an ongoing activity which permeates all aspects of decision making as new data are received and processed.

At some point in the data management process there is enough information to conclude the investigations and establish goals. This is not a linear process (as some models suggest) since tentative goals and treatment decisions are considered from the initial contact and refined throughout the data management process. However, goals are finalized and treatment decisions are made after identification of the client's major problems, or confirmation of a diagnosis. In practice, the treatment plan is designed to meet the long and short term goals established in relationship to the client's defined problems.

The plan of action is implemented early. We usually start some treatment on the first visit based on initial hypotheses and early data gathering. The formal plan of action can be defined as an externally observable behaviour which evolves from a decision. It may be the decision to perform a particular evaluation procedure, to initiate treatment, or to refer the client to another therapist. Implementation requires further judgements as we interpret client feedback and revise actions accordingly.

Finally we evaluate the outcomes. Outcome evaluation provides feedback for further and more refined judgements and a continuation of the process. Clinical decision making is really a feedback loop system which requires ongoing determination of whether or not the outcomes are desired. Use of feedback has been shown to be problematic for some decision makers and will be explored further later in this chapter. The evaluation of outcomes has an effect on the decision maker's mind set or pattern for this type of problem which in turn will influence subsequent decisions about similar clinical situations.

There is much overlap and mental movement between the 'steps' outlined above depending on the clarity of the pattern. As stated before, in familiar situations and in many standardized situations, decisions are almost automatic and are based on existing decision rules. In unfamiliar and open decisions we may have no pattern or conflicting patterns.

Decision rules

How much of the reasoning process is actually involved in practice depends on the complexity of the situation. Many familiar and standardized decisions are actually made on the basis of decision rules (i.e. 'if–then' relationships between cue and inference or information and action). Such rules have been developed through past experiences and education and are modified by new knowledge and experiences. For instance, if a client has at least grade 3 quadriceps strength, then we know to progress to active exercises and to begin to introduce some resistance. If the strength is less than a 3, then we know to concentrate on quadriceps setting exercises.

Decision rules can be given, discovered or extrapolated. We give many decision rules to our students. Practitioners seek decision rules through continuing education courses, articles or books. One of our responsibilities is to help students learn when decision rules are appropriate and when they are not.

Elements which affect decision making

The decision making process is affected by many elements. Understanding the effect of the many factors influencing the process is helpful in designing learning experiences as well as helping students become skilled in self evaluation. The process takes place within the decision maker's mind and is subject to interpretation by the decision maker's past experiences, values and attitudes. Although usually not taught to students directly, faculty can seek opportunities to help students understand the effect of these elements. For example, if a student justifies a decision on the basis of 'the patient I saw in the clinic yesterday', the faculty can alert the student to the limitations of basing decisions on a small number of instances.

Cue perception

Each of us frames a situation differently. Our past experiences, attitudes or beliefs and the extent to which cues are linked in our memory can influence our perceptions and the cues to which we attend. Students working with actual or simulated clients in an orthopaedic course will focus on musculoskeletal cues and may overlook cues related to other problems. Differentiating between critical and non-critical cues is an important part of the learning experience which helps the student make necessary links to form useful clinical pictures.

Representativeness

Representativeness refers to making a decision on the basis of case similarity (Kahneman et al, 1982). This concept is especially useful for management decisions, but may also apply to diagnostic decisions or problem identification. Decisions are frequently made on the basis of class membership, e.g. 'the typical arthritic.'

Availability

Availability refers to the ease with which associations come to mind and are used by the decision maker as an estimate of frequency or probability (Kahneman et al, 1982). Availability is highly influential in an individual's perception of the world and is acquired by exposure to the task. Availability helps us handle routine decisions with minimal mental effort, particularly with classes of problems which occur frequently. The strong associative bonds between cues and memory help us easily recall what to do. A problem arises when the strength of these cue–memory associations prevents us from seeing other non-familiar components of the familiar problem. This can result in an inappropriate use of routine treatments and a lack of individual emphasis. We may even interpret a problem as familiar by selectively attending to the 'available' aspects and ignore the unfamiliar thereby possibly misdiagnosing the causal elements or mismanaging the problem.

Law of small numbers

Isolated and unusual incidents have a stronger influence on our thinking than is statistically appropriate (Kahneman et al, 1982). We remember unusual situations and outcomes more than routine events. When considering treatment options, outcomes experienced with two or three clients may lead us to expect all clients with similar problems to function in the same manner.

Protocols

The term 'protocol' is variously used in practice. Semantically, a protocol is a procedural document specifying the course of action to be followed under certain circumstances. Protocols are useful guides to efficiency in our evaluations and treatments. A protocol may guide us through a complex evaluation step by step or explain what to do if we find symptoms 'a', 'b', and 'c', but not 'd'. Protocols provide a structure for students. However, protocols can be limiting if used too rigidly, in that they can lead to a circumscribed data base and inappropriate general decisions, which are not designed for individual circumstances. The use of treatment protocols, particularly with students, can discourage the consideration of alternative approaches.

Order effects

A number of studies have documented the influence of information received first or last on the decision outcome (Hogarth, 1980). Initial information often makes a lasting impression as does the source of the information. Students need to understand this factor as they obtain information from a variety of sources, particularly when they start in the clinic. It is difficult to fully overcome the effects of the first impression. Subsequent thinking takes place from a particular starting point and is tempered accordingly.

Decision maker factors

The knowledge of the decision maker and how it is encoded in memory is of major importance in the attention to cues and in the development of initial hypotheses. Studies of experts and novices have suggested that the rich networks of relationships in the memory of the expert allows information to be structured and restructured, with many permutations and combinations of the same data to suggest several different hypotheses (Elstein et al, 1978; Hogarth, 1980; Gale and Marsden, 1980). Errors that stem from knowledge base deficiencies include failure to generate the right hypothesis because the cues available did not trigger the appropriate schema, or because the actual disease schema is not encoded in the memory. However, knowledge itself has no value unless it can be used. In guiding the student's acquisition of knowledge we need to help the student make the necessary linkages. The use of case studies and decision making processes can help the student in this process.

A person's ego, self concept, and emotional state all influence decision making. A student who is tense and frustrated may not structure the task environment as effectively as when feeling relaxed and integrated. Does the student value the decision making role? Similarly, a person's value system and socio-cultural background influences the structuring of the task environment.

Problem selection

Teaching clinical decision making requires the use of client problems in the learning experiences. Whether in the clinic or classroom, the type of client problem selected or designed is critical. There are a variety of methodologies which can be used to stimulate decision making activities. Discussing all possible teaching methodologies is beyond the scope of this chapter. Rather we will focus on the use of client-oriented problems in the classroom and the clinic.

Selecting the client situation

There are a number of guidelines which will help the faculty in client selection.

1. Select a prototypical problem

It is very important that the client problem be typical rather than atypical. As indicated above, working through the problem helps the learner make connections between data and cues. The problem helps the learner develop the clinical picture which enhances efficient decision making. Therefore, it is necessary for the problem to include the critical cues which are most frequently seen. There is a tendency, particularly in the clinical setting, to expose the student to the unusual client, the person presenting with a combination of symptoms or problems not usually seen. While interesting to the experienced clinician, the unusual client serves only to confuse the novice who has not yet developed a strong clinical knowledge base.

2. Set complexity according to student needs

It is never too early to involve students in clinical decision making. There is no magic knowledge level necessary to be able to begin the process. Rather, being involved in a decision making task may enhance the acquisition and retention of knowledge as students determine what they need to know to make decisions, then go and learn it. Problem situations in the early part of the educational program need to be structured relatively simply to allow the student to concentrate on the key elements. Complexity in a client situation is related to the number of unknowns and the extent to which the situation can be classified as unfamiliar or open. When developing a simulated problem, the faculty has the opportunity to make it as complex or simple as desired. An uncomplicated total hip replacement for an otherwise healthy individual, with single joint degenerative joint problem and with no complicating financial or family problems, allows the student to concentrate on the clinical picture, the medical and surgical management, and therapeutic interventions without becoming lost in a wide array of complications. On the other hand, a final year student close to graduation should be given the opportunity to make decisions in highly complex situations. Adding complications, such as cardiorespiratory disease, diabetes, living alone and limited financial resources can turn a simple musculoskeletal problem into a complex decision making task.

In the clinical setting client selection is more restricted, but even a complex client situation can be made simple for the student by focusing the student's decisions regarding evaluation and therapeutic management. Student supervision is another method which can be used to control complexity. In an early clinical situation, the student can be asked to develop an evaluation plan focusing just on the musculoskeletal problem, for example, then have the opportunity to discuss the plan and its rationale with a supervisor prior to implementation. The actual evaluation can be done under supervision. A student near graduation would be expected to perform a complete and accurate evaluation independently, which is a more complex decision making task.

3. Select client situations that allow the integration of previously learned concepts

Clinical decision making activities can be effective tools for the integration of concepts learned in previous or concurrent courses. For instance, a client for the study of pulmonary problems which follow a musculoskeletal course, can be recovering from total hip replacement and encounter a respiratory emergency. The same simulated client can be used in adjacent or subsequent courses. In the clinical setting, it is more difficult to find clients that exactly match student needs. It is important for the educational program to maintain very open communication to ensure that the clinical supervisor knows exactly what didactic courses the student has completed and what the expectations are for that clinical experience.

4. Use course objectives to guide problem development

Desired behaviours are commonly outlined in course objectives. Problem situations are then designed to elicit those behaviours. The faculty needs to decide clearly the focus of the case. Are the decisions related to assessment or to selecting treatment interventions? Is the purpose of the problem to help the student correlate various pathophysiology concepts? Is this a single

step case or a series that will guide the student through the total management of the client? It is important that the decision making skills are delineated in relation to the types of problems to be solved as clearly and specifically as possible.

Problem construction

There are many ways decision making tasks can be presented to students. Paper and pencil simulations, video tapes, computer programs, simulated clients, or actual clients are probably the most common. Since there are similarities in developing a case study or problem situation, non-computer methods are considered together and referred to as the case study. Computer problems are addressed separately. Although a case study can be totally a paper and pencil activity, integrating the use of slides, videos, simulations and role play will enhance the learning situation.

Identifying critical concepts

While the focus of the case is on the behaviours the student will exhibit, the concepts to be learned must also be identified. It is very important to differentiate between essential concepts and information which is nice to know but not necessary to achieving the objectives. It is difficult for many faculty to avoid trying to 'cover the material'. The case study approach guides the students to identify essential concepts which must be learned and helps them learn these concepts in a relevant environment. It does not, however, support the learning of large laundry lists of data. A well designed case study will elicit the major concepts considered important by the faculty and can be used to reinforce selected basic science concepts.

Developing case specifics

Once the objectives and major concepts have been specified, the dimensions of the case must be determined. Case studies may focus on one particular aspect of practice such as selecting an appropriate treatment option in the initial stages of postoperative care. They may also be sequenced to carry the student through a series of experiences, starting with assessment, then working through the interpretation of assessments to the implementation of treatment. Case information does not need to be limited only to the critical concepts. To the contrary, including some non-critical data will help the student learn to differentiate between critical and non-critical cues.

Keeping the decision making model in mind, the faculty defines the task universe in whatever degree of detail is deemed necessary to the attainment of the objectives. What information does the student need to be given and how will the student access the information? Such questions are best answered in relation to the purpose of the problem. If the focus is on developing assessment skills, for example, the initial information might be limited to that generally available on a referral or directly from the client on a self-referral. The student might then access the information by asking appropriate questions simulating an evaluation session. Such a format works well with computer problems, simulated clients and role playing but can also be done in a paper and pencil case study by having the student develop an evaluation plan before the evaluation results are provided. The rationale for including or not including each part of the assessment can be reviewed in a debriefing session thereby further reinforcing differences between critical and non-critical data.

Selecting stimulus questions

Stimulus questions are open ended and are answered by explanation, justification, and extrapolation. They guide learning in a desired direction. Questions such as 'What do you need to know about the surgical management of this problem to appropriately select assessment processes?' are designed to help students focus on important concepts rather than trying to 'learn it all'. 'What do you already know about this problem which you can apply to this situation?' helps the student relate information learned in another course or through past experiences to the current situation and reinforces such learning. It also provides the student with the opportunity to review past learning and expand partial concepts or discard outdated or inaccurate concepts. 'How will the symptoms affect current and future function?' helps students consider critical cues and guides them to a more holistic view of the problem. Too many questions can be overwhelming. A few key stimulus questions keeps the case study manageable.

Role of faculty

The faculty has three major roles in the case study process: designing the learning experience, implementing it, then evaluating the results. We have already discussed something of the designing activities. Case studies, computer simulations, and decision making activities of all types can be used in classroom, laboratory, or clinical activities. They can also be used with large groups, small groups, and as individual learning experiences. Case studies can be the major learning experiences in a course or unit with lectures used to provide key information when the students are ready for that information. The way the case study is used will have considerable influence on its ability to elicit the desired behaviours.

Providing feedback

Feedback is necessary for the student to become skilled in decision making. Feedback can be in terms of client outcomes, the process of therapeutic management and the process of decision making. Through feedback, the student can gain insight about her or his decision making style and can learn what decision maker factors influence the process. Through feedback and in the process of exploring the decision making activity, the student can learn more about how to structure the task environment.

Feedback activities may also include reflective sessions, journals and small group discussions (Jensen and Denton, 1991). The focus can be on the outcome of the client evaluation and management sessions or on the process of decision making. Students can be encouraged to review their personal cognitive style or preference and relate those characteristics to effectiveness in decision making.

Debriefing sessions

Debriefing a case study in a large group can be used to provide feedback. In a debriefing, it is important to create an open environment in which the student feels comfortable exploring what might be an erroneous concept. The environment needs to foster student independence of thinking rather than reinforce what the teacher thinks is the 'right' answer. Often there are no 'right' answers and exploration of alternatives becomes the key to learning.

Stimulus questions are an important tool for debriefing the learning experience. Student groups reporting on their assessment and treatment approach to the case study can be guided to compare and contrast their approach with that of other groups. The faculty can use such an opportunity to illustrate the 'art' of physical therapy. It is important to correct misconceptions which may occur in the debriefing process particularly if the class is large and several student groups are presenting. During the debriefing, faculty actively listen to ensure that desired linkages and associations are drawn.

It is helpful to summarize key concepts following a debriefing session. A summary can come from the class itself. It is useful to focus on linking key concepts or clarifying advantages and disadvantages of certain approaches, depending on the focus of the discussion. Care must be taken that the summary does not become a lecture on the 'right' answer, particularly if controversial topics have been discussed.

The case study in the laboratory

A case study is an excellent tool to focus lab activities. If there are separate guidelines for the patient and therapist role, each lab partner can be guided to play the part as accurately as possible. The case study can guide the student to practise different skills around the realistic framework of an actual patient problem. The student playing the patient learns many aspects of the patient's condition. There is also effective spontaneity in the patient–therapist interaction.

Computer programs

Computerized patient problems have been used to teach decision making. More sophisticated technology-based learning experiences are also available. For example, positive learning outcomes have been reported with the use of intelligent simulations requiring decision making (Breuer and Kummer, 1990) and case-based decision support systems (Kolodner and Simpson, 1988; Turner, 1989). Others recommend the use of hypertexts to develop flexible knowledge structures that are well suited to

making decisions about ill-structured problems (Nix and Spiro, 1990; Lyon et al, 1992). Patient problems encountered by a physiotherapist are typically ill-structured.

Computerized problems

Computerized problems have several advantages over the use of non-computerized case studies. Students can pace themselves and process as many case studies as are available. They can select the types of cases they feel the greatest need to practise and explore evaluation without fearing judgement. Students will not become experts without experience, and the opportunity to work on a large number of similar, but slightly different cases might help to expand the students' schemata and assist the learning of the process of patient assessment. Students generally report enjoying computerized patient problems (Harless et al, 1990; Xakellis and Gjerde, 1990; Kulik and Kulik, 1991).

There are many variations on the theme of patient management problems available on computer. We have developed a shell affording comprehensive evaluation of any patient presenting for physiotherapy evaluation (Dennis and David, 1992). The shell has advantages over programs designed around individual cases. The first advantage is efficiency since the teacher does not have to design the program, but merely enter coded responses into a text file that is accessed by the computer when the student selects that case. The second advantage is that the shell has been designed from a cluster analysis of physical therapists' classification of a large number of evaluation procedures and their report of the frequency of use of these procedures. These data contributed to a menu design that can be assumed to reflect the way practising therapists cognitively group evaluative procedures. It is expected that returning again and again to the same environment will predispose students to learning the components of the evaluation process.

Developing computerized problems

1. The learner

Results of studies on the links between individual learning and cognitive styles and success in computerized learning environments are inconclusive (for further discussion see Pocius, 1991). Students who are unused to computers for learning need to be well prepared for the computer environment and early exposure should not be assessed summatively. It is wise to beta test and evaluate carefully the form of feedback given within a stand-alone program since feedback that is given in an environment without non-verbal language is easily misinterpreted.

2. *Human factors engineering*

Interaction between the individual learner and the computer system should be designed to minimize the effects of individual differences and maximize enjoyment. The more 'invisible' the technology the better the learner can focus on the task. This may be achieved through attention to screen design, methods of interaction, use of colour and typeface. Optional methods of interaction, for example choices between 'click on' versus command keys, touch screen technology and voice activated systems allow for individual preferences among users. The more comfortable students are with the computer interface, the freer they are to become excited and involved in the problem without experiencing frustration with the technology. Physical therapy educators are advised to seek the assistance of an instructional technologist when designing computerized problems. Technology has a life cycle that involves design, prototyping, ongoing testing, modification, and the evaluation of learning outcomes with reference to the project's objectives.

Using computer programs

Computer programs can be used in a number of ways. Individual students can access the simulator for personal study. Small groups of students (4–6) may work together on a problem, thus benefiting from group discussion and the sharing of ideas. The teacher might use a single case in the classroom to demonstrate specific points about evaluation. The teacher might require students to do one or more case studies in their own time and bring them to class for discussion.

It is important to recognize that providing students with control over their own learning in a technology-based environment does not replace the teacher. Instead, the role of the teacher might change to include more facilitation of reflection and less didactic input.

Providing feedback

Some authoring systems allow tracking of the decision path. Individuals can compare their decision paths with those of other students and with decision paths of content experts. Reflection on the path taken and the implications of different paths may heighten students' awareness of their decision processes. Frequent rehearsal of client evaluations for different problems may help students identify context issues that influence their inquiry processes.

Outcomes of decision making can be compared among classmates or with the decisions of one or more content expert's decisions. Reflection on the connections between the most critical pieces of information accessed and the decision outcomes can help students develop an appreciation of the value of different pieces of information. Specific areas that students do not follow up and areas of redundancy become obvious.

Educator concerns

We have many questions that we are planning to evaluate as we continue to work in this area. Some of these questions and concerns are discussed below.

1. What is the effect of the task structure on learning? We are concerned about the influence of the structure of the hierarchical menus of the evaluation simulator on clinical decision making processes. As yet little is known about the way clinicians store clinical information in memory. At the same time we assume that students will learn process skills as they work through the content of different tasks. Identification of how information and procedures are stored could be helpful in developing better structured learning tasks.

2. What is the role of observation and palpation in clinical decision making? Is it legitimate to work on the cognitive dimensions of decision making without the opportunity to 'see' how the client looks or to 'feel' the part? How does practising the cognitive component of decision making, independent of direct client interaction, influence the

development of decision making skills? This raises the question of when and how knowledge develops into a schema. Is the list of suitable evaluations, instantiated at an appropriate time, a fledgling schema or a simple rule, i.e. if 'evaluation situation', then recall 'list of procedures'? And, does the 'list of procedures' need to be in place for the schema to develop? There are no definitive answers. The basic questions remain: Will students learn a generic schema for evaluation from the structure of the menus of the simulator? Will students learn more context specific schemata if they explore items within one submenu, given that these items are strongly associated in the minds of practising clinicians?

The juxtaposition of related items together in a menu system has been the subject of criticism as it cues students about what to select and does not require them to process information. It has been of great concern in the field of medical education where computerized patient management problems have been used as evaluation tools (for discussion see Swanson, 1992). In the past, strong cueing effects were blamed for the discrepancies between performance on patient management problems and real world problem solving in different fields. This is certainly a problem for outcome measurement, but for learning purposes cueing might be an advantage rather than a hindrance (Lyon et al, 1992). An unpublished study of physical therapy students showed that those who practised evaluations on computer simulation felt more confident than those who practised in labs on one another, but there was no objective difference in their performances (Bork, 1992, personal communication).

Conclusion

The process of teaching decision making is challenging but rewarding. Students initially may be resistant to trying to 'figure it out' for themselves rather than relying on the expertise of the faculty. Faculty may become frustrated trying to find the path which will guide the student to make necessary connections rather than just tell them 'the answer' . Students may look for formulas or protocols rather than respond to

each situation individually. Experience has taught us that real clinical problems can be the most effective way to engage students in the learning process. Facilitating learning rather than imparting knowledge is an exciting role for faculty. Newer technologies can expand that role to further creative dimensions.

References

Bork,C. (1992) Personal communication, June

Breuer, K. and Kummer, R. (1990) Cognitive effects from process learning with computer-based simulations. *Computers in Human Behavior*, **6**, 69–81

Dennis, J.K. (1992) Scheme and technologies: Designing computerised case studies. *Journal of Physical Therapy Education*, **6**, 64–65

Dennis, J.K. and David, C.L. (1992) *Physical Therapy Patient Simulator*. Medical College of Georgia, Center for the Study of Physical Therapy Education, Atlanta, GA

Elstein, A.S., Shulman, L.S. and Sprafka, S.A. (1978) *Medical Problem Solving: An Analysis of Clinical Reasoning*. Harvard University Press, Cambridge, Massachusetts

Gale J. and Marsden P. (1980) *Medical Diagnosis: From Student to Clinician*. Oxford University Press, Toronto, Ontario

Harless W.G., Duncan, R.C., Zier, M.A., Ayers, W.R., Berman, J.R. and Pohl, H.S. (1990) A field test of the TIME patient simulation model. *Academic Medicine*, **65**, 327–332

Hogarth R. (1980) *Judgement and Choice: The Psychology of Decisions*. John Wiley and Sons, New York

Jensen G.M. and Denton B. (1991) Teaching physical therapy students to reflect: A suggestion for clinical education. *Journal of Physical Therapy Education*, **5**, 33–38

Jensen G.M., Shepard K.F. and Hack L.M. (1990) The novice versus the experienced clinician: insights into the work of the physical therapist. *Physical Therapy*, **70**, 314–323

Jensen G.M., Shepard K.F., Gwyer, J. and Hack, L.M. (1992) Attribute dimensions that distinguish master and novice physical therapy clinicians in orthopedic settings. *Physical Therapy*, **72**, 711–722

Kahneman, D., Slovic, P. and Tversky, A. (1982) *Judgement Under Uncertainty: Heuristics and Biases*. Cambridge University Press, New Cambridge, CT

Kolodner, J.L. and Simpson, R.L. Jnr (1988) *The Mediator: A Case Study of a Case-based Problem Solver*. GIT-ICS-

88/11. School of Information and Computer Science, Georgia Institute of Technology, Atlanta, GA

Kulik C.C. and Kulik J.A. (1991) Effectiveness of computer based instruction: An updated analysis. *Computers in Human Behavior*, **7**, 75–94

Lyon, H.C., Healy, J.C., Bell, J.R. et al (1992) PlanAlyzer, an interactive computer-assisted program to teach clinical problem solving in diagnosing anemia and coronary artery disease. *Academic Medicine*, **67**, 821–828

May, B.J. (1992) Classroom strategies: The case study method. *Journal of Physical Therapy Education*, **6**, 61–62

May, B.J. and Dennis J.K. (1993) Clinical decision making. In *Home Health and Rehabilitation: Concepts of Care* (ed. B.J. May). F.A. Davis Co, Philadelphia, PA

Nix, D. and Spiro, R. (1990) *Cognition, Education, Multimedia*. Lawrence Erlbaum Associates, Hillsdale, NJ

Patel V.L., Groen G.J. and Frederiksen C.H. (1986) Differences between medical students and doctors in memory for clinical cases. *Medical Education*, **20**, 3–9

Pocius, K.E. (1991) Personality factors in human–computer interaction: A review of the literature. *Computers in Human Behavior*, **7**, 103–135

Swanson, D.B. (1992) Authentic assessment of clinical skills: A psychometric perspective. Paper presented at the Annual meeting of American Educational Research Association, San Francisco

Turner, R. (1989) *A Schema-Based Model of Adaptive Problem Solving*, GIT-ICS-89/42. School of Information and Computer Sciences, Georgia Institute of Technology, Altanta, GA

Xakellis, G.C. and Gjerde, C. (1990) Evaluation by second year medical students of their computer-aided instruction. *Academic Medicine*, **65**, 23–26

26

Facilitating the use and generation of knowledge in clinical reasoning

Angie Titchen and Joy Higgs

One important reason, perhaps, for our failure to realize how much knowing there is in caring is our habit sometimes of restricting knowledge arbitrarily to what can be verbalized. We do not consider implicit knowledge, knowing how, and direct knowledge as ways of knowing. Restricting the meaning of knowledge in this way is as arbitrary as assuming that only words can be communicated and restricting the meaning of communication to what can be put into words. (Mayeroff, 1971, p. 15)

Throughout this book the strong link between knowledge and clinical reasoning has been emphasized. In particular, Chapter 10 discusses the role of propositional, professional and personal knowledge in clinical reasoning. In this chapter, the focus is on fostering the development of students' and practitioners' knowledge bases and on increasing their awareness of how they use their knowledge in clinical reasoning. Educational strategies and milieux, underpinned by a theoretical framework of three themes of concern for curriculum planners, are suggested. The themes relate, firstly, to facilitating the construction and generation of knowledge, secondly, to studying conceptions of knowledge, and, thirdly, to the climate within the organization. The educational strategies described are observing, listening and questioning, story-telling, keeping reflective diaries, conceptual mapping, and studying and expressing knowledge through literary texts, visual art and drama. The strategies are founded upon a wide view of clinical reasoning in which all types of knowledge are valued and integrated.

The relationship of sources of knowledge is seen as interdependent, rather than hierarchical, and the whole person and the contexts of practice are also taken into account. The milieux include the classroom, but the focus is upon inservice education and clinical supervision programs which help practitioners to articulate the knowledge they use in their clinical reasoning. Ultimately, learners are likely to benefit from this emphasis because it will help educators to ground theory in practice and help practitioners to talk about their practice in richness and in detail. We begin with some background and an examination of the theoretical framework.

Background

The quest for professionalization has led to the development of health science curricula in which rational models of decision making and de-contextualized knowledge have been preferred. Education in clinical reasoning ignored the exigencies and constraints of the workplace (Benner, 1984), the person as a whole and the social, political, cultural and historical contexts of practice. A hierarchical relationship has also grown up between propositional knowledge and professional and personal knowledge. As health professions sought to establish their schools in higher education, propositional knowledge became the most valued type of knowledge, supplanting craft and artistry which were no longer considered to have a place in rigorous practice (Schon, 1983). Health science educators now recognize that other types of knowledge also play an important part in practice, and that inattention to them could have profound effects on the development of students' clinical reasoning skills. Alongside this recognition, the traditional notion that new knowledge is generated solely by researchers in academic institutions is being challenged and many now believe that practitioners have the potential to generate knowledge through their practice (see for example Schon, 1983; Eraut, 1985; Carr and Kemmis, 1986; Elliott 1991).

The theoretical framework

Given the above background, we have developed a theoretical framework along with educational strategies and milieux to address the challenges faced by educators and practitioners, as they strive to realize in their practice, these new values and ways of thinking. These educational strategies are based on a coherent, theoretical framework in which concepts are clarified and rigour demonstrated. The three themes within the framework were derived from the discussion in Chapter 10.

1. Facilitating the construction and generation of knowledge

This theme builds on three assertions: firstly, that learners construct knowledge from experience; secondly, that knowledge can be generated by practitioners, as well as by researchers; and, thirdly, that educational strategies designed to promote the construction and generation of all types of knowledge should offer experiences located in practice contexts and should attend to the whole person (in order to strengthen links between knowledge and the contextual factors influencing its interpretation and use).

The first assertion that learners construct their knowledge from experience has significant implications for curriculum planners. Opportunities need to be made available for learners to experience and construct their own realities through critical reflection upon, and theorization of, their practice. There are a variety of suitable approaches, for example, experiential learning, inquiry learning, problem solving, co-operative group learning and negotiating curricula with students. A deep approach to learning is also very desirable and can be promoted by helping students to search actively for meaning, for an understanding of what they are learning and for links within their knowledge bases. Discussion of ideas with others and individual reflection upon experiences enables students to own the knowledge acquired and to use it in their clinical reasoning in a way that is compatible with autonomous behaviour. Such learning becomes a personal process.

Reflection upon experience is a key element in helping learners to construct their own realities and, according to Engel (1991), for promoting a deep approach to learning. Reflection is a concept that describes the action of consciously reviewing experience, and is seen as a means of processing and making sense of learning experiences. This conscious review is thought to be necessary because learning experiences of themselves do not guarantee learning. Instead, it is the processing of experiences and the search for meaning within them which promotes learning. Boud (1988) suggests that reflection is a critical element of experience-based learning, both as a behaviour of learners which occurs throughout learning experiences and as a structured component of experiential learning programs (e.g. via debriefing sessions). Similarly, Schon (1987) asserts that there is a need to educate reflective practitioners whose actions and learning are influenced by their ability to reflect upon their thoughts and behaviour both during (i.e. 'reflection-in-action') and after the learning activity. In addition, the importance of preparing students well, before learning experiences, and recognizing and reflecting upon their existing knowledge and previous learning experiences is an important part of knowledge development (Boud and Walker, 1991).

Reflection is also a component of the complex concept of metacognition or 'thinking about thinking'. Metacognition is reflective self-awareness and thinking which is over and above normal conscious thinking (cognition). It refers to having knowledge of, and examining one's own cognitive processes and is concerned with control and the organization of the thinking process. It is, therefore, a vital element of clinical reasoning and is an important factor in the construction of knowledge (Higgs, 1992). Research into this area identifies the value of metacognition in helping learners to develop learning and problem solving skills (Biggs and

Telfer, 1987). Fostering the use of both cognitive and metacognitive skills will help learners to learn to conceptualize, test and construct their knowledge. In developing a greater awareness of their mental processes, for example, clinical reasoning, learners are better able to use them. By prompting learners to use, articulate, critique and review their cognitive skills, they are able to raise their awareness of their thinking and develop an enhanced capacity for responsible self-direction of learning. Through their awareness and management of the learning process, learners are better able to conceptualize, test and construct their knowledge. Both reflection and metacognition are means of reviewing knowledge and they underpin the educational strategies we describe later in which learners are helped to reflect critically upon their own and others' experiences and thinking.

We now examine the second assertion, namely, that practitioners outside the higher education system can generate knowledge from their practice. Whilst ways of generating propositional knowledge have been well advanced by academic communities, Eraut (1985) suggests there has been little attention paid to developing and enhancing the ways individuals and professional communities create professional and personal knowledge. We have attempted to redress this imbalance.

Taking the knowledge creation ability of the individual first, Higgs (1992) suggests that a practitioner can generate clinical knowledge, new to that practitioner, through a clinical experience. For example, when practitioners encounter a puzzle or find that what normally works is not working in this particular case, they stop and reflect in order to develop an idea of what might work. The idea is then tested, and if it succeeds, new knowledge is generated. Schon (1983) calls this process 'on-the-spot experimentation' and describes it as a form of 'reflection-in-action'. If we accept that Schon's empirical evidence is transferable to the health care professions, the implications are that knowledge creation skills could be enhanced by critical reflection and debate and that students should be taught by practitioners, as well as by academics, so that these skills can be demonstrated.

To enhance the knowledge creation ability of academic and professional communities, new kinds of partnerships and relationships with each other could be formed. Academics/educators, adequately prepared, could help practitioners to articulate their tacit knowledge and together there could be a systematic attempt to generalize the knowledge by looking for recurring patterns and themes, within and between cases (Titchen and McIntyre, 1993; Titchen and Binnie, in press). Thus, professional and personal knowledge would become propositional knowledge and others would be able to debate and test it. Such a partnership was developed by Titchen and Binnie (1993a; 1993b).

We turn now to the third assertion; that educational strategies, designed to promote the construction and generation of all types of knowledge and thinking used in clinical reasoning, should offer experiences located within the contexts of practice and should engage with the whole person.

Traditional educational strategies tend to decontextualize knowledge and to break the person into component parts. In addition, by tending to focus on linear, rational models of clinical reasoning, they have neglected holistic thinking and intuition (Rew and Barrow, 1987; Benner and Tanner, 1987). We argue that attention to contexts and the person will enhance the construction and generation of all types of knowledge and thinking, but that the construction of professional and personal knowledge and the development of holistic and intuitive thinking, will require a further step. Propositional knowledge and rational thinking can be acquired through such means as reading, literature review, case studies, essays, discussion, lectures and seminars, but the other types of knowledge and thinking cannot be easily acquired in these ways, either because they remain embedded in practitioners' accumulated experience or cannot be expressed in words.

So far, the interpretive research methodologies used by Benner (1984), MacLeod (1990), Mattingly (1991), Titchen and Binnie (1993a) and Brown and McIntyre (1993) suggest effective ways of facilitating experienced practitioners' communication of professional and personal knowledge. These researchers used phenomenological approaches to develop an understanding of the lived experience of practice and to see the situation through the eyes of the actors in the situation. The research methods included observing, listening and questioning, story-telling and keeping reflective diaries. We propose that building on these methods in the design of educational strategies will enable contextual and experiential integrity and wholeness to be retained. It will facilitate exploration of the meanings and significance which people attach to events and situations. Finally, it will foster the development of holistic and intuitive thinking because learners are able to watch, and/or listen to, an expert making clinical judgements (Benner and Tanner, 1987).

2. Studying conceptions of knowledge

The second theme in the theoretical framework is that studying conceptions of knowledge (or acquiring 'knowledge about knowledge') will lead to effective learning and clinical reasoning. Research is now showing that the relevance and depth of knowledge content, the structure of individuals' knowledge bases (Bordage and Lemieux, 1986; Grant and Marsden, 1987; Norman, 1988), and the learners' ability to organize knowledge in a meaningful way (Grant et al, 1988; Norman, 1988) are of major importance to clinical reasoning ability.

This evidence has influenced the design of our strategies. Firstly, the relevance of knowledge is made explicit, in the classroom or clinical setting, because the knowledge is described, reflected upon and analysed in relation to a specific experience or case. Secondly, different types of knowledge are valued and made explicit through analysis of the experience and the thinking. Thirdly, the structure of individuals' knowledge bases can be articulated through this analysis which will help learners to develop an understanding of the structure of knowledge of their field. Benner's (1984) domains of practical knowledge in nursing offer a framework for analysis, but as far as we are aware, domains of such knowledge have not yet been inductively derived in other health professions. They may, therefore, find Carper's (1978) empirical, personal, aesthetic and ethical ways of knowing helpful (see Boykin and Schoenhofer, 1991 for an example). This kind of analysis is very different from the way traditional case studies focus on the medical, psychological, sociological, and epidemiological features which makes articulation of the structure and essence of the particular discipline knowledge very difficult. Fourthly, the integration of the different types of knowledge used in a particular concrete case may lead to meaningful organization of knowledge. Fifthly, the depth and complexity of knowledge is demonstrated to learners, and sixthly, by understanding the content and structure of knowledge, learners can more easily judge its validity.

3. A climate of challenge, open-mindedness and critical debate

The third theme describes the climate in which the educational strategies need to be located, if they are to be successful. For instance, if educators and practitioners are genuinely to value the different types of knowledge used and generated in clinical reasoning, a climate of challenge, open-mindedness and critical debate is essential. Within this climate, there is a belief that different types of knowledge have equal status, are generated in different ways and will require a variety of ways of learning including reflection, conceptualization, theorization from practice, and experimentation. Learning experiences are facilitated within relationships which build on the humanness and wholeness of relationships and learners are helped to examine how their own beliefs, values, perceptions and interpretations influence their clinical reasoning. Self-evaluation and an understanding of the need to test and re-test knowledge and to justify knowledge claims are promoted.

It is likely that, in some schools and clinical settings, this kind of climate does not exist, due to previous socialization. Those who wish to examine the climate in their institution might start by asking themselves, 'What do we really believe?' 'What really matters?' 'What is the philosophy underpinning what we do?' 'Is there a "hidden" curriculum?' 'Are we giving out hidden messages?' 'Are there differences between my beliefs and values and those of the institution?'.

Having discussed the theoretical framework underpinning the educational strategies and milieux, we are now ready to explore these strategies in some detail.

Educational strategies

The educational strategies are derived, not only from empirical work, but also from our experiences of facilitating learning.

Observing, listening and questioning

The 'observing, listening and questioning' strategy is particularly useful for two purposes. Firstly, it can enable practitioners to deepen, refine and generate professional and personal knowledge through verbalization, interaction and communication with colleagues. Secondly, it makes their knowledge available for learners to reflect upon and to critically debate, with particular reference to its use in clinical reasoning.

In a study where teachers' professional craft knowledge was accessed effectively, Brown and McIntyre (1993) observed teachers going about their ordinary everyday activities in the classroom. After the observation, they asked the teachers to tell them about the aspects of their practice which they thought had gone particularly well. The researchers found that teachers who, through the research, had been thoroughly inducted into a recognition of the richness and nature of their professional craft knowledge were able to share it effectively with novice teachers (see also McAlpine et al, 1988). Titchen and Binnie's (1993a) work with nurses in an acute care setting supports this finding. To help practitioners make their knowledge accessible, we suggest that their professional and academic colleagues could use the guidelines in Table 26.1. These guidelines could also be used by experienced practitioners to facilitate students' or less experienced practitioners' learning from their own practice. Staff nurses in Titchen and Binnie's (1992) study found that being observed and questioned by an expert nurse enabled them to articulate and generate professional knowledge in a way that excited and empowered them.

The success of this educational strategy depends upon time being set aside for pre- and post-observation discussion and analysis of the knowledge revealed. Engaging in such activities is not part of the culture in most professional work contexts and Eraut (1985, p. 130) argues that 'knowledge development receives little attention in an action-oriented environment'. However, Titchen and Binnie (1993a) found that a strong commitment to facilitating learning and generating knowledge made it possible to find time within the working day in a busy, acute ward.

Table 26.1 Guidelines for helping experienced practitioners articulate their professional and personal knowledge

After observing the experienced practitioner in the clinical setting, an opportunity is sought to talk with the practitioner, as soon as possible after the observation and to:

- focus questions to the practitioner on the events just observed
- avoid framing questions in a generalized form
- concentrate on what had gone well during the observation period and avoid adverse criticism of the practitioner
- aim to probe and find out what the practitioner had done in achieving his or her success
- enquire about how the practitioner made his or her various judgements
- phrase questions in open rather than closed ways
- be supportive and willing to accept the practitioner's responses
- allow plenty of time for the practitioner to respond to questions

Adapted from McAlpine et al (1988)

Story-telling

Narrative approaches or story-telling in qualitative research (see for example, Benner, 1984; Sandelowski, 1991; Mattingly, 1991; Uden et al, 1992; Titchen and Binnie, 1992), and in education (Boykin and Schoenhofer, 1991; Smith, 1992) have re-opened perhaps the oldest way in which human beings make sense of themselves and their worlds. Stories concern action and are dynamic accounts of things changing as a result of people taking action. Although stories are unable to capture the whole of the lived experience of the situation, the story-teller conveys the essence of the experience, leaving out unnecessary detail (Boykin and Schoenhofer, 1991). The focal point of concern is the motives and intentions of the actors (Mattingly, 1991). Narrators recount and connect events in their lives, chronologically, thematically and teleologically, using a very different kind of thought to the logico-scientific mode of thought. Rather than attempting to reach empirically validated truth, narratives seek to give meaning to events. Lives in health, illness and transition can be revealed, understood and transformed through stories and story-telling (Sandelowski, 1991). Boykin and Schoenhofer (1991) also found that the value of story is the insights and deepened understanding practitioners can achieve into the meaning of their own practice. As well as helping us to understand past events, Mattingly (1991, p. 237) suggests that they also provide a 'forward glance, helping us to anticipate meaningful shapes for situations even before we enter them'.

Mattingly (1991), in her action research study of occupational therapists, found that what she called 'chart talk' (language used during presentations of case studies to colleagues), revealed their clinical reasoning as it relates to the physical body. This 'chart talk' was in marked contrast to the genre of the therapists' ordinary, everyday story-telling which conveyed their reasoning about how they were helping people to deal with disabled lives. Mattingly also facilitated reflective story-telling by videotaping the clinical work of individual therapists. She showed a video to a group of therapists and asked them to 'tell the story' of the clinical event recorded on the video. The invariably multiple interpretations of what had happened facilitated reflective thinking. The therapists reported that this experience was empowering and Mattingly suggests that this feeling of empowerment sprang from their stories being able to capture a level of complexity in their clinical work that biomedically-oriented accounts of practice could not capture. Mattingly's work suggests then that video can be useful in providing a shared experience for analysis where learners do not work with the same patients.

Benner (1984) facilitated story-telling by preparing guidelines for nurses to record critical incidents. For example, nurses were asked to describe an incident in which they felt that they had made a positive difference to a patient or where things went unusually well. Benner found, however, that using the term 'critical incident' resulted in the majority of stories being about critical care incidents, rather than everyday nursing. In contrast, Titchen and Binnie (1992) accessed nurses' stories about their day to day care of patients, by asking them to talk about the patients they were looking after, or had recently cared for.

Building on ideas and concepts emerging from Benner's (1984) work, clinical judgement seminars have been developed, as part of a career development program for nurses (Dolan, 1984). These seminars use a formalized story-telling approach. Practitioners with similar experiential backgrounds meet to describe a

case and to articulate their clinical judgements in relation to that case. Dolan found that the formal, often sterile language of case presentation was abandoned as the nurses began to use a more expressive style that included the context and a holistic grasp of the situation. Evaluations by the practitioners showed that the seminars enriched their nursing practice and sense of self as a nurse.

We propose that story-telling will facilitate the construction and creation of knowledge and the study of the conceptions of knowledge. It will also offer practitioners' clinical reasoning for exploration and critical debate. We conclude that story-telling can be facilitated both informally in the staff room and formally in the classroom and in inservice education programs. Spontaneous story-telling will become more reflective if colleagues and students ask 'why?' and seek and offer interpretations. Formally, it can be used in seminars, group work and clinical supervision, using the three processes of representing, interpreting and envisioning (Smith, 1992). Facilitators may ask learners to write or tell their stories, help them to analyse and interpret these stories and widen learners' horizons by offering alternatives, helping them to think ahead or think through the consequences of a clinical decision. Interpretation might include looking for differences, similarities and themes emerging from an analysis of all the stories told by group members.

Keeping reflective diaries

People often find it difficult to start writing or to sustain a reflective diary and educators may find that learners' diaries do not demonstrate critical thinking, analysis or evaluation of practice (see for example, Brown and Sorrell, 1993). However, given support and preparation, writing enables individuals to theorize their practice, to test their ideas, to explore, integrate and generate the different types of knowledge used in their clinical reasoning and to evaluate their clinical judgements in relation to the outcomes. Research has shown that reflective diaries can reveal the taken-for-granted, raising it to explicit, reflexive consciousness (for example, Ersser, 1991) and facilitate learning from practice (for example, Titchen and Binnie, 1993a; Johns and Butcher, 1993). In Titchen and Binnie's (1993a) study, staff nurses wrote about their experiences of looking after patients and they found that writing helped them to go further in their understanding of themselves, as people and as nurses, and to understand the thinking behind their decisions. Aesthetic or personal knowledge can also be expressed in a diary through poems, drawings or analogies. In addition, diaries can be used to help learners to reflect upon their observations and questioning of expert practitioners' clinical reasoning and upon others' stories of clinical experiences.

Holly's (1989) book *Writing to Grow: Keeping a Personal–Professional Journal* offers some exciting ways to help people get started and suggests ways that diaries can be structured. Johns' (1993a) model of structured reflection, empirically derived by reflecting upon his own supervision process, may also be helpful, and Brown and Sorrell (1993) suggest ways that students can be guided to analyse a particular event systematically. Some people may find sharing their diary entries with a peer or their clinical supervisor stimulates further reflection and broadens their horizons. It is our view, however, that people promoting the use of diaries should keep one themselves!

Conceptual mapping

Conceptual mapping provides another way of processing clinical reasoning experiences and prior knowledge, and subjecting these to conscious appraisal. A concept (or cognitive) map is an external representation of internal ideas. The term commonly refers to a visual representation of one or more areas of an individual's unique knowledge base. Cognitive maps can be formulated in many ways such as flow charts, annotated diagrams, images or maps illustrating interconnected ideas (Novak and Gowin, 1984). They represent the way individuals conceptualize and organize their knowledge about their environment, their discipline and their experiences and offer an opportunity for learners to think about their thinking (metacognition) and to analyse their clinical reasoning.

Involvement of learners in conceptual mapping enables them to analyse, explore and discuss their own concepts and the way their concepts are linked and their knowledge is organized (Gowin, 1981). Learners can assess and revise their knowledge bases in terms of accuracy, comprehensiveness and organization and

learn how to organize and access their knowledge more effectively. Cognitive maps enable others to appreciate and evaluate what the learner knows, how the student has organized his/her knowledge and to provide feedback to the learner.

Deshler (1990) discusses the role of concept maps in helping students to appraise their own knowledge, to evaluate and/or validate their concept maps through critical self-reflection and/or discussion with others, and to reconstruct this knowledge. In addition, these maps can be used as a device for communication and evaluation of knowledge, which Deshler relates to Habermas' (1984; 1987) idea of explicative discourse, using language and explanations to attempt to clarify the validity of knowledge claims and to question and reconstruct the language used to communicate this knowledge.

Conceptual mapping could be used to analyse stories and articulations of practice, both the learners' and others', individually or in groups where they can compare their knowledge with others (Higgs, 1992). In our experience, students' initial attempts tend to emphasize propositional knowledge, possibly because of their socialization. The facilitator may, therefore, have to encourage the inclusion of other types of knowledge.

Studying and expressing knowledge through literary texts, visual art and drama

Literary texts, visual art and drama can be used to help learners to explore, experience and express aesthetic, personal and ethical knowledge and the place of this knowledge in clinical reasoning.

It is likely that each health profession has rich sources of insights hidden away in reflective accounts in the form of stories, poems, diaries and anecdotes. These accounts could offer material for analysis and interpretation. For example, there are increasing numbers of published narratives (e.g. Benner, 1984; Dyck, 1989; Miller, 1992; Hedges, 1993) which focus attention on the characteristically human aspects of health care and which offer opportunities to explore our own practice, selves and relationships with others (Holmes, 1992) and to explore our clinical reasoning in relation to the person receiving our care. Robb and Murray (1992) and Thow and Murray (1991) explore the use of literary texts, films, plays, novels, short stories, newspaper articles, drawings, paintings and photography to help learners to engage with a variety of experiences, to analyse attitudes, values and ethics, to encourage reflection and to promote self awareness.

As well as analysing and reflecting upon other people's accounts, various media (for example, creative writing and documenting practice stories) can be used for the expression of learners' tacit knowledge. However, a reliance on verbal expression alone assumes that we believe that we can know and speak all that we are. Aldridge (1991, p. 149) in his discussion of aesthetic knowledge in medicine, suggests that knowledge generation can be achieved by encouraging people to 'develop an articulacy of self based on their own expressive realizations' through the use of sounds, pictures, image, gesture, visual arts and music.

An example of the use of drama to help nurses to learn about themselves is described by Pearson (1992). In his action research study, he used professional actors as lay teachers and gave them patient profiles, constructed from real patients, from which to develop their characters. The aim was to help the nurses to relate to their patients through empathizing with them. The 'play' was performed with nurses playing themselves and responding to the situation played out by the actors. After the role-play, the actors, in and then out of role, discussed their experiences with the nurses. Pearson reports that, in the group discussion which followed, deep and sensitive issues emerged and painful and personal stories were shared by the group. Evaluation of the experience was entirely positive and resulted in significant personal learning and change in behaviour.

On a visit to the School of Nursing at Deakin University, Victoria, one of us (A.T.) observed paintings and sculptures by students displayed along the corridors. Visual art, play writing, production and performance were used in this school to help students to express their knowledge of nursing.

We conclude that these approaches could be developed in the school setting and inservice education. Individuals could document (and perhaps publish) clinical practice stories, drawn from their diary entries, or produce pictures, videos or plays to generate or express their personal or aesthetic knowledge which they cannot describe in words. Through expressing the experience of, say, empathy, it may be possible for someone else to engage with or experience it too. For example, A.T. created a display of photographs of nurses with their patients to convey nurses' aesthetic and personal knowledge. Visual art forms could be used to illustrate stories, to stimulate others' storytelling (for example, 'what does this picture mean to you?') or be presented as assignments.

Having looked at the educational strategies in the light of the theoretical framework, we now put them in context by discussing the milieux in which they could be used.

Milieux

Although we limit our discussion to the milieux of inservice education programs in the clinical setting and clinical supervision, we emphasize that all the strategies, except 'observing, listening and questioning' (of real clinical interactions), can be used in the school setting. In this final section, we propose some principles for an inservice program which aims to bring a scholarly approach to practice. The program is designed to develop practitioners' expertise in articulating both their knowledge and their knowledge creation skills, so that they can become effective clinical supervisors for students and less experienced colleagues.

In the past, inservice education in the health professions has often been based on a 'deficit' approach which does not make it easy for practitioners to recognize their own skilfulness or to feel that they have valuable expertise to share with others. It is unusual for experienced practitioners to invite less experienced colleagues to observe and discuss their practice and their clinical reasoning. In addition, Benner (1984) observed that inservice programs for nurses commonly neglected the professional development of expert nurses, being more focused on teaching isolated skills and procedures. She proposes that nurses at proficient and expert levels will benefit from clinical case studies and participation in research programs investigating clinical problems. We support these initiatives and, in addition, propose that inservice programs could be built upon the principles of focusing on participants' strengths, and on collaborative learning and knowledge generation by academics/educators and practitioners.

A 'strengths' notion would centre around a commitment, firstly, to exploring what went well in the observation, story, or reflective account in the diary and so on, and, secondly, to understanding the events from the perspective of the actor in the situation. The notion springs from Brown and McIntyre's (1993) work. They found that a deliberate emphasis on collecting data on the positive aspects of practice was appreciated by teachers who were more used to the focus being on their weaknesses. This emphasis appeared to have a motivating effect and engendered confidence in the teachers to talk about and explain their actions in the classroom. A similar effect was found in a nursing study (Titchen and Binnie, 1993a).

This kind of program would enable academics/educators and practitioners to learn from each other, thus setting up a new kind of relationship between academic and professional communities, as described in Theme 1. The emphasis in the program would be on the two communities working *with* each other and recognizing each other's strengths, rather than the perhaps more traditional approach of academics setting up programs *for* practitioners. Practitioners are likely to benefit from the expert facilitation of educators, and educators from being able to access practitioners' expertise. Moreover, this kind of program would give students on clinical placements, the fruitful experience of watching experienced practitioners and educators learning from practice and analysing their knowledge generation and knowledge use in clinical reasoning.

Clinical supervision is well-established in health science curricula in both basic and post basic education. In nursing, clinical supervision is also being established as a means of staff development and two distinct, yet overlapping, models of supervision have been developed. Johns (1993a; 1993b; Johns and Butcher, 1993) has developed a formal model of supervision in which sessions take place outside the ward, whilst Titchen and Binnie (Titchen, 1993; Titchen and Binnie, 1992) have developed informal, opportunistic patterns of supervision which take place within the hurly-burly of the ward.

In Johns' approach, the supervisee keeps a diary, using a model for structured reflection (Johns, 1993a). During the supervision session, the supervisee shares diary entries of his or her own choosing with the supervisor. Titchen and Binnie (1992) developed three patterns of supervision. In the first pattern, the supervisor facilitates the supervisee's story-telling about patients he or she is looking after. In the second, the supervisor articulates her or his knowledge through story-telling or through post-observation discussion, and in the third, the supervisor and supervisee work together, so that each has the opportunity to observe, listen and question the other and to reflect upon their own, each other's and their joint experiences. In each model, the supervisor attends to the whole person, supports, questions, and challenges. Open questions are used to probe, for example, 'why?', 'what were you doing?', 'what were you thinking?, feeling?' The supervisor questions assumptions, provides vision, facilitates theorization of practice, offers appropriate knowledge of all types to match the supervisee's experiences and gives constructive feedback and criticism. Learners are also encouraged to question, criticize and doubt their own perceptions, look for personal meaning, interpret the data and examine their beliefs and values.

Critical friendships are another form of clinical supervision. They can be established between peers who negotiate the ground rules for such a friendship, for example, rules on confidentiality. Peers might agree to observe each other's practice, review assessments and professional records and give constructive criticism. They may decide to share reflective diary entries. But critical friendships will only be helpful if practitioners have learned the art of giving constructive criticism to peers and receiving it non-defensively from them. In A.T.'s experience with nurses, there is a danger that peers will be 'too nice' to each other unless an open climate has been established in the work setting, where honesty, challenge and debate are valued and criticism is seen as a learning opportunity, rather than as a reprimand.

Conclusion

The idea that we have developed in this chapter is that critical communities of practitioners and academics/educators should be formed in which students can access practitioners' knowledge structure, creation and use in clinical reasoning, and compare it with the theories, models and rules that they need as novices. The aim is that by giving students a sense of practitioners' knowledge and ways of thinking in relation to specific, concrete cases, these students will be better able to develop and organize their own knowledge bases. Within such a community, practitioners would be able to deepen, refine and generate knowledge by making it available for self-reflection and evaluation and for debate and critique by colleagues.

We have presented a theoretical framework to help educators and practitioners realize new values in their practice. Three themes of concern to curriculum planners were discussed, that is, facilitating the construction and generation of knowledge, studying conceptions of knowledge and creating a climate of challenge, open-mindedness and critical debate. Educational strategies and milieux were described and located in an experiential learning approach.

Putting these ideas and their underlying values into practice will involve a number of steps (not necessarily in chronological order). Firstly, the climate in schools and clinical settings will need to be examined and people's beliefs and values about the different types of knowledge, their use and generation should be made explicit. Dissonance between individuals' and the institution's beliefs and values will need to be addressed. Secondly, practitioners will need help from colleagues and educators to become clinical supervisors who can make their professional and personal knowledge accessible to learners, and who can facilitate learners' knowledge use and generation through reflection and metacognition. Thirdly, learning opportunities will be designed to retain experiential and contextual integrity and wholeness. Fourthly, practitioners and educators will be helped to develop their expertise and knowledge through collaborative inservice education programs, through clinical supervision by a more experienced clinician or through critical friendship with peers.

There are four conclusions to our discussion. Firstly, we suggest that our proposal will enable learners, practitioners and educators to work towards a self-critical process of professional development and self-discovery. Practice will be improved and knowledge will be constructed and created more effectively. Secondly, it will enlarge learners' views of their discipline knowledge content and structure and will foster the development of their knowledge bases and increased awareness of how they use their knowledge. Thirdly, our proposal is a response to the call for liberating educational strategies that are underpinned by connoisseurship, critical consciousness and scholarly collaboration (Bevis and Murray, 1990, cited in Smith, 1992). And finally, we argue that the enhancement of clinicians' knowledge base and their understanding of this knowledge will improve their clinical reasoning capacity and performance.

References

Aldridge, D. (1991) Aesthetics and the individual in the practice of medical research: discussion paper. *Journal of the Royal Society of Medicine*, **84**, 147–150

Benner, P. (1984) *From Novice to Expert: Excellence and Power in Clinical Nursing Practice*. Addison-Wesley Publishing Company, London

Benner, P. and Tanner, C. (1987) Clinical judgment: How expert nurses use intuition. *American Journal of Nursing*, **87**, 23–31

Bevis, E. and Murray, J. (1990) The essence of curriculum revolution: emancipatory teaching. *Journal of Nursing Education*, **29**, 326–331

Biggs, J.B. and Telfer, R. (1987) *The Process of Learning*, 2nd edn. Prentice Hall, Sydney

Bordage, G. and Lemieux, M. (1986) Some cognitive characteristics of medical students with and without diagnostic reasoning difficulties. *Proceedings of the 25th Annual Conference of Research in Medical Education of the American Association of Medical Colleges*. American Association of Medical Colleges, New Orleans, pp. 185–190

Boud, D. (1988) How to help students learn from experience. In *The Medical Teacher*, 2nd edn. (eds K. Cox and C. Ewan) Churchill Livingstone, Edinburgh, pp. 68-73

Boud, D. and Walker, D. (1991) In the midst of experience: developing a model to aid learners and facilitators. *A Quarterly Experience*, **27**, 5–9

Boykin, A. and Schoenhofer, S.O. (1991) Story as link between nursing practice, ontology, epistemology. *IMAGE: Journal of Nursing Scholarship*, **23**, 245–248

Brown, H.N. and Sorrell, J.M. (1993) Use of clinical journals to enhance critical thinking. *Nurse Educator*, **18**, 16–19

Brown, S. and McIntyre, D. (1993) *Making Sense of Teaching*. Open University Press, Milton Keynes

Carper, B.A. (1978) Fundamental patterns of knowing. *Advances in Nursing Science*, **1**, 13–23

Carr, W. and Kemmis, S. (1986) *Becoming Critical: Education, Knowledge and Action Research*. Falmer Press, London

Deshler D. (1990) Conceptual mapping: drawing charts of the mind. In *Fostering Critical Reflection in Adulthood* (eds J. Mezirow and Associates) Jossey-Bass, San Francisco, pp. 336–353

Dolan, K. (1984) Building bridges between education and practice. In *From Novice to Expert: Excellence and Power in Clinical Nursing Practice* (ed. P. Benner). Addison-Wesley Publishing Company, London, pp. 275–284

Dyck, B. (1989) The paper crane. *American Journal of Nursing*, 824–825

Elliott, J. (1991) *Action Research for Educational Change.* Open University Press, Milton Keynes

Engel, C.E. (1991) Not just a method but a way of learning. In *The Challenge of Problem-Based Learning* (eds D. Boud and G. Feletti). Kogan Page, London pp. 23–33

Eraut, M. (1985) Knowledge creation and knowledge use in professional contexts. *Studies in Higher Education*, **10**, 117–133

Ersser, S. (1991) A search for the therapeutic dimensions of nurse–patient interaction. In *Nursing as Therapy* (eds R. McMahon and A. Pearson). Chapman & Hall, London pp. 43–84

Gowin, D.B. (1981) *Educating.* Cornell University Press, New York

Grant, J. and Marsden, P. (1987) The structure of memorized knowledge in students and clinicians: an explanation for diagnostic expertise. *Medical Education*, **21**, 92–98

Grant, R., Jones, M. and Maitland, G.D. (1988) Clinical decision making in upper quadrant dysfunction. In *Physical Therapy of the Cervical and Thoracic Spine* (ed. R. Grant). Churchill Livingstone, New York, pp. 51–79

Habermas, J. (1984) *The Theory of Communicative Action,* Vol. I (T. McCarthy, trans.). Beacon Press, Boston

Habermas, J. (1987) *The Theory of Communicative Action,* Vol. 2 (T. McCarthy, trans.). Beacon Press, Boston

Hedges, J. (1993) Into new life: a reflective account. *Journal of Clinical Nursing*, **2**, 194–195

Higgs, J. (1992) Developing knowledge: a process of construction, mapping and review. *New Zealand Journal of Physiotherapy*, **20**, 23–30

Holly, M.L. (1989) *Writing to Grow: Keeping a Personal–Professional Journal.* Heinemann, Portsmouth, New Hampshire

Holmes C.A. (1992) The drama of nursing. *Journal of Advanced Nursing*, **17**, 941–950

Johns, C. (1993a) Professional supervision. *Journal of Nursing Management*, **1**, 9–18

Johns, C. (1993b) On becoming effective in taking ethical action. *Journal of Clinical Nursing*, **2**, 307–312

Johns, C. and Butcher, K. (1993) Learning through supervision: a case study of respite care. *Journal of Clinical Nursing*, **2**, 89–93

MacLeod, M. (1990) Experience in everyday nursing practice: A study of 'experienced' ward sisters. Doctoral Thesis, University of Edinburgh, Edinburgh

Mattingly, C. (1991) Narrative reflections on practical actions: two learning experiments in reflective storytelling. In *The Reflective Turn: Case Studies In and On Educational Practice* (ed. D. Schon). Teachers College Press, London, pp. 235–257

Mayeroff, M. (1971) *On Caring.* Harper & Row, London

McAlpine, A., Brown, S., McIntyre, D. and Haggar, H. (1988) *Student-Teachers Learning from Experienced Teachers.* The Scottish Council for Research in Education, Edinburgh

Miller, A. (1992) From theory to practice. *Journal of Clinical Nursing*, **1**, 295–296

Norman, G.R. (1988) Problem-solving skills, solving problems, and problem-based learning. *Medical Education*, **22**, 279–286

Novak, J.D., Gowin, D.B. (1984) *Learning How to Learn.* Cambridge University Press, Cambridge

Pearson, A. (1992) *Nursing at Burford: A Story of Change.* Scutari, Harrow

Rew, L. and Barrow, E.M. (1987) Intuition: a neglected hallmark of nursing knowledge. *Advances in Nursing Science*, **10**, 49–62

Robb, A.J.P. and Murray R. (1992) Medical humanities in nursing: thought provoking? *Journal of Advanced Nursing*, **17**, 1182–1187

Sandelowski, M. (1991) Telling stories: narrative approaches in qualitative research. *IMAGE: Journal of Nursing Scholarship*, **23**, 161–166

Schon, D.A. (1983) *The Reflective Practitioner: How Professionals Think in Action.* Temple Smith, London

Schon, D.A. (1987) *Educating the Reflective Practitioner.* Jossey-Bass Publishers, London

Smith, M.J. (1992) Enhancing esthetic knowledge: a teaching strategy. *Advances in Nursing Science*, **14**, 52–59

Thow, M. and Murray, R. (1991) Medical humanities in physiotherapy: education and practice. *Physiotherapy*, **77**, 733–736

Titchen, A. (1993) Engaging with the whole person as a person: Professional craft knowledge in patient-centred nursing. Paper presented at a seminar on 'Patient-Centred Health Care', Green College, Oxford

Titchen, A.C. and Binnie, A. J. (1992) Developing the art of clinical supervision. Paper presented at the Art & Science of Nursing Seminar Series. National Institute for Nursing, Oxford

Titchen, A. and Binnie, A. (1993a) A 'double-act': co-action researcher roles in an acute hospital setting. In *Changing Nursing Practice through Action Research* (ed. A. Titchen). National Institute for Nursing, Oxford, pp. 19–28

Titchen, A. and Binnie, A. (1993b) Research partnerships: collaborative action research in nursing. *Journal of Advanced Nursing*, **18**, 858–865

Titchen, A. and Binnie, A. (in press) Action research: A strategy for generating and testing theory. *International Journal of Nursing Studies*

Titchen, A. and McIntyre, D. (1993) A phenomenological

approach to qualitative data analysis in nursing research. In *Changing Nursing Practice through Action Research* (ed. A. Titchen). National Institute for Nursing, Oxford, pp. 29-48

Uden, G., Norberg, A., Lindseth, A. and Marhaug, V. (1992) Ethical reasoning in nurses' and physicians' stories about care episodes. *Journal of Advanced Nursing*, **17**, 1028–1034

Section Five

Directions for the future

27

Future directions

Mark Jones and Joy Higgs

In this chapter we aim to consider future directions for developments in clinical reasoning within the contexts of research, education and clinical practice. We have canvassed ideas from the authors contributing to this book to compile our suggestions for future directions.

Emergence of a shared field of study

From the literature referenced throughout this book it can be seen that clinical reasoning has only been researched and formally addressed in health sciences education for around 20 to 30 years, and for a much shorter time in some professions. Relative to other fields of research and learning the collective understanding of clinical reasoning is therefore only in its infancy. It is clear from the accounts provided in Section Two of this book, regarding the varying perspectives of clinical reasoning from medicine, nursing, physiotherapy, and occupational therapy, that each of these professions has undergone an evolution in their understanding and practice of clinical reasoning. Further, all professions represented in this book have described their conceptualizations of the nature of clinical reasoning as incomplete and still evolving. While this would be the case with any area of study, the understanding of clinical reasoning is perhaps slower than others because of the inherent difficulty associated with investigating a largely internal phenomenon which is influenced by a multitude of personal and contextual factors.

We suspect the advancement of our understanding of clinical reasoning and how best to facilitate it in our students, has also been hampered to some degree by the self-imposed isolation the different health professions too often exist within. While the medical perspective is perhaps most familiar to all the professions due to its early inroads into this area, there tends to be a limitation of exchange of other disciplines' literature between the various health professions.

The future development of the study of clinical reasoning we believe involves a growing sharing of ideas and understanding across the health professions and related disciplines. This book is unique in this respect since it aims to provide an impetus to promote this collaboration and does provide a wealth of experience, insights and research from across the disciplines. We hope that further developments in the field of clinical reasoning will be enhanced by the collaboration which has occurred during the writing of the book and from the transdisciplinary collaboration and communication which we hope will arise from it.

Research

Further research is clearly needed to clarify the nature of expertise in general and the nature, role and expert characteristics of clinical reasoning in particular. The different aims and responsibilities of the respective health professions require continued investigation within each discipline. Similarly, as clinicians' roles, clients' needs and worksite constraints also vary across practice and professional settings these too must be considered in future research.

Hypothetico-deductive reasoning and forward reasoning or pattern recognition represent the cognitive or reasoning strategies most commonly referenced to describe clinical reasoning in medicine. While these modes of reasoning are similarly acknowledged in the other health professions, a notable feature in recent theories of clinical reasoning espoused in the occupational therapy, nursing and (more recently) physiotherapy professions is the identification of additional dimensions to reasoning strategies. One example is the phenomenological mode of reasoning where the focus is on understanding the meaning that clients' problems hold for them personally. These professions see this non-diagnostic aspect of clinical reasoning as central to the understanding and management of clients' problems, in that this phenomenological perspective contributes to formulating the aims, perceptions, inquiry strategies and clinical decisions associated with managing the clients' problems.

Additional dimensions to reasoning strategies presented across the professions include cognitive processes and inquiry strategies such as intuition, interactive reasoning, conditional reasoning and ethical reasoning (Carper, 1978; Sarter, 1988; Fleming, 1991). Whether these dimensions truly represent different processes and strategies from hypothetico-deduction and pattern recognition or whether they simply reflect a different focus of attention within the clinical reasoning of different health professionals in line with their varying roles and responsibilities, could be debated. Nevertheless, these differing perspectives on the nature of clinical reasoning reflect the need for further and broader research in this area. Ryan (Chapter 20) for instance, has suggested the need for research regarding the applicability of weighting of different types of reasoning in different practice areas.

Further research is also needed to investigate relationships between contextual factors and modes of clinical reasoning. Contextual factors associated with clinical cases include: clinician characteristics (e.g. knowledge organization, cognitive or reasoning strategies, experience and expertise, values, attitudes, beliefs), setting variables (e.g. the clinician's work setting) and client characteristics (e.g. needs, illness experiences). Another priority area for research is investigation of modes and strategies of clinical reasoning in relation to client outcomes.

Of the clinician characteristics, differentiation of expertise is most frequently linked to knowledge depth and organization (see Chapter 2 by Boshuizen and Schmidt). As presented throughout this book, expert clinicians possess a superior organization of knowledge that includes specific patterns which can be explicitly and intuitively recognized and more general abstract sets of semantic relations which reflect clinically meaningful links between aspects of the problem. Patel and Kaufman (see Chapter 9) have provided significant insights into the role of biomedical knowledge in clinical decision making. Studies conducted at their centre have suggested that basic science does not contribute directly to clinical reasoning for experienced clinicians, although they do note that biomedical knowledge is used by clinicians confronted with difficult tasks or uncertain diagnoses. These researchers have also shown that expert clinicians utilize basic science knowledge to a lesser extent than medical researchers (Patel et al, 1989). The latter observation raises a series of very interesting questions. To what extent is the clinical reasoning of expert clinical practitioners optimal? Can clinical reasoning of experts as well as novices be enhanced through the development of understanding and skills of clinical reasoning? What can clinicians and educators learn from researchers and other scholars (e.g. psychologists, philosophers) about effective reasoning?

The issue of how and where various forms of knowledge (including biomedical, ethical, professional craft knowledge) are utilized is of obvious relevance for all the health professions. The discussions presented by Higgs and Titchen (in Chapter 10) and Patel and Kaufman (in Chapter 9) suggest that clinical and biomedical knowledge serve the situation-specific purpose of enabling the clinician to understand the clinical phenomena present, and that other types of knowledge including the personal knowledge of the clinician and the client are essential to gaining a deep understanding of the clinical problem within the context of the client's particular situation.

Further research is needed to clarify the contexts where different forms of knowledge facilitate clinical reasoning and the level and nature of knowledge which is needed. In such investigations researchers need to proceed beyond studies of novice/expert differences in relation to biomedical knowledge and beyond diagnostic reasoning. As highlighted throughout many chapters in this book, diagnosis represents only one focus of clinical reasoning, and in some professions or work settings within a profession, diagnostic reasoning is arguably less important than other types of reasoning or other reasoning priorities such as understanding the clinical problem from the client's perspective. This highlights the need for a broader range of outcome measures which include diagnostic accuracy and management effectiveness. In measuring management effectiveness consideration needs to be given to perspectives of clients, clinicians, professions, the public, and health care financiers.

While attempting to clarify the knowledge required for optimal clinical reasoning, further research is also needed to understand the growth of knowledge structures used in clinical reasoning. Boshuizen and Schmidt (see Chapter 2) have proposed a theory to account for the encapsulation of biomedical knowledge into clinical knowledge. While this may provide an account of how some biomedical knowledge comes to be integrated into clinically usable patterns, findings cited by Patel and Kaufman of the different role basic science knowledge plays in different clinical domains and the misconceptions and inaccuracies present in some physicians' biomedical explanations (Kaufman et al, 1992), highlight the need for further investigation of development of knowledge structures. This is needed for the development of all types of knowledge structures including propositional knowledge (e.g. biomedical knowledge), professional craft knowledge (e.g. clinical knowledge) and personal knowledge (e.g. individual frame of reference and knowledge of self).

Knowledge retained in either its original form or integrated into clinical knowledge will be influenced by the context in which it was initially acquired. This argument is used to support problem-based teaching strategies which appear to have an important place in future teaching to facilitate clinical reasoning. However, regardless of how it was learned,

knowledge which is not required or regularly activated in clinical decision making is likely to become more difficult to recall or even inaccessible. Perhaps the question to ask is not whether biomedical knowledge, or any other type of knowledge, is required for clinical decision making, but rather, what is the level of the various types of knowledge required in different practice settings. For example, it is not necessary for a physiotherapist treating a patient with 'musculoskeletal pain' to know the names and structure of the various neuromodulators that contribute to the expression of pain. But knowledge of the mechanisms by which pain is manifested is necessary as different pain mechanisms suggest different management alternatives and assist in recognition of patterns of prognosis. Various levels of professional craft knowledge and personal knowledge are also required in different circumstances. For instance, knowledge of how patients cope with dying, gained from experience of nursing a variety of such patients is invaluable in helping the nurse deal effectively and compassionately in these circumstances. In addition, greater clarification of the relative proportions and levels of knowledge required in different clinical contexts would assist our understanding of clinical reasoning.

Much emphasis in clinical reasoning is currently being placed on the interdependence of knowledge and reasoning. Similarly, there is a long history of research and scholarship into the areas of values, attitudes and beliefs. There is a very real need to examine the interrelationships between these two fields, to extend the studies of Carper (1978) and others into clinical reasoning which deals with ethical and human issues. In addition, it is necessary, in the search for scientific credibility and justification of our professional roles and decisions, to deal with the human side of clinical reasoning. Beyond the focus on finding the (scientifically) acceptable answer(s) clinical reasoning education and practice needs to prepare and enable clinicians to deal with the human dilemmas of decision making, including its controversies (e.g. euthanasia), its conflicts (e.g. clinician/ institution differences of values/judgements), its ambiguities and its differences in preferences and perspectives. Further research in this area is very necessary.

Errors in reasoning occur across all levels of expertise and in all aspects of clinical reasoning including clinicians' perceptions, interpretations, inquiries, planning, analysis and self appraisal. That is, errors can be cognitive, meta-cognitive, knowledge-related or the result of poor information gathering strategies and technique. 'Errors' may also be more subtle in the sense of decisions made by the clinician who fails to take into consideration the values of the client or the prevailing ethos or 'ground rules' of the institution and/or the particular health care team. Research to date that has de-emphasized the significance of process or reasoning strategies, has limited its outcome measures to diagnostic 'accuracy'. Further research is required to assess the type and frequency of errors that occur and their relationship to context variables (e.g. practice settings, and patient characteristics) and both diagnostic and non-diagnostic outcome measures. This information would allow specific errors to be targeted in educational efforts to facilitate effective clinical reasoning.

In addition to expanding the scope of factors/variables investigated, the methodology for future research in clinical reasoning must be considered. Patel and Arocha (see Chapter 3) have provided an excellent overview of the range of methods used to study clinical reasoning. They cite 'a multiplicity of methods ranging from the more traditional psychometric-based methods . . . to the newer developments such as the phenomenological approach . . . the interpretive approach . . . and research based on traditional experimental psychology . . . '. We support their view that this 'methodological pluralism' is healthy and that through this diversity of approaches, deeper understanding of the nature and development of clinical reasoning expertise should emerge. Clinical reasoning is becoming understood as being more than just diagnostic reasoning, and no single method of investigation is likely to be sufficient to depict and clarify its full dimension. Qualitative research methods can provide evidence and insight for the existence of the clinical reasoning phenomena investigated, and quantitative research methods can facilitate prediction and generalization.

Both artificially-designed research conditions and real life situations can contribute to our understanding of the numerous aspects of clinical reasoning. Patel and Arocha (Chapter 3) point out that the results of research in artificial environments should not be judged for their real life validity; rather it is the theoretical conclusions that are logically connected to those results which are being tested. Research in this fashion allows for an increase in the number of tightly controlled studies and exploratory/illuminatory investigations of theoretical constructs, and for subsequent exploration of these constructs within the complexities of the real life clinical setting. In contrast, the variance in clinician behaviour and cognition which is likely to exist when reasoning occurs in 'real life' situations, necessitates concurrent efforts to investigate the dimensions of clinical reasoning discussed in real life settings.

As an example, Doyle (Chapter 18) has called for longitudinal studies over 5–10 years to empirically describe and track the clinical reasoning of graduating students over a specified set of clinical problems. This could assist to clarify clinician, context and outcome relationships as they vary over time. Doyle also advocates further investigations of the contribution of clinician reasoning and clinician–client interaction towards client outcome, including both client and clinician outcome expectations. She also proposes research into client reasoning in relation to the client's perceptions of the presenting problem, its management, and outcomes. Such investigations could contribute significantly to examining the actual and potential role of clients in clinical decision making. In many contexts today there is a growing emphasis on 'customer-focused' health care. Doyle's proposals could contribute to the education and understanding of health care practitioners in relation to this practice.

Education

Educational research and development

It has been argued in this book that clinical reasoning can and should be taught. However, it is important for educators to clarify what it is that they are teaching and to critically examine the goals, process and outcomes of their teaching programs to provide support for their claims or aspirations for these programs.

A significant trend in clinical reasoning teaching and research relates to clinical reasoning 'process' skills. Norman and Schmidt (1992) note little support exists for the concept of general problem-solving or inquiry skills which can be taught, improved and generalized through education occurring out of context. They relate this largely to the lack of adequate measures of such skills and in part to the debate regarding the very existence of such skills. This perspective is understandable in light of findings such as the importance of 'content specificity' (Elstein et al, 1978) and the inability to differentiate levels of expertise using any of the clinical reasoning process measures investigated to date. For instance, hypothesis-related variables (e.g. number of hypotheses, time of hypothesis generation, number of questions related to hypotheses) and data gathering variables (e.g. thoroughness, efficiency, activeness, accuracy) do not correlate with level of expertise or quality measures of the final diagnosis and management plan in studies undertaken within the medical profession (Feltovich and Barrows, 1984). However, it is our hope that the broader perspectives of reasoning as portrayed through this book will broaden future research of clinical reasoning process skills. With the knowledge that the above measures have not yielded any differentiating results in the medical setting, analogous research should be extended across the other health professions and additional measures of process skills sought.

As Norman and Schmidt (1992) point out, it is too extreme to assume that no general characteristics of clinical reasoning exist. There are no doubt some discipline-specific and setting-specific strategies which can be generalizable for some context and problem categories. Such examples might include the various reasoning strategies discussed by Chapparo and Ranka (see Chapter 7) or other non-discipline-specific aspects of the clinical reasoning process such as metacognition.

Research and developments such as those described above in the area of clinical reasoning education should proceed alongside research into understanding and enhancing the practice of clinical reasoning. Both fields of investigation can serve to influence the future of clinical reasoning in action. In the educational area, it is desirable that ongoing research be conducted into the effectiveness of educational programs, learning approaches, methods and strategies used to teach/facilitate clinical reasoning. Evaluation serves several purposes including program improvement, program justification and comparison with other programs or methods maintaining similar objectives (Boud and Feletti, 1991). While program improvement and justification may be required by the broader educational institution, the search for optimal approaches to facilitate clinical reasoning should also include comparison across approaches.

We propose that principal targets of research into the teaching of clinical reasoning include a study of what is being taught about clinical reasoning, the outcomes of clinical reasoning learning programs in relation to teaching strategies, and research into ways of teaching clinical reasoning. Based on the discussions and models presented in this book we encourage educators to study through research and teaching practice, ways of teaching clinical reasoning in context, ways of enhancing the integration of knowledge and reasoning and the transfer of this integration from classroom to clinical practice, ways of promoting the development of metacognitive skills including an awareness of how the clinician reasons, ways of helping the student to learn how to learn (including the ability to acquire and generate knowledge and evaluate his/her own performance), ways of effectively evaluating reasoning performance, and ways of combining many of these factors into integrated programs which promote the development of clinical reasoning expertise.

The scope of research dealing with the outcomes of clinical reasoning teaching programs needs to take into account the intended learning goals of the program in question as well as related influences which may occur in both the educational milieu (e.g. student, faculty and institutional effects) and the health service delivery settings (e.g. expected client and service outcomes). That is, a broad range of dependent variables need to be included if any evaluation is to capture the full impact any learning program will have.

Educational practice

In terms of future trends in the teaching of clinical reasoning it is hoped that teaching practices will be informed by research conducted along the lines discussed above and by publications, such as this textbook, which present teaching strategies in operation and evaluate the effectiveness of these strategies. A number of trends in the teaching of clinical reasoning have emerged from the work presented in this book and personal communications provided by authors of the book. These include:

- designing programs which are relevant to local needs
- teaching clinical reasoning in the context of clinical problems
- utilizing experiential modes of teaching/learning
- increasing the focus of teaching in relation to understanding the reasoning process and the incorporation of higher level reasoning skills
- emphasizing the learner's role in knowledge generation
- reviewing curriculum content and adjusting curriculum priorities
- adapting teaching to changing clinical practice priorities and patterns
- teaching the teachers
- using new technologies
- improving assessment strategies.

Relevance of programs to local needs

From the numerous examples of approaches to teaching clinical reasoning which are provided throughout Section Four in this book it is evident that a major factor influencing the teacher's choice of teaching strategy is the need to make the learning program relevant to local needs. In particular, the choice of learning approach and setting appears to be strongly influenced by consideration of many factors including teacher preference/ability, norms and traditions of the institution, venue capacity and resources, and the capabilities, learning styles and personal objectives of students. These factors combined with a focus of reasoning which differs in accordance with the aims, roles, and practice philosophy of the respective professions has led to the implementation of a wide variety of approaches to teaching clinical reasoning.

Many of this book's contributing authors have emphasized the importance of learning clinical reasoning skills within the relevant disciplinary framework. It has been repeatedly argued that expertise in reasoning is associated with a rich discipline-specific knowledge base, that clinical reasoning occurs within and needs to be relevant to the framework of the reasoner's profession, that different modes of reasoning are more practised in different professional settings and that decision making needs to consider the actual context of clients and their management.

Teaching clinical reasoning in the context of clinical problems

There is strong support in this text and from its authors for teaching clinical reasoning in context. Boshuizen and Schmidt (personal communication) describe this as follows:

> In traditional curricula students . . . know which findings go with which disease, but have major difficulties in applying this knowledge in practice. This requires that knowledge acquisition takes place in a problem-solving setting. Learning with practical cases will help a great deal. Finally, practical experience has to be incorporated in a curriculum as early as possible. The role of practical experience will change during a curriculum. First it will serve the purpose of adding reality to book stuff and giving students the opportunity to practise uncomplicated skills, later on it will serve as a means to (re)organize the knowledge in such a way that it becomes easily accessible in practical situations and can become encapsulated.

For many authors and educators the concept of problem-based learning, where teaching/learning aims to integrate the learning of knowledge (propositional, professional craft and personal knowledge) as well as clinical reasoning skills, provides a valuable approach to teaching clinical reasoning. The term 'problem-based learning', in its broadest sense, can encompass many teaching/learning strategies including small group learning where students solve hypothetical or real pen-and-paper clinical problems, the use of simulated patients to enrich clinical cases which students are asked to manage, and a variety of classroom formats including role plays, panels (etc.) which centre around solving clinical problems.

Ongoing research and experience with many modes of problem-based learning (PBL) is desirable to test the claims of supporters of this teaching/learning approach that it is effective in achieving such goals as the development of clinical reasoning skills, enhanced acquisition, retention and use of knowledge, enhanced self-directed learning and motivation to learn, and the even wider goals of problem-based learning supported by Engel (1991, p. 25):

- adapting to and participating in change
- dealing with problems, making reasoned decisions in unfamiliar situations
- reasoning critically and creatively
- adopting a more universal or holistic approach
- practising empathy, appreciating the other person's point of view
- collaborating productively in groups or teams
- identifying own strengths and weaknesses and undertaking appropriate remediation, e.g. through continuing, self-directed learning.

While theoretical and research-based arguments to support the above claims of PBL are numerous throughout the literature (e.g. Barrows and Tamblyn, 1980; Willems, 1981; Schmidt, 1983; Schmidt and De Volder, 1984; Barrows, 1986; Boud, 1985; Walton and Matthews, 1989; Boud and Feletti, 1991), direct empirical evidence of superiority of PBL over conventional curricula is still incomplete. In review articles by Schmidt et al (1987) and Norman and Schmidt (1992), for instance, mixed results were presented in studies where various modes of problem-based learning (PBL) and traditional curricula were directly compared. Norman and Schmidt (1992) reported 'fairly conclusive' results from both experimental results and findings from PBL graduates that 'they find the learning environment more stimulating and humane than do graduates of conventional schools' and found that students in PBL curriculum acquired more self-directed learning skills which were sustained beyond the length of the curriculum. In relation to the development of clinical reasoning skills per se, Norman and Schmidt (1992) summarized their findings by stating that 'there were small or negative differences between the overall knowledge or competence of students trained by PBL and by conventional curricula. However, there are substantial differences, related to the retention of knowledge and learning skills, that may be attributable to PBL. There is also a strong theoretical basis for the idea that PBL students may be better able to transfer concepts to new problems, and there is some preliminary evidence to this effect'.

The issue of knowledge structure development is also dealt with in Patel and Kaufman's chapter (Chapter 9) with specific reference to biomedical knowledge. These authors acknowledge that problem-based learning successfully promotes integration of basic science knowledge into clinical structure, but also point out the problem of PBL students' inability to decontextualize this knowledge once it has been integrated. In brief, Patel and Kaufman caution regarding attempts for the basic sciences being totally taught in the context of clinical problems and suggest a compromise 'such that there is some core basic sciences taught at the beginning of the curriculum followed by an early introduction of clinical problems, where early basic science will produce some form of anchor and early clinical problems will provide the structural support'.

Experiential learning

A fundamental aspect of skill acquisition is experience. By participating in learning activities which incorporate experience of the process of clinical reasoning, and by learning how to appreciate these skills and become conscious of the utilization of reasoning skills, students in the health sciences gain first-hand knowledge of what clinical reasoning is and how to use it effectively. In Section Four numerous chapters present experiential learning as the focus of clinical reasoning learning programs. Experiential learning strategies represented include simulated patients, role plays, hypothetical panels and drama.

Understanding the process of clinical reasoning – using higher level cognitive skills

In Chapter 1 metacognition is presented as one of the three key elements of clinical reasoning. It is seen as the means of integrating knowledge and cognition. Without this higher level of attention being utilized to monitor and manage clinical reasoning, reasoning is less skilled, less responsive to the dynamics of clinical reasoning contexts and less capable of dealing effectively with the complexity of clinical problems. Throughout this text the importance of metacognition and strategies for the promotion of such higher level cognitive skills are presented, particularly in Chapters 1, 10, 19 and 26. Related topics such as the process of categorization (Chapter 11), decision analysis (Chapter

16) and the process of self-monitoring (Chapter 14), are also explored.

An important aspect of the use of higher level cognitive skills is the capacity of the clinician/student to detect and redress errors in reasoning. Not only is the overall effectiveness of clinical intervention influenced by the capacity of the clinician to avoid reasoning and decision making errors, the current health care environment is increasingly demanding a high level of performance characterized by cost-efficiency and accountability. To address this need educational programs need to teach students to understand, avoid, detect and redress reasoning errors. Helping students to develop metacognitive skills (as discussed above) is one method of achieving this outcome. Another is to improve learners' understanding of and capacity to employ the skills of decision analysis.

For example, Elstein (personal communication) notes that everyday clinical reasoning in medicine frequently departs from the principles embodied in decision theory. Clinicians order unnecessary tests, even when there is no economic incentive to do so, and sometimes withhold treatments that are beneficial for fear of potential losses (e.g. hormonal replacement therapy for menopausal women). That is, decisions are occasionally made by minimizing anticipated regret rather than by maximizing expected utility. To combat this situation Elstein (see Chapter 4) has called for a broader use of decision support statistical methods as instructional tools and for use in clinical practice. Chapter 16 by Watts provides an illustration of how decision analysis can be taught.

Knowledge generation

In Chapters 1, 2, 9 and 10 knowledge is presented as an essential element of effective clinical reasoning and the growth of knowledge is considered to be a key part of the development of clinical reasoning expertise. For the clinician therefore, the capacity to learn and to generate is very important.

In Chapter 10 knowledge is portrayed as a dynamic phenomenon undergoing constant change and testing through both personal and public validation. Both propositional (theoretical/scientific) and non-propositional knowledge are accorded validity, and knowledge is envisioned as a construction of the human mind. That is, individuals create unique constructions or interpretations of the world around them and of their own experiences, and knowledge is the product of a dynamic and indeed difficult process of knowing, or striving to understand. As a result, learners need to learn how to generate knowledge and to assimilate this through testing and experience, into their knowledge bases, in order to develop a rich knowledge base to underpin clinical reasoning.

Review of curriculum content

Increasing student numbers often combined with disproportionate resources (e.g. staffing/teacher time, student placements/patient availability, and general funding) and self-imposed as well as external demands for accountability and optimal effectiveness are ongoing forces which drive the search for improved approaches to facilitate student learning. With respect to clinical reasoning, our challenge is to develop and evaluate effective strategies to enhance students' reasoning and associated knowledge acquisition. It is no longer plausible to simply add more content or practice (e.g. in the form of extended learning apprenticeships) to our present curricula. Efforts need to be directed toward using the existing content-intensive period of education more effectively. In the process of re-examining the knowledge/content/subject matter necessary for respective professional responsibilities it would be desirable to address the question of the optimal use of limited time in the curriculum in relation to desired outcomes. For instance, greater priority could be given to enhancing knowledge structure development and accessibility, self-directed learning behaviours, reasoning strategies, educator preparation, teaching strategies, utilization of higher technology, and continued efforts at developing effective and user-friendly methods for assessing clinical reasoning.

Adapting teaching to changes in clinical practice

Current and future trends in health service delivery will also require ongoing changes to educational programs in order to ensure that all graduates are well prepared to be able to operate effectively and appropriately within changed circumstances (e.g. in a community-based, community-focused health care system).

Clinicians will also increasingly need to learn how to involve clients in the reasoning process. This learning can commence in undergraduate programs. In addition, postgraduate and continuing education programs can play a significant role in helping clinicians adapt to changes in the health care system and also changes in their individual roles. They may need to develop reasoning skills and strategies associated with practice management and planning roles, family counselling, the role of family advocate and so on.

Teaching the teachers

The effectiveness of any strategy employed in an effort to facilitate learning is significantly affected by the knowledge and skills of the educator involved. Not only do educators need to have a reasonable understanding of the nature of clinical reasoning, but they also need to be able to design and implement strategies which make this complex skill understandable to and achievable by their students.

In clinical education the lack of teacher preparation can be a particular problem. Full time staff who engage in clinical supervision may lack current clinical experience while part time clinical facilitators are often practising clinicians with little or no formal education background. As such, they may lack teaching and facilitatory skills and may be unfamiliar with clinical reasoning theory. That is, expert clinicians are clearly not necessarily expert educators. If their awareness of their own clinical reasoning is deficient then their ability to make that reasoning explicit for students will be hampered.

To facilitate teachers' capacity to teach clinical reasoning (and also to improve students' opportunities to learn) preparation of teachers for this task is necessary. Ryan (see Chapter 20) argues in favour of more postgraduate courses to prepare health science teachers for their teaching role, and specifically emphasizes the area of fieldwork education. At the very least, she contends, clinical supervisors should be given opportunities to learn clinical reasoning theory and educational strategies which promote learning with emphasis on supervised practical experience as any other learner would receive.

Clinical supervisors are also disadvantaged when they are not directly associated with the selection or delivery of the classroom subject matter. Without knowledge of the depth and sequence of information students receive, clinical supervisor expectations may be misplaced. Even more challenging for clinical supervisors is the difficulty in maintaining their own knowledge base to keep up with the latest information which students are continually receiving. Personal motivation may not always be sufficient and institutions should assist with ongoing 'knowledge' updates. Analogous efforts to incorporate new knowledge and learning strategies should clearly also be expected of classroom educators.

The use of new technologies

While new and varied learning strategies and educator proficiency will contribute to optimizing students' clinical reasoning, advances in educational technology and innovative resources such as the use of simulated patients also represent future directions to achieving this end. Ongoing advances in technology will continue to make new opportunities available to understand, access and communicate clinical reasoning. It is desirable for educators to keep in touch with these developments and to identify and adopt technologies which will enhance their teaching programs.

Computer-assisted interactive learning activities, decision support systems and data base knowledge resources are examples of technology currently available to assist students' development of clinical reasoning skills (see Chapter 12). Simulated patients have successfully been used for both learning and assessment of clinical reasoning (see Chapter 22). Whether it be simulated patients, videotaped patient problems or more sophisticated interactive computer programs, resources such as these offer numerous advantages including control over problem selection and design, diminished ethical and safety risks that accompany learning activities with real patients and economical benefits derived from more efficient use of student and teacher time.

However, while increasing student numbers and corresponding reductions in teacher availability/resources will necessitate greater use of technological resources, utilization of these resources will only be successful if they are strategically integrated into existing programs. That is, resources and technology which are only used because they are the latest educational 'toy' available will not succeed. The same care and thought is needed in the selection and design of educational resources and technology as would occur with any teaching material or strategy to ensure the desired knowledge and process skills are addressed in accordance with the intended students' respective stage of learning.

Assessment developments

Concurrent with the above efforts to proceed with the use and exploration of teaching strategies, teacher preparation and educational technology, future directions within education must also take up the challenge put forward by Newble, van der Vleuten and Norman (see Chapter 13) to continue experimentation with different methods of assessing clinical reasoning. Their view expressed in that chapter that 'it is hard to imagine a credible assessment of clinical competence which does not attempt to evaluate clinical reasoning skills' is particularly challenging when many programs across the health professions would still lack specific assessment methods which target reasoning skills. It is clear from their chapter that there is no single best method of assessing clinical reasoning. However, Newble et al offer useful suggestions to minimize known problems which frequently occur with existing assessment methods.

Clinical practice

Clinical reasoning in practice is influenced by a mixture of external and internal factors. External factors include client needs/expectations, professional and institutional canon, community needs/expectations, resource availability and funding, while internal factors include personal values and beliefs, general and domain-specific knowledge and individual cognitive or reasoning strategies. All of the above factors will contribute to future directions of reasoning in clinical practice with a major external influence emanating from changes in the health care market. An investigation by the Pew Health Commission in the United States (1992) identified the following trends within the health care environment in America. This is provided as an example of some of the types of trends which face health care worldwide. These trends include:

1. Acute-care hospitals becoming a collection of intensive care units
2. The increasing prevalence of self-care facilities and a move to greater consumer self-reliance
3. An increasing public pressure for public disclosure, consumer information, and involvement
4. A burgeoning home health industry
5. The demographic shifts with accompanying expectations of elder care and chronic illness
6. The adoption of clinical practice guidelines that create a more prescriptive practice and at the same time increase the opportunity for autonomous practice
7. Limited financial, technical and human resources
8. Increased competition in the marketplace.

These precise trends do not affect all countries. Some countries face very different trends or challenges such as coping with the health care needs in the face of insurmountable economic difficulties, population explosions, widespread drought, famine or war. Yet, in each case it could be argued that the following common themes exist: attempting to provide the best possible care within the limited resources available and the need for health care workers to be adept at coping with rapid change and complex situations. In each case therefore, it could be argued that health workers need to rely heavily upon, and need to develop further competence in, their ability to reason effectively, to be able to make sense of the mass of conflicting and complex information, constraints and opportunities available to them within the context of their work environment and the client's situation, and to learn to make relevant and defensible decisions for the given situation.

In many countries there is a trend towards increased lower-cost, community-based, community-focused health care services where the client is an increasingly informed participant in decisions affecting his or her care. These changes in practice are already occurring in a number of settings and influence all health care practitioners (Moccia, 1993). A move to different work settings means practitioners will encounter clients at different stages of development of their clinical problems and will need to deal with different contextual considerations. For example, the location of clinical practice services in work settings enables direct access to environmental analysis and greater opportunity for monitoring and management of prevention or rehabilitation efforts. Similarly, in community-based rehabilitation programs a greater depth of understanding of cultural and socioeconomic influences occur which can be a decided advantage in designing and implementing relevant clinical management programs.

With these changes in practice settings, some individuals will adopt broader perspectives of client management than previously held, with greater attention to individual contexts of client problems necessitating acquisition of new knowledge structures and greater inclusion of clients themselves in the decision making process. Rather than being passive recipients of the clinician's decisions about 'this is what's wrong with you' and 'this is what you need to do', health care consumers will be given responsibility for applying their own problem solving skills to preventative and rehabilitative health care. This may be a challenging and even uncomfortable situation for those practitioners who consider they know what is best for their clients but the advantages of paying greater attention to clients' views, feelings and personal analysis is clear to those practitioners who already practise in this manner. Involving clients in decision making is valuable because it utilizes insights available from the clients' first hand knowledge of their own problems. This leads to an increased potential for positive outcomes due to better matching between client preferences and treatment methods and greater ownership by the client of treatment choices and outcome responsibilities.

Increasing health care costs have precipitated numerous governmental measures which directly impact on clinicians' latitude to practice. Increasing use of health care or rehabilitation managers through national and private health care programs encourages greater interdisciplinary communication while demanding greater accountability and quality assurance from practitioners involved. Cost ceilings and clinical practice guidelines are forcing practitioners to re-analyse cost and outcome effectiveness of treatment strategies. While self-appraisal can promote improved services, the danger exists that outcomes, particularly with regard to quality of life, may suffer at the expense of cost efficiencies. Extreme cost reduction measures such as creation of 'generic health care workers' may be suitable in some situations where economic limitations and access to basic health care are of paramount importance. However, it is essential that such measures do not proceed without detailed consideration of the limitations they could create in terms of quality of service available. In terms of clinical reasoning effectiveness, which involves integration of reasoning and discipline-specific knowledge within a disciplinary framework of philosophy, attitudes and operation norms, multidisciplinary health care worker models are likely to sacrifice depth of knowledge, expertise and quality care for limited apparent functional advantages.

With respect to the internal factors (e.g. personal values, beliefs, knowledge and reasoning strategies) influencing clinical reasoning in practice, we can anticipate that through shared perspectives as emerge in books such as this, the future will include improved strategies for facilitating knowledge acquisition and knowledge accessibility, increased open mindedness, and greater breadth of thinking styles.

Clinical reasoning will be increasingly more cognitively demanding as the body of professional knowledge continues to grow. In light of this and the errors of reasoning which humans make, Elstein (see Chapter 4) highlights the need for greater use and evaluation of computer-assisted decision support systems to aid clinicians to reason, to make decisions about appropriate actions and to evaluate their impact on client outcomes.

Where practice is dominated by reasoning-deficient adherence to routines or politically-motivated allegiance to one approach, we would hope for an increase in critical thinking and theoretical pluralism. Rule-governed behaviour may be able to contribute to efficiency and effectiveness of health care, but it must be accompanied by attitudes of curiosity and strategies of critical and reflective thinking. Where practice is dominated by critical thinking, we would hope for greater creative and lateral thinking (as per De Bono, 1970).

Conclusions

Future directions for developments in clinical reasoning have been considered within the contexts of research, education and clinical practice. With understanding of clinical reasoning being in its relative infancy, there is considerable scope for further research. We anticipate future directions will utilize a multitude of research designs to investigate relationships amongst a broad range of variables including clinician characteristics (e.g. knowledge, reasoning strategies, values, beliefs, etc.), client characteristics (with respect to both the person and the problem), practice settings, and outcomes (with consideration given to perspectives of clients, clinicians, professions, the public, and health care financiers). From an educational perspective research should continue to investigate growth of individuals' knowledge structures with additional efforts to clarify the level of the various types of knowledge (e.g. propositional, clinical, personal) required in different practice settings. Principal targets of research into the teaching of clinical reasoning could include what is being taught about clinical reasoning, the outcomes of clinical reasoning learning programs in relation to teaching strategies, and research into ways of teaching clinical reasoning.

Future directions in the teaching of clinical reasoning are reflected in a number of the trends which have emerged from the work presented in this book. These include: designing programs which are relevant to local needs, teaching clinical reasoning in the context of clinical problems, utilizing experiential modes of teaching/learning, increasing the focus of teaching on promoting understanding of the reasoning process and the incorporation of higher level reasoning skills, emphasizing the learner's role in knowledge generation, reviewing curriculum content and adjusting curriculum priorities, adapting teaching to changing clinical practice priorities and patterns, teaching the teachers, using new technologies, and improving assessment strategies.

Clinical reasoning in practice will continue to be influenced by external factors such as client needs/expectation, resource availability and funding and internal factors including personal values and beliefs, general and domain-specific knowledge and individual cognitive or reasoning strategies. Future worldwide trends influencing health care such as increasing financial constraints, changing health care settings, and greater consumer involvement will require clinicians to adopt broader perspectives of client management that include greater attention to individual contexts of client problems and greater involvement of clients in the decision making process. Clinicians of the future will benefit from flexibility and breadth of thinking styles and are likely to make greater use of computer-assisted decision support systems to manage the ever increasing growth of knowledge.

References

Barrows, H.S. (1986) A taxonomy of problem-based learning methods. *Medical Education*, **20**, 481–486

Barrows, H.S. and Tamblyn, R.M. (1980) *Problem-Based Learning: An Approach to Medical Education.* Springer, New York

Boud, D. (ed.) (1985) *Problem-Based Learning in Education for the Professions.* HERSDA, Sydney

Boud, D. and Feletti, G. (eds) (1991) *The Challenge of Problem-Based Learning.* Kogan Page, London

Carper, B.A. (1978). Fundamental patterns of knowing. *Advances in Nursing Science*, **1**, 13–23

De Bono, E. (1970) *Lateral Thinking.* Penguin Books, London

Engel, C.E. (1991) Not just a method but a way of learning. In *The Challenge of Problem-based Learning* (Boud, D. and Feletti, G., eds) London: Kogan Page, pp. 23–33

Elstein, A.S., Shulman, L.S. and Sprafka, S.S. (1978) *Medical Problem Solving: An Analysis of Clinical Reasoning.* Harvard University Press, Cambridge, MA

Feltovich, P.J. and Barrows, H.S. (1984) Issues of generality in medical problem solving. In *Tutorials in Problem-Based Learning* (eds H.G. Schmidt and M.L. De Volder). Van Gorcum, Assen/Maastricht, pp. 128–141

Fleming, M.H. (1991) Clinical reasoning in medicine compared with clinical reasoning in occupational therapy. *American Journal of Occupational Therapy*, **45**, 988–996

Kaufman, D.R., Patel, V.L. and Magder, S.A. (1992) Development of conceptual understanding of biomedical concepts. Technical Report # CME92-CS4. Centre for Medical Education, McGill University, Montreal, Quebec

Moccia, P. (1993) *A Vision for Nursing Education.* National League for Nursing, New York.

Norman, G.R. and Schmidt, H.G. (1992) The psychological basis of problem-based learning: a review of the evidence. *Academic Medicine*, **67**, 557–568

Patel, V.L., Evans, D.A. and Kaufman, D.R. (1989) A cognitive framework for doctor–patient interaction. In *Cognitive Science in Medicine* (eds D.A. Evans and V.L. Patel). MIT Press, London, England, pp. 257–312

Pew Health Commission (1992) Executive Summary from the Pew Health Commission. 'Healthy America:

Practitioners for 2005'. *Journal of Allied Health*, **Fall**, 3–22

Sarter, B. (ed.) (1988). *Paths to Knowledge: Innovative Research Methods for Nursing*. National League for Nursing, New York

Schmidt, H.G. (1983) Problem-based learning: a rationale and description. *Medical Education*, **17**, 11–16

Schmidt, H.G. and De Volder, M.L. (eds) (1984) *Tutorials in Problem-based Learning*. Van Gorcum, Assen/Maastricht

Schmidt, H.G., Dauphinee, D.G. and Patel, V.L. (1987) Comparing the effects of problem-based and conventional curricula in an international sample. *Journal of Medical Education*, **62**, 305–315

Walton, H.J. and Matthews, M.B. (1989) Essentials of problem-based learning. *Medical Education*, **23**, 542–558

Willems, J. (1981) Problem-based (group) teaching: a cognitive science approach to using available knowledge. *Instructional Science*, **10**, 5–21

Index